Skin Disease and the History of Dermatology

This text is both a history of skin disease and a history of dermatology, telling the human historical experience of skin disease and how we have come to know what we know about the skin and its myriad diseases over the course of four millennia, looking at key figures in life and literature and key events such as the Black Death and the eradication of smallpox. The text:

- Examines how the history of skin disease fits into the larger picture of the history of each age
- Provides dermatological insight into major events and personalities from history
- Offers a unique perspective on the history of each age

Skin Disease and the History of Dermatology
Order out of Chaos

Scott M. Jackson, MD

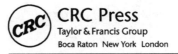

CRC Press
Taylor & Francis Group
Boca Raton New York London

CRC Press is an imprint of the
Taylor & Francis Group, an **informa** business

First edition published 2023
by CRC Press
6000 Broken Sound Parkway NW, Suite 300, Boca Raton, FL 33487-2742

and by CRC Press
4 Park Square, Milton Park, Abingdon, Oxon, OX14 4RN

CRC Press is an imprint of Taylor & Francis Group, LLC

© 2023 Taylor & Francis Group, LLC

ISBN: 9781032226606 (hbk)
ISBN: 9781032226637 (pbk)
ISBN: 9781003273622 (ebk)

DOI: 10.1201/9781003273622

Typeset in Times
by KnowledgeWorks Global Ltd.

Contents

Preface

I have never regretted my choice. There is only one more beautiful thing in the world than a fine healthy skin, and that is a rare skin disease.[1]

Erasmus Wilson

I feel fortunate to reliably find comfort in the past. For the better part of my life, I have received everything I needed spiritually and intellectually—wisdom, knowledge, entertainment—in history. Whether we are talking about my personal history—reminiscing about my life experience with my late father or recalling my mentor, Dr. Lee T. Nesbitt, for a clinical question—or world history, for example, ancient Rome, it does not matter to me. I look backward.

Some of my fondest memories come from the years I spent carrying out the major coursework in the Department of History at Tulane University, where the eminent Dr. Kenneth Harl, a world-renowned expert on Roman and Byzantine History, made evident the excitement in studying and discussing history. I encountered the first significant fork in the road of my life in 1997 when I was forced to choose either a career in medicine or a career in history. While I chose the former and remain convinced today it was the right choice, I am still drawn by the allure of the past. Know that I am not a historian, but I almost tried to be one.

I started practicing dermatology in 2007 after completing a dermatology residency at Louisiana State University in New Orleans. My residency had been a tumultuous time in my life because it was interrupted by Hurricane Katrina in 2005. I was one of the last physicians to train at Charity Hospital, its doors closed due to catastrophic flooding from the hurricane. "Big Charity" was the second oldest hospital in the United States by just a few weeks; it opened on May 10, 1736, while Bellevue Hospital opened on March 31, 1736. With a large indigent patient population, the full breadth of pathology, some brilliant physician educators, and an "in the trenches" autonomy-promoting culture, Charity Hospital was one of the most incredible places in the world to get a medical education.

Dermatology is an outstanding specialty of medicine in which to practice. I see the full range of age-groups, from one-day-old babies to centenarians; sometimes four generations of the same family; clinic patients and hospital patients; patients who are very sick and ones who are quite well; patients with skin tumors and ones with rashes; and ones with valid complaints, others with imagined problems. I get to act as internist, rheumatologist, pediatrician, surgeon, psychiatrist, infectious disease doctor, allergist, and immunologist every single day. I use my brain to diagnose interesting rashes and my hands to excise worrisome skin cancers. I literally look at disease, my eyes intently focus on it, inspecting its nuances, patterns, severity, and distribution, watching it evolve or spread or disappear with treatment or time. The intellectual stimulation of the field is extraordinary, with the seemingly infinite ways a disease can present on the surface of our bodies and the great uncertainty that remains about the cause of many of our skin diseases. Formulating a differential diagnosis—and selecting the best possible diagnosis from over 2000 different skin diseases—is the most intellectually rewarding part. So is applying a career of memories of previous cases to the present case. Finding the proper treatment for the given problem in front of me is also a challenge that I relish. I am regularly intrigued by seeing uncommon diseases as well as unusual presentations of common diseases. I employ cool instruments—microscopes, dermatoscopes, cautery needles, and liquid nitrogen canisters that look like blowtorches. Dermatology is a science that has its own unique subdisciplines—dermatopathology, dermoscopy, and mycology—that deepen the intellectual challenges of the profession.

With most of my patients healthy at the point of our encounter, I can make some wonderful relationships with many different types of people. I love getting to know my patients—where they are from, where they've traveled, what they are reading, what they do for a living, what they are celebrating, and what they are worried about. I get humbled every day, kept in check by the mysteries of medicine, the pitfalls, the fact that I am human and make mistakes, and the challenges of trying to fix what seems unfixable. That same day, I can get an ego boost from making an elusive diagnosis or curing a troublesome rash after attempts elsewhere had failed. I am practicing at a time when most of the skin problems faced in the office do have a reliable solution. This was not the case when I started my career. The difference is attributed to the miraculous technological advancements in this specialty over the last 15 years.

Yet, after just seven years of practice, I entered into "a pattern of a relentless downward spiral" in response to cumulative work stress—a mode that, unlike everyday stress, is not relieved with time off from work or monetary compensation and is best known as *burnout.*[2] The painful truth is that I only had myself to blame; difficulty with "no" plus inadequate coping mechanisms for dealing with chronic stress will lead one there every time. The stress in part resulted from taking on too many patients, the incorporation of the electronic health record into my practice, being perpetually understaffed, and the increasingly complex challenges of practice, such as having to go to great lengths to get patients the medications they need. While *burnout* is apparently taboo for the majority of healthcare institutions, it was comforting to know that I was not alone: 42–50 percent of physicians at any given time experience *burnout,* and 29–32 percent of dermatologists experience the same. But, in addition to the classic symptoms of exhaustion, cynicism, and helplessness, I had lost my passion for the work itself.

In 2018, desperate for some spark to reignite my interest in dermatology, I naturally went to the past. I stumbled upon a British surgeon named Daniel Turner, whose work straddles the seventeenth and eighteenth centuries (see Chapter 9). I found his life and career fascinating, and I wanted to know more and more about him. I realized at this point that I had little knowledge about the history of my specialty, and I found that the last complete survey on the topic was written in 1933. And then it dawned on me: could I write a history of dermatology for myself? Could studying the history of my field and writing about it inspire me again and help me with my burnout? Would gaining knowledge about the history of the specialty reconnect me to the specialty itself? Could individual figures in the past inspire me? These are the questions I had back in those early days when I started this quest for knowledge. The answers to the above questions are a resounding yes, yes, yes, and yes! I am living proof that studying history can help with burnout. What follows is the end product of my deeply personal, four-year-long journey that began at the depths of physician burnout and ended with my exit from that terrible downward spiral.

The following history of the skin and its diseases is preceded by several successful attempts by others to tell all or part of this story. The first history of dermatology, entitled *Geschichte* (History) *der Dermatologie,* was written in German by Paul Richter and was published in 1928 as the first 240 pages of Jadassohn's multi-volume *Handbuch der Haut und Geschlechts Krankheiten* (Handbook of Skin and Sexually Transmitted Diseases). William A. Pusey (1865–1940) authored the first and only complete history of dermatology, *The History of Dermatology* (1933). John T. Crissey and Lawrence C. Parish penned a well-researched and entertaining history of dermatology of the nineteenth century, entitled *The Dermatology and Syphilology of the 19th Century* (1981). The four biographical encyclopedias of the great historical contributors to dermatology are as follows: Herman Goodman's *Notable Contributors to the Knowledge of Dermatology* (1953); Walter Shelley and John T. Crissey's *Classics in Clinical Dermatology with Biographical Sketches* (1953, 2003); John T. Crissey, Karl Holubar, and Lawrence C. Parish's *Historical Atlas of Dermatology and Dermatologists* (2002); and possibly the greatest work ever produced on the history of the specialty, *Pantheon of Dermatology* (2008 in German, 2013 in English), edited by Christoph Löser, Gerd Plewig, and Walter H.C. Burgdorf. My work is not a cultural history of skin, but there are cultural aspects of skin discussed throughout the work. Cultural histories of the skin do exist; these include *The Book of Skin* (2004) by Steven Connor; *Skin: A Natural History* (2006) by Nina Jablonski; and *Skin* (2002) by Claudia Benthien. Kevin Siena's anthology of essays, *A Medical History of Skin* (2013), is an important work that contains discussions of specific topics in the history of skin disease starting at the beginning of the modern era. I referred to all of these works, except for the inaccessible Richter work, in my research, and I know that the shoes I need to fill are not lacking in size.

I had two main goals as I set out to tell this story. My first goal was to describe how the skin and skin diseases were viewed throughout history by the most significant natural philosophers, surgeons, and physicians who wrote about these topics. Most importantly, I paid particular attention to exactly what was said and attempted to compile each writer's own words in one place, this book. Dozens of contributors to the history of dermatology are highlighted in this text, and while it was impossible to record every word, what follows is an attempt to give the reader a selection of some of the most interesting things that these great men and women wrote. The second goal was to examine the possibility that skin disease caused more suffering over the millennia than any other type of disease. With a focus on leprosy, plagues and pandemics, syphilis, and smallpox, I hope it will be obvious to the reader at the conclusion of this book that the possibility was a reality.

For supplemental material, the reader is referred to my website: www.historyofderm.com.

I want to thank the following people for assisting me with the preparation of this text, supporting my endeavor, or for inspiring me in some way to write it: my anchor and always-supporter, my wife Svetlana; my sons Stephen and Timothy, who give me reasons to seek idealism every day; my dear friend, Latin tutor and proofreader, and former neighbor, Dr. Althea Ashe, for her tireless sunday morning proofreading sessions, translation assistance, and moral support; my wonderful editor, Dr. Holly Caldwell; Evelyn Duffy, for helping me through the painful process of writing a book proposal; Jenni Fry, for her exceptional knowledge of the Chicago citation format; the ever-mindful and compassionate Dr. Francinne Lawrence; the brilliantly insightful Todd Atkins; the only person I know who likes history more than I do, my dear friend, Alan Comer; the venerable Dr. George Karam, one of the most influential persons in my life; my mother, Carolyn, for her unending care; Dr. Stephen J. Greenberg at the National Library of Medicine, for answering my unsolicited questions; Robert Peden at CRC Press, for believing in my project; persons otherwise dear to me: Barbara Jackson, Tenicia Tucker, Tony Parker, Dr. Wayne Binning, Jim Siebolt, Mike Liffman, and Dr. Douglas Lewis; and the two mentioned above, the illustrious Dr. Kenneth Harl, who showed me how, and the late Dr. Lee T. Nesbitt, who was to me in his role as chairman of the department of dermatology at LSU a modern-day Besnier. I would like to thank my colleagues at Ozark Dermatology Clinic for the opportunity for a fresh start. Finally, I recognize the figures in this book whose lives inspire me or taught me something along this journey, especially Samuel Plumbe, in whom I see so much of myself, and the freelance Paul Unna, the melancholic Thomas Addison, the neurasthenic Louis Duhring, and the incomparable Robert Willan, whom I aspire to emulate every day when I enter the clinic. And for the physician who knows burnout as well as I do: history is therapy and love thyself.

Scott M. Jackson, MD
Bentonville, Arkansas

Introduction

For all but the last one or two hundred years, skin disease was poorly understood by societies and equally confusing to the physicians who were tasked with dealing with it. Knowledge of the skin and skin disease by medical communities evolved over time, as did the identification, classification, and treatment of these diseases. Characters in the following story—the contributors to the knowledge of dermatology—include the Babylonian *âsû*, the ancient Egyptian *swnw* (soo-noo), the ancient Greek ιατρός (iatros), the Roman *medicus*, the Anglo-Saxon *laece* (leech), the Islamic physician, the medieval surgeon, the Renaissance *physicus*, and the modern-era physician and surgeon. Thus, the story of how we came to know what we know about the outer surface of our bodies and its myriad diseases is a long and winding one that spanned at least four millennia. It will be shown that the achievement of the collective physicians of history to get order from the absolute chaos that was the identification, classification, and understanding of these diseases is one of the greatest and most underappreciated achievements in the history of medicine. Specialization in the skin by physicians and surgeons was ultimately necessary to reach our modern understanding of skin disease, and the formation of that specialty—dermatology—is, too, a subject of this book.

As skin disease has been on the mind of physicians dating back to the earliest days of medicine, evidenced by the fact that many of the medical texts have large portions devoted to skin disease, the main narrative of this book is centered around these texts and begins in ancient Mesopotamia and Egypt (Chapters 1 and 2). Then we examine what Hippocrates, Galen, and the ancient Greek and Roman medical writers had to say about the skin and its diseases (Chapters 3 and 4). Next is a long section on the Middle Ages, addressing the viewpoints of medieval scholars, the Byzantine compilers, the Anglo-Saxons, the great physicians of the Islamic Golden Age, and the medical and surgical writers of Western Europe (Chapters 5–7). Subsequently, the dermatology of the Renaissance, the Scientific Revolution, and the Enlightenment are covered within individual chapters (Chapters 8–10). Finally, in the most important chapters of this book, the drawn-out story of the nineteenth century is told and divided into five chapters (Chapters 11–15). The last chapter—on the twentieth century and beyond—brings the reader up to date on the more recent events in the history of dermatology. In addition, when one thinks of the major diseases that have afflicted man dating back to the beginning of history, many of them are skin diseases or disease states with major skin manifestations such as leprosy, plague, syphilis, and smallpox. Each of these diseases has a rich history and is dealt with in their individual sections, or "Interludes," that break up the main historical narrative at regular points.

For those who lack a basic familiarity with the skin and its disease, let us answer the question, what do we now know? We know that the skin is the largest organ of the human body and covers an area of approximately 21 square feet (2 square meters), accounting for 15 percent of body weight. It has three layers: the waterproof *epidermis*; the sturdy, collagenous *dermis*; and the cushioning *hypodermis* (subcutaneous layer). The skin varies in thickness with the skin of the feet the thickest in the body, and the skin of the eyelids the thinnest. It can also thicken itself in places where external forces such as friction and pressure are acting regularly against the skin. The skin has a remarkable capacity to heal itself after traumatic, thermal, or chemical injury. Only if the dermis is injured do scars form. Whether an injury happens or not, however, a new epidermis is generated every 28 days as cells rise from the bottom layer (basal layer) and migrate up to the surface of the skin (stratum corneum), only to reach their fate to slough off as dead skin cells. We shed 30,000–40,000 of these skin cells every minute, and dead skin cells make up at least half of the dust in our homes. The surface of the skin is home to some 1000 species of bacteria, yeast, and viruses—the skin's permanent and transient microbial residents.

The skin has many functions. It protects structures underlying it—the muscles, bones, and internal organs—from outside infectious agents and external trauma. The skin is an organ of sensation with five different types of receptors within its layers for pain and touch. It is an impermeable barrier to prevent

DOI: 10.1201/9781003273622-1

water from leaving the body (except through the pores dedicated for this purpose in the sweating mechanism). The skin is an immunologically active organ that contains immune cells called Langerhans cells whose purpose is to recruit other immune cells from the blood in response to the presence of foreign invaders or substances against which one's immune system is primed to react (allergens). The skin has sebaceous glands that secrete sebum, a substance that keeps the skin smooth and waterproof. The subcutaneous layer, serving as a padding for the muscles and bones to protect them from injury, varies in size from person to person. The skin regulates body temperature by means of two mechanisms. First is the evaporation of excreted sweat, up to a quart a day, off the surface of the skin to remove heat from the body (evaporative cooling). Second, temperature is regulated by the alteration of vascular tone in the skin, in which vasodilation of cutaneous blood vessels causes dissipation of heat from inside the body to outside to cool the body, while vasoconstriction of these vessels causes retention or movement of warm blood to the core to warm the body. The generation of hair and the erection of hair (by smooth muscle contraction) are vestigial mechanisms for warmth. Everything has a purpose in the skin.

The surface of the human body has undergone three major evolutionary changes over the millions of years that have passed from the emergence of the first bipedal species four to seven million years ago; it has become less hairy, able to sweat, and varied in color. In concert with the ability to walk upright on 2 feet came the reduction in body hair and the development of the thermoregulatory system of sweating, a uniquely human system. Both of these modifications gave early hominids better capacity to dissipate heat. The advantage allowed by this cooling system may have been the promotion of daytime foraging and hunting for food, when other predators were hiding from the heat.

The different shades of skin color are determined simply by the type and quantity of melanin one has in their epidermal cells. Microscopically speaking, however, everyone's skin is otherwise exactly the same. Melanin, the natural sunscreen produced by the melanocytes of our epidermis, provides an SPF (sun protection factor) of up to 13 in the darkest skin types. Melanin is a pigment that protects the DNA of epidermal cells from the sun's harmful ultraviolet (UV) rays; under the microscope, it looks like a little brown cellular umbrella covering the cell nucleus.

The color of the skin of the first *Homo* species was dark. As the first species emerged in equatorial Africa, the quantity of melanin in the skin was necessary for protection from the high UV index found in that part of the world. Melanin "afforded protection against photodegradation of cutaneous and systemic folate," an important vitamin in fertility, DNA and RNA production, and blood cell formation.[1] As early humans migrated away from the equator, the exposure to UV light dropped progressively with distance from the equator, and human skin color lightened. The selective force for this change is widely believed to be the need for vitamin D, generated in the skin in response to UV light exposure. With its UV-absorbing capacity, melanin limits the generation of vitamin D; therefore, in latitudes where UV light is at a premium, less melanin in the skin is beneficial to the goal of maintaining a healthy level of vitamin D. In sum, the darker skin tones of equatorial Africa were driven by folate protection, and the lighter skin tones of northern and southern latitudes result from pressures to keep the vitamin D levels up.[2]

Given its external placement, the skin is the most vulnerable organ in the human body—vulnerable to disease as well as injury. Diseases of the skin, i.e., itching, infestations, infections, rashes, and tumors, are extremely common, with over 2000 different diseases affecting the skin, hair, or nails. More than 85 million Americans sought medical attention for a skin problem in 2013—a third of these cases were managed by a dermatologist. In modern dermatology clinics, the most common reasons for visits are acne, sun damage and skin cancer checks, benign growths, moles, itching, dry skin, eczema, dermatitis, psoriasis, skin infections, rosacea, drug eruptions, ulcers, seborrheic dermatitis, vitiligo, hives, wounds, and disorders of the hairs and nails. The demand for dermatologic care in the United States is extraordinary. A person with an unsightly and/or itchy rash or skin lesion is more likely to seek medical attention than one with elevated blood pressure; the difference is in the patient's awareness of the problem and the social stigma assigned to skin disease. These diseases have a tremendous capacity to affect a person's quality of life, not just from the standpoint of physical discomfort, but also from a psychological or social standpoint. Some skin diseases can be fatal, like melanoma or toxic epidermal necrolysis, the latter of which kills up to 50 percent of persons afflicted.

Skin disease can occur as *primary* disturbance of the skin's structure, properties, or function—that is, a disease of the skin itself, such as in the case of psoriasis—or it can occur as a feature *secondary* to an internal disease process, such as jaundice. In both categories, there are skin diseases that have an infectious, inflammatory, autoimmune, neoplastic, vascular, neurological, metabolic, endocrinological, or genetic etiology or result from external (physical) forces working against the skin. While changes in the skin can sometimes indicate a problem or change in internal medical health, emotional and psychological health plays a major role in the status of the skin. The peripheral nervous system connects the brain and the skin, enabling psychological stress to influence the skin through stress hormones, neurotransmitters, cytokines, and inflammation.

Skin diseases have affected people of all societies, all epochs, all ages, and all skin colors; they are thus a universal human experience. Physicians have been trying to explain skin diseases since the beginning of history. Presumably this is due to the visible nature of these diseases, requiring no testing to discover them since they are always there for the eyes to inspect. The mystery is not in the *where* but in the *why* and the *how*. Perhaps the urgency to explain and successfully treat was driven by the great number of people afflicted by these diseases. We have no way of estimating the prevalence, but without any reliable treatments, the many infectious diseases of the skin—as well as the ones dependent on hygiene and the diseases that tend to worsen without treatment (such as eczema)—were very prevalent for the duration of human history, and they were severe.

Finally, a few words about the subtitle, *Order out of Chaos*. The phrase is not the author's but a phrase that was commonly used in the nineteenth and early-twentieth centuries by dermatological writers. The phrase describes the attainment of understanding and arrangement (order) concerning diseases of the skin that were—for all but the last 200 years—completely disorganized, confused, conflicted, and misunderstood (chaos). It is precisely this *Order out of Chaos* that represents, in the author's opinion, one of the greatest achievements in the history of medicine. And it will be shown that it was not one or even a few people that brought this order, but many individuals, over centuries if not millennia, from many different lands.

Part I

Chaos

Diseases of the body which separately afflict and devour each limb and each part, and which also rack and torture it all over with fevers, and chills, and wasting consumptions, and terrible rashes and scrofulous diseases and spasmodic convulsions of the eyes, and putrefying sores and abscesses, and cutaneous disorders extending over the whole of the skin, and disorders of the bowels and inward parts, and convulsions of the stomach ....[1]

Philo of Alexandria

That disease [smallpox], over which science has since achieved a succession of glorious and beneficent victories, was then the most terrible of all the ministers of death ... and the smallpox was always present, filling the churchyards with corpses, tormenting with constant fears all whom it had not yet stricken, leaving on those whose lives it spared the hideous traces of its power, turning the babe into a changeling at which the mother shuddered, and making the eyes and cheeks of the betrothed maiden objects of horror to the lover.[2]

Thomas Macaulay

The great number and the diversity of cutaneous diseases, the obscurity of their causes and differences, as well as the difficulty of treating them, have made this branch of medicine one of the most difficult and most incomprehensible for those initiating in medicine. The authors whom we are able to consult up until this point are few. Some authors describe the kinds of diseases common to every age, unless there is divine intervention; others use vague and inconsistent diagnostic names, and they formulate an uncertain reason for the cure. These are the things which have spurred me to labor to reduce this vast and disparate pile of diseases into a system.[3]

Joseph Jacob Plenck

DOI: 10.1201/9781003273622-2

1

Ancient Mesopotamia

Derived from Greek, the term *Mesopotamia* means "between rivers," referring to the Tigris and Euphrates Rivers of the Middle East. The area is the large eastern part of the Fertile Crescent, the boomerang-shaped, fruitful region where civilization—or in simple terms, an urbanized society that has achieved writing—began to emerge during the Bronze Age (3300–1200 BCE). Civilization rose there simultaneously with the advanced communities in Egypt, India, China, and Peru. It is no coincidence that each of these "cradles of civilization" was centered around rivers (the Nile, Hindus, Yellow, and Fortaleza Rivers, respectively), which provided rich sediment that fueled agriculture, leading to food surpluses and resultant economic, cultural, and technological development. Ancient Mesopotamia was not dominated by a single culture; one group would control the region for several centuries, then another culture would rise to predominance. The first of these dominions was the Sumerian civilization, which flourished roughly from 4100 to 2300 BCE, centered around the ancient city of Uruk. After 2300 BCE, there was more frequent turnover of the ruling culture, as demonstrated by this oversimplified timeline (see Table 1.1).

The Sumerians are credited with one of the first written language systems; it was called cuneiform. The first libraries were established during the Old Babylonian period, which peaked during the reign of King Hammurabi (1810–1750 BCE). A body of literature, including the Epic of Gilgamesh (ca. 1800 BCE), was also developed during this time. Astronomy, mathematics, and science were strong suits of the Mesopotamian peoples, and our sexagesimal number system for time and the seven-day week originated with the Sumerians and Babylonians. More detailed research into the history of this region would reveal that it was home to polytheistic, magic-based religions and to peoples capable of producing impressive demonstrations of music, art, and architecture.

Mesopotamian Medicine

The last great Assyrian king, Ashurbanipal (r. 668–627 BCE), was an enlightened, literate man who assembled a great library at his capital of Nineveh, near modern-day Mosul, Iraq. When Nineveh was burned by its successor kingdom forces, clay tablets were baked and fortuitously preserved for perpetuity. Approximately 30,000 of these clay tablets were uncovered in the 1850s by archeologists there, many of which were collected from Old Babylonian sources and were devoted to medicine. The Assyrians saved the ancient medical information of the Babylonians and other preceding kingdoms, resulting in a scholarly focus termed Assyriological study. The majority of these tablets are today housed today at the British Museum, London. Another source of information is the Code of Hammurabi (1754 BCE), which regulated Babylonian society, including its occupations. Physicians were not immune to the code's famous retaliatory punishments. For example, a physician who erred in the care of a high-born patient suffered the penalty of amputation of his hands. However, less is known about Mesopotamian medicine than that of other ancient peoples like the Egyptians because the cuneiform language source material—the only source material in existence for this type of study—has not yet been fully researched.[4]

The most extensive and important single work of Mesopotamian medical information is the *Sakikkū*, written by Esagil-kīn-apli, the head scholar of the Babylonian King Adad-apla-iddina (r. 1067–1046 BCE). Even in its damaged and incomplete state, this "Treatise of Medical Diagnoses and Prognoses" (also referred to as the "Diagnostic Handbook") is a treasure trove of information, describing the medical practices of the pre-Greek ancient world. Written in Akkadian cuneiform, it addresses a number

TABLE 1.1

Ruling Cultures of Mesopotamia

2334–2154 BCE	Akkadians
2004–1763 BCE	Amorites
1763–1595 BCE	Old Babylonians
1595–1155 BCE	Kassites
1200–900 BCE	Transition Period
911–609 BCE	Assyrians
612–539 BCE	New Babylonians

of ailments, including stomach pains, ear diseases, hemorrhoids, and toothaches. There are two tablets describing the interpretations of omens at the patient's bedside, twelve tablets on the different parts of the body in a head-to-heel order, seven tablets based on the prognosis of different diseases, one on epilepsy, and three on pregnancy and infants.[5] According to Majno, the treatise was "a handbook of the sorcerer, not a manual of medicine" and as its correct translation is in a constant state of flux, "the printed translation has no value."[6]

Historians have pieced together an understanding of ancient Mesopotamian medicine, which was primarily religious in nature, from the *Sakikkū* and other archaeological and textual proof.[7] Contrary to Herodotus' claim that there were no physicians in ancient Babylon, there is evidence of three types of healers practicing as early as the third millennium BCE:[8]

1. *bârû* (seers): The experts in divination, omens, diagnoses, and prognoses;
2. *âshipu* (exorcists): Experts with incantations used for expelling demons;
3. *âsû* (physician-priests): Experts in charms, drugs, and operations.

The *âshipu* manipulated the supernatural; the *âsû*, the natural. Both men filled a need, and the two types of healers more likely worked together than competed with one another, but it is not known how patients decided which to see for their ailment.[9]

Ancient Mesopotamians viewed illness as retribution from the gods for sins committed against them, gods who should be appeased at all times with worship and offerings. Demons could also bring about disease; amulets and charms were worn as special protections from these evil spirits, which descend upon a person because that individual did not heed certain omens, had been subject to the spells of a black magic sorcerer, or had contact with a diseased person, such as a leper, who already carried an evil spirit. The interventions of the healers, e.g., exorcism and incantations, were directed with the primary purpose of driving the evil spirit from the afflicted or making things right with the furious god. In addition to an elaborate pharmacopeia containing herbal (including poppy, hemp, and mandrake), mineral, and faunal medicaments, healers also used fumigations, suppositories, enemas, and therapeutic baths. Wound care was not primitive, and they performed surgical procedures like the draining of boils and abscesses. These practices have led scholars like Teall to argue that while Mesopotamian medical and surgical treatments could not be separated from religious interventions such as divination and healing ritual, Mesopotamian medicine was more sophisticated than once thought by scholars.[10] And the physical treatments would eventually win, supplanting the supernatural interventions in the last millennium before the common era.

Skin Disease in Ancient Mesopotamia

There are more lines in the Mesopotamian medical literature devoted to the signs and symptoms of skin disease than disease of any other organ, indicating that evaluating abnormalities or changes in the skin was a major focus of the ancient physician.[11] There were over 50 terms for different types of skin lesions and conditions, including terms for dryness, oozing/dampness, redness, wind-burned appearance, swollen, indurated, relaxed, sweaty, hairless, scratched, dark, black, thermal burn, bruised, spot, petechiae, white spots, red spots, bright red spots, dark spots, spots of any color, pinpoint spots, generalized dark spots, generalized red spots, scale, wheal, nodule, dark nodule, vesicle, generalized red vesicles, pockmarks, evolving lesion, whitehead, ulcer, and individual black spots.[12]

The Mesopotamians had their own original dermatological nomenclature. For example, *girgišu* is the term for a "sore that is hot like a burn but does not contain fluid"; *bubu'tu* is the term for a "sore that is hot like a burn that does contain fluid"; *išītu* refers to a "sore that is hot like a burn that does not contain fluid and is full of little *bubu'tu*."[13] From these references, it can be inferred that morphology, distribution, and color of skin lesions (especially red and black, but also yellow-green) were important diagnostic information to the Mesopotamian physician.[14] References to surface and dimension (flat versus elevated lesions), as well as distinction among elevated lesions by their consistency (solid or containing liquid, such as serum or pus), also appear.[15]

The dermatologic nomenclature of this ancient culture was detailed and extensive, as were the prescriptions, such as the one below, indicating an almost scientific approach to the evaluation of skin diseases:

> If a person's head is full of *kibsu* (favus), *kissatu* (hairless patches), and *gurastu* (ringworm), to cure him, you dry together in the shade, crush, and sift these nine items: *kibritu* (sulfur), *uhhulu qarnanu*, *rikibti arkabi*, *tittu* (fig cuttings), *e'ru* (tree cuttings), *mussukanu* (tree), *binu* (tamarisk bark), *aktam*, and gazelle droppings. You mix it with urine from a black cow. You wash his head with it. If the *kibsu*, *kissatu*, and *gurastu* are extinguished, he should recover.[16]

Any divergence from normal represented a bad omen and was subjected to observation, interpretation, and study.[17] Skin conditions were deemed a sign of impurity, and they were particularly disturbing to the afflicted because they reflected some type of guilt—of a criminal or sinful act. The "guilty" unnerved their peers, who in turn distanced themselves from the afflicted or sought their isolation, as proclaimed in the following quote:

> If the skin (or) the flesh of a man exhibits white spots and is full of nodules, such a man has been rejected by his gods, and such a man is to be rejected by mankind.[18]

The specific pattern of a skin eruption correlated with the act that caused the person to become affected by the ailment, and it also suggested the god responsible for bringing it. The moon god Sîn was particularly effective at producing skin diseases in the impure, but so were the sun god Shamash and the god of Venus, Ishtar. Generalized vesicular (blistering) rashes were caused by "getting in bed with a woman" and brought about by "the hand" of a god. If the person had from head-to-toe red vesicles on white skin, Sîn was responsible for the eruption, but if they were white vesicles on dark skin, the rash was the doing of Shamash.[19] In addition to suggesting the transgression and the god who delivered the punishment, a skin eruption signaled a prognosis to the physician, e.g., a rock-hard sore that was located on the neck, armpit, or abdomen would mean death after three days.[20]

The Babylonians referred to the skin disease that reflected the most impurity as *saharšubbû*. It shared much in common with the Hebrew skin disease of ritual impurity, *tsara'at*, and might be the Mesopotamian equivalent of Biblical leprosy (see Interlude 1). One source describes a curse that invoked the god Sîn to cover the victim's whole body with *saharšubbû*, which will never leave the body before death, forcing the targeted one to "lie as a wild ass outside the walls of his own city."[21] Contrary to the incurable status of this disease implied in the curse, there were treatments available for it, and a cure could be achieved. Treatment entailed crushing or fumigating herbals and applying them to the surface of the skin or onto the surface of the unroofed vesicles.[22]

PROTECTION FROM ABANDONMENT

The Code of Hammurabi, published during the reign of Hammurabi (1810–1750 BCE), included a law that prohibited a man from abandoning his wife if she became afflicted with *la'bu*:

> If a man has married a wife and she falls ill with the la'bu disease, and he has made plans to marry someone else, and does marry, he shall not leave the wife who has fallen ill with the la'bu disease. She shall live in the house which he has built and he shall support her as long as she lives.

> If that wife does not agree to live in her husband's house, he shall pay back the gift she brought from her father's house and she shall depart.[23]

According to the Chicago Assyriological Dictionary, there is "clear evidence that *la'bu* (and the verb *la'abu*) denote a skin disease."[24] In the ancient sense of the word, leprosy is the most likely skin disease referred to as *la'bu*, and the law reflects governmental compassion for and protection of women with a skin condition that would otherwise result in her being ostracized.

It is apparent from the Akkadian texts that the Mesopotamians experienced a wide variety of skin diseases. The sun and wind exacted acute and chronic tolls on the skin. Bites from an assortment of fleas, lice, and crabs caused intense itching. Scorpions and snakes were abundant in the region. Personal hygiene was emphasized in the culture as a way to prevent illness, and there are numerous references to the use of medicated and non-medicated soaps and shampoos as both preventatives and treatments. The Mesopotamians recorded a number of skin diseases, including superficial fungal infections such as ringworm, burns, traumas, petechial eruptions, vitiligo, scarlet fever, hives, venereal warts, herpes, chickenpox, measles, smallpox, plague, acne, erysipelas, favus, skin cancer, hair loss, hair graying, leishmaniasis, onchocerciasis, and loiasis.[25] They wrote extensively about mycetoma, a deep fungal infection of the foot. Eruptions (exanthems), which we now know to be viral in etiology, were placed together in a grouping called *ašû* (different from *âsû*).

These ancient texts make no reference to the skin's functions, indicating that Mesopotamian peoples did not give any specific respect as an independent structure to the part of the body we call the skin. There was not even a specific vocabulary word for the concept of living skin in the Mesopotamian written record. The terms *mašku* and *pāru* meant skin and hide, respectively, but they refer to human skin only in cases where it has been removed from the body (the flayed skin).[26] And the term for the body, *zumru*, has the same cuneiform symbol as *mašku*, indicating that at least in the textual sense, the Mesopotamians saw no point in distinguishing the two, as the skin ailments were typically described in the context of where they occurred on the body.[27] We indeed still do this today, i.e., a dermatologist might say, "measles spreads all over the body" instead of "measles spreads all over the skin."

Wounds, in particular, were discussed extensively in the *Sakikkū* tablets, suggesting the knowledge contained within the tablets may have been useful in military medicine. The person who suffered from a mysterious lesion called *liptu* could receive the supernatural approach of the *âshipu* (the first remedy) or the natural protocol of the *âsû* (the second remedy):

> If a man has a blow [bruise] on the cheek: *Lolium* … in water from the well of the Temple of Marduk thou shalt bray, dust of four crossroads therein thou shalt col[lect], … seven and seven times his mouth shalt cleanse, with the water from the well of the Temple of Marduk his mouth [thou shalt wash].

> If a man is sick with a blow on the cheek, fir-turpentine, pine-turpentine, tamarisk, daisy, flour of *inninnu*, together thou shalt pound, strain, in milk and beer in a small copper pan thou shalt mix, spread on skin, bind on him, and he shall recover.[28]

The Mesopotamians demonstrated a knowledge of the three most essential steps in caring for a wound: cleansing, plastering, and bandaging. Even the world's oldest medical manuscript, a small clay tablet written in Sumerian around 2100 BCE, correctly described this approach; it contains the world's oldest poultices, and 12 of 15 prescriptions on the tablet are for external use, 8 of which are plasters.[29] It appears these prescriptions were intended not only for wounds but also for skin diseases, such as ulcers, sores, and lesions. One prescription on the Sumerian clay tablet read:

> Pound together: dried wine dregs, juniper and prunes; pour beer on the mixture. Then rub [the diseased part] with [sesame] oil, and bind on as a plaster.[30]

Beer and sesame oil were two ingredients commonly used in both wound care and the management of ulcers. Our current formulations of beer contain too low an alcohol content to have effective antiseptic properties, but perhaps ancient Mesopotamian beer was stronger than our modern brew. Or maybe its thick, porridge-like consistency allowed it to double as a poultice.[31] The sesame oil ingredient has been proven to have natural anti-streptococcal and anti-staphylococcal properties.[32] Many of the plants used in the poultice prescriptions have also been shown to have antibiotic properties. Willow bark, the natural source of salicylates, was used medicinally. It would be incorrect to assume that Mesopotamian medicine was ineffective and wholly based on placebo.

Summary

The Mesopotamian *âsû* and his religious colleague, the *âshipu*, offered a variety of natural and supernatural remedies for dealing with what appeared to be an abundance of skin problems in their society. The presence of a skin disease provided the Mesopotamian healer with much information. It indicated not only the diagnosis but also the prognosis—and the sin that caused the affliction and the god deemed responsible for the punishment. While there is no written record that the skin itself was respected as a functional structure or even a protective coating, or that the skin was even assigned its own word, the Mesopotamians can be singled out for their ancient form of dermatology, as judged by their extensive nomenclature for skin diseases, which in many ways was superior to their successors. It is worth repeating that there are more lines in the Mesopotamian medical literature devoted to the signs and symptoms of skin disease than disease of any other part of the body.

2

Ancient Egypt

At the western end of the Fertile Crescent resided another great civilization of the Bronze Age, Ancient Egypt. Humans began to settle along the fruitful banks of the Nile River by the sixth millennium BCE, but the Upper (southern) and Lower (northern) parts of this region did not become unified until circa 3100 BCE when a monarchy was established there by the first pharaoh. The pharaohs reigned supreme until the Persians conquered Egypt in 525 BCE. The Persians subsequently handed over Egypt to Alexander the Great in 332 BCE, thus starting the Hellenistic kingdom of the Greek-speaking Ptolemies, who ruled Egypt until the Romans annexed it in 30 BCE. Egypt then belonged to the Roman Empire until it was conquered by the Muslims in 641 CE.

Thirty-four different dynasties ruled Egypt over the course of 3000 years (3150–30 BCE). The Sphinx and the great pyramids at Giza were constructed during the Old Kingdom (2686–2181 BCE). The zenith of Egyptian civilization took place during the period of the New Kingdom (1549–1069 BCE), also called the Egyptian Empire, when the famous pharaohs of the 18th Dynasty such as Hatshepsut, Akhenaten and his wife Nefertiti, and Tutankhamen ruled the land. The Library and the famous Lighthouse of Alexandria were built during the Ptolemaic period (332–30 BCE), the former symbolizing Alexandria as the intellectual center of the known world.

In addition to its spectacular architectural achievements, ancient Egyptian civilization is famous for its thriving agriculture, polytheistic religion which emphasized the afterlife, its mummification practices, and numerous other accomplishments in art, science, and technology, including sculpture, mathematics, and shipbuilding. The Frenchman Jean-François Champollion deciphered the hieroglyphic writing system of the ancient Egyptians in 1822, some 23 years after an officer in Napoleon's army discovered the Rosetta Stone. Carved in 196 BCE, the stone contained a code-breaking Ptolemaic decree written in both ancient Egyptian and Greek.

Ancient Egyptian Medicine

Like that of the Mesopotamians, Egyptian medicine was advanced for its time, and it had more influence on the medical traditions that followed it than did its Middle Eastern counterpart. The Egyptians left a lengthy corpus of primary source material—medical papyri—from which we learn about their medical practices. Papyrus (pl. *papyri*) is a paper-like material used by the Alexandrians as a writing surface that came from the papyrus plant, *Cyperus papyrus*, which was once prevalent in the Nile River delta. Papyrus was the major writing material of the ancient world until the plant from which it was derived became harder to obtain, either because it was harvested to the brink of extinction or because of the Ptolemaic monopoly in charge of its export. The rise in price of papyrus led to the widespread acceptance of cheaper alternatives called parchment and vellum (a finer quality of parchment), made from animal skins. Parchment and vellum were the principal writing surfaces of the late ancient and medieval periods, although papyrus continued to be used at the Vatican until the eleventh century.[1] Paper, incidentally, was invented in China in the second century CE but did not reach the Western world until a thousand years later.

The papyri were discovered during the heyday of modern Egyptology that occurred in the latter half of the nineteenth century. There are 12 important medical papyri, but 5 are noteworthy for our study: Edwin Smith Papyrus, Ebers Papyrus, Kahun Gynaecological Papyrus, London Medical Papyrus, and the Hearst Papyrus.[2] Named for the American Egyptologist (1822–1906) who first

DOI: 10.1201/9781003273622-4

acquired it in 1862, the Edwin Smith Papyrus dates to 1600 BCE and is the most scientific and least magic-based of the papyri. This extraordinary document is almost entirely a trauma surgery text. The Ebers Papyrus was named after Georg Ebers (1837–1898), a German Egyptologist who purchased it in 1872. It dates to 1550 BCE, and as the longest of the papyri, it encompasses a variety of medical disciplines including gastroenterology, urology, dermatology, ophthalmology, and cardiology. The oldest of the papyri, The Kahun Gynaecological Papyrus, dates to 1800 BCE. It was discovered at El-Lahun (not Kahun) in 1889 by the great British archeologist Flinders Petrie (1853–1942) and is devoted entirely to women's health. The London medical papyrus gives significant attention to skin and eye disease. The last one is named after the newspaper magnate William Randolph Hearst's mother, Phoebe, and is in superb condition; it contains a chapter in which 13 remedies for diseases of the skin and nails are presented.

From these papyri, we can learn much about the nature of Egyptian medicine. The Egyptian approach to disease and its treatment combined elements of the natural and the supernatural while sharing many features with Mesopotamian medicine. Disease was generally believed to be caused by the entrance of demoniacal spirits into the body, and health could be restored with spells, amulets, and rituals meant to rid the body of the spirit or to make things right for the patient with the gods. The line between religion and medicine was blurred. The papyri reveal an emphasis by the Egyptian healer on the use of herbal, vegetable, animal, and mineral substances deemed to have healing properties in the form of pills, ointments, poultices, fumigations, inhalations, gargles, and suppositories.[3] Honey, frankincense, and salt were the most prevalent ingredients.[4] These healers, equipped with both spells and remedies, were "magicians contending with a demon-infested world."[5]

Enemas were particularly revered and frequently used, often on a scheduled basis, in ancient Egypt. Writing in 450 BCE, Herodotus noted that the Egyptians designated three days of every month for purging the bowels, as they believed that corruption (*purulency*) emanating from excrements in the bowels (termed *whdw*, pronounced *uhkedu*) could be absorbed into the body and end up anywhere in the body, leading to suppuration, blood coagulation, and destruction.[6] The absorption of *whdw* into the body from the bowels continued with age and was the cause of senescence and death. Thus, the ancient Egyptians were obsessed with the bowels, anus, feces, and bowel movements.[7] The use of purges and enemas to evacuate toxic material from the bowels was picked up by the Greeks and incorporated into their humoral theory of disease, and purging the bowels became a mainstay of treating disease until modern times.

The Egyptians, too, had three types of healers, though their functions were rather nebulous: (1) the *swnw*; (2) the priest (of Sekhmet); and (3) the sorcerer.[8] *Swnw*, the Egyptian word for doctor and conventionally pronounced "soo-noo," referred to a healer who prescribed natural medicine and performed surgery, analogous to the *âsû* of Babylon. There was a hierarchy of *swnw* with court physicians at the top, and there was a division of generalists and specialists as we have today. Herodotus famously stated that there were many doctors in Egypt and that "one treats only the diseases of the eye, another those of the head, the teeth, the abdomen, or of the internal organs."[9] The historical record shows that while there were other specialists, such as proctologists, dentists, and eye doctor, there was no specialty of dermatology. With no fee for service in ancient Egyptian medicine, the *swnw* worked for and was funded by the state.[10]

The priests of Sekhmet, a goddess of healing and the patron of doctors, were a type of skilled doctor that administered magical remedies and incantations. Sekhmet was not the only god of healing. The most significant of these deities was Horus, the falcon-headed god and the son of Osiris and Isis, who was often invoked in exorcisms to drive the demons out of the ailing patient. The Eye of Horus was an ancient symbol of protection and good health, particularly in the afterlife. The Rx symbol used on prescriptions, traditionally believed to come from the Latin word for recipe, may have actually been derived from the eye of Horus.[11] Other important Egyptian gods in the realm of health include Thoth and Serket. Thoth, the ibis-headed god of writing and scribes, also gave physicians the healing art; he was also the all-important inventor of the enema. Serket, the scorpion-headed goddess of venomous bites and stings, was revered because the Egyptian people were susceptible to a myriad of bites from snakes, scorpions, crocodiles, and even hippos. If a *swnw* or priest was not available, the afflicted could seek the services of a sorcerer.

IMHOTEP, THE TRUE FOUNDER OF MEDICINE?

The most celebrated physician in ancient Egyptian history was Imhotep (twenty-seventh century BCE), whose name means "he who cometh in peace" and who served as chief vizier to the Pharaoh Zoser and high priest at Heliopolis. He designed the Step Pyramid of Sakkara. Imhotep is considered the first polymath in history, but is most renowned for being a physician, and due to a scarcity of sources about his life, it is impossible to suggest exactly where to put him in the pantheon of the history of medicine. Perhaps if his tomb is finally discovered, his actual accomplishments in medicine will become known to us. Varied are the scholarly opinions of this man. James Breasted, the translator of the Edwin Smith papyrus into English, conjectured that Imhotep authored the document, but there is simply no proof of this assertion.[12] Others, such as the great William Osler, have tried to designate Imhotep as the true "Founder of Medicine" and even argue that the Hippocratic Oath was taken from his philosophy. On the other hand, Prioreschi questioned whether Imhotep was ever a physician.[13] Indeed, there is no historical evidence linking Imhotep to medicine until he was deified 2000 years after his life.[14] The cult of Imhotep, akin to that of Asclepius (see Chapter 3), did not peak until around 300 BCE, when healing shrines in his honor arose. Patients slept overnight at these temples, and they would be visited in their dreams by a god or a snake; upon awakening, their illness was resolved.[15] The other famous Egyptian physicians were: Hesy-Ra, the oldest known physician in world history who was famous for his dentistry; Peseshet, one of the first female physicians; and Iri, whose tomb was found at Giza and who was a physician specialist who lived in the mid-third millennium BCE and was known as the "keeper of the royal rectum."

The embalming practices and mummification techniques imparted a level of knowledge about anatomy that far surpassed that of the Mesopotamian or Greek doctor.[16] The viscera were removed entirely and inspected at the beginning of the embalming process. Their specialization of various medical disciplines reminds us of our modern distinctions of the different fields of medicine. Inscriptions revealing various surgical instruments indicate that surgical intervention was available, albeit in a limited capacity. Circumcision was widely practiced. Contraceptives and abortifacients were written about extensively. Dentists could fill carious teeth. Parasitic illnesses, especially ones caused by worms, were rampant, as were various maladies such as blindness, heart attack, fractures, and dislocations; all of these things had treatments. Prosthetic limbs have been uncovered by archeologists. Bloodletting was not yet practiced— the Egyptians saw no reason for doing so as they did with the enemas.[17] The medicine that the Egyptians practiced was logical and coherent in keeping with their understanding of the world around them.

Skin Disease in Ancient Egypt

The ancient Egyptians left ample material that can be analyzed for the purposes of describing their view of the skin and its diseases, and the natural place to start is the most significant medical document of ancient Egypt, the Ebers Papyrus. It was written during the reign of Amenhotep I in the 1500s BCE in the Egyptian hieratic, a cursive form of hieroglyphic writing. The papyrus that Ebers first saw was a long roll, 12 inches in width and 68 feet in length.[18] It was later cut into 110 pages, each about 20 lines long; modern scholars have divided its content into 877 sections. It reads from right to left. The Ebers Papyrus is so complete that it meets the true definition of a book, and its completeness and perfection inspire awe upon viewing the plates as the scribe who wrote it made no mistakes anywhere throughout the work; no line, word, or letter is missing from the text.[19] The translation of this ancient text is not without difficulty, if not impossible; several scholars of the last century have staked their reputations on that endeavor.[20]

The Ebers Papyrus contains 811 prescriptions for a number of ailments, in addition to sections on diagnosis and symptoms, the physiology of the heart and its vessels, and the surgical management of wounds and sores. Treatments described include salves, plasters, poultices, snuffs, inhalations, gargles, draughts, confections, pills, fumigations, suppositories, and enemata.[21] Many of the remedies have been shown to have therapeutic value. An entire chapter is dedicated to a discussion of castor oil, a laxative found in over 100 of the prescriptions. Natron, a salt found in Lower Egypt, was used for its dehydrating and astringent benefits. Moldy bread or fresh onions were placed on infected wounds; antibiotic substances in these materials may have provided an anti-infective effect.[22] Human excrement as a treatment for disease—termed *drekapotheke*—sounds downright bizarre to the modern student of ancient medicine, but it was a commonplace practice in the ancient world. Plant, mineral, and organic ingredients, including human and animal bodily fluids and excrements in various combinations, make up the concoctions. In addition to medical therapies, spells and incantations are interspersed throughout the work.

The skin is given substantial attention in the Ebers Papyrus, not only as it relates to its diseases but also to the enhancement of its cosmetic appearance. Personal hygiene was crucial to the ancient Egyptian as were esthetics and cosmetics. The Egyptians, unlike the Mesopotamians, did have a well-attested word for the skin—*inm*.[23] Of the 877 sections in the papyrus, 168 (19 percent) deal with acute and chronic wounds, injuries, skin, and hair disorders.[24] The dermatologic conditions addressed in the Ebers Papyrus include dermatitis, pustules, scabies, excoriations, sores, ulcers, buboes, moles/skin tumors, stings/bites, facial eczema, itching, and alopecia areata.[25]

The Ebers Papyrus is heavy on practice and light on theory. The only theory gleaned from the papyrus regarding skin disease is the idea that inflammation of the skin (such as that in erysipelas) and itching were considered manifestations of disease inside the body due to corruptive substances in the abdomen.

The Egyptian treatments for skin disease were, for the most part, bizarre and based more on magical beliefs than scientific principles. Most skin diseases were treated externally with poultices and internally with laxatives or enemas to remove the *whdw*.[26] Itching was treated according to the affected area of the body. For generalized itching, onion and honey added to beer was ingested. Neck itching was treated with "chopped up bat" applied as a poultice, while a poultice consisting of onions, dried beads, red natron, sea salt, and sour milk healed itching of the thigh "at once."[27] For more severe itching accompanying "blood corrosion," a concoction of elderberries, linseed, wormwood, natron, and various native plants was rubbed into a poultice with "semen of a man, yeast of wine, and juice of the wild date."[28] The same plaster was advised for the common scurf (dandruff), and for more severe cases, the dung of the cat and dog was applied.[29]

For the "stinking ulcer in a man or woman," the wound was anointed with powdered onion or a mixture of warm ostrich egg and tortoise shell, with the admonition, "don't get tired doing it."[30] Numerous other therapies for wounds, burns, and ulcers are described, such as cold meat applied to hot, infected wounds.[31] There are several different remedies for "eliminating heat from the anus" or "cooling the anus," suggesting that the ancient Egyptians were plagued by anal pruritus.[32] Crocodile bites are addressed in Section 436. In Section 869, a description of a sebaceous cyst and its excision can be found, with the all-too-true statement, "if anything remains in its pocket, it will recur."[33] The first extant description of how to properly extract the Guinea worm (*dracunculiasis*), after impaling it with a stick, can be found in Section 875. Other skin issues addressed include ingrown toenails, scalp eczema, herpes of the face, perspiration-related rashes, and body odor. When all else failed, a panacea to completely rid the skin of any disease could be ingested: ass's milk, resin of acanthus, indigo, duat plant, turpentine nuts, and honey.[34]

The Ebers Papyrus also deals with the cosmetic concerns of wrinkles, "renewing the skin," "causing the face to stretch," and "eliminating spots of the face."[35] Honey, natron, and alabaster flour were rubbed on the skin daily to promote a youthful appearance. The author promises, "Do it, you will witness success."[36] Several of the recipes call for milk; it is known that Cleopatra used sour milk, high in lactic acid, which can achieve the same effect as a modern-day chemical peel.[37] Many of the artifacts discovered in royal tombs are bottles containing lotions and oils that were used for cosmetic purposes. Sandpaper, still used today for that exact purpose, was used by the Egyptians to abrade scars for the purposes of improving their appearance. The Egyptians were apparently as obsessed with eliminating gray hair as we can be today, and another ten remedies are listed for stimulating hair growth in the balding person.[38] The papyrus mentions alopecia areata, and the bald spots were anointed with unguent containing "hedgehog bristle, burnt, dipped in fat."[39] Remedies for removing hair were described, but not for the reasons you would typically think. Instead, they were used for the sake of revenge, "to be poured over the head of the hated woman."[40] In spite of this abundant content about the skin, some scholars have argued that the book is actually deficient in its dealings with skin diseases, which must have been a rampant problem at the time.[41]

THE PRICE OF BEAUTY

According to evidence from a CT scan of her mummified corpse, Hatshepsut (1507–1458 BCE) allegedly died of bone cancer, which ended lifelong suffering from a chronic skin disease that may have been familial. Suspect diseases include the congenital ichthyoses, pemphigus, psoriasis, and other disorders of keratinization. Researchers at the University of Bonn claim that a bottle of skin lotion found among her artifacts was shown to contain a hazardous carcinogen called benzopyrene, leading several modern scholars to question whether Hatshepsut's skin cream killed her.[42] Per these investigators, the residual substance inside the bottle contained hydrocarbons derived from creosote and asphalt and was apparently very greasy, making it the perfect type of vehicle for someone with a hyperkeratotic skin disease.

And speaking of cosmetics, when one thinks of Cleopatra, one might first imagine her eyes and the heavy makeup she applied to them. It turns out this ritual was not just for beauty but also for medical reasons. Ancient Egyptians applied to their eyelids the dark soil from the Nile region, which, in some instances, contained a plant-based substance called *kohl* in order to ward off diseases or other dangerous forces that could damage the eyes. Other motives behind the use of *kohl* were to reduce the glare from the bright Egyptian sun and to keep disease-causing flies out of the eyes. Modern scientists who have studied the effectiveness of this practice have shown that the substance Egyptians applied to the eyes contained lead sulfide—a compound that is toxic in high doses but in low doses invokes nitric oxide production from the skin and an immune response to infection.[43]

Hatshepsut and Cleopatra were not the only famous monarchs in history to dabble in potentially deadly makeup. Queen Elizabeth (1533–1603) was so self-conscious about her smallpox scars that she wore a layer of "clown white" makeup up to an inch thick on her face and may have used a lead-based makeup (Venetian ceruse) to lighten her skin, a substance that may have ultimately killed her (lead poisoning). And while we are on the topic of deadly cosmeceuticals, we cannot ignore Giulia Tofana (1620–1659), the seventeenth-century Italian inventor of *aqua tofana*, an arsenic-based, poisonous liquid sold in innocuous cosmetic bottles. Before she was finally caught and executed, over 600 Roman wives killed their abusive husbands with just a few drops of the concoction.

But unlike the Mesopotamians, who were "splitters" and crafted a descriptive nomenclature of skin lesions, the Egyptians were apparently "lumpers"—they did not have a wide variety of terms for different lesions or diseases. The categories of skin ailments dealt with by the Egyptians were broad topics such as itching, ulcers, wounds, swellings, etc. This less scientific approach to dermatologic concerns is evident in the Ebers Papyrus, but it seems that the *swnw* would have been able to find something in the book to treat any skin disease he was asked to address.

Absent from the Ebers Papyrus is any categorical description of leprosy. Although the case delineated in Section 870 was long held to be a discussion of that disease, it is more likely to represent tuberculosis.[44] The first solid evidence of leprosy in Egyptian medicine dates to the Ptolemaic period.[45] Contrary to what most dermatologists are taught about the history of phototherapy in residency and in review articles, there is no mention in the Ebers Papyrus of the Egyptians having used sunlight to treat vitiligo.[46]

The Edwin Smith Papyrus provides little information about Egyptian dermatological practices. The document is dated to the seventeenth century BCE, but "the original author's first manuscript was produced a thousand years earlier."[47] The work contains surgical cases as opposed to the therapeutic recipes of the Ebers Papyrus. The cases were copied by a scribe 3500 years ago who, unlike the writer of the Ebers Papyrus, "had been none too careful in his copying, and he made many errors."[48] All 48 cases deal with trauma to the body, arranged starting with injuries to the head and working down the body. The brutality of the wounds discussed, such as a broken nose, gaping wound, and fracture of the humerus, would suggest that the author was a military surgeon. The physical examination performed by the surgeon, as it still is today, is an instrumental step in the evaluation of the patient in these cases. In addition, the Edwin Smith Papyrus has the earliest evidence of an inductive process involving observation and conclusions.[49] Review by the present author of these cases in the Breasted translation failed to reveal any substantive information about the skin or skin disease.

But there is a section of dermatologic interest in the Edwin Smith Papyrus: the somewhat random insertion of material regarding cosmetics at the end of the document. As in the Ebers Papyrus, we see the recommendation of a simple topical application of ingredients seen previously: honey, red natron, and salt (in 1:1:1 ratio) for the purposes of "transforming the skin."[50] The more compelling portion is the last section of the entire work entitled "Recipe for Transforming an Old Man into a Youth." A different scribe added these last 26 lines at a later date and described the recipe for an ointment that can "become a beautifier of the skin, a remover of blemishes, of all disfigurements, of all signs of age, of all weaknesses which are in the flesh. Found effective myriads of times."[51] The main ingredient in this rather propitious ointment was called by the Egyptians hemayet fruit. Originally thought to be a type of legume called fenugreek, more recently it has been suggested that the term instead refers to bitter almonds.[52] Bitter almonds, unlike sweet almonds, contain prussic acid (also known as hydrogen cyanide), which can cause lethal cyanide poisoning upon ingesting just 50 nuts on average for adults and much less for children. Boiling and baking the almonds, as the papyrus suggests, extricates the prussic acid and makes them safe to eat. The bitter almond also contains mandelic acid, and it is this chemical that has been purported to have cosmetic benefits for the wrinkled face, as well as improvement in acne. Authors of a recent research article claimed that elasticity of the skin improved by 25 percent and firmness by 24 percent after just four weeks of application.[53] Perhaps the Egyptians were on to something.

Paleodermatology: The Mummies

In addition to the literary documents, the Egyptians also left behind unusual physical evidence which informs us about skin disease: the mummies. The study of disease through the examination of ancient remains is called paleopathology, and the evaluation of the skin in these remains is termed paleodermatology.[54] Although it is dehydrated, brittle and heavily pigmented, mummy skin is often surprisingly well preserved, and the tissue must be rehydrated before staining can ensue.[55] Only a few thousand of the estimated 70 million Egyptian mummies have been discovered, with more being exhumed every year.[56] The Egyptians were not the only culture to practice mummification. In fact, mummies have been found on six continents.

The Egyptian mummification process was an elaborate effort to preserve the body in order to increase the chances that the dead would experience the afterlife. They believed that the soul, known as *Ka*, left the body upon death but would return to a properly embalmed body, and the afterlife would ensue. The custom of embalming was initially only available to the royal or wealthy families, but eventually it became a universal practice.[57] There were several different methods of mummification; the choice depended on what the dead could afford. The earliest routine involved dehydrating the body in a shallow grave pit in the hot sands by a process known as natural mummification. The more famous, two-phase intentional method dates to the early New Kingdom (1549–1069 BCE). In the first phase, which lasted 40 days, the internal organs—except for the heart—were eviscerated and placed in ceremonial jars. The brain was extracted piece by piece from the skull by a hook inserted through a nostril (excerebration) and discarded. The body was then washed, fragranced with spices, and stuffed and covered with natron in order to dehydrate the body. In the second phase, lasting 30 days, the remaining substances inside the body were removed, and the corpse was anointed with oils, coated with a protective resin, wrapped with strips of linen, and decorated with masks and shrouds. After 70 days, the mummy was ready for burial.

THE ORIGINS OF THE WORD "MUMMY"

The word "mummy" can be traced back to its root words *mum*, *mumya*, and *mumiya* which referred to a black bituminous resin (asphalt) that was found, albeit rarely, in Egypt, the Dead Sea region, and the Middle East. Beginning in the first century CE, it was believed to have medicinal properties. While some of the mummies of later ancient Egypt were indeed coated with this natural *mumiya*, Europeans in the Middle Ages assumed the blackened exudate on the surface of the skin of all mummies to be this medicinal bitumen, which they called *mumia* in Latin.[58] As a result of this mistaken belief, Egyptian mummies became valuable commodities which were exported from Egypt to Europe until the eighteenth century, and broken pieces or powder from mummies could be found in bottles in European apothecaries as a prescription medication starting in the sixteenth century.[59] After that century, the word *mumia* evolved into the English word mummy, to represent the entirety of the remains of the dead, not just the material scraped off its surface. There was eventually a crackdown on the mummy trade, and a resulting black market ensued. Derived from the desiccated bodies of travelers and animals, numerous faux mummy products appeared in pharmacopeias all over Europe and were mainly used in the treatment of falls and bruises throughout the Enlightenment; in 1905, it was still listed in a German pharmacist's handbook.[60]

What remains today of these Egyptian mummies can be studied not only with the naked eye, but also histologically and molecularly in order to determine the presence of skin disease. With varying degrees of quality, the epidermis, pilosebaceous structures, collagen, elastic tissue fibers, blood vessels, and subcutaneous fat are preserved in mummies, but the detail of keratinocyte nuclei and hair follicles is lost, as well as many dermal details.[61] The biopsy findings of several dermatologic diseases have also been described.[62] In their published research, Jones et al. identified 230 proteins in the skin of three 4200-year-old mummies and, based on the protein composition in the skin, drew conclusions about the cause of death of the mummies.[63] At a molecular level, enzyme-linked immunosorbent assays (ELISA), electron microscopy, and polymerase chain reaction (PCR) have been used, with varying degrees of diagnostic certainty, to establish the presence of certain infectious agents such as treponemes, mycobacteria, and smallpox. Nits and head lice have been identified on mummies.[64] While no tattoos have been found on the skin of Egyptian mummies, eye paint has been identified, as well as makeup.[65] Baldness is not an uncommon finding among Egyptian mummies, but, when found, hair is generally in excellent condition for study and is considered "the keeper of history," as its color and style is typically preserved over time, allowing for description of ancient Egyptian styling practices.[66]

The most famous example of Egyptian paleodermatology was documented by Donald Hopkins, who was able to inspect the well-preserved mummy of the pharaoh Ramses V (twelfth century BCE) in 1979.[67] Ramses was suspected of having smallpox by gross inspection of the facial scarring and pustules found on his skin, but this has not been substantiated with molecular studies.[68] According to Hopkins, elevated pustules that are 2–4 mm in size are found on Ramses' face, neck, shoulders, and arms. He could not examine the palms and soles where smallpox lesions would be expected. As the lesions were not present on his chest or upper abdomen, the classic centrifugal pattern (see Interlude 4) of smallpox is confirmed.

Examination of mummy hair led to one of the great mysteries in modern archeological research. In the 1990s, a team of German scientists led by Svetlana Balabanova claimed to have found evidence of nicotine and cocaine residue in the hair of the Henut Taui mummy from the 21st dynasty (ca. 1000 BCE). Henut Taui was dubbed one of several "cocaine mummies."[69] Cocaine and nicotine came from the New World plants coca and tobacco, respectively, so the claims were obviously antithetical to the commonly held belief that there was no contact between the New World and Old World until the Age of Exploration beginning in the fifteenth century CE. The story of the "cocaine mummies" was picked up by the media and popular science magazines but failed to gain any traction in archeological circles, where contamination of the mummies with these substances is the prevailing explanation for this asynchronous finding.

Summary

The Egyptian *swnw* left his mark on the history of medicine and, in some minor ways, on the history of dermatology. Several informative documents, such as the medical papyri, as well as human remains enable us to identify disease "in the flesh" from their era. The Egyptians did have a name for the skin—*inm*—but they lacked a detailed nomenclature for skin diseases comparable to the one developed by the Mesopotamians. Personal hygiene was crucial to the ancient Egyptian as were esthetics and cosmetics. While there seemed to be specialists in virtually every field but dermatology, skin disease was on the mind of the general *swnw*, and almost 20 percent of the most famous Egyptian medical papyrus, the Ebers, was devoted to skin disease. The Egyptians saw the skin as a reflection of internal health, particularly in the case of inflammatory skin diseases and itching. Many of the therapeutic interventions of the *swnw*, such as purgation, influenced the Greeks, Romans, and beyond. Although the papyri contain glimpses of a preference for a natural view of disease and its treatment, Egyptian medicine could not shed its supernatural influences.

3

Classical Greece

It is hard to argue that there was ever a more impactful period in human history than the fifth and fourth centuries BCE, when the ancient Greeks experienced their Classical Age (510–323 BCE). This spectacular period of nearly 200 years was sandwiched between the Archaic period, which began with the first Olympic games in 776 BCE and ended with the deposing of the last Greek tyrant in 510 BCE, and the Hellenistic period, which started with the death of Alexander the Great in 323 BCE. The Greek Classical Age is represented by Socrates, Plato, and Aristotle—philosophers who undoubtedly left a great legacy. It was also a period marked by three domestic wars: the 50-year-long conflict with the Persian Empire (499–449 BCE) that ended with the defeat of the Persians and their ousting from the Aegean region, as well as two internal wars between the dominant city-states of Athens and Sparta in the Peloponnesian Wars (460–445 BCE and 431–404 BCE). Though the First Peloponnesian War ended with a truce, Athens clearly had the upper hand, and the period after the first war is called the "Golden Age of Athens." Led by the statesman Pericles (495–429 BCE), the economic and political successes of the Athenian Empire allowed for a quintessential cultural flourishing, so typical in history for this level of stability.

During this "Age of Pericles," the Athenians dominated Greece and produced many of its enduring cultural legacies, e.g., the tragedies of Aeschylus (523–456 BCE), Sophocles (497–406 BCE), and Euripides (480–406 BCE); the comedies of Aristophanes (446–386 BCE); the histories of Herodotus (484–425 BCE) and Thucydides (460–400 BCE). Despite the construction of the Parthenon and a demonstration of the democratic form of government, Athenian hegemony was short-lived. In 431 BCE, Athens entered into a Second Peloponnesian War with Sparta and Pericles, and tens of thousands of Athenians were decimated by a plague just two years into the conflict (see Interlude 2). While their dominance lasted until 404 BCE, the Athenians never recovered, and they were finally defeated by the Spartans, whose power also eventually waned after the turn of the fourth century BCE. That century saw the rise of the Macedonian Empire, begun by Philip II (382–336 BCE) and expanded all the way to India by his son Alexander (356–323 BCE), whose still-unsurpassed accomplishments occurred over such a short life.

The Greek achievements throughout the fourth and fifth centuries BCE in philosophy, literature, architecture, and government were accompanied by commensurate successes in the realm of natural philosophy (science), but these accomplishments preceded this period and would continue well afterward. Starting in the sixth century with Thales of Miletus (624–546 BCE), a string of philosopher-mathematician-astronomer types—the pre-Socratic philosophers—attempted to explain the world around them with a scientific approach instead of the entrenched mythology. Anaximander (610–546 BCE), possibly a pupil of Thales, was the first to develop a systematic cosmology using mathematical principles. His student, Pythagoras of Samos (570–495 BCE), whose actual contributions have been debated intensely by modern historians, was credited with many discoveries in mathematics, music, astronomy, and philosophy. He was among the first in the West to promote the idea of reincarnation with his belief in the transmigration of the soul: the immortal soul leaves the body at death and enters another. Also attributed to Pythagoras is the glorious theory of *musica universalis*, "universal music," the idea that the heavenly bodies move around one another in a mathematics-based, musical—albeit inaudible— symphony. Next in line was Xenophanes of Colophon (570–475 BCE), one of the first skeptics; he viewed religious beliefs as human constructs. Democritus (460–370 BCE), who proposed the atomic theory of the universe, and Empedocles (494–434 BCE), who originated the idea of the four elements—earth, air, fire, and water—were among the last of the great pre-Socratic philosophers.

Socrates, Plato, and Aristotle were the three greatest philosophers of the Classical Greek period; all three are considered founders of Western philosophy. Although he never wrote any books, Socrates (470–399 BCE) was an enigmatic figure written about extensively by his pupil, Plato (428–348 BCE) in

DOI: 10.1201/9781003273622-5

his *Dialogues*. Socrates' greatest contributions are in the fields of ethics and epistemology (the study of knowledge). Plato is famous for founding the first institution of higher learning in the Western world—the Academy at Athens. He is also known for his Theory of Forms, which proposes that ideas (forms) are more absolute than physical objects, which are mere physical interpretations or representations of an idea. To Plato, observation of these objects occurred through sensation, and because the senses could not be trusted, one's observations could not be trusted. His contribution to the history of medicine was his *Timaeus*, an influential text that focused on medicine, health, philosophy, and politics.[1]

Of the Greek philosophers, the career of Plato's most famous student, Aristotle (384–322 BCE), was the most consequential in the history of medicine. As the true father of natural philosophy (science), Aristotle wrote influential works on logic, physics, metaphysics, astronomy, biology, and zoology. Of these, his contributions in logic are his most outstanding achievement. Aristotle's philosophy was more concrete than that of his mentor; for Aristotle, direct observation was the key to understanding the natural world. Some have argued that Aristotle is one of the founders of evidence-based medicine as his teachings were the driving force that steered medicine away from supernatural methods and toward the scientific method.[2] According to Aristotle, in the human body, "nature did nothing in vain;" therefore, each part of the body had a purpose. The heart was the seat of the soul and the source of innate heat, while the brain functioned to cool the blood and bring about sleep.[3] Views of the natural world such as this, as well as his approach to investigating and analyzing the natural world, dominated Western discourses in natural philosophy until the Scientific Revolution of the seventeenth century.

While the aforementioned achievements represent a small sampling of the many accomplishments of the Greeks during the Classical and Hellenistic periods, they symbolize a transition point in the history of Western civilization. In many ways, the Greeks represent a shift from the ancient to the pre-modern because they laid the foundations for modernity. Their contributions in the history of medicine are prime examples.

Classical Greek Medicine

All histories of Greek medicine begin with Asclepius, venerated by the Greeks as the god of medicine and mentioned in the first line of the Hippocratic Oath. The son of Apollo, Asclepius learned the healing art from Chiron, the centaur, but because of fears that he might make all men immortal, Zeus had Asclepius killed with a thunderbolt; from that time forward, he was known as the god of medicine and physicians. Asclepius carried a staff encircled by a single snake. The Rod of Asclepius is the correct symbol of medicine, not the *caduceus*—the staff of the god Hermes (Mercury)—which has two wings at the top and is intertwined with two snakes. The confusion began when the US Army Medical Corps mistakenly adopted the *caduceus* in 1902.[4]

In seeking relief from their illnesses, the ailing would flock to healing temples called asclepeions throughout the Greek world, named in honor of Asclepius. After a night spent in the snake-laden asclepeion, the infirm would report their dreams to the temple priest (asclepiad), who would perform a ritual appropriate for the dream, often involving non-venomous snakes. Or the patient could donate to the asclepeion votive offerings of pottery or metal, depicting the organ or disease of concern.[5] The asclepeions thrived for hundreds of years and would remain a popular destination for healthcare well into the Roman period.

It was within one of these asclepeions that the seeds of scientific medicine were sown. The most crucial figure in the history of Greek medicine was an Asclepiad named Hippocrates (460–370 BCE) from the Greek island of Kos. While there was indeed a physician (ἰατρός, iatrós, Greek for "physician") of this name who practiced medicine during the Age of Pericles, our knowledge about his life is limited to information from biographies written about him hundreds of years later and is, in large part, the stuff of legends. What we do know about the man is that he was mentioned by Plato and that he practiced medicine, taught what he knew for a fee, and had a son.[6] The eponymous writings were composed between 420 and 350 BCE and assembled at Alexandria around 280 BCE.[7] Hippocrates himself wrote none of them, including the famous oath bearing his name. This collection of 60 works that represent the accumulation of classical Greek medical knowledge is called the "Hippocratic Corpus." The different texts that make up the corpus do not share a uniformity of viewpoints. In fact, it is sometimes very challenging to make any generalizations from the corpus because it contains many theories, many of which conflict with one another.[8] So, the Hippocratic medicine that we know today was both an amalgamation of the many different points of view in the corpus and a cherry-picking of sorts of the most agreeable features of the corpus to Galen (129–210 CE), the first and most influential advocate of Hippocratic medicine. Thus, Hippocratic medicine is a historical construct, i.e., concepts put together in a framework that was unknown by the writers of the corpus.[9]

Hippocratic medicine was, above all else, holistic medicine; the Greeks emphasized diet and exercise, "nothing in excess," and refrained from intervention in order to "let nature run its course."[10] In addition to their preference for treating the whole patient, rather than focusing on a specific disease state, the Hippocratics differed from other ancient physicians in that they understood disease as a natural phenomenon, and they deemphasized religion. The Hippocratics appealed to rationality and argument and viewed disease as resulting from natural phenomenon, not supernatural interference.[11] Inspection and observation of the patient were important to the Hippocratics. While priests administered a religion-based type of healing at shrines that continued to flourish during the classical period, Hippocratic medicine developed as an alternative to the arcane, non-rational sanctums.[12]

Underlying the entirety of Hippocratic medicine was the humoral theory of disease, which would become the principal means by which disease was explained for the next 2000 years.[13] The Greeks believed that the body was composed of four humors: blood, produced by the heart; phlegm, by the brain; yellow bile, by the liver; and black bile, by the spleen. As there is no such thing as "black bile" in the human body, the ancients had to completely fabricate it to make their scheme work. Each humor had a corresponding element, respectively: air, water, fire, and earth. It was held that disease was caused by an imbalance of these humors, and therapeutic interventions—such as purgation to remove excessive amounts of bile—were expected to restore the natural balance of humors that varied according to the age of the patient. No longer were diseases such as epilepsy, which had been referred to as the "Sacred Disease," explained as being brought about, or relieved, by divine intervention.[14] In addition, the Hippocratics differed from the Mesopotamians and Egyptians in other, distinctly modern points of emphasis. They preferred practice over theory, experience over precedent, speculation over acceptance, bedside over classroom, balance over imbalance, less over more. Finally, Hippocratic medicine was ethical medicine. In reference to the Oath, it is evident that the Hippocratics held themselves to the highest moral and professional standards the Western world had yet seen. With all of these differences in mind, it can be said that the history of modern medicine begins with Hippocrates. The Hippocratics left a legacy emphasizing the natural cause of disease and providing guidelines for the practice of medicine by a selfless and ethical physician.[15]

But how much exactly did the Greeks borrow from the medicine of neighboring cultures of the Near East? It is a complex question, but according to Vivian Nutton, one of the world's foremost authorities on ancient medicine, the Greeks knew of the "sophisticated medical culture of Egypt," and Greek medicine shared many features with that of its Egyptian predecessors, especially their emphasis on bodily fluids.[16] But there are many aspects of Greek medicine that cannot be found in ancient Egyptian medicine. The main weakness of Hippocratic medicine was its limited knowledge about the inner workings of the human body.[17] Dissection was a cultural taboo of the Greeks, and in the Hippocratic corpus there is no conclusive evidence that the Hippocratic physicians had any experience with dissection of the human body.[18]

Not quite three years after Aristotle's most renowned student, Alexander of Macedon, completed his conquest of the eastern territory up to the Indus River, Alexander abruptly died in Babylon at just 32 years of age. His empire was eventually partitioned into several different kingdoms; the three most important were in Macedonia, Ptolemaic Egypt (centered around Alexandria), and the Seleucid empire (centered around Antioch in modern-day Turkey). The nearly 300 years of history after Alexander's death (323 BCE) are called the Hellenistic period, a period that ended with the Roman conquest of Egypt in 31 BCE and the death of Cleopatra a year later. The ancient Greeks called themselves Hellenes, and the word Hellenistic refers to the adoption of Greek language, philosophy, art and architecture, and political ideals across the Mediterranean and Middle East. Like the preceding Classical period (510–323 BCE), the Hellenistic period was an age rich in the arts, architecture, literature, astronomy, mathematics, and science. This Hellenistic period saw the writing of *Elements* by Euclid (ca. 325–265 BCE), the most influential mathematics book in human history, and the "Eureka!" moment of Archimedes (287–212 BCE), as he discovered his principle of buoyancy. Eratosthenes (276–194 BCE) correctly estimated the circumference of the earth. It was the era of competing philosophical schools of the Epicureans, founded by Epicurus (341–270 BCE); the Cynics, founded by Diogenes (412–323 BCE); and the Stoics, founded by Zeno (334–262 BCE). There is no greater symbol of the Hellenistic period than the Library at Alexandria, most likely constructed during the reign of Ptolemy II (283–246 BCE). Other aspects of Hellenistic culture combined elements of classical Greece with the ancient Near East and Egypt.

Medicine after Hippocrates diverged into competing sects (schools) which differed in their doctrines regarding the origins of disease and the manner in which knowledge about disease and its treatment should best be obtained. The direct descendants of Hippocrates, including his physician-son Thessalus, belonged to the Dogmatic school, so-called because they viewed the rational leanings of the Hippocratic corpus as dogma. The Dogmatics believed that hidden disease explained symptoms and that evaluation of the patient should be directed toward revealing that disease, which would then suggest a treatment. Animal dissection was valued as a means by which an understanding of the inner workings of the human body could be attained. The two most important members of this medical sect were Diocles of Carystus (ca. 375–295 BCE) and Praxagoras of Cos (b. 340 BCE). The former is particularly noteworthy, as he authored the first textbook on animal anatomy and is also acknowledged for his writings on human health. Scholarship by van der Eijk has elevated Diocles, "the younger Hippocrates," to a level second only to Hippocrates on the influence scale of ancient Greek physicians.[19]

The Dogmatic school dominated Greek medicine for much of antiquity; competition from the Empiric school and Methodic school began in the Roman period. Led by Heraclides of Tarentum (fl. third to second century BCE), the Empiric school argued in favor of observation, history, and experience over the Hippocratic reasoning and speculation.[20] Rather than focus on the hidden disease state, Empirics used their past experience with the observed symptoms to determine the proper treatment for the patient. In contrast, the Methodic school, founded by Themison of Laodicea (fl. first century BCE), shunned both knowledge of disease and past experience in favor of a more "cookbook" type of medicine; the symptoms quickly suggested the treatment.[21]

The intellectual center of medicine shifted to Alexandria during the Hellenistic period, when two very influential physicians in Alexandrian medicine, Herophilus of Chalcedon (335–280 BCE) and Erasistratus of Chios (304–250 BCE), came to the fore. The writings of both have been lost, but we know of their contributions through later writers. Herophilus carried forth the work of his mentor Praxagoras who made contributions in the field of human anatomy and was perhaps the first to dissect a human for scientific purposes in ancient Greece. He dissected cadavers in public and may have performed vivisections on condemned criminals. Herophilus was able to trace the path of each of the nerves back to the brain, which he believed—rather than the heart—to be the source of intelligence, movement, and sensation, as well as the seat of the soul.[22] Furthermore, while the Hippocratic school saw no association between the lungs and breathing, Herophilus believed that air entered the body through the lungs. He proved that arteries are different from veins and were not air tubes but conduits for blood and *pneuma*, the term used for the vital "air" or "spirit" that maintained the living state or consciousness. In addition to several other findings, such as the discovery and naming of the prostate and the duodenum, Herophilus worked with the pulse and was able to measure it with a portable water clock.[23]

Erasistratus, too, experimented on humans, both dead and alive, and echoed Herophilus' conclusions that the brain was the organ of intelligence. The main distinction was his belief that nerves were hollow tubes containing *pneuma*, which was also contained in the arteries.[24] He explained that the blood squirted out of cut arteries because it was drawn into those vessels as in a vacuum.[25] Erasistratus, as well as Herophilus before him, promoted bloodletting to remove sanguine humor from the body, as he thought excess blood, in particular, was responsible for many diseases. The practice, which the Hippocratics wrote about but did not put forth as a principal treatment approach, entered mainstream medicine in the Roman period.

In the centuries that followed, medicine was further subdivided into sects (the Herophileans and the Erasistrateans) based on these differences in understanding the nature of the human body. Another school, the Pneumatic school of the first century CE, led by Athenaeus of Cilicia (fl. first century CE), emphasized *pneuma* as the vital substance and the cause of disease; this belief can be traced back to the discoveries of Herophilus and Erasistratus in the third century BCE.

By the time the Romans began to dominate the Greek-speaking world, Hippocratic medicine had been established as the primary basis of medical knowledge for the ancient physician. Hippocratic medicine emphasized rational theory and the wisdom that comes from the experience of practice, and it promoted ethical and moral behavior in its practitioners. And medicine after the Hippocratics was well on its way to being completely severed from the supernatural. By the end of the period, the Greeks had a rudimentary understanding of the anatomy of the nervous and circulatory systems, and although they had yet to figure out precisely the physiology of those systems, they recognized the place of the brain, not the heart, as the seat of intelligence. Based on imbalances of the four humors, the Greeks had developed a sensible explanation for the roots of disease. Still, there was no unity of belief as Greek medicine splintered into several aforementioned competing schools of thought. Only after the career of Galen (see Chapter 4), who rectified, codified, and solidified all of the different viewpoints, did the Greco-Roman world have its singular workable system.

Skin Disease in Classical Greece

The dermatologist pays homage to the Greeks every single day in practice. *Epidermis. Rhinophyma. Pityriasis lichenoides.* The language of the field of dermatology was in part built by the Greeks. One of the joys of being a dermatologist is speaking the antiquated language that perpetually recognizes the influence of the Greeks (and Romans) in the specialty. Although the meanings of the words may have changed, the dermatologist uses words today that were used by physicians 2000 years ago. The language of dermatology, like the language of medicine, did not stray from its roots as it evolved. Ninety percent of the technical terms used today in medicine have Greek, Latin, or Greco-Latin origins.[26]

The Greeks had a word for human skin—*derma* (δέρμα)—which meant "skin." Prior to the time of Homer, this word meant "animal hide."[27] It came from the ancient Greek verb, *dero* (δέρω), which means to skin or to flay. Hippocrates was the first to refer to the epidermis, which meant "on top of the skin," but it did not become an English word until 1626.[28] Later, Latin writers would refer to the dermal layer as the "true skin" because the dermis gives the skin its strength and texture and is very much the substance of the skin. No microscope was required to discover the two main layers of the skin; the lesson is learned through the blistering experience of a burn or aggressive cupping. The word "dermatology" is derived from the Greek *derma* and *logia* (δέρμα-λογία)—the study of the skin. Incidentally, the word "skin" is derived from the Norse word *skinn* and entered into Old English sometime after the Vikings settled in Britain, after 800 CE.

Many of the dermatological terms that are still in use today were first found in the pages of the Hippocratic corpus; Galen and the later Latin authors modified or added to the terminology. Many of the terms derive from the botanical, agricultural, or zoological fields, terms that were by the process of metaphorization transformed into "medicalisms."[29] A dermatologic word of Greek derivation that was developed with botanical metaphorization is "lichen" (*leichen*, tree moss). Other important dermatologic words of Greek origin include herpes (*herpo*, to creep or move slowly), eczema (*ekzeo*, to boil up), alopecia (*alopex,* fox), erythema (*eruthrós*, red), condyloma (*condylos*, knuckle), hyperhidrosis (*hidros*, sweat), scleroderma (*skleros*, hard), exanthem (*anthema*, flower, blooming), and pityriasis (*pityron*, scurf or bran).

SKIN DISEASE IN GREEK MYTHOLOGY

In Greek mythology, skin disease is mentioned frequently. For example, in the myth of Melampus as told by Hesiod (ca. 750–650 BCE), the daughters of King Proetus of Argos angered Dionysius and were afflicted with hysteria and two dermatologic problems: *alphos* (vitiligo) and hair loss. Melampus, a healer and soothsayer, cured the girls using hellebore in exchange for taking one of the daughters as his wife. White hellebore, a plant called *Veratrum album,* was believed to be discovered by Melampus and was used as a purgative in ancient Greco-Roman medicine. It can have a somewhat toxic effect, and recently a researcher argued that the same agent may have been responsible for the poisoning death of Alexander the Great.[30] The story reflects a unique circumstance when natural medicine was incorporated in the supernatural stories of the ancient Greeks.

Although the Greeks had a rich vocabulary to describe the layers and diseases of the skin, the organ itself received little scientific attention in the Hippocratic corpus. They simply viewed the skin as a surface envelope, encasing the structures underneath it and containing pores from which sweat emanated. Prior to the anatomic discoveries of Herophilus and Erasistratus, some non-Hippocratic Greek thinkers, e.g., Empedocles, Plato, and Diocles, considered the skin an essential structure in the process of breathing. This concept can be found in the origins of the word perspiration, Latin for "breathing through." Empedocles wrote of people having "bloodless tubes of flesh extended over the surface of their bodies; and at the mouths of these the outermost surface of the skin is perforated all over with pores closely packed together, so as to keep in the blood while a free passage is cut for the air to pass through."[31] In the *Timaeus*, Plato quoted Empedocles and offered a similar explanation of the skin as the interface between the inside of the body and the outside air, which is absorbed through the skin into the blood. Plato viewed the skin as a fishnet—a structure that was woven together tightly enough to keep together the parts it contained but porous enough to allow for the exchange of air and heat. This porous, fishnet interpretation of the skin would persist well into the Renaissance.[32] Diocles also subscribed to the skin-breathing theory; in a passage on caring for the skin, he wrote that "cleaning makes the pores less clogged and better capable of breathing."[33] The concept died, however, with the writings of Aristotle, who criticized their theories, ignored the skin, and saw the breath as having the sole purpose to cool the heart by entering and exiting the body through the lungs.[34] The Alexandrian anatomists would provide evidence that Aristotle's system of breathing was more accurate than that of his mentor, Plato.

The ancient Greek physician was unaware of sweat glands, which were not discovered until the seventeenth-century microscopists started viewing the skin with their instrument. Nor did they understand the function of perspiration as a cooling mechanism. Instead, the Greeks appreciated sweat as a mechanism by which the body could be rid of superfluous humors, and sweat's association with pollution and stench made its elimination seem crucial to the Greek physician, believing the failure to sweat out such pollution could lead to disease.[35] Thus, sweat baths and medicines that promoted sweating (sudorifics) were widely used, with the caution that too much sweating could also be dangerous.[36] In Hippocrates' *Prognostics*, sweats in the setting of illness varied by type and prognostic value. Sweating during acute diseases, especially sweats over the whole body, were considered beneficial and believed to carry off the fever, but cold sweats confined to the head, face, and neck along with an acute fever predicted death.[37]

The Greeks were ignorant of the details of the tactile functions of the skin. The most influential writer on the subject of the sense of touch was Aristotle, who held that the organ of touch was not the brain, nor in the skin or flesh, but in the area around the heart.[38] Unaware of both the cutaneous nerves and the sensory function of the peripheral nervous system, Aristotle believed that wave-like undulations of the blood conducted sensation from the skin to the heart, but he never investigated the anatomical basis of sense perception in the skin itself.[39] While Galen advanced somewhat the understanding of tactile sensation, the basic premises of the Aristotelian theory of touch remained dogma until the discovery of the cutaneous nerves by the great anatomists of the Renaissance and early modern period.

In the *Timaeus*, Plato offered a rather elaborate explanation for how the integumentary structures were formed by his creator.[40] Driven by the moisture and heat from the brain, the skin first formed around the head by shaping into a sort of rind and detaching itself from the flesh and then covering the head entirely. Then the liquid heat escaped from the head and became the ingredient for the skin of the rest of the body, released onto the surface by punctures in the flesh. Hairs were formed in the same way, but hairs were harder and denser than the skin. The creator made hair to protect the brain by providing shade in the summer and warmth in the winter. Women and beasts were later born from men, and the presence of nails reflects the first attempt at creating talons in man that would later be used by the diverse creatures derived from man.

Aristotle also believed the skin itself was excreted by the flesh:

> The skin, again, is formed by the drying of the flesh, like the scum of boiled substances; it is so formed not only because it is on the outside, but also because what is glutinous, being unable to evaporate, remains on the surface.[41]

In Aristotle's *Problems*, a work of questionable authenticity and possibly compiled by followers at Aristotle's Peripatetic school, there is a lengthy discussion about comparative anatomy between man and animals, and in particular, the differences in hair between man/animal and man/woman. Aristotle was utterly fascinated by hair, even more so than skin. For example, the work addresses such questions as "why can hair grow out of scars in horses and asses, but not in man?" or "why are thick-haired men and birds with thick feathers lustful?" or "why is it that sheep hair gets harder as it gets longer, but in man it gets softer?" or "why does man have no mane?" The reader is referred to the source of these and other fascinating questions upon which Aristotle or his followers speculated.[42]

In his *On Generation of Animals*, Aristotle demonstrated a typical ancient Greek perspective on hair in his theory on hair loss and graying in older persons:

> The skin becomes harder and thicker due to the failing of heat and moisture, so many hairs become disconnected at the base and fall out. Similarly, the failing heat is unable to properly concoct the nutriment that replenishes the hair, so it begins to decay and lose its colour.[43]

According to Aristotle, lice were believed to arise from the flesh of animals, in keeping with a prevailing theory of his time which stated that living things could arise from any substance that contained vital energy (*pneuma*) or even from non-living things. The theory of spontaneous generation went untested until the seventeenth and eighteenth centuries, when it was challenged and finally debunked.

The ancient Greek physician did not consider the skin to have its own specific diseases. Changes on the skin were, instead, a consequence of internal humoral pathology. Plato devoted many pages of his *Timaeus* to disease in general, but there is only one short, albeit rather revealing, passage about skin disease:

> Thanks to air in its bubbles, white phlegm is dangerous when arrested, and although less harmful if it finds a vent to the outside of the body, it still stipples the body with its offspring—white pustules and cysts, and similar skin conditions.[44]

This idea of the skin as a "vent to the outside of the body" where humors would accumulate is at the heart of Greek understanding of skin disease, and one that would dominate medicine for the next two millennia.

We can look to the archaeological record to gain an understanding of the various dermatologic complaints that were managed at the asclepeions. The votive offerings found at ancient Corinth depicted diseases of the breast and penis, such as breast abscess, eczema, phimosis, and balanitis. A more striking example for a dermatologist is a votive offering that depicts a nodule on the back of the hand, which may represent squamous cell carcinoma, a type of skin cancer common in that location.[45] The asclepeion at Epidaurus was perhaps an ancient "center of excellence" for skin disease, as ample historical evidence in the form of inscriptions exists that persons with such conditions were treated there. For example, a boy was healed of a leg wound after the temple dog licked it, and a man with no hair on his head was given a divine salve from the temple priest, and his hair grew again.[46]

THE DERMATOLOGICAL TALE OF PANDAROS AND ECHIDOROS[47]

Pandaros went to the asclepeion at Epidaurus to have some marks (possibly tattoos indicating he was once a slave) removed from his forehead. He was commanded by the temple priest to apply a cloth to his forehead and remove the cloth upon exiting the temple in order to dedicate the fabric to the temple. When he did this, he noticed the marks were gone. His friend Echidoros went there for similar marks, with the expectation he would donate to the temple money that Pandaros had given to him for that purpose. Instead of donating the money, Echidoros slyly pocketed it for himself. The slighted gods commanded that he, too, wear a cloth on his forehead—Pandaros' cloth—and upon exiting the temple, he noted that his forehead had retained the old marks and developed new ones, the ones that Pandaros had lost.

The case histories presented in the Hippocratic corpus mention numerous dermatological signs and symptoms, but they disappoint the modern reader in projecting any sense of exactly which aberrations the authors were referring to when discussing skin diseases. This lack of detail about the skin is in keeping with the concept that if the skin was connected to a given syndrome, this was only a complication of some internal process. As a result, skin conditions were not managed directly; it was believed that correcting any internal imbalances was all that was required to address most dermatologic situations. The most commonly discussed dermatologic problems, according to the present author's review of the corpus, are erysipelas, ulcers, and itching. Other notable inclusions are exanthems, especially pustular and vesicular ones, as well as boils, buboes, and anthrax. Hippocrates may have been the first to describe trichotillomania; he cited cases of people who pulled out their hair in response to stress.[48] The reader is referred to a list of dermatologic conditions mentioned in the corpus as compiled by Goodman and reviewed later by Alsaidan.[49]

Indeed, the vocabulary of dermatology has its origins in these pages: *herpes, exanthema, ecthyma, phyma, edema, alopecia, psora, lepra, lichen, phagedena, gangrene,* and *bubo.*[50] *Herpes* in the time of Hippocrates referred to any skin disease that "crawled" (spread). *Exanthema* referred to a skin rash that erupted from within, outward onto the skin; these eruptions were considered a sign of healthy expulsion of imbalanced humors from the body. To Hippocrates, *psora* probably meant an itchy condition such as eczema or scabies or impetigo; *lepra* likely referred to what we today call psoriasis.[51] The leprosy we know today was referred to as *elephantiasis,* to which Hippocrates may have been referring when he mentioned the "Phoenician disease." *Alphos* and *leuce,* characterized by white patches on the skin, were likely in most cases vitiligo or morphea and deemed very serious by the Hippocratics. Perhaps some of these cases were tuberculoid leprosy, which can have areas of the skin of a lightened tone. The terms were used loosely, and it is not possible to identify what exactly the Greeks were talking about in today's terms. The Greeks did not place enough emphasis on the skin to be precise and descriptive in their dermatologic dealings. To some extent, the dermatology of the ancients was unscientific because the focus was on inside the body, and skin diseases were viewed as a symptom of some internal process.

Every dermatologist has to withstand the indignity of hearing this jocular phrase, which pokes fun at the specialty: "Dermatology is simple. If it's wet, dry it, and if it's dry, wet it." It turns out that Hippocrates was the originator of this simplified approach to treating skin disease.[52] It is woefully disappointing to the present author that even the entirety of Hippocratic skin therapeutics can be distilled down to this catchy phrase. The topical oils, fats, and lards they used and the vegetable and mineral remedies did not differ much from those used by the Egyptians.[53]

DERMATOLOGICAL MYSTERY IN THE HIPPOCRATIC CORPUS

The most oft-cited dermatologic case in the corpus involves the itchy Athenian man in Hippocrates' *On Epidemics* (Book V, Section 9):

> A man at Athens was seized with an itching all over, especially in his testicles and forehead, which proved exceedingly troublesome. His skin was thick from head to foot in appearance like that of a leper; and could not be taken up any where for the thickness of it. This man could receive no benefit from any body; but upon using the hot-baths at Melus, got rid of his itching and his thick skin. He died, however, of a dropsy afterward.[54]

The case reveals an important teaching point endorsed by the Hippocratics: treating only the skin and not the inside of the body was a fatal mistake. The case presents a medical mystery for the modern dermatologist to sleuth. The skin condition described in the passage could have been atopic dermatitis or neurodermatitis, both of which are very pruritic and chronic and can lead to skin thickening all over the body due to long-term rubbing and scratching.[55] Because the baths at Melos were sulfur baths, known to be therapeutic against scabies, the patient may have been suffering with severe, crusted scabies. The dropsy (anasarca) may have resulted from post-streptococcal glomerulonephritis brought about by streptococcal skin infection, a known complication of scratching chronic skin diseases such as scabies.[56]

Hippocrates' name has been given to two dermatologic findings: the Hippocratic facies and Hippocratic nails. The former refers to the changes that occur in the face immediately before death. He describes the face as having the following appearance: sharp nose, hollow eyes, collapsed temples; the ears cold, contracted and their lobes turned out; the skin about the forehead being rough, distended and parched; the color of the whole being green, black, livid, or lead-colored.[57] Hippocratic nails refer to clubbing, defined as the widening of the fingers and an increase in the angle between the nail fold and nail plate. Clubbing is associated with pulmonary diseases, and Hippocrates was the first to describe it.

The Greeks, especially Diocles of Carystus, appreciated skin hygiene as a means by which the skin could be kept healthy. The Greeks worshipped the human body and sought the ideal form of it for themselves through athletics and regular bathing. They emphasized cleanliness achieved in the Greek and Roman bath, massages with fresh oil, the routine use of the gymnasia, and exposure to sunlight and fresh air; pleasant salubrious surroundings had both preventative and therapeutic value.[58]

Summary

The Greek *iatros*, as shown in the writings of the Hippocratic corpus, gave us many of the terms—like *epidermis*, *eczema*, and *psoriasis*—still used today in modern dermatology. Many of these words were derived from botanical or vegetable terms. The *iatros* saw the skin primarily as a fishnet encasing for its underlying structures, and while he was unaware of the tactile functions of the skin, he appreciated the skin as having a breathing function. He considered sweating an important process whereby the body could rid itself of excessive humors. Above all, the Hippocratics gave us the art of clinical inspection and observation, essential skills for the dermatologist. Although the descriptions of skin diseases in the Hippocratic corpus are incomplete, there is no doubt that the ancient Greek individual suffered greatly with them, judging from the archaeological record of the asclepeions. These healthcare facilities, such as the one at Epidaurus, incorporated both natural and supernatural medicine and served as ancient dermatologic "centers of excellence." Skin diseases were never viewed as primary problems. They were considered secondary to internal humoral imbalance and managed not with skin-directed treatments— which could be fatal because they theoretically drive the morbid matter into the body—but instead, they were managed with systemic therapies such as purgatives or medicinal herbs. The emphasis on hygiene indicates that a skin disease in the ancient Greek culture was something best prevented. The most significant aspect of Hippocratic medicine in the history of skin disease was its influence on later medical writers, starting with Galen and virtually every physician following him until the nineteenth century.

4

The Roman Empire

The Roman Empire (27 BCE–476 CE) was the 500-year-long period in the history of ancient Rome when the Romans ruled the territories surrounding the Mediterranean Sea with an imperial system of government. The republican system of government of the preceding 500 years, marred by perpetual civil wars, ended not long after the assassination of Julius Caesar (100–44 BCE) in 44 BCE. The roughly 200-year period of relative peace and stability from the establishment of imperial rule with the reign of Augustus (r. 27 BCE–14 CE) until the death of Marcus Aurelius (r. 161–180 CE), the last of the "Good Emperors," is called the *Pax Romana* (The Roman Peace). The Roman Empire reached its zenith in land area in 117 CE during the reign of the emperor Trajan (r. 98–117 CE) when the Roman Empire encompassed modern-day Italy, Greece, Turkey, the Middle East, Egypt, North Africa, Spain, France, southern Germany, and Britain. The emperors ruled over the entire empire as autocrats, backed by the powerful and well-organized Roman military, while the territories were controlled by provincial governors. Despite wars of expansion and revolt, this steady period of firm central authority mirrored the Greek Classical Age in terms of the stability needed for significant cultural and scientific advancements. The Roman Empire nearly collapsed with the "Crisis of the Third Century" when barbarian invasions, a series of incompetent rulers, disease, and economic depression, pushed the empire to its brink. While peace was achieved again during the reign of Aurelian (r. 270–275 CE) and the Roman Empire lasted another 200 years, it had seen its best days in the first 200 years of its existence.

Rome's cultural accomplishments are in no way inferior to those of the Greeks. In literature, the Romans are most celebrated for their poetry; they gave us the works of Lucretius (99–55 BCE), Catullus (84–54 BCE), Vergil (70–21 BCE), Horace (65–8 BCE), Ovid (43 BCE–17 CE), and Martial (38–102 CE). In the discipline of history, the Romans contributed the works of Julius Caesar (100–44 BCE), Livy (64 BCE–12 CE), and Tacitus (56–120 CE), and in rhetoric, the works of Cicero (106–43 BCE). The Romans invented satire, exemplified in the works of Persius (34–62 CE) and Juvenal (fl. first to second century CE). In natural philosophy, Pliny the Elder (23–79 CE) wrote the *Naturalis Historia*, an encyclopedia that compiled much of the knowledge of his time; his nephew Pliny the Younger (61–113 CE), who witnessed and reported on the eruption of Mt. Vesuvius in 79 CE, wrote a series of letters that contained invaluable descriptions of everyday Roman life and administrative history. The two most important philosophical schools of ancient Rome were the closely related schools of Cynicism and Stoicism, both of which were inherited from the Greeks and expanded upon by influential Roman philosophers such as Seneca (4 BCE–65 CE) and Epictetus (55–135 CE). The Romans also left tremendous legacies in the fields of art, music, architecture, sports, and entertainment. In addition, it would be impossible to estimate the value of the Roman contributions in law and language (Latin), or, for that matter, in the subject of medicine.

The history of medicine in ancient Rome is a series of biographies of men who made prodigious contributions largely constructed upon the foundation of knowledge laid by the Greeks. Three main principles guided the field of medicine at this time: humoralism, an emphasis on botanical medicaments, and a secular approach to disease. The Greek physicians of the Hellenistic territories that were initially incorporated into the Roman Republic brought their Hippocratic principles to Rome.[1] The average Roman, however, was wary of these immigrant physicians. Roman sensibilities included a matter-of-fact stoicism and xenophobia; consequently, Greek physicians were deemed worthless, fraudulent, and more likely to hasten death than thwart it. The Romans, instead, believed in a regimen of health that promoted frequent exercise and moderation in the consumption of food and beverage.[2] These barriers did not prevent the emergence of a new era of physician, called *medicus*, who, in generating a body of medical literature—a

DOI: 10.1201/9781003273622-6

consolidation of and an expansion upon Hippocratic medicine—provided succeeding physicians the underpinnings of medical knowledge until the nineteenth century. By the time Galen emerged in the second century CE, Greek medicine and Roman medicine were synonymous. The following medical writers of ancient Rome each made significant contributions in the history of medicine and, in particular, the history of dermatology.

Celsus (25 BCE–50 CE)

Aulus Cornelius Celsus was among the earliest of the classical Roman medical writers. Little is known about his life; his *nomen*, Cornelius, suggests high birth. Even though he demonstrated impressive knowledge about the practice of medicine in his texts, he was likely not a physician but an encyclopedist who authored *Artes*, "The Sciences." His section *De medicina* (ca. 47 CE), "On medicine," survived when all other portions of his encyclopedia did not. Celsus' lost texts, which were referenced by later writers, covered agriculture, law, philosophy, and military science. While some scholars call him a *philiatros*, "friend of physicians," others refer to him as the "Cicero of Physicians," in reference to his elegant Latin writing style.[3] He flourished during the reigns of Augustus (r. 27 BCE–14 CE) and Tiberius (r. 14–37 CE). A minority view of some scholars is that he was only a translator of Tiberius' Greek physician, Tiberius Claudius Menecrates (fl. first century CE), who wrote 156 books.[4] Celsus' work summarizes the medical knowledge of the Roman world. Lost for over 1300 years and discovered in the Vatican Library in 1426 by the future pope Nicholas V, it was the first medical book printed with the Gutenberg printing press (Florence, 1478).[5] Revered to the same degree as the Hippocratic corpus, *De medicina* is a vital work in the history of medicine as well as the history of dermatology. Celsus' masterpiece has had more editions produced than any other medical text.[6]

After offering the first detailed history of medicine until his time, Celsus lamented in his introduction the clashing sects of dogmatism, empiricism, and Methodism, promoting instead a type of medicine that combined experience and reason, and morality and virtue.[7] Celsus expressed a "distinctively Roman point of view": rationality above everything else and more decency and moderation.[8] *De medicina* is divided into eight books; Book V (descriptions of various drugs; bites/ulcers) and Book VI (diseases of the skin, eyes, ears, and mouth) are the most relevant to our study. In the other books, there are many discoveries that can be attributed to Celsus. For example, Celsus was the first to identify the four cardinal features of inflammation: *dolor* (pain), *tumor* (swelling), *calor* (warmth), and *rubor* (redness). He also took the Greek word for carcinoma (*karkinos*) and translated it into the Latin word *cancer*. He coined the Latin word for insanity (*insanus*).[9]

Among Celsus' greatest legacies is his work with skin disease. He wrote extensively about the skin in *De medicina,* describing 40–50 skin diseases.[10] Skin afflictions remained a feature of internal disease in Celsus' time. It is true that much of the information is in the Hippocratic corpus or was gleaned from the influx of Alexandrian physicians, but Celsus built upon the language of dermatology that was founded by the Greeks and translated many Greek medical terms into Latin. In the process, he offered a more complete description of the skin diseases than can be found in the Hippocratic corpus and may have inspired the objective morphologists of the nineteenth century (see Chapter 12).[11]

Elephantiasis, which he noted was unknown in Italy, is the only disease with skin involvement addressed in Book III, and he gives a lengthy description of the natural course of that disease— which we know today to be leprosy. In Book V, he dealt with wounds, ulcers, gangrene, and various growths and cancers. His exposition on the fluids that seep from wounds is elaborate; he classified these fluids into broad categories of blood, *sanies*, and pus, and he further subdivided *sanies* and pus into the now-extinct terms of *ichor, melicera,* and *elaoides*, the presence of which reflect the overall healthiness of a wound. For example, Celsus reported that blood, *sanies*, pus, and *elaoides* are visible in healthy wounds, but *ichor* and *melicera* are produced by unhealthy ones.[12] *Ichor*, incidentally, is a term that was originally used in Greek mythology to name the ethereal fluid that flowed in the veins of the Greek gods. Celsus continued to describe these wound fluids in even greater detail in the succeeding paragraph, demonstrating the extreme focus on detail in his task.

There are multiple pages on different types of wounds and how to care for wounds in various stages, from the healthy to the gangrenous. Several words of caution that stand out in this chapter include his comment on *erysipelas*, which can complicate wounds or occur without wound; the latter "carries with it considerable danger, especially if it fix itself near the neck or head."[13] He discouraged bathing gangrenous wounds "because the wound softened by this means is attacked with a renewal of the same malady."[14]

On bites, he advocated extracting the fluid in the bite with a cupping glass for every type of bite because "every bite has most commonly some venom in it."[15] His approach to treating hydrophobia after "bite of the mad dog" is horrifying:

> But from this kind of wound, if ineffectually treated, a dread of water is the usual result: the Greeks call it υδροφοβίαν (hydrophobia), a most heart-rending malady, in which the patient is at once tormented with thirst, and a dread of water. When thus afflicted, there is scarcely a shade of hope. The sole remedy consists of throwing him unawares into a pond; and if he cannot swim, he should be allowed to drink in the water as he sinks, and to be elevated alternately; if he can swim, he should be repeatedly kept under water, that he may be compelled to drink: for this is the way to remove both the thirst and the hydrophobia.[16]

Of the skin lesions that "arise internally from corruption of some internal part ... there is none worse than the carbuncle," and "the best plan is to cauterize without loss of time."[17] On the other hand, carcinoma "is not so dangerous, unless exasperated by imprudent treatment" and "chiefly occurs in the upper parts, about the face, nose, ears, lips, and the breasts of females."[18] Celsus noted stages of skin cancer: first an early, curable stage called a *cacoethes*, next a cancer without ulcer, then an ulcer, and finally a thymium (warty mass). He discouraged treatment of any stage but the first. Celsus' *ignis sacer* (see Interlude 2) sounds more like an ulcerative disease such as pyoderma gangrenosum or shingles than erysipelas, which does not ulcerate. Celsus was among the first to describe scrofula (*struma* in Latin), a cutaneous presentation of tuberculosis:

> Scrofula is a tumor in which certain concretions below the skin, consisting of pus and blood, arise like small glands: these are particularly troublesome to the medical attendant; for not only do they excite fever, but they scarcely ever maturate without difficulty; and whether treated by the knife, or by medicaments, they again make their appearance near the old cicatrix, but much more frequently after being treated by the last; add to these, they are of long continuance. They principally occur in the neck, but in the armpits also, the groins, and sides.[19]

For scrofula, he prescribes white hellebore and drawing salves, noting that some use caustics to corrode the skin overlying the glands to the point of inducing an ulcer, while "certain rustics" have discovered that "one affected with a strume is freed from it by eating a snake."[20] He explained the different types of warts and used the term *myrmecia,* derived from the ancient Greek word for ant, for a certain type of plantar wart with a broad base and narrow apex, like an ant-hill.[21] His description of what he called *acrochordon*, a term used today for the skin tag, actually resembles the molluscum wart. Book VII delves into genital warts. Celsus described in great detail pustular eruptions, and after reading Celsus' descriptions of scabies and impetigo, the latter of which has four types—including a red type and a black type—one can surmise he was talking about various types of eczema or psoriasis, with Celsus' red type of impetigo possibly the first description in history of true psoriasis. Impetigo, incidentally, derives from the Latin word, *impeto,* to rush upon, in reference to that condition's sudden onset. Celsus was the first to use the term *vitiligo* to refer to three species of skin conditions that whiten the skin (the term that today refers to immune-mediated depigmentation of the skin):

> Leprosy [the original Latin is *vitiligo*] also, although in itself not dangerous, is nevertheless a loathsome disease, and arises from a bad habit of body. There are three species of it. That called *alphos* is of a white colour, usually roughish, and not confluent, looking as though scattered in drops: sometimes spreading more widely, and with interspaces. The *melas* is black, and shadowy, but in other respects like the last. The *leuce* is in some respects similar to the *alphos*, but whiter,

and penetrates more deeply; and it has white downy hairs on it. All these spread, but some cases more rapidly than in others. The *alphos* and *melas* both come and go at various periods. The *leuce* does not easily quit him whom it has once attacked. The two former are cured without very great difficulty: the last is all but incurable.[22]

Alphos, *melas*, and *leuce* are dermatologic diagnoses that would recur in medical writings for the next eighteen centuries. The *alphos* and *melas* of Celsus resemble guttate psoriasis; his *leuce* is almost certainly true vitiligo. The ancient and medieval medical writers, including Celsus, considered these conditions related to *lepra*, a term that is conspicuously absent in *De medicina*. The origin of the word *vitiligo* is debated but most likely derives from the Latin word for blemish, *vitium*.

In Book VI, he covered rashes of the head. He was the first to describe *kerion*, a type of fungal infection of the scalp in children, known today as *kerion Celsi*. For alopecia that was not due to old age, he recommended frequent shaving of the affected area "because, when the cuticle has thus been gradually cut away, the roots of the hair are laid bare."[23] Shaving did not work for male pattern baldness, and he stated, "We have no remedy." His explanation of *porrigo*, what we today call seborrheic dermatitis, gives us a glimpse into his view on the pathogenesis of skin disease:

> It generally occurs in the hair of the head, more rarely in the beard, now and then in the eyebrows. And neither does it take place except there be some disorder in the system, nor is it altogether without its beneficial effects, for it never appears during a perfectly healthy condition of the head; and when disease is existing there, it is advantageous; for it is better that the surface be occasionally corrupted, than that the nocent matter be translated to another part more essential to life. The better plan therefore is to clear it away by repeated combing, and not to suppress it entirely.[24]

Celsus admitted some reluctance to discuss cosmetic issues in his great work; still, he proceeded with information regarding the removal of pimples, freckles, and age spots:

> It is almost folly to adopt any method of cure for *vari* [pimples], *lentils* [age spots], and *ephelidae* [freckles]; but the fair sex are not to be divested of their natural anxiety for the preservation of their personal charms.[25]

Other topics of dermatologic interest are Celsus' accurate dealings with styes and chalazia, scalp cysts, phimosis, and perianal itching and fissures, the latter of which he treated with hot boiled pigeon eggs.[26] Aware of the modesty of a typical Roman male, he described the challenges of dealing with "affections which belong to the privities":

> One who is desirous of at once expressing himself with delicacy, and at the same time of plainly delivering the precepts of the art, to afford a description of such diseases is no easy matter. Not that this should deter me from writing an account of them: first, because I would omit nothing that may prove conducive to the recovery of health; and, secondly, because there are no diseases whose cure ought to be more generally known than those which one man has the greatest reluctance to submit to the inspection of another.[27]

Such is the dermatology that can be found in *De medicina*; there is much more on skin disease in this greatest of works, but it can be left for the reader to explore. Celsus' descriptions are more accurate and provide more detailed treatment information than those found in the Hippocratic corpus. His influence on the future of the history of medicine is questionable, however, as *De medicina* was lost soon after Celsus' life ended, not to be rediscovered until the fifteenth century. Only Isidore of Seville (seventh/ eighth centuries CE) made any mention of his book.[28] Thus, Celsus "made no impression on his contemporaries or the medieval writers."[29] However, his redemption eventually came during the Renaissance, when physicians of that era, convinced "that older is better, welcomed it as an authoritative medical textbook" and an invaluable representation of Roman medicine before Galen.[30] For our purposes, the very fact that Celsus' *De medicina* is the oldest Latin medical text in the history of medicine, with its full attention to the language and descriptions of skin diseases during the ancient Roman period, gives it incalculable value in the history of dermatology.

Scribonius Largus (1–50 CE)

Scribonius Largus was one of several medical writers who flourished during the Roman Empire and was among the first to author a major medical treatise in Latin. After serving as a physician in the Roman army, he was the court physician during the reign of Claudius (r. 41–54 CE), whom he accompanied to Britain in 43 CE; little else is known about the details of his life.[31] Scribonius was not the court physician who, according to Tacitus, allegedly murdered Claudius by poison at the behest of Claudius' fourth wife, Agrippina; that was Xenophon (10 BCE–54 CE). Scholars believe Scribonius was born in Sicily, but even this assertion cannot be confirmed with historical evidence.

Scribonius wrote his *Compositiones medicamentorum,* "The Composition of Remedies," circa 47–48 CE. From his writings, it can be inferred that he was a general practitioner with a busy practice, not merely a theoretician, and he took care of a wide social range of patients with varied medical problems.[32] His philosophy toward his craft, laid out in his preface, was one of moral and ethical professionalism; he distrusted amateurs and believed that good doctors should help even their enemies to the best of their abilities. He referred to medications as "divine hands" and thought that physicians should try them on themselves before administering them to patients.[33] Scribonius rightly believed that physicians need a heart full of *misericordia* (compassion) and *humanitas* (humanity). He was the first to invoke the Hippocratic oath and interpreted it to mean that abortions were not the business of physicians. Although Hippocrates specifically opposed physicians giving an abortive suppository (pessary), interpretation of Hippocrates' intention with this portion of the oath remains controversial to this day.[34]

The text contains 271 recipes for prescriptions, arranged for conditions affecting the body from the head to the feet. *Compositiones* contains antidotes against bites, stings and poisons, as well as salves, dressings, and plasters for various wounds, and a host of fascinating medical tidbits. For example, Scribonius was the first to prescribe the shock of the torpedo ray (an electric eel-like ray) to manage both headache and gout; later writers even used the ray's jolts for treating prolapsed anus![35] And unlike his contemporary Celsus, Scribonius opposed the common practice of ingesting the fresh blood of a gladiator for the purposes of treating epilepsy.

Scribonius wrote about several skin diseases, e.g., *papula, porrigo, ignis sacer, impetigo*, and *scabies* in *Compositiones*, and, in particular, their treatment. He conscripted the term *zona*, a Latin word for a belt or girdle worn by women, to refer to the disease we call shingles. It would be used in medical writing to refer to shingles until the nineteenth century. On three separate occasions, Scribonius pointed out that what he was referring to as *zona*, the Greeks called *herpes* (today shingles is known as herpes zoster).[36] Incidentally, the word shingles evolved from the Latin *cingulum,* a type of girdle worn by the soldiers of the Roman legions, and its English counterpart, "schingles." The first recorded mention of the word shingles was in a medieval encyclopedia written by Bartholomaeus Anglicus called *De Proprietatibus Rerum* "On the Property of Things" (1398).[37]

Pliny the Elder (24–79 CE) and *Mentagra*

Gaius Plinius Secundus, better known as Pliny the Elder, was another Roman encyclopedist who attempted to provide his readers with a comprehensive summary of the knowledge current for his time in all matters relating to the natural world. Unlike the similar project of Celsus, Pliny's *Naturalis Historia*, "Natural History," is intact. It was published two years prior to his death in 79 CE; he died in Herculaneum while he was there to rescue a friend from the eruption of Mt. Vesuvius. His nephew, Pliny the Younger (61–113 CE), attributed to his uncle the quote, "fortune favors the brave." Modern scholars believe he died of a heart attack.[38] In addition to his literary pursuits, Pliny the Elder was also a lawyer, military commander, provincial governor, and friend of the emperor at various times throughout his career.

Naturalis Historia is a massive work, consisting of 37 books that cover such fields as astronomy, meteorology, geography, anthropology, zoology, and many others.[39] Like Celsus, Pliny should be remembered as a great compiler, not an original thinker. His lofty purpose, as laid out in the preface, is to do something that has never been done before: describe "the nature of things, and life as it actually exists."[40]

Books 20–29 deal with medicine and pharmacology; Book 26 is most relevant to our study because Pliny's comments found therein, especially in his discussion of *mentagra*, reveal much about Roman views toward skin disease:

> The face of man has recently been sensible to new forms of disease, unknown in ancient times, not only to Italy, but to almost the whole of Europe. Still, however, they have not as yet extended to the whole of Italy, nor have they made any very great inroads in Illyricum, Gaul, or Spain, or indeed any other parts, to so great an extent as in Rome and its environs. Though unattended with pain, and not dangerous to life, these diseases are of so loathsome a nature, that any form of death would be preferable to them.[41]

This is the first reference illustrating the social and psychological effects of skin diseases. The appearance of one's skin mattered much in Roman society, and for the average Roman, the presence of skin disease on the face was absolutely devastating—because of vanity, embarrassment, and social stigma—to the point of suicide. The worst of these diseases, according to Pliny, was known as *lichen* to the Greeks and *mentagra* to the Romans (from the Latin word for chin [*mentum*] and the Greek word for catching [*agra*]). Pliny wrote the following description of that malady:

> In consequence, however, of its generally making its first appearance at the chin, the Latins, by way of joke, originally—so prone are mankind to make a jest of the misfortunes of others—gave it the name *mentagra;* an appellation which has since become established in general use. In many cases, however, this disease spreads over the interior of the mouth, and takes possession of the whole face, with sole exception of the eyes; after which, it passes downwards to the neck, breast, and hands, covering them with foul, furfuraceous eruptions.[42]

Since it started on the chin, *mentagra* was believed to be spread by kissing, the customary greeting for the Romans. Pliny stated that *mentagra* first came to Italy from Asia during the middle years reign of Tiberius (r. 14–37 CE). First a disease of male nobles, it was "communicated even by the momentary contact requisite for the act of salutation," and it spared women, slaves, and the lower orders.[43] Tiberius issued an edict against everyday kissing for salutation; it has been suggested that the emperor may have suffered with the disease himself and may have been the reason for his departure from Rome in 26 CE.[44]

In his *Epigrams*, the Roman satirist and poet Martial (41–104 CE) lamented all the kissing:

> Rome gives, on one's return after fifteen years' absence,
> such a number of kisses
> as exceeds those given by Lesbia to Catullus.
> Every neighbour, every hairy-faced fanner,
> presses on you with a strongly-scented kiss.
> Here the weaver assails you, there the fuller
> and the cobbler, who has just been kissing leather;
> here the owner of a filthy beard,
> and a one-eyed gentleman; there one with bleared eyes,
> and fellows whose mouths are defiled with all manner of abominations.
> It was hardly worth while to return.[45]

A solution to the problem, per Martial, was to feign a skin disease in order to avoid kisses from others:

> Do you ask, Philaenis, why I often come abroad with plaster
> on my chin, or with my lips covered with salve
> when nothing ails them? I do not wish to kiss you.[46]

Still, avoiding the kissers was no easy task, even in cases when you had a skin disease:

It is impossible, Flaccus, to avoid the kissers.
They press upon you, they delay you, they pursue you, they run against you,
on all sides, from every direction, and in every place.
No malignant ulcer will protect you from them,
no inflamed pimples, or diseased chin, or ugly tetter,
or lips smeared with oily cerate,
or drop at the cold nose.[47]

Mentagra was treated with cautery, which demonstrates that the Roman man would go to any depths to get rid of it:

Many of those who persevered in undergoing a course of remedial treatment, though cured of the disease, retained scars upon the body more hideous even than the malady itself; it being treated with cauteries, as it was certain to break out afresh, unless means were adopted for burning it out of the body by cauterizing to the very bone.[48]

Interestingly, Pliny wrote that many physicians from Alexandria came to Rome and "devoted themselves solely to this branch of medicine [managing *mentagra*]; and very considerable were the profits they made."[49] Perhaps these Alexandrian skin specialists were the first dermatologists. Skin was a lucrative business; a man of noble birth, according to Pliny, spent "no less a sum than two hundred thousand sesterces upon his cure."[50] The value of a single Roman sestertius has been estimated to be from one to three of today's US dollars. Pliny suggested several plant-based remedies that were alternatives to cautery, the most interesting of which was the use of actual lichens, also in use for the effacement of brand marks. The skin disease *mentagra* (*lichen*) was probably what we today call *tinea* (ringworm), *sycosis barbae* (staphylococcal infection of the beard follicles), or perhaps *impetigo contagiosa*, but none of these conditions "spread over the interior of the mouth" as claimed by Pliny in his description.

He also described or provided remedies for carbuncle, elephantiasis, scrofula, erysipelas, boils, warts, and ulcers. Pliny was the first to record the term *zoster*—instead of Scribonius' term *zona*—for what we today call shingles. Derived from Greek, the original meaning of the word *zoster* was a waist-belt worn by Greek soldiers, analogous to the *zona* worn by women; Pliny wrote:

There are several kinds of erysipelas, one in particular which attacks the middle of the body, and is known as zoster: should it entirely surround the body, its effects are fatal.[51]

But modern-day shingles does not attack only the middle of the body, nor does it surround the body entirely, nor is it commonly fatal. Finally, Pliny offers countless options for beautifying, clearing, or softening the skin and removing blemishes, sunspots, freckles, and pimples.

In conclusion, Pliny devoted a considerable amount of space in his *Naturalis Historia* to describing the appearance and treatment of several skin diseases. The diseases covered differ somewhat from those listed in Celsus' *De medicina;* therefore, the two books complement each other if the purpose is gaining an understanding of the skin diseases plaguing the typical person living in ancient Rome. Pliny's comments on the psychologically devastating effects of skin disease on the Roman shed light on the deep concerns for skin beauty and health during his time. While Pliny has been criticized for his lack of evidence-based medicine, he was heavily referenced by later medieval writers such as Isidore of Seville. It is important to remember that he, like Celsus, was not a physician, when it comes to judging his contributions to the history of medicine.

Dioscorides (40–90 CE) and *De Materia Medica*

Pedanius Dioscorides was a Greek physician and pharmacologist who wrote one of the most influential works in the history of medicine, *De materia medica,* "On Medical Material" (ca. 77 CE). Written in Greek and fully translated into Latin probably by the sixth century, the five-volume work became the principal source of pharmacological information for physicians for the next 1500 years. Though the details of his life are murky, we know that he was from Anazarbus in southern Asia Minor (modern-day Turkey) and studied medicine in the nearby town of Tarsus, known for its strong tradition of pharmacological teaching.[52] He briefly served as a surgeon in the army of Nero (r. 54–68 CE). Other works, such as *Ex herbis feminis*, "On Herbs for Women," that were attributed to Dioscorides have been determined to be apocryphal and given the authorship by "pseudo-Dioscorides."

It is difficult to place Dioscorides in one of the competing schools of the time, as his views developed out of the rational Hellenistic medical tradition.[53] He obviously promoted pharmacological intervention and rejected Methodic principles, which downplayed medications. In his text, he did not entertain the controversies of his time; he even ignored the concept of the four humors.[54] In fact, there was no discernable theory of disease in the work.[55] His interest was the medicinal value of the individual remedies, not providing a list of remedies for a given condition.[56] Each chapter adheres to the following order of information: name and picture of the substance; habitat; botanical description; drug properties; medicinal usages; harmful side effects; quantities and dosages; harvesting, preparation, and storage instructions; adulteration methods and tests for detection; veterinary usages; magical and non-medical usages; and specific geographic locations or habitats.[57] There are approximately 1000 substances in *De materia medica*, some 600 of which are plants.

By simply flipping through the pages of *De materia medica,* one can appreciate that many of Dioscorides' treatments had dermatologic applications. Diagnoses mentioned under the remedies include *erysipelas* (mentioned in 39 remedies), *herpes* (23), *impetigo* (11), *lichen* (22), *lepra* (50), *elephantiasis* (5), *vitiligines* (30), *favus* (6), *carbuncle* (19), *alopecia* (20), and lice (11). There are substantially more suggestions for general skin ailments such as ulcers, bites, and scabs; 20 remedies promise to remove freckles, while 7 promise to smooth wrinkles. Remedies verified today to be effective that were known to Dioscorides include amygdalin, belladonna, opium, wild cherry, aloe, tragacanth, castor oil, croton oil, and cassia.[58]

Dioscorides considered barley a cure for lepra but thought that when it was brewed into beer, it could actually cause the same disease.[59] He recommended "grime from gymnasium walls" for the purpose of "warming and dissolving inflammed growths" (phymata).[60] After pointing out that by Dioscorides' *phymata* was likely referring to what Galen or Celsus would have called anthrax or carbuncle, and this "grime" (as in mold) may have had some antibiotic property.[61] Dioscorides' use of amygdalin for cancer may have had some positive effect.[62] Dioscorides was the first to write down the usefulness of coal tar for the treatment of inflammation, a therapy that dermatologists still recommend today for skin inflammation.[63] Sea urchins were burned to generate quicklime, which was mixed with water to make calcium hydroxide. This caustic had three main uses: it was rubbed on *psora*, used to cleanse ulcers, and applied to "halt excrescences of the flesh."[64] Dioscorides' entry on zinc oxide (cadmia) lists numerous beneficial properties for skin disease: it stops discharges of the pores; it dries, draws to a scab, and represses abnormal growths of the flesh; and it creates a new skin on malignant ulcers.[65] This represents a small sampling of the seemingly countless entries of dermatologic therapies in *De materia medica*.

According to the Hippocratics, medications had four basic effects on the body: warming, cooling, drying, and moistening. In *De materia medica,* Dioscorides expanded the effects to include softening, astringent, diuretic, concocting, sharpening, thinning, dilating, gluing, sleep-inducing, relaxing, sweat-inducing, and stopping of pores, among others.[66] It is not always clear how a certain property would be useful in Dioscorides' mind for a given problem, as he assumes his reader already understands the pathophysiology of the diseases he listed, on which he provides little-to-no information.

Dioscorides' *De materia medica* is a fascinating tour of the pharmacological armamentarium available to the ancient and medieval physician. Its main contribution is the way in which Dioscorides elevated pharmacy by focusing on the mechanism of action of the medications.[67] His emphasis on dermatologic issues is not surprising, as skin diseases were a major concern of his reader, the *medicus*.

INSIDE THE HANDBAG OF THE *MEDICUS*

The ancient world had a variety of instruments of dermatologic interest, and the size and variety of the assorted findings suggest an outright obsession with the skin by ancient peoples.[68] Small sticks, spatulas, and brushes were available as early as the Egyptian period for the application of oils, cosmetics, poultices, colors, and powders. Vessels made of ceramic, clay, leather, wood, and glass have been found containing creams, ointments, and powders. Stones for abrading calluses have been used since ancient times. With its ancient Greek origins, the *strigil* was a favorite in ancient Rome, especially among gladiators. This boomerang-shaped device was used to scrape away the accumulated ointments, oils, or unguents that were applied to the skin for the purposes of cleanliness. In a surgeon's bag could be found the predecessor of the scalpel, known as the *bistoury*, as well as the *pincer*, the *cautery*, the *terebrum* (small drill), the cupping glass, and the *specillum* (probe). These instruments did not change much over the centuries for the medieval and early modern surgeon; only in the late nineteenth century did surgical instruments begin to resemble the variety used today.

Galen (129–216 CE)

Claudius Galenus, called Galen, was a Greek physician from the city in western Asia Minor known as Pergamum or Pergamon (Pergamos to the modern Greeks); he was arguably the most important and most discussed figure in the history of medicine. He was both a gifted physician with great experience and observation skills, and an egotistical, infallible dogmatist.[69] The impact of his writings lasted until the nineteenth century. Galen is most famous for transmitting the Hippocratic legacy to the West and doing so through a corpus of writings containing more words than any other ancient writer of any discipline.[70] He left us some 350 titles; his most important works are listed in the endnotes.[71] *On Anatomical Preparations* was his principal text on anatomy; *On the Affected Part*s was the most important on pathology; *On the Usefulness of the Parts* contained Galen's physiological doctrines; and *On the Medical Art* was a summary of Galen's knowledge that became known as *Articella* in the Middle Ages (see Chapter 7).

The son of an architect, Galen began his career with a well-rounded education at Pergamum, a flourishing city and intellectual center in the Greek-speaking portion of the Empire. He traveled far and wide to many cities of the Greek world, including Alexandria, where he absorbed regional medical knowledge, particularly in regard to pharmacological interventions. After about ten years abroad, he returned to Pergamum to become physician to the gladiators.[72] Galen went to Rome in 162 CE, where he performed for large audiences in public debates against Methodists. He was a master of one-upmanship and chastised his opponents as fools.[73] His fame enabled him to become a court physician for the emperor Marcus Aurelius (r. 161–180 CE).[74] At the beginning of the Antonine Plague (see Interlude 2), Galen fled Rome in 166 to return home to Pergamum. The cause of his departure might have been fear of the epidemic.[75] He was recalled to Rome by the Emperor three years later, when his prolific writing years ensued. He died at 87 years of age in Palermo, Sicily.

Galen believed that an understanding of anatomy could untangle the mysteries of the human body and its diseases. Because human dissection was forbidden during his time, he used pigs, apes, and other animals for his investigations and demonstrations. He performed experiments to work out problems posed by his predecessors.[76] Without any qualms, he assumed that animal anatomy was equivalent to human anatomy. His inference led to numerous errors, the most significant of which was his doctrine that blood moves between the ventricles of the heart through tiny pores in the ventricular wall. Still, his experimental work with anatomy and physiology led to numerous accurate descriptions, and it is this work that is considered his greatest achievement.

Galenic medicine, set forth in the ten million Greek words of the corpus authored by Galen—three million of which survive today—would become the type of medicine that was practiced until the nineteenth century. Galenic medicine was essentially an updated version of Hippocratic medicine, with relatively few changes in the areas of disease explanation (humoralism) and therapeutics. Its emphasis remained on diet before drugs and drugs before surgery.[77]

However, Galen did make several important modifications. He linked the four humors to the four elements, thus creating "a highly metaphysical theory of disease."[78] His choice of treatment was usually a remedy with attributes that would oppose the qualities of the disease, e.g., the application of a warming salve to the abdomen of the patient with a bellyache from ingesting too much cold food. He promoted the practice of bloodletting to correct surpluses of humors, particularly in fevers, which were deemed to be caused by an excess of blood or other humor type. Galen developed an elaborate "pulse lore"; he wrote at least 16 books on the pulse, which he considered the most important aspect of the physical exam.[79] He erroneously furthered the concept that certain types of pus indicated healing and were, therefore, "laudable" (see Chapter 7). Galen disregarded the concepts of contagion and miasma, the latter an idea that bad air could cause disease. While not outwardly opposing supernatural interventions, he did not promote them or write about them. Dreams of the patient mattered to Galen; they could change the course of treatment.[80] He advanced Hippocrates' work on stress-induced disease and even addressed the topic of malingering. He disagreed with the use of human and animal excrements and secretions, a practice that saw a decline in late antiquity and the medieval period. He described close to 500 plant, animal, and mineral medicaments; of these, Galen's theriac is the most famous.

According to a book entirely devoted to the subject, Galen's theriac contained over 70 ingredients. One of the first theriacs was originally an antidote to poison associated with Mithridates VI (132–63 BCE), the King of Pontus, a kingdom on the Black Sea coast of Asia Minor. The poison-fearing Mithridates had over 40 ingredients compounded into a daily antidote for every poisonous substance. Andromachus the Elder from Crete (fl. first century) was physician to the emperor Nero and was the first physician given the designation *archiater* (chief physician to a monarch) thanks to his invention of a very successful theriac that contained some 64 ingredients, including opium.[81] Not just an antidote for poisonous bites, the Theriac of Andromachus was purported to treat asthma, colic, dropsy, inflammation, and plague. By Galen's time, theriac had become known as a heal-all, and Galen tweaked the recipe to his satisfaction but retained the name in honor of Andromachus. It could be taken orally or applied topically to draw out poisons or abscesses. Galen's theriac was expensive, enjoying a long run as a popular treatment among the elite. Theriac was prescribed until the nineteenth century, undergoing many permutations, with some recipes even containing the aforementioned mummy.

Galen believed, on the one hand, that to be successful, a physician should master logic, physics, and ethics and should be a philosopher as well. On the other hand, ever-so-proud of his own knowledge, Galen believed that a physician should accept the knowledge contained within his writings rather than the teachings of a particular school. He was certainly not a Methodic, nor was he an Empiric or Dogmatic, but something in between—he was a master of direct observation (an Empiric principle) but also emphasized his understanding of the inner workings of the human body (Dogmatic principle). Galen saw himself and the ideal physician as one who displayed logic, argument, experiment, reason, experience, book learning, personal skills, anatomical knowledge, speculation, intuition, and sound judgment.[82]

He listened carefully to his patients, examined them thoroughly, and after gathering as much information as possible, he established both a diagnosis and prognosis, all while trying to gain the confidence of the patient.[83] Only then would treatment be instituted. Diet, exercise, sleep, and environment were important to Galen, as food and drink had properties that could affect the four humors, and moderate exercise and adequate sleep promoted a healthy body. When these simple measures failed, Galen would then prescribe medication to restore the body's balance, such as a purgative to rid the body of excessive bile. Surgery was a last resort, except for venesection, which he employed without hesitation when he deemed it necessary. Galen did not say much about the popular Roman tradition of bathing, other than to warn against overbathing, or risk the "moist diseases that are found in women."[84]

Galenic medicine became incontrovertible dogma for several reasons. First, it developed from a foundation of Hippocratic principles that the learned physicians who followed him held in high regard. Second, Galen's verbal and written language was forceful and his readers were easily persuaded by his claims. Third, Galen accepted the *pneuma* as the spirit of life and was a pagan with monotheistic leanings, believing that one God designed the human body and ordered the world.[85] Galen's doctrines coincided with Church teachings, and the Church's seal of approval was the support that explains the dominance of his doctrines for the next 1500 years; it was heretical to question his theories.[86] Finally, there was a general decline in intellectual curiosity in the centuries that followed, and people preferred to accept dogma rather than discuss or criticize it.[87]

Modern historians have given the enigmatic Galen mixed reviews. Nuland's summation of the man is unsurpassed: his career was simultaneously medicine's best and worst influence as he was both the founder of experimental medical investigation and "the obstructing force" that prevented growth of knowledge for the next 1500 years.[88]

Galen and Skin Disease

If Galen is the most influential figure in the history of medicine, then it might be inferred that he is the most influential figure in the history of dermatology. After all, medicine and dermatology were insepa-rable until only 200 years ago. Yet, as someone with a keen interest in anatomy, Galen did not consider the skin itself worthy of investigation; in fact, there is no mention of the skin in his dissection manual.[89] He did suggest that the skin was the organ of touch.[90] His anatomical research with peripheral nerves led him to conclude that skin all over the body transmitted various information about an object, but Galen believed the hand, in particular, was the central organ for the perception of all tactile qualities.[91] He theorized that sweating was a natural phenomenon and that the failure to sweat because of blockage of pores in the skin could lead to disease, as opposed to Diocles, who considered it unnatural. Galen also equated beauty with health; the "harmony of bodily proportions and perfect complexion" indicated bal-ance of the four humors.[92]

Galen's views on diseases of the skin can be found scattered throughout his corpus, but the majority of his dermatological dealings are published in *De tumoribus praeter naturam,* "On Swellings that are Contrary to Nature." Galen's information is not as detailed on skin disease as the sixth book of Celsus' *De medicina,* but it is worthy of our attention nonetheless, especially in light of the fact that it is consid-ered by some to be the first book devoted entirely to skin diseases.[93]

Galen's understanding of skin disease is summarized in Table 4.1.[94]

Galen continued to promote the idea that all skin diseases resulted from internal humoral imbalance. Few details are given as to the morphological appearance or differential diagnosis of the skin lesions themselves, and there is no effort undertaken in Galen's corpus to categorize skin lesions according to morphology. Elsewhere in the Galenic corpus, it is evident that Galen viewed two broad categories of skin disease: those involving the hair-bearing areas, especially the head; and those involving the non-hair bearing areas. This system had its roots in the Aristotelean assertion that the skin of the head dif-fered from the skin of the rest of the body.[95] Future medical writers would utilize this highly simplistic classification system until the eighteenth century. Although there was little new information in Galen's commentary on skin lesions, it had "a flavor of newness and originality" because of the way Galen incor-porated skin disease into his theoretical framework.[96]

Finally, Galen deserves recognition for several other contributions to the history of dermatology. He was the first to use the term *psora* to name an itchy, scaly skin condition that affected the eyelids and scrotum, which was more likely a description of seborrheic dermatitis than psoriasis.[97] He was the first to describe a pustular disease of the mouth called *febris pemphigodes*, which some have suggested was pemphigus vulgaris. The word "Galenical" refers to his pharmacological prowess for concocting medi-cations with plant or animal ingredients, and Galenic formulation is a term still used today that means the process by which a topical medication is formulated to optimize absorption. Galen is also credited with inventing the cold cream used for skin beautification.

In sum, Galen took Hippocratic medicine, put his own spin on it, and gave it an authoritative stamp. His corpus then became canon for the next 1500 years. His major contributions concerned the discovery of the skin as the medium of the sense of touch and a theory of humoral pathology to explain the origins of skin afflictions. His system of organizing skin diseases by hair-bearing and non-hair-bearing areas

TABLE 4.1

Dermatological Terms Used by Galen and Their Meaning

Phlegmon	Caused blood collecting in spaces under the skin. Over time, this blood becomes "concocted" and turns to pus, and due to "acridity," it eats through the skin and forms an *abscess*. Some abscesses do not contain pus but contain mud, urine, clots, mucous, honey-like juice, bones, rocks, stones, nails, hair, or even living things
Sinuses or *fistula*	Occur when abscesses tunnel through the adjacent tissue
Atheroma	Contains something like porridge and can be covered by a "membranous tunic"
Steatoma	Contain fat
Melicerides	Contain something like honey
Gangrene and *carbuncle*	Develop when the blood boils and scorches the skin. These are both covered with a black eschar, which must be distinguished from the black color of cancers, which contain pure unboiled black bile. Gangrene results from the "mortification of the affected part" and is very deadly
Herpes	When pure yellow bile accumulates in the skin, leading to ulceration
Erysipelas	From yellow bile mixed with blood accumulating and swelling the tissue. *Erysipelas* is on a spectrum with *phlegmon*—more blood than yellow bile in the skin leads to *phlegmone erysipelatodes*; more yellow bile than blood results from *erysipelas phlegmonodes*
Edema	Results from the accumulation of phlegm and does not throb and sinks in when the fingers press on it
Ecchymomata/melasmata	Occurs in old people with bruised veins, which are black in color and occur for the slightest reasons
Ulcer and cancer	Black bile can eat through the skin and cause an *ulcer*; if mild, it causes *cancer* without ulceration
Phagedenic ulcer	An ulcer that feeds on the underlying tissue and spreads
Elephantiasis	Results when blood contains too much black bile
Satyriasis	The first stage of elephantiasis, as the patient takes on the appearance of a satyr
Achor	A small ulcer on the head containing salty and nitrous phlegm
Ceria	An ulcer slightly larger than an achor that drains a honey-like humor

proved to have much staying power. Although he promoted observation and experiment, he, for the most part, did not observe the skin or its lesions in any great detail. Stagnation followed Galen, and for that, do we blame Galen who positioned himself with persuasive authority? Or do we blame the uncurious, unimaginative medical writers of the next millennium and a half who resolved to keep him in such a position?

Crito (First/Second Centuries CE)

Titus Statilius Crito (first/second centuries CE), also known as Crito, Criton, or Kriton, was a Greek physician who served as the personal physician of the emperor Trajan and his wife, Plotina. His only contribution to the history of medicine was his now-lost work, "On Cosmetics," which we only know about because Galen, Aetius (see Chapter 5), and a few later medical writers referenced it. Crito's work was drawn from a treatise on cosmetics that has been attributed "almost certainly wrongly" to Queen Cleopatra.[98]

Galen stated that Crito's popular four-volume book was "known to everybody" and listed Crito's topics in his *De compositione medicamentorum secundum locos,* "On the composition of medications by affected areas [of the human body]."[99] The following list of remedies discussed by Crito enumerates the cosmetic concerns of a second-century Roman patient: treatments for preserving hair, increasing hair, protect hair, for whitening hair, to make hair blond or golden, for removing wrinkles, to make the face bright and clean, to blacken the eyebrows, for foul smell of the nose, toothpastes, to combat axillary foul smell, for halitosis, for blackness of the neck, for axillary perspiration, creams for the breast, laxatives, soaps to make the hands clean and pleasant, for the pigmentations of pregnancy, for pregnancy wrinkles, for pregnancy stretch marks, for protrusion of the umbilicus, for retarding puberty in boys, for preserving virginity for girls, lubricants for frigid women, for pigmented scars, for removing hair, creams for the whole body, cleaning laxatives, perfumes for clothes, fumigations of all kinds, lotions and unguents of all compositions, for all kinds of scaly affections of the skin, for eruptions of the scalp, for chronic ulcers, for lice and their eggs, for alopecia, for scabies of the face, for birthmarks, for freckles, for face cosmetics, for tattoos, for bruises, for discolorations, for pimples, for overnight pustules, for tuberous lesions of the chin, for chin impetigo (mentagra), for removing skin, for abrasions, healing white plasters, emollient medicaments to be rubbed on impetigo, for black and white leprosy, for white scars, for scaly skin, for scaly nails, for itchy conditions, for blisters and excoriations, for serpiginous ulcers, for scabies, for passions, for pediculate and non-pediculate warts, for swelling of the umbilicus, for prolapse of the intestine, for hydrocele, for areas missing skin, for procidentia ani (rectal prolapse), for chilblains, and for cracked feet.[100]

The list of topics addressed by Crito gives us a revealing look at the cosmetic "chief complaints" of the affluent Roman citizen, who was seemingly obsessed with his or her appearance and scent. How exceptionally similar this list is to a list of patient complaints in a modern dermatology practice! And how tragic it is that Crito's text has been lost forever.

Cassius Felix (fl. Fifth Century)

Cassius Felix is the last of the important authors from the period of the Roman Empire. Hailing from Roman Africa (from Cirta, renamed Constantina, in modern-day Algeria), Cassius Felix authored a medical treatise in Latin, based on Greek medical sources, entitled *De medicina* in 447 CE.[101] The text is a handbook, with each entry containing a short paragraph about the diagnosis, and another paragraph on the treatment. Roughly one-quarter of the 82 chapters in *De medicina* are devoted to skin diseases, thus providing us with an excellent reference point for the status of the understanding of skin disease in the late Roman Empire. The book is particularly valuable because Cassius Felix gave both the Latin and the Greek terms for some of the skin diseases he discussed (see Table 4.2).[102]

Within the pages of *De medicina* can be found the first use of the term, *tinea*, the medical term used today for the fungal infection that the layperson calls ringworm. The word *tinea* in Latin translates to a type of worm that puts holes in books or clothing. Since the condition frequently presents with ring-shaped lesions, it is easy to see how ringworm developed as the term for this condition. Cassius Felix's description of *tinea*, however, sounds more like what is known today as favus in that it describes a thick and viscous humor, similar to honey, emitted by the skin from holes in the skin.

TABLE 4.2

Cassius Felix and His Latin-Greek Clarification

Latin Term	Greek Term
Tinea capitis	Achor
Pediculosis	Phthriasis
Maculas albas (white spots)	Alphus leucas
Maculas nigras (black spots)	Alphus melaenus
Impetigines/zernas	Lichen
Scabies	Lepidas/Lepra
Collectiones	Aposthemata
Carbunculus	Anthrax
Ignis sacer	Erysipelas
Aranea	Herpes

De medicina contains fairly comprehensive dermatologic information.[103] Felix stated that pediculosis (lice) was a disorder of cachectic (wasted) persons. He correctly understood that *capillorum defluxionem,* a hair-shedding problem which we today call telogen effluvium, could be caused by having a debilitated body, prolonged illness, or labor. His description of *cantabriem capitis* equates to our description of seborrheic dermatitis. His term for acne is *ionthi,* which can occur from the time of puberty to middle age. His description of *ignis sacer* coincides with a modern understanding of erysipelas: redness, swelling, and pain of the face, neck, or chest. He states that the layperson (common) Latin term for *impetigines* is *zernas,* and for *herpes* is *aranea* (spider). His description of elephantiasis is the same as that of leprosy in the modern sense.

Miscellaneous Roman Contributors

This history of dermatology would not be complete without mentioning briefly a few other important Roman writers who contributed to a growing body of literature that later medical writers referenced in their works. The first distinct and noteworthy Roman physician was Asclepiades of Bithynia (124–40 BCE), who enjoyed a stupendous reputation in Rome and was the first to introduce the Hippocratic ideals to the Romans during the era of the Roman Republic. Though none of his writings survive, we do know that Asclepiades dismissed history and physical exam to instead focus on symptoms, and he rejected the humoral theory of disease. He espoused an atomic theory, likely inspired by Democritus, which involved health being related to the proper arrangement of atoms and the spaces in between them.[104] Blockage of these spaces could lead to increased tension in the body and disease, so health was "the balance between tension and relaxation," and cure was achieved by opening or closing these spaces, with massage, exercise, and cold-water baths.[105] Preferring less intervention than the average Greek physician, Asclepiades prescribed wine and safe medications and promoted relaxation and stress reduction. He used enemas to relieve indigestion, which he believed to be the source of disease, and he employed music therapy as a means to calm his patients. His principles, carried forth by his pupil Themison of Laodicea (fl. first century BCE), found followers in the so-called Methodic School over the next several centuries. It is worth noting that Themison was the first documented physician to promote the use of leeches in medicine. His contributions to the history of dermatology are minimal, with his most significant bequest the Methodic concept of tightness versus looseness, particularly as it relates to the skin and the effect of this quality of the skin's pores. These ideas were mentioned frequently in the medical writings about the skin until the sixteenth century.

Titus Lucretius Carus, called Lucretius (99–55 BCE), was a Roman poet and philosopher who wrote the "the most beautiful scientific work of classic Latinism," the *De rerum natura*, "On the nature of things."[106] Within the lines of this extraordinary six-volume poem can be found many innovative statements about anatomy, physiology, and disease. The last book contains a famous account of the Plague of Athens (430–426 BCE). This poem is a must-read for any student of the history of science, the history of medicine, or philosophy.

Publius Ovidius Naso, known as Ovid (43 BCE–17 CE), was a Roman poet most famous for the narrative poem *Metamorphoses*. He also authored a 100-line poem entitled *Medicamina faciei femineae,* "Remedies for Female Faces." Scholars have debated whether the text represents a legitimate medical document, or whether Ovid is merely playing a literary game with Roman-era cosmeceuticals.[107] In the text are the poet's recipes for whitening and smoothing the face, removing blemishes and freckles, and two recipes for removing makeup. Of the many ingredients mentioned for his four recipes, barley, vetch, egg, antler of a stag, bulb of narcissus, acacia, spelt, honey, lupine, faba bean, white lead, scum of red natron, orrisroot, alcyonium, incense, myrrh, fennel, rose petals, frankincense, salt from Libyan desert, mucilage of barley, and poppy, most could be found in other medical texts of the period and have either therapeutic value (17), cosmetic value (14), or both (13), leading us to conclude that *Medicamina faciei femineae* is based on bonafide medical information of his time.[108]

Rufus of Ephesus (70–110 CE) was another great Greek physician of the Pax Romana. His most important publication, "On the Names of the Parts of the Human Body," is a summary of Roman anatomic knowledge as of the early second century CE. Rufus recognized that Guinea worm disease was contracted through contaminated drinking water and may have been the first Roman writer to mention the bubonic plague that was reported to be occurring in the Near East.[109] The encyclopedic work of the great Byzantine compiler, Oribasius, includes Rufus' description of "pestilential boubónes" (buboes).

Archigenes of Apamea (54–114 CE) was an ancient Greek physician from Apamea (Syria) who practiced in Rome during the reign of the emperor Trajan (r. 98–117 CE). He is most famous for being one of the founders of the Eclectic School, a group of physicians who did not follow any particular school such as Dogmatism or Methodism but instead cherry-picked doctrines from the different systems which worked the best for them. Archigenes had strong Pneumatistic leanings and maintained that the heart was the seat of memory and mentation.[110] His most important writings dealt with the pulse and with surgery; he believed that cancer should be excised from the body, even in its advanced stages.[111] He amputated limbs. He wrote about the necessity of filling dental cavities, for which he used a paste containing roasted earthworms and crushed spider eggs.[112] Although none of his writings survived, he was referenced by writers such as Aretaeus, Galen, Aetius, and Rhazes.[113] He was also mentioned in the *Satires* of Juvenal.

Archigenes' legacy in the history of dermatology is twofold. First, he is remembered for his excellent description of elephantiasis (leprosy) and was among the first to believe that elephantiasis was transmitted by contagion (see Interlude 1). The prevailing notion in the ancient world, even by the esteemed Galen, was that leprosy was *not* a contagious disease. But the Pneumatists, with their emphasis on the breath, naturally reached the conclusion that it was. Archigenes observed that breathing in air infected by a leper could result in the disease, so he advocated segregating these persons from the rest of society.[114] Second, his writings on cosmetics and particularly hair are noteworthy; Goodman referred to him as among the first of the "physician-cosmetologists."[115]

Aretaeus (fl. first/second centuries CE), a Greek physician from Cappadocia in the Roman province of Asia Minor, was "an Eclectic by practice and a Pneumatist by training."[116] His dates are unknown, but his works were probably written between the mid-first century and early second centuries CE. After his death, his writings disappeared until 1552.[117] His eight-volume treatise is broken into two equal parts: "On the Causes and Indications of Acute and Chronic Diseases" and "On the Treatment of Acute and Chronic Diseases." Within these volumes can be found several seminal descriptions of diseases: celiac disease, diphtheria, and heart murmur, as well as vivid descriptions of angina, asthma, dysentery, epilepsy, headaches, pneumonia, tetanus, and uterine cancer. He observed that a patient could experience both mania and depression.[118] Also noteworthy is that he was the first to give diabetes its name and is, therefore, the ancient physician most associated with that diagnosis. His work contains some of the clearest and most accurate descriptions of disease given by any ancient Greek physician.

Aretaeus should be remembered for his accurate description of leprosy (see Interlude 1), which he, like his mentor Archigenes, believed was a contagious disease. Aretaeus stated that the breath of one person can infect another, who can then transmit it to others.[119] In the treatment of skin disease, Aretaeus wrote one of the first comments on topical vehicle preference: he preferred ointments over liquid preparations, believing them to be more agreeable, effective, and better absorbed.[120] Dermatologists of today would agree with Aretaeus—his understanding of the itch associated with jaundice as being caused by "prickly bilious particles" was on the right track.

Highly regarded by his peers and called the "prince of the Methodists," Soranus of Ephesus (fl. first/second centuries CE) was yet another Greek physician who thrived in Rome during the reign of Trajan.[121] Considered the ancient father of gynecology and neonatology, Soranus wrote "On the Diseases of Women," the most authoritative textbook on both gynecology and newborn care for the next fifteen centuries. He also was the first to pen a biography of Hippocrates. His other influential work, "On Acute and Chronic Diseases," survived in a Latin translation by Caelius Aurelianus (unknown dates, possibly fifth century) from Roman Africa, who translated it from the Greek. Two chapters in that work are devoted to diseases that feature the skin: *elephantiasis* (leprosy) and *phthiriasis* (lice). The former discusses the different ways in which the condition was treated, and the noteworthy part of this chapter is Soranus' merciful commentary on segregating lepers. He questioned the practice of imprisoning foreigners with elephantiasis and exiling citizens with the same, noting that this practice was abandonment and "foreign to the humanitarian principles of medicine."[122] Soranus' comments on lice reveal the classical understanding of this peculiar affliction. Brought about by a "run-down state," it can lead to loss of sleep, appetite, and hair, as well as itching and pallor, and the tiny animals arise from reddish bile excreted from the pores.[123] Caelius' translation of Soranus became a critical reference work for the medical writers who followed him.

Julius Pollux (fl. second century CE) was born in Naukratis, Egypt, and appointed chair of rhetoric in Athens by the Roman emperor Commodus (r. 180–192). He compiled a long dictionary of Attic Greek words entitled *Onomasticon* that survives as several incomplete ninth-century epitomes. He cataloged in Book IV many Greek words that pertain to dermatology, which include (in English) *edema, ulcer, abscess, eschar, phyma, terminthos, tylosis, anthrax, achor, pityriasis, alopecia, ophis, alphos, leuce, lichen, lepra, psora, psydrakia, ephelis, ionthi, phakos, thymos, acrochordon, myrmecia, helos, epinyctis, chironium, ganglion, meliceris, carcinoma, chelae, kerion, erysipelas, bubo, condyloma, steatoma, herpes, phagedena,* and *gangrene.*[124]

MORBUS CAMPANUS, THE CAMPANIAN DISEASE

Quintus Horatius Flaccus (65–8 BCE), known today as Horace, was a Roman poet and contemporary of Vergil and Ovid during the golden age of Roman poetry in the last century BCE. While he did not contribute any knowledge on skin disease, he did give us one of the great dermatological mysteries of ancient Rome. The mystery began in the seventeenth century when the Dutch editor of Horace's *Satires*, Jacobus Cruquius, transcribed that Sarmentus, a member of Maecenas' entourage, joked about the ugly appearance of his opponent, Messius Cicirrus, and referred to Messius as having *morbus Campanus.* Sarmentus mocked him, noting "foul scar has disgraced the left part of Messius's bristly forehead" and ridiculed him that the scar must have been the remnant of a horn that used to be there.[125] Named after the Campania region of ancient Italy, Horace's *morbus Campanus* has since been described as horns or warts on the forehead in persons from this region.[126] Knorr argued that even in the text itself, there is no connection between a horn or scar and *morbus Campanus*, and to the Romans *morbus Campanus* is a "comic allusion to the proverbial Campanian arrogance."[127] Yet, much has been made of these horns, and the easiest association for horns on the forehead has been satyrism—a state most commonly linked with leprosy, in which a person takes on the appearance of a satyr. But there is no reference in ancient sources to the Campanians having been regularly associated with any disease, including warts, venereal diseases, or leprosy. Perhaps the inhabitants of sunny, ancient Campania did grow true horns, which can actually happen on human skin, in the case of the heavily sun-damaged farmer who develops a skin cancer (squamous cell carcinoma) that forms enough keratin that a horn develops. Messius' "bristly forehead" might have been a reference to his actinic keratoses. Or perhaps translational confusion and liberal interpretation of ancient Latin have buried the original intent of the ancient author.

Dermatological Latin

While many of the words used today in the field of dermatology have roots in the Greek language, others stem from Latin, the language of the Romans. Although the majority of medical writers highlighted in the previous sections wrote in their native Greek, and while no Latin medical book exists from the Republican period (509–27 BCE), the Roman Empire did see a few important medical works in classical Latin, such as those of Celsus, Scribonius Largus, and Pliny. However, for much of the period covered by this chapter, Greek remained the unofficial language of medicine, as the Roman Empire encompassed many Greek-speaking lands. Greek doctors, while initially mistrusted in Rome, were eventually held in high regard throughout the Roman Empire. Medicine under the Roman Empire was "an exclusively Greek science, practiced and written about almost exclusively by Greeks in Greek."[128]

A large proportion of the Latin words in the texts of Celsus and the other Latin writers were borrowed from the Greek through a process known as transliteration—the swapping of Greek letters for

TABLE 4.3

The Meaning of Suffixes in Latin Medical Terminology

-igo	Skin diseases; e.g., *impetigo*, *lentigo* (lentil-like freckle), *porrigo* (seborrheic dermatitis), *prurigo* (itch), *vitiligo*, and *aurigo* (jaundice)
-ies	Formed abstract nouns on a verbal or adjectival base, respectively: *scabies* (from *scabere*, "to scratch") and *canities* (from *canus* gray)
-lus, -li, -la, -lae, -lum	Diminutives, meaning small or little: *pediculus, furunculus, panniculus, vermiculi, carbuncula, papillae, tuberculum*

Latin letters that make similar sounds. Other words are original Latin ones, such as the three words that were used by the Romans to denote "skin": *pellis*, *cutis*, and *corium*; each initially meant something that covered and protected. The high number of occurrences of the word *cutis* in Celsus may have elevated that word to be the sole designation for "human skin" in medicine, and *pellis* or *corium* both eventually referred to "animal hide."[129] *Cutis* later morphed into *cutaneus* (Latin) and *cutaneous* (English). Integument derives from the Latin *tego*, "to cover."[130] "Tangible" and "tactile" come from *tango*, "to touch." The words "follicle" and "sebum" come from the Latin, *folliculus*, meaning "pod," "small bag," or "shell," and *sebum*, meaning "grease" or "tallow."[131] "Perspiration" comes from *perspiro*, "to breathe through."

Many words related to skin maladies are derived from Latin. Scabies derives from the Latin word *scabo*, "to scratch." "To itch" was *prurio* in Latin and *psorao* in Greek; these words give us pruritus and psoriasis, respectively. The Latins took *herpo* from the Greeks and made it *serpo*, "to creep," which led to "serpiginous." Carbuncle was a diminutive form of *carbo*, which means "coal" and is the root of the English word "carbon." The Greek counterpart of carbuncle was *anthrak*, meaning "coal," from which we get the word "anthrax." Carbuncles looked and felt as if hot coals were under the skin. Molluscum (soft), verruca (wart), clavus (nail), and purpura (purple) are examples of direct borrowings from the Latin. The suffix of a Latin medical term could indicate something about the type of affliction to which it was attached, as shown in Table 4.3.[132] It should be pointed out that the commonly seen word endings in medicine, "-osis," "-iasis," and "-itis," are of Greek derivation.

Biblical Skin Disease

As mentioned in the section on Pliny, skin diseases were considered a fate worse than death in the ancient Roman world, and the damage a person experienced was threefold: physical, psychological, and social. Ancient skin diseases were frequently described as very painful or severely itchy, presumably because effective treatment was unavailable; conditions such as staph infections or scabies progressed and spread over the body to extremes that are hard to fathom today. Skin disease was also psychologically devastating because of the stigma attached to these conditions, which frequently led to ostracization. Persons with severe skin diseases were assumed by society to have committed sins of vice or lust, and the disease was seen as a punishment from God. Consequently, one can find numerous references to skin diseases in both the Old Testament (Hebrew Bible) and New Testament of the Holy Bible.

The most famous story in the Bible involving skin disease occurs in the literary masterpiece, that is, the Old Testament's Book of Job. Job was a pious, upright man, happy with his life, until God put him to the test by allowing Satan to curse him:

> So went Satan forth from the presence of the Lord, and smote Job with sore boils from the sole of his foot unto his crown.[133]

The Hebrew word for this affliction is *shechin*, generally translated as "boils," but is derived from the word for "heat."[134] The term is used elsewhere in the Old Testament: In Isaiah 38:13–14, the King of Judah, Hezekiah, suffered acutely with a life-threatening form of *shechin*. The sixth plague of Egypt, as narrated in the Book of Exodus (9:8–12), was a plague of *shechin* brought down upon the Egyptians.

Affecting man and beast, this plague was described as causing *ababouth*, "swellings"; one may imagine an outbreak of staphylococcus, anthrax, or even smallpox.[135] In the Book of Samuel, a plague of boils known as the Plague of Ashdod was used as retaliation against the Philistines for capturing the Ark of the Covenant.[136] Afflictions of skin disease are a recurring subject in the Bible.

WHAT SKIN DISEASE DID JOB HAVE?

It is impossible to classify Job's affliction as one distinct syndrome. Medieval commentators considered Job's affliction to be leprosy, and a few writers in the early modern period believed that Job suffered from syphilis and even named him the patron saint of syphilitics. Modern scholars have determined that neither diagnosis is likely the case. Staphylococcal disease presenting as multiple abscesses is also improbable, as this type of "boils" is unlikely to occur on non-hair bearing regions such as the sole of the foot. Using clues from the rest of the chapter of Job, his symptoms of progressively ulcerating skin lesions from the top of his head to the soles of his feet, intense itching that worsens at night and unrelieved by scratching with a piece of broken glass, cracked and blackened skin infested with worms, a wasted, disfigured appearance, bone pain, bilious vomiting, and confusion indicate that Job was likely suffering from scabies and superinfection of the skin with staph and resultant sepsis.[137] Scabies is one of the most miserable skin diseases a person can have, as is dermatitis herpetiformis, the cutaneous eruption caused by gluten insensitivity and associated with celiac disease. Severe atopic dermatitis (eczema) or psoriasis can cause this symptomatology as well. Incidentally, to emphasize the degree of suffering experienced by affected patients, Job's name was assigned to a syndrome (Job's syndrome) in 1966 that was characterized by eczema, itching, staph infections, lung infections, and markedly elevated IgE levels.[138]

Skin disease in the Bible was considered either a punishment for an individual's sins or as a test or trial that a person must experience to prove one's faith in God. Moses warned of incurable hemorrhoids, scabs, and itching as a punishment for disobedience.[139] The only outcomes were resolution after proving one's faith, being shown mercy by God, or worst-case scenario, exile. It is certain that biblical leprosy was not leprosy in our modern understanding but could have been vitiligo, psoriasis, or even more likely, a designation for a whole host of different skin diseases that indicated impurity. Diagnosing biblical characters *a posteriori* is an interesting undertaking for the modern medical sleuth, but it is a task that is impossible to achieve with any degree of certainty.

HEROD'S HORRID AFFLICTION

Herod the Great (73–4 BCE) was the Roman-appointed King of Judaea, the kingdom in which Jesus of Nazareth was born. From the writings of Josephus (37–100 CE), a Roman-Jewish historian of the first century CE, we know that Herod the Great suffered from a severe skin disease in the last year of his life. Herod frequented the Dead Sea seeking relief from his many ailments. As the world's saltiest lake and the earth's lowest non-oceanic point, the Dead Sea is today a popular destination for what is termed climatotherapy. The salinity, the minerals, the warmth, the low humidity, and the filtered ultraviolet light (high in UV-A and low in UV-B) permit extended exposure without sunburn, and numerous reports argue for its efficacy and safety in such conditions as psoriasis and eczema.[140] But it does not sound like the Dead Sea could ever cure what ailed Herod. Josephus wrote:

> Now Herod's distemper greatly increased upon him after a severe manner, and this by God's judgment upon him for his sins; for a fire glowed in him slowly, which did not so much appear to the touch outwardly, as it augmented his pains inwardly; for it brought

upon him a vehement appetite to eating, which he could not avoid to supply with one sort of food or other. His entrails were also ex-ulcerated, and the chief violence of his pain lay on his colon; an aqueous and transparent liquor also had settled itself about his feet, and a like matter afflicted him at the bottom of his belly. Nay, further, his privy-member was putrefied, and produced worms; and when he sat upright, he had a difficulty of breathing, which was very loathsome, on account of the stench of his breath, and the quickness of its returns; he had also convulsions in all parts of his body, which increased in strength to an insufferable degree.[141]

In another work, Josephus included "intolerable itching over all the surface of his body" as a feature of this syndrome.[142] Herod's affliction may have started with diabetes and renal failure, the latter of which caused the reduced appetite, itching, and generalized edema. The severe skin breakdown of his genital area was most likely due to infection, possibly from chronic scratching, and Fournier's gangrene, a necrotizing skin infection of the genital area, has been postulated as the specific name for this ailment.[143] Another possibility is severe candida intertrigo caused by diabetes, obesity, or edema. The claim that worms infested his wounds may either have some validity or signify exaggeration by his contemporaries in order to paint a picture of extreme end-of-life justice for a tyrannical ruler. Note that worms in putrefying tissues in the setting of an agonizing demise were a recurring theme in the death sagas of the cruel tyrants of antiquity.[144]

Summary

Lichen, lepra, and *lentigo*; *melas* and *mentagra*; *achor, alphus, elephantiasis, erysipelas, herpes,* and *impetigo*; *pediculosis, porrigo,* and *prurigo*; *psora, scabies, scrofula,* and *zona* were the skin diseases diagnosed by the Roman *medicus*. Skin diseases at this time continued to be thought of not as primary diseases of the skin, but instead a reflection on the skin of an internal humoral imbalance. The treatment of skin disease during the Roman Empire involved a variety of measures to correct this imbalance, such as bloodletting, which really entered the mainstream of medicine during this era. There was also an elaborate mix of topical and oral medicaments, as outlined by Dioscorides in his masterpiece on pharmacology, *De Materia Medica*. The Romans were extremely vain and valued hygiene, and the typical cosmetic concerns of the Roman man and woman available for our review are virtually identical to concerns expressed today by patients to dermatologists. A distinctly Roman skin disease—*mentagra*—was a disease of the face that invoked so much fear that Pliny the Elder once wrote "that any form of death would be preferable" to it. Medical writers of the Roman imperial period, especially Celsus, Pliny, Scribonius Largus, Galen, Caelius Aurelianus, and Cassius Felix, authored many chapters on skin diseases, but their final product—the body of knowledge about the skin and its diseases from the ancient world—was full of disorder and confusion for the future learned medical men to apply in their own times. Galen's approach to classifying skin disease by those of the hairy parts of the body and those of the non-hairy parts of the body was set in stone as the only way to classify diseases until the sixteenth through seventeenth centuries. The Roman *medicus* knew the skin to be a protective coating, but, after Galen, there was an awareness of the skin's function in tactile sensation. The Romans deserve credit for taking the nomenclature of the Greeks and translating it into Latin, the future language of medicine. The *medicus* had a more elaborate terminology for skin diseases from which to choose a diagnosis than did his Hippocratic predecessors. Judging from the volume of content, the efforts of the Roman Empire's medical writers to make sense of skin diseases must have been timely and pertinent for their readers, and the chaotic knowledge bequeathed was nonetheless appreciated as dogma for more than 1300 years after the empire's collapse.

Interlude 1

Leprosy (Hansen's Disease)

To name a single disease with a more fascinating history than leprosy might be an impossible task. Leprosy dates back to ancient times in its existence, but the legacy of confusion left by the ancients regarding the word *lepra*—and its affiliated terms *elephantiasis, alphus, leuce,* and *melas*—creates challenges when studying the history of leprosy in the ancient and medieval periods. We now know that what the ancients called *lepra* is different from the infectious disease we know today as leprosy. In the modern sense of the term, leprosy, also known as Hansen's disease (HD), is an infectious disease caused by the bacterium *Mycobacterium leprae.* HD is a chronic, indolent condition that is spread by respiratory secretions from infected persons to persons who are genetically susceptible to acquiring the infection. The countries with the highest incidence of HD in today's world are India, Brazil, and Indonesia. From 100 to 200 new cases are reported in the United States each year, in states such as Arkansas, California, Florida, Hawaii, Louisiana, New York, and Texas.

Significant, long-term, close contact with the infected is necessary to acquire the illness; thus, HD is actually quite difficult to contract from a person with the disease. Conjugal leprosy (the spread by cohabitation) accounts for only 3 percent of all cases of modern leprosy.[1] With estimates as high as 1 in 30 persons in Europe with leprosy during the Middle Ages—and up to 30 percent in some parts of southern Scandinavia—Europeans were clearly more susceptible to the disease at that time. However, centuries of genetic modifications in the capacity for humans to resist the infection account for the reduction in susceptibility to the point that today only 5 percent of the world's population can get HD. One's risk to contract HD is genetically determined and higher among familial clusters; the offspring—not the spouse—of a person with HD is more likely to get it. But for the last several decades, the epidemiology of leprosy has been changing; sporadic cases, without familial or geographic connections, are more common—suggesting a potential natural or zoonotic source, such as the nine-banded armadillo.

There are two different clinical presentations of HD; the form a person gets is determined by the individual's immune response to the infection. If the person develops a good immune response against the bacterium, then the relatively benign, *tuberculoid* form of the disease manifests, characterized by few or many patches of skin with a lightened skin color that exhibit anesthesia because of damage to the peripheral nerves. Anesthesia is a unique feature of this disease, and when medical writers of the ancient and medieval periods discussed anesthesia, it is easy to infer they were talking about HD. Because of the healthy immune response, the pathologist's task of finding the bacteria on the skin biopsy is difficult because the organisms are scarce; another term for this form is *paucibacillary,* "few bacilli."

On the other end of the spectrum is the *lepromatous* form of the disease, characterized by widespread nodules and plaques, nasal congestion and nosebleeds, loss of eyebrow hair, progressive infiltration of the face with the eventual development of leonine facies, lymph node and internal organ involvement, and nerve damage and resultant neuropathy so severe that ulceration, infection, and amputation of digits—or even limbs—might ensue. Neurological symptomatology is very frequently the first sign of the disease since the organism shows a tendency to thrive in the Schwann cells of peripheral nerves. Ample organisms are seen on the biopsy of these patients' skin lesions because the host response is poor and the organism thrives; another term for this form is *multibacillary* disease. The most common form of the disease is actually somewhere in the middle of the spectrum between tuberculoid and lepromatous, which has been termed *borderline* leprosy, as it presents with features of both. Today, HD is an illness that can be treated successfully with antibiotics. Due to the

DOI: 10.1201/9781003273622-7

rapid development of antibiotic resistance with single-agent regimens, multi-drug treatment is recommended with rifampin, clofazimine, and dapsone.

The Origins of Leprosy

The literary history of HD begins in ancient India, China, and Mesopotamia, with our current knowledge about the origins of HD suggesting that the condition had its origins in India. In contrast, there is no literary record of HD in pharaonic Egypt. The earliest, widely accepted literary evidence of the illness dates to 600 BCE in the South Asian text *Sushruta Samhita*. In 2009, however, archeologists identified leprous skeletal stigmata on remains found in India dated to 2000 BCE and contended that the following Sanskrit hymn of the *Atharva Veda,* composed before the first millennium BCE, is the actual earliest literary evidence of leprosy:

> Born by night art thou, O plant, dark, black, sable. Do thou, that art rich in colour, stain this leprosy, and the grey spots! ... The leprosy which has originated in the bones, and that which has originated in the body and upon the skin, the white mark begotten of corruption, I have destroyed with my charm.[2]

It is believed that the ancient Chinese people also wrote about leprosy in an ancient Chinese medical text written on bamboo slip (a writing media that preceded paper) entitled *Feng zhen shi* 封診, "Models for sealing and investigating" (266–246 BCE). Scholars believe leprosy was under a generic term for skin disease called *li* 癘. In that work, a person was suspected of having *li*, with easily recognizable features of leprosy: sores on the head; swollen brows; loss of eyebrow hair; destroyed nasal bridge and collapsed nose; suppurating elbows, knees, and soles; and hoarse voice.[3]

A literal interpretation of the Old Babylonian Omen Text, quoted in Chapter 1, argues that leprosy may have been even older. Believed to have been written before or during the reign of Hammurabi (eighteenth century BCE), the text suggests the presence of leprosy in ancient Babylon and even a knowledge of its two different forms. The consensus among historians, however, is that leprosy originated in the Indian subcontinent, then spread to Europe after the fourth century BCE, but it did not become a severe public health problem in Europe until the Middle Ages.

The English word leprosy was derived from the Latin word *lepra,* which came from the Greek noun λέπρα (lepra), which was itself originally derived from the Greek verb λέπω (lepo, to peel). By the time of the Hippocratics, the word *lepra* referred to any skin condition that had scaling or flaking; neither are major features of HD. In other words, Hippocrates' *lepra* was not HD, but it was a benign skin condition, such as psoriasis, which Hippocrates attributed to poor hygiene.[4] To the Hippocratics, *lepra* could be acute and self-limited, or chronic; "a simple surface reaction on the skin" or "a disease in the fullest sense."[5] *Lepra* was frequently associated with *leuce* and *alphus* in the Hippocratic texts, both terms that refer to skin conditions that lighten the skin color. Vitiligo and morphea are two diseases that both lighten the skin tone and are excellent candidates for either of these terms.[6]

Biblical Leprosy

The "leprosy" of the Bible was also not HD. In the Hebrew Bible, a skin condition associated with ritual impurity called *tsara'at* (tsaraath) is described; it was essentially mistranslated twice and eventually became known during the Middle Ages as leprosy. When the Hebrew Bible was first translated into the Greek Septuagint around 250 BCE, there was no equivalent for *tsara'at* in Greek, and the author(s) chose the word closest in meaning, λέπρα. This word survived as *lepra* in the Latin translation of the Bible (the Vulgate). It may have been the scholar John of Damascus (fl. seventh to eighth centuries CE) who first used lepra to exclusively denote what is now called HD, instead of the traditional term for HD, *elephantiasis.*[7] In 1382, *lepra* was later transliterated in the first English translation of the Bible as *leprosie.* And so the word leprosy became forever linked to *tsara'at*, the "leprosy" of the Bible.[8]

The words *tsara'at* in the Old Testament and *lepra* in the New Testament appear 68 times.[9] Based on the description of the condition in the 13th chapter of the Book of Leviticus, *tsara'at* was unlike HD as we understand it today, as seen in this abridged excerpt:

> And the Lord spake unto Moses and Aaron, saying, when a man shall have in the skin of his flesh a rising, a scab, or bright spot, and it be in the skin of his flesh like the plague of leprosy; then he shall be brought unto Aaron the priest, or unto one of his sons the priests: And the priest shall look on the plague in the skin of the flesh: and when the hair in the plague is turned white, and the plague in sight be deeper than the skin of his flesh, it is a plague of leprosy: and the priest shall look on him, and pronounce him unclean.[10]

The description continues for many more verses; the affliction is curiously described as also damaging the clothing and the walls of the house. The whitening of the skin is a consistent feature in other parts of the Bible; Moses' daughter Miriam was "made leprous as white as snow."[11] Naaman, in the Book of Kings, dipped himself in the Jordan River seven times to rid himself of his leprosy, and his "flesh was restored," while Gehazi, after stealing Naaman's silver, became afflicted with leprosy: "his skin had become as white as snow."[12]

Thus, the essential features of biblical leprosy include white spots with white hairs, swellings, scabs, scales, or ulcers. Some scholars have broadened the definition of *tsara'at* to refer to skin disease collectively as it is impossible to arrive at one diagnosis which includes each of these skin lesions.[13] Vitiligo classically presents with widespread white patches and white hairs, but the patches are not depressed below the level of the surrounding skin. Psoriasis causes widespread silvery-white scaly or scabby plaques that bleed when picked at or scratched but do not change the hair color. Note that it is not rare for patients to have both vitiligo and psoriasis at the same time. Fungal infection, impetigo, lupus, and scabies are unlikely candidates for biblical leprosy. True leprosy in its early stages can present with skin patches with a lightened tone, but it is not as white as vitiligo. It is safe to say that biblical leprosy was not our modern understanding of leprosy when considering the fact that there is no historical, archeological, literary, or artistic evidence for true leprosy in Palestine or Syria before the return of Alexander's armies from India in 325 BCE; the Old Testament was written much earlier (ca. sixth century BCE).[14]

In the biblical Hebrew culture, any significant skin disease could be reason enough to have you brought in front of the priest, as skin disease was a sign of impurity. The priest determined whether the person's condition was *tsara'at* (biblical leprosy), and if so diagnosed, the diseased person was excluded from the community so their impurity could not be passed on to others. If a person was suspected of having *tsara'at*, they were first placed in a seven-day quarantine, and if the skin condition improved or resolved after ritual purification and an offering, that person could return to society.[15] But if the skin disease persisted beyond the seven-day window, the afflicted had to leave their family and join communities of similarly ostracized individuals outside the village.

Leprosy in Ancient Times

The Greek physicians of the Roman Empire such as Galen and Dioscorides discussed λέπρα in their writings, but the Latin writers Celsus and Cassius Felix ignored the Latinized form of the word *lepra* in their texts. They instead used scabies and impetigo to refer to the scaly eruptions the Greeks called *lepra*. The word *lepra* remained in use, however, because both the Greek and Latin (St. Jerome) translations of the Bible had used the term.

In ancient times, historians believe that the term used by the Greeks and Latins for HD was *elephantiasis* or "Elephant's disease." Note that the term elephantiasis is still in use today but has nothing to do with leprosy. In the modern sense, elephantiasis is a filarial parasitic infection that causes severe edema and skin thickening, particularly of the lower legs. The initial awareness in the Western world of *elephantiasis* is believed to have occurred in the third century BCE, when the Alexandrian physicians began to see an increasing number of cases as a result of a portion of Alexander's armies returning to Egypt from India, bringing the disease with them.[16] According to Rufus of Ephesus (first century CE), the first to mention what Rufus called *elephantiasis* was a student of Erasistratus named Straton, who called the condition *kakochymia*, which meant "a mixture of bad humors."[17] Hippocrates did not specifically use the term *elephantiasis*, but it is widely held that he called the same condition the "Phoenician disease." Galen concurred in his commentary on Hippocrates' *Prorrhetics* that the "Phoenician disease" was *elephantiasis*.[18]

Pliny the Elder penned the following about the Roman experience of the Elephant's disease:

> We have already stated that elephantiasis was unknown in Italy before the time of Pompeius Magnus [Pompey]. This malady, too, like those already mentioned, mostly makes its first appearance in the face. In its primary form, it bears a considerable resemblance to a small lentil upon the nose; the skin gradually dries up all over the body, is marked with spots of various colours, and presents an unequal surface, being thick in one place, thin in another, indurated every here and there, and covered with a sort of rough scab. At a later period, the skin assumes a black hue, and compresses the flesh upon the bones, the fingers and toes becoming swollen. This disease was originally peculiar to Egypt.[19]

Pompey (106–48 BCE) was a Roman general and statesman who returned from war in Asia Minor in 62 BCE, indicating that elephantiasis was introduced into Italy in the first century BCE. Pliny went on to say that the outbreak of *elephantiasis* in Italy was short-lived.

Galen wrote about *elephantiasis* and noted that Alexandria was a hotbed for the disease. He did not describe it as contagious; instead, he blamed the origins of the disease on a diet of foods that generated black bile (lentils, snails, brine-preserved foods, and donkey) combined with the heat of the region, which caused "a thick melancholic humor that entered the blood and eventually rose toward the skin."[20] Galen treated *elephantiasis* with bloodletting and purgatives to remove the black bile, along with a diet rich in vegetables, fish, fowl, and a unique addition—viper flesh. Since snakes shed their skin, it was believed that ingesting snake meat would cause the skin lesions of elephantiasis to slough off.[21]

Aretaeus of Cappadocia wrote the most detailed description of *elephantiasis* of any Greek or Roman medical writer; the Adams translation is an extraordinarily eloquent read. After opening his chapter with an unusually lengthy description of an elephant, he then noted that this disease had other names:

> The disease is called *Leo*, on account of the resemblance of the eyebrows, as I shall afterwords explain; and *Satyriasis*, from the redness of the cheeks, and the irresistible and shameless impulse *ad coitum*. Moreover, it is also called the *Heracleian* affection, insomuch as there is none greater and stronger than it.[22]

He described the condition as arising in the bowels, spreading to the internal organs, and then erupting out of the body onto the face and around the joints:

> … but lurking among the bowels, like a concealed fire it smolders there, and having prevailed over the internal parts, it afterwards blazes forth on the surface, for the most part beginning, like a bad signal-fire, on the face, as it were its watch-tower; but in certain cases from the joint of the elbow, the knee, and knuckles of the hands and feet.[23]

He then notes that the physician must be alert to these early signs or risk the situation becoming hopeless. Aretaeus then offers the following details of the skin itself:

> Tumours prominent, not continuous with one another anywhere, but thick and rough, and the intermediate space cracked, like the skin of the elephant. Veins enlarged, not from abundance of blood, but from thickness of the skin; and for no long time is the situation of them manifest, the whole surface being elevated equally in the swelling. The hairs on the whole body die prematurely, on the hands, the thighs, the legs, and again on the pubes; scanty on the chin, and also the hairs on the head are scarce. And still more frequently premature hoariness, and sudden baldness; in a very short time the pubes and chin naked of hair, or if a few hairs should remain,

they are more unseemly than where they are gone. The skin of the head deeply cracked; wrinkles frequent, deep, rough; tumours on the face hard, sharp; sometimes white at the top, but more green at the base. Pulse small, dull, languid, as if moved with difficulty through the mud; veins on the temples elevated, and also those under the tongue; bowels bilious; tongue roughened with *vari*, resembling hailstones; not unusual for the whole frame to be full of such (and thus also in unsound victims, the flesh is full of these tubercles resembling hail). But if the affection be much raised up from the parts within, and appear upon the extremities, *lichens* occur on the extremities of the fingers; there is pruritus on the knees, and the patients rub the itchy parts with pleasure. And the *lichen* sometimes embraces the chin all round; it reddens the cheeks, but is attended with no great swelling; eyes misty, resembling bronze; eyebrows prominent, thick, bald, inclining downwards, tumid from contraction of the intermediate space; colour livid or black; eyelid, therefore, much retracted to cover the eyes, as in enraged lions; on this account it is named *leontium*. Wherefore it is not like to the lions and elephants only, but also in the eyelids "resembles swift night." Nose, with black protuberances, rugged; prominence of the lips thickened, but lower part livid; nose elongated; teeth not white indeed, but appearing to be so under a dark body; ears red, black, contracted, resembling the elephant, so that they appear to have a greater size than usual; ulcers upon the base of the ears, discharge of ichor, with pruritus; shrivelled all over the body with rough wrinkles; but likewise deep fissures, like black furrows on the skin; and for this reason the disease has got the name of *elephas*. Cracks on the feet and heels, as far as the middle of the toes; but if the ailment still further increase, the tumours become ulcerated, so that on the cheeks, chin, fingers, and knees, there are fetid and incurable ulcers, some of which are springing up on one part, while others are subsiding on another. Sometimes, too, certain of the members of the patient will die, so as to drop off, such as the nose, the fingers, the feet, the privy parts, and the whole hands; for the ailment does not prove fatal, so as to relieve the patient from a foul life and dreadful sufferings, until he has been divided limb from limb. For it is long-lived, like the animal, the elephant.[24]

There can be no doubt after reading this description that Aretaeus' section on *elephantiasis* is a discussion of HD. Aretaeus' Pneumatist leanings led him to conclude that inhaling the corrupted air either exhaled by persons with leprosy or emitted from their ulcers could cause a person to get the disease. However, Aretaeus was not as widely read in the Middle Ages as Galen; therefore, Aretaeus' assertions about the contagiousness of the disease were likely never heard.[25] Finally, he concludes, as does Galen, with a discussion of the use of viper flesh, which he advocates for this disease.

HD was not common in the Roman Empire until the fourth century; both medical and Christian writings support this statement.[26] Eventually, more and more persons with leprosy trickled into the eastern part of the Roman Empire from the Middle East, and by the middle of the fourth century CE, the Byzantines saw the prevalence of leprosy increase to the point that asylums had to be constructed outside Constantinople. The first leper asylum arose around Rome in 400 CE, the first in France circa 550 CE.[27] The isolation of these infected persons from the rest of society, mandated in the Book of Leviticus, became the standard protocol; they were deemed a threat to society both because of their perceived corruption and immorality and because of an increasing sense that the diseased person was contagious.

Medieval Leprosy

During the Middle Ages, the Latin word *lepra* became explicitly associated with what we today call HD, increasingly replacing *elephantiasis*. While the influence of the Christian writers—with their Bibles containing the word *lepra* and not *elephantiasis*—cannot be overstated, perhaps most influential of all was Gerard of Cremona, the translator of Avicenna's *Canon*, who chose *lepra* for Avicenna's *elephantiasis*, thus sealing the fate of the latter, and elevating the status of the former.[28]

The classic "leper"—the frail, disfigured beggar, missing digits, limbs, or his or her nose, traveling on foot alone or with a group, ringing his ominous bell—migrated throughout Western Europe, invoking in the healthy populace responses ranging from utter disgust and outrage to sympathy and moral obligation to assist; the latter was the view increasingly promulgated by the Catholic Church. The prevalence of leprosy rose throughout the Middle Ages in Western Europe; at its peak at the end of the twelfth century, there were an estimated 19,000 leper houses throughout Europe.[29] The leper house was also known as a leprosarium, leper hospital, or a lazar house, after Lazarus, the patron saint of lepers.

A common theory to explain the twelfth-century leprosy epidemic involves the influence of the Crusades. One association of the Crusades with leprosy involves the Military Order of Saint Lazarus of Jerusalem. This was a Catholic military order established at a leper hospital in Jerusalem in 1119. The term *lazar house* originated with this order. These so-called Knights Hospitallers demonstrated a life-style that stressed chivalry, monastic piety, and charitable concern for the infirm and indigent while continuing to participate in military operations in the region. After Jerusalem fell to Saladin and the Muslims in 1187, the Crusaders returned home; eighteenth- and nineteenth-century historians stated that the Crusaders brought back leprosy with them from Palestine. The return of the Crusaders accounts for some of the cases, but modern scholars contend that the epidemic was already ongoing and that the increase in leper hospitals is attributed to a new enthusiasm for charitable institutions that took care of the poor and sick.[30] Other factors include increased urbanization and the proliferation of trade with regions where leprosy was endemic.

THE LEPER KING

Leprosy will always be associated with the Crusades because of the life of one of the Crusader kings, Baldwin IV of Jerusalem (1161–1185), "the Leper King," who had suffered with the disease since he was a child. His first symptom was insensitivity to pain in his right arm. His intelligence, bravery, and strong leadership abilities allowed him to overcome his disability and rule with the respect of his subjects. Baldwin was the last successful Christian king of the Holy City, having defeated Saladin on the battlefield on several occasions.[31] But his physicians could never cure him. After a life of much suffering, eventual blindness, and disability, he died at age 24 when leg ulcers and presumed sepsis overwhelmed him. His death left the kingdom divided and contributed to the decline of Crusader power in the territory and the conquest of Jerusalem by Saladin. Baldwin may just be the most famous person to ever have leprosy.

Efforts to identify and isolate persons with leprosy reached a fever pitch in the thirteenth through fifteenth centuries; the Leprosy Plot of 1321 represents the peak of hysteria surrounding this disease. In France, rumors erupted that the lepers were allegedly conspiring with the Jews and Muslims of that region to poison the water supply, and fear of the plot widened to the Kingdom of Aragon. Lepers in both France and Aragon were arrested, interrogated, and examined by laypersons; if found "guilty" of having leprosy, they were then tortured and burned alive.

After this horrendous event, physicians got involved with the medical diagnosis of leprosy. With so much skin disease rampant during this time, it must have been difficult to determine who had the disease and who did not. Courts were set up for the purpose of convicting or exonerating lepers. Physicians were asked to testify in court whether a person in question had leprosy; if convicted of leprosy, they were condemned to be isolated.[32] This "due process" was known as the *iudicium leprosorum*, "judgement of the lepers," and included an *ordo examinandi*, "order to examine."

The degree of knowledge of this disease in the examining physician—or medieval surgeon—was the most crucial aspect in determining the fate of the accused. Much of the ability to make the correct decision came from experience with the disease, but there were several essential texts to which the medieval physician could turn. Three of the most significant medieval writers on leprosy are addressed in other chapters: Paul of Aegina (Chapter 5), Avicenna (Chapter 6), and Guy de Chauliac (Chapter 7). However, there was possibly one more important than these: Bernard de Gordon (fl. 1270–1330), also known as Gordonius.

Gordonius was a physician and professor of medicine at the medical school in Montpellier, France. Compiling information from the writings of Galen and Avicenna, he completed an encyclopedic medical textbook entitled *Lilium medicinae*, "The Lily of Medicine" (1305). His canonical book was cited frequently in both court depositions and scholarly treatises, and because of its comprehensiveness and lucidity, the Lily of Medicine became the gold standard text on leprosy in the Middle Ages.[33] Later known as the "Liliator," Gordonius appreciated the seriousness of the situation facing his fellow physicians, concluding that even after inspecting the patient for all of the nuances of the disease that he had laid out in his lengthy treatise, a person should not be judged leprous unless disfigured by the illness.[34]

A person with leprosy throughout the Middle Ages and up until the twentieth century was seen by laypeople and physicians alike as a grotesque monster, and the collective group of lepers reached almost mythical status. They were portrayed in both cultural and medical literature as terrifying, foul, wretched, fetid, hideous, putrid, and abominable; these exaggerated terms described the overall physical appearance, the ulcerated skin lesions, and the breath. The leonine appearance of the face is accurate and a term still in use today when the lepromatous nodules infiltrate the face, especially the brow and periorbital skin. There is no evidence that leprosy causes the hypersexuality of a satyr, as the myth suggested.[35]

The medieval medical writers explained leprosy in the framework of Galenic medicine as a disease caused by an abundance of black bile, which corrupted various parts of the body, especially the skin. With the availability of both Galen's writings and Avicenna's *Canon of Medicine* for later medieval writers to explore, a controversy developed from the fact that Galen and Avicenna differed in their view of whether leprosy was a disease of those affected parts, i.e., the skin (the Galenic view), or a "cancer of the whole body" (the opinion of Avicenna).[36] This discussion in the medieval literature is the first example of the debate about whether an affliction involving the skin was a disease of the skin or a disease of the whole body manifesting on the skin.

Medieval medical writers also struggled to blend Galenic medicine with the proliferating notions that leprosy was a contagious disease. There was no easy, rational way to explain the contagiousness of disease within the Galenic framework. But the fact that leprosy was contagious was increasingly undeniable, even without a microbial theory of disease, which did not come until the nineteenth century. It was believed that one could acquire leprosy by breathing the exhaled air or vapors emitted by a leprous person or a rotting corpse. Intercourse was another route of transmission; it was widely held that women were more likely to transmit leprosy to men by intercourse than men were to transmit it to women.[37]

There were several other notable causes of leprosy, according to the medieval physician. While the traditional belief was that leprosy was more common in higher-temperature regions, later medieval writers noted an increased prevalence of leprosy in northern, cold-temperature areas, especially coastal ones.[38] Leprosy was particularly common in Scandinavia. It was also believed that a person's diet could increase susceptibility to leprosy. Numerous foods were suspect over the centuries, and while there was no consistent viewpoint, the ones that were believed to generate abundant black bile, such as donkey meat and lentils, were among those to avoid.[39] Overeating was also thought to cause an excess of black bile, as did the blockage of pores of the skin; baths to cleanse the pores were frequently recommended as a treatment. Medieval literature cited both the condition referred to as "suppression of the menses" (amenorrhea) and intercourse during menstruation as risk factors for leprosy. In addition, medieval physicians believed that conception during menstruation would lead to leprous offspring. Medieval writers emphasized that both too much sleep and too much activity could be problematic, as could too much sex or too little sex. Finally, emotional states such as anger, fear, and sadness (melancholia) could lead to leprosy.[40]

Several skin conditions were discussed along with *lepra* in the medieval medical texts: *alphus, leuce, scabies, psora, impetigo, vitiligo, albaras, white morphea, and black morphea. Albaras* and *morphea* may have been synonyms. Morphea, a term used today to denote an uncommon skin condition characterized by localized or generalized skin thickening and loss of pigmentation, was generally believed to be a precursor of *lepra* in late medieval and Renaissance texts.[41] Morphea is unrelated to HD, however; it is an autoimmune skin disease. As the modern dermatologist can attest, skin diseases such as psoriasis, eczema, and scleroderma can be severely disfiguring. And the following entry from later editions of Samuel Johnson's *Dictionary of the English Language* (first edition, 1755) suggests that psoriasis was clearly confused with leprosy as late as the nineteenth century:

Leprosy: A loathsome distemper, which covers the body with a kind of white scales.[42]

As true HD has no tendency to cover the body with white scales, there is no doubt that persons with severe skin diseases such as psoriasis were condemned to leprosaria well into the nineteenth century.

For the certification of a subject as having been afflicted with *lepra* or not, the medieval physician obtained in detail the personal and family history of the subject and then performed a comprehensive physical examination of the subject from head to toe, looking for specific findings: nodules on the forehead, chin, and cheeks; livid, dark face; frowning brow; thinning of eyelashes and eyebrows; unwavering, terrifying stare; round eyes; dark, bloodshot eyes; dilated nostrils; nasal voice; corroded nasal cartilage; strained breathing; hoarse voice; granules under the tongue; thick, livid lips; contracted earlobes; rough, bumpy, thickened skin; oily skin; darkening of the skin; scabs, pustules, and morphea; fetid breath and sweat; hideous appearance; bad conduct; high libido; insomnia and nightmares; atrophic muscles; swollen extremities; thick cloudy urine; slow, weak pulse; and clotty, sandy blood.[43] Two results were particularly important: if the examination of the face revealed no changes, a diagnosis of leprosy was less likely to be given; and anesthesia of the extremities—a major feature of HD which Galen, Aretaeus, and Avicenna did not address.[44]

Curing leprosy in the Middle Ages was generally considered an impossible task by the medieval physician with the available treatment approaches. Therefore, this time period saw a return to supernatural healing as the afflicted beseeched God and the saints for a miraculous cure or, more importantly, salvation. Medical treatment for leprosy entailed a combination of preventative and therapeutic interventions, such as the avoidance of salty, acidic, and spicy foods and sexual activity.[45] Castration was utilized as a means of ensuring the elimination of sex and seen as therapeutically beneficial to the patient. Prescribed for evacuating the melancholic humor from the body, bloodletting and purgatives were the mainstays of treatment. Physicians also recommended baths of various kinds and unguents of different concoctions as well as other medicaments that included gold, antimony, snake meat, and human or animal blood.

The Decline of Leprosy

Leprosy disappeared from most of Europe by 1600. Scientists have proven that there is no difference in the genome of medieval and modern *M. leprae* to suggest that the organism mutated to a less virulent or contagious form.[46] While a simple explanation for the demise of leprosy in Western Europe is the improvement of socioeconomic conditions in the aftermath of the Black Death, some scholars believe that it was cross-immunity against other mycobacterial diseases in the population that caused the decline. Tuberculosis, a highly contagious mycobacterial disease, reached its climax in Europe between 1750 and 1850. Scientists have proven that infection with tuberculosis can provide a person with relative immunity against leprosy, and it seems probable that the rise of tuberculosis in the West led to the decline of leprosy.[47] Another theory contends that people with lepromatous leprosy are actually more susceptible to the already-more-contagious tuberculosis, and that co-infection and a markedly shorter life expectancy with both diseases, led to leprosy's decline.[48] Thus, it is possible that both the cross-immunity and co-infection hypotheses could explain the decrease in leprosy. Or perhaps it was the Second Pandemic of Plague (see Interlude 2) that really caused the decline of leprosy; the plague took the lives of the more vulnerable, i.e., those with leprosy.

A long-held view to explain the rise of tuberculosis was that the urbanization of the European population brought about by the Industrial Revolution—and the resultant demographic density and crowded living quarters—promoted easy communication of the disease from person to person. It was not just crowding that led to the European endemic of tuberculosis but the poor living conditions—"the failure of the native and immune resistance to protect against infection in the face of physiological and social misery."[49] The social circumstances allowed for tuberculosis to ultimately become the most successful infectious disease of all time. Tuberculosis peaked as a cause of death in the nineteenth century, when it was responsible for the death of as many as one in four people, and it killed more people in human history than any other infectious disease.

TUBERCULOSIS AND THE SKIN

Tuberculosis is a disease with significance in the history of dermatology. Known prior to the late nineteenth century as *phthisis* and then as *consumption*, it has a variety of dermatologic manifestations, and in the era of epidemic tuberculosis (eighteenth to nineteenth centuries in Europe), it was not uncommon for patients to present to the physician's office with cutaneous signs of tuberculosis. Scrofula (the King's evil) was a chronic form of tuberculosis in which the lung infection spread to lymph nodes in the neck; the condition subsequently breaks down the skin overlying and drains onto the neck. Lupus vulgaris, which is very different from the lupus most people think of today, was a chronic ulcerative and deforming form of tuberculosis of the face, especially the nose and cheeks. Caused by hematogenous spread of the infection from the lungs to the skin, the condition was the "common" type of lupus in this era, particularly in Central Europe and Scandinavia, and it was a favorite of the nineteenth-century medical writers, easily found in virtually every dermatologic atlas in this period. In 1903, inventor and father of phototherapy, Danish-Faroese physician Niels Finsen (1860–1904), won the Nobel Prize in 1903 for his research into the use of phototherapy as a treatment for lupus vulgaris. Pathologists performing an autopsy of a tuberculosis victim were at risk for the "prosector's wart," which refers to infection of the ungloved finger with the mycobacterium. Other forms of cutaneous tuberculosis include miliary tuberculosis, tuberculous gumma, and orificial tuberculosis. Before the era of antibiotics, tuberculosis caused all kinds of skin problems.

Tuberculosis was known as the "white death" or "white plague" because of the pallor caused by the wasting and anemia of chronic disease induced by the infection. Perhaps the most fascinating fact about this disease was the romance culturally assigned to it—the idea that there was something romantic about the slowly progressive suffering and "good death" associated with this condition. The White Death took the lives of many famous artists, poets, and writers of the artistic period known as Romanticism, such as John Keats (1795–1821) and Frédéric Chopin (1810–1849), thus sealing the link between the disease and the movement. The association with Romanticism eventually resulted in a fad in which young women of the period up until 1850 disposed of the desire for the corpulent figure that shaped the Enlightenment and instead sought a "tubercular" appearance—pale skin, blushed cheeks, delicate figure, and a general fragility—all which made them somehow more appealing than the healthy-appearing competition.[50]

Hansen's Disease

Although leprosy declined in most of Europe after the sixteenth century, pockets of the disease continued to permeate in Scandinavia, Iceland, and England. The center of leprosy research in Europe moved north in the eighteenth century to Uppsala, Sweden, where Isaac Uddman, a Finnish doctoral student under the famous physician and biologist Carl Linnaeus (1707–1778), published a dissertation in 1765 entitled *Lepra*, in which he claimed that leprosy was caused by animalcules smaller than what could be seen with the microscope.[51] His claim was not taken seriously, and he fell into obscurity. Then the story of leprosy moved due west to Bergen, Norway.

Norway saw a spike in cases of leprosy in the nineteenth century, eventually becoming a public health issue. In the 1850s, 2 per 1000 persons in Norway had leprosy; in Bergen, the prevalence was as high as 25 per 1000 persons.[52] Research into the epidemic ensued at a leprosy hospital that had been established 600 years prior in the thirteenth century in Bergen. In 1847, a physician named Daniel Cornelius Danielssen (1815–1894) and a dermatologist named Carl Wilhelm Boeck (1808–1875) published their research in *Om Spedalskhed* "On Leprosy," a landmark book and first authoritative publication to distinguish leprosy from other similar diseases affecting the skin. In that work, the authors concluded that the condition was indeed hereditary and not contagious, challenging the prevailing notion of their time. The "proof" of their theory was Danielssen's failure to acquire the disease after inoculating himself with material from leprous patients. To Danielssen, anesthesia of the extremities was a particularly important diagnostic finding of leprosy, which it is to this day; this finding was given the name "Danielssen's sign" in his honor, even though anesthesia had been known to be a feature of leprosy since the career of the medieval Flemish surgeon Jehan Yperman (1260–1331). Danielssen and Boeck are also credited with being the first to describe a severe variant of scabies infestation termed Norwegian crusted scabies.

Danielssen's junior colleague and son-in-law, the Norwegian physician Gerhard-Henrik Armauer Hansen (1841–1912), challenged Danielssen with a hypothesis that leprosy was an infectious disease. Hansen went to Vienna in 1870 for training in staining and histopathology, training which gave him the skillset he needed to find the infectious material. After sitting for days and days at the microscope looking at leprous tissue, Hansen's efforts paid off when he finally found the rod-shaped *M. leprae*.[53] It was the first human bacterial pathogen ever discovered.

In 1873, Hansen's published findings shocked Europe's medical community, who could not accept this finding as the cause of the disease. Hansen needed to somehow prove that his discovered bacterium was indeed the culprit. In an 1879 experiment, Hansen attempted to inoculate the bacillus into a non-consenting female patient's eye using a cataract knife. Naturally, she pressed charges against him. Meanwhile, a German bacteriologist, Albert Neisser, went to Bergen, studied Hansen's research, and took some specimens with him back to Germany for his own investigation, where he performed experiments with better stains. He published his findings in 1880, which contained definitive proof that *M. leprae* was the cause, without giving any credit to Hansen.[54] While Hansen was in court fighting for his professional life for violating medical ethics, *M. leprae* became known as "Neisser's bacterium." Once news of Neisser's alleged plagiarism reached Bergen, the Norwegian medical community vehemently defended Hansen, and when the truth was unveiled at a leprosy congress in Berlin, he was officially recognized as the true discoverer of *M. leprae*.[55] Leprosy was renamed HD in the 1930s in honor of his discovery. Hansen, who had suffered a stroke in 1877, was disabled for the remainder of his life and died of heart disease in 1912; it has been rumored that both his stroke and heart disease were the result of infection with syphilis, a condition that took the life of several of the characters in this story.[56]

Leprosy in Modern Times

In the almost 70-year period between the discovery of the bacillus and the discovery of effective antibiotic therapy, one treatment gained attention and became commonplace in the late nineteenth and early twentieth centuries: chaulmoogra oil. Extracted from the seeds of the chaulmoogra tree (*Hydnocarpus wightianus*), this oil had been used in Eastern medicine as a treatment for leprosy for hundreds of years.[57] It was introduced into Western medicine by British physician Frederic John Mouat in 1854, but it would be another 50 years before the oil entered the mainstream in Europe and the United States. While the oral version was most effective, nausea was a limiting side effect. Intravenous, intramuscular, and subcutaneous injections were instead tried but led to varying degrees of complications such as pain and abscess formation. Esters of the fatty acids in the chaulmoogra oil were extracted and given, also with mixed results. The drug reached its peak use in the 1920s and 1930s, before falling out of favor when the first antibiotic for leprosy, promin, was developed in the 1940s.[58] Promin is the pro-drug of dapsone, which became the mainstay of treatment until antibiotic resistance was noted in the 1960s; that same decade saw the introduction of clofazimine and rifampicin. When each drug is used alone, all three can develop resistance, but the combination of these three drugs, called multi-drug therapy and advocated since 1981, can now effectively cure a person of this disease in 6 to 12 months. Isolation of infected patients is no longer necessary as antibiotic treatments erase the infectiousness of a person with this disease.

There is no solid evidence that HD existed in the Americas prior to the arrival of the European explorers in the late fifteenth century. The strain of *M. leprae* in the Americas—the North African/European strain—was brought by European settlers along with several other infectious diseases (e.g., smallpox) in what has been termed the Columbian Exchange (see Interlude 3).[59] African slaves were likely another vital source of the infection in the New World. While a leper asylum had to be established in the sixteenth century in Mexico soon after Cortés' arrival, the first writings on leprosy in the present-day United States come from the eighteenth century; it was initially stereotyped as a problem of the African slaves. The first leper asylum in the United States, called *La Terre des Lepreux*, "Leper's land," was established in New Orleans in 1785 when Louisiana was still a Spanish colony, but after Louisiana was acquired by France in 1800, the asylum fell into neglect and was abandoned soon after the Louisiana Purchase (1803) in 1806.[60]

CARVILLE

By the 1880s, 4.5 out of 100,000 persons had leprosy in south Louisiana, and the Louisiana State Board of Health decided to act.[61] A decision was made in 1892 to quarantine persons with leprosy and provide them with humane medical care, administered by the Catholic Daughters of Charity of St. Vincent de Paul and led by Dr. Isadore Dyer (1865–1920). The site chosen was a plantation known as Indian Camp along the banks of the Mississippi River some 70 mi west of New Orleans, outside of Baton Rouge. The first seven leprosy patients were relocated there from New Orleans in 1894. This area was renamed Carville in 1909, and the leprosy hospital became known as "Carville." The incidence of leprosy in south Louisiana continued to rise to 12 per 100,000 in the 1920s, and seeing the need for a nationalized HD program where persons could be sent from all over the country, the federal government purchased Carville and took over the program in 1921.[62] The National Hansen's Disease Program was initially involuntary; Carville was enclosed by a barbed-wire fence. The largest census Carville ever had at one time was 400, and the site became a research center as well as a hospital and refuge.[63] Much of the research into the antibiotic treatments of leprosy took place there. Study of the disease itself and decades of experience with patients led to an understanding that the contagiousness of HD was not nearly what was once suspected. The 1950s saw a call to end compulsory isolation, which finally occurred in 1960.[64] The funding for Carville dwindled over the next several decades, and the leprosarium was closed in 1999. The research program was moved to Baton Rouge, where it remains today.

The reason Louisiana, even to this day, has a higher incidence of leprosy than most states is a matter of debate. Because more cases of the disease were identified in the twentieth century in "cajun" parishes than any other, a long-held view is that it was brought there by the Acadians (French Canadians; cajuns) when they were deported from Acadia (modern-day Nova Scotia, New Brunswick, and Prince Edward Island) by the British military in 1755. It is also likely that leprosy became endemic in Louisiana from the influx of Spanish-speaking peoples and African slaves who settled there and were brought there, respectively. The nine-banded armadillo, which is not native to Louisiana but colonized the region by 1957, is a probable source of the disease today. According to numerous surveys of frozen armadillo specimens, infection rates of the armadillo with *M. leprae* were as high as 16 percent as early as 1961. A history of contact with armadillos among present-day patients is often elicited.[65]

Carville was not the only settlement for persons with HD in the United States; the other was in Hawaii. Leprosy was brought to Hawaii by Chinese workers in the first half of the nineteenth century. An isolation law was enacted during the reign of King Kamehameha V (1830–1872) that led to the sequestration of leprosy patients in 1869 in the community of Kalaupapa on the northern coast of the island of Moloka'i. This remote region of the island is a flat peninsula that is geographically separated from the rest of the island by a beautiful ridge of sea cliffs. Compulsory isolation existed there from 1866 to 1969, during which period approximately 8000 persons were segregated, with a peak at one time of nearly 1200. Its most famous resident was St. Damien of Molokai (1840–1889, canonized in 2009), a Roman Catholic priest from Belgium who served as a missionary there in the 1870s and 1880s. He demonstrated compassion and leadership in the community and ultimately contracted leprosy himself while working with the lepers. Today, there are a few remaining residents with HD in Kalaupapa on a voluntary basis. Kalaupapa has been designated a National Historical Park since 1980.

In the era of antibiotics, the number of cases in the world of all forms of HD has declined, but the disease persists among the 5 percent of the world's population who are susceptible to it. According to data published by the World Health Organization, which is striving to eradicate HD with its Global Leprosy Strategy, 14 million cases of leprosy have been cured since 1980.[66] But there were still 178,371 persons worldwide registered with the disease and on treatment at the end of 2019, and 202,256 new cases were detected in 2019.[67] India accounts for 60 percent of patients across the globe, and there has been no decline in the number of new cases there in the last ten years.[68] Efforts to eradicate the disease in India have been frustrated by factors such as delay in self-reporting/presentation for treatment because of persistent social stigmas, discrimination, and superstitions; delay in diagnosis because of deficiencies in trained manpower and leprosy expertise; drug availability issues; and inadequate surveillance of patients for the duration of treatment.[69] The situation in India and around the world may improve as two different leprosy vaccines are rolled out.

Summary

Leprosy, or HD, is the most famous of the historical skin diseases. We now know that the "leprosy" of the Bible was not actually leprosy; it was probably psoriasis and other severe skin diseases. Leprosy did exist in ancient or Biblical times, but it was called *elephantiasis* in that period. Leprosy should be thought of as a medieval disease because its prevalence and contagiousness peaked during this era (one in thirty Europeans). During the Middle Ages, the reaction of the healthy population to the leper ranged from disgust to compassion, and measures implemented by the governments to control the spread of the disease included sequestration, hospitalization, and execution. Courts were set up where physicians had to testify as to whether a person suspected of having leprosy indeed had it or not. The incidence of leprosy waned in the early modern period, as populations in the cities of Europe rose and tuberculosis became more prevalent. Since tuberculosis and leprosy are both mycobacterial diseases, one theory holds that having tuberculosis is protective against leprosy, and since tuberculosis is more contagious than leprosy, leprosy declined. Another theory argues that persons with tuberculosis are actually more likely to get leprosy and that co-infection and a more rapid death reduced the transmission of leprosy through European societies. While the incidence of leprosy waned in the early modern period, it continued to be studied fervently, and in the nineteenth century, the mycobacterial agent responsible for the disease was discovered. Leper colonies were established in the late nineteenth century in the United States, and on the grounds of the campus of Carville, Louisiana, research led to the successful development of antibiotics capable of ending the infection. Leprosy remains a public health concern today in India, and efforts are ongoing to eradicate the infection entirely from the world.

5

The Early Middle Ages

The Crisis of the Third Century for the Roman Empire ended with the stabilizing efforts of the emperor Diocletian (r. 284–305 CE). Not only did he secure the borders of the empire with several successful military campaigns, but Diocletian, believing the empire too large to be ruled by one man, divided it into eastern and western halves and established a new imperial system known as the Tetrarchy. After this time, the Eastern Empire rose in power and eminence as the West faltered. The Roman Emperor Constantine I (r. 324–337), the first Christian emperor, reunited the empire in 324 but moved the capital of the Roman Empire from Rome to Byzantium in 330, renaming the city after himself: Constantinople. In 395 CE, Theodosius I (r. 379–395) again divided the rule of the empire between his two sons into a western half and an eastern half. The Western Roman Empire deteriorated for the next 80 years due to financial troubles, overextension, corrupt and/or incompetent leadership, relentless barbarian invasions, the weakening of the legions, and the demise of traditional Roman values coinciding with the rise of Christianity. The Western Roman Empire ended in 476 CE with its last emperor deposed. The eastern half did survive, and because of stronger finances and a nearly impregnable capital, the Eastern Roman Empire, later known as the Byzantine Empire, would thrive for another thousand years, only to finally collapse in 1453 at the hands of the Ottoman Turks. There were efforts in the sixth century by the Byzantines to reunite the western provinces, but these efforts ceased after 600. The Byzantine emperors in the East saw themselves as Roman emperors, but once Rome was lost forever, an era had ended, and the Middle Ages had begun.

The Middle Ages was the vast epoch stretching between the decline of the Western Roman Empire in the fifth century CE and the Renaissance, which began in the fourteenth century. The early Middle Ages, which spans from roughly 500 to 1000 CE, has been referred to in the past as the Dark Ages, but this moniker has fallen out of favor because modern-day scholars deem it an inaccurate descriptor of the period. While some historians have tried to cast light on this mysterious period, others have stubbornly defended the term "the Dark Ages." References to the period as "dark" disregard the numerous scholarly and cultural achievements of the Byzantines, the Anglo-Saxons, and the Carolingians (see Chapter 7). It is to the dermatological knowledge of the first two of these historical groups that our attention now turns. After covering these Western societies, there will be a brief digression to the East in order to explore the ancient and medieval dermatology practiced in China and India.

Isidore of Seville (560–636 CE)

Learned medical writers in the former Western Roman Empire were in short supply in the first few centuries of the Middle Ages. However, Isidore of Seville was one man who made some important contributions at this time, a man who has been referred to as the "last great scholar of the ancient world" by some, or the "first great scholar of the medieval world" by others. In addition to his ecclesiastical occupations of converting the Visigothic kings of Spain to Catholicism and serving as archbishop of Seville for the last three decades of his life, Isidore was a true medieval polymath and compiler of classical learning. His greatest literary achievement was the *Etymologiae*, "Etymologies," which contained the definition of some 5500 words from a wide range of topics, including grammar, history, mathematics, law, science, and medicine. He compiled and summarized all of the known factual information about the world; it was so comprehensive that it became a starting point for learning for hundreds and hundreds of years. Book IV, *De medicina*, and Book XI, *De homine et portentis*, "On Man and Portents," which includes a discussion of anatomy, were landmark summaries of existing medical knowledge, dominated by the learned medicine of Caelius Aurelianus, Soranus of Ephesus, and Pliny, as well as Galen and Hippocrates.

DOI: 10.1201/9781003273622-8

It echoed the teachings at the medical school in Alexandria. Isidore of Seville was declared the most learned man of his age at the Council of Toledo (653), and he shared with Gregory the Great the title "schoolmaster of the Middle Ages."[1] Isidore's Latin style is "the very opposite of Ciceronian—unpolished, jerky, and repetitious," but *Etymologies* enjoyed enormous popularity well into the Renaissance.[2]

Isidore stated that *medicina* protects the body or restores health.[3] He pointed out that Apollo founded and discovered medicine and that his son Asclepius expanded it, and when Asclepius died, the art of medicine ceased and was unknown for 500 years until Hippocrates brought it back.[4] Isidore explained that there were three schools of medicine: the Methodists who used remedies and charms; the Empirics who relied on experience alone; and the Logical, who used rational thinking.[5] Isidore described the four humors of the body, then listed the acute and chronic diseases. He knew of bubonic plague and characterized it as a contagion passing quickly from person to person, brought forth from corrupt air and not without the will of God.[6] He discussed diseases of the skin and concluded the section with summaries of three different types of treatments (dietetic, pharmacy, and surgery), described different types of surgical instruments, and commented on scents and unguents.

In Book XI, Isidore addressed the etymology of the Latin words for hair and skin. In Isidore's time, the skin was thought of as a protective covering, and the hair was recognized for both its decorative and protective properties. According to Isidore, *capilli* (hair) is derived from *capitis pili* (hairs of the head) and is present to decorate the head, keep the brain warm, and protect the head from the sun. The skin is called *cutis* from the Greek κυτις (incision—cut), and it is also called *pellis* because it protects from external injuries (*pellit*—as in repel or expel), rain, wind, and the sun.[7] Connor noted that there was no single word for skin in Latin; *cutis* was the word for living skin, whereas *pellis* was the word for dead skin (as in the flayed skin or animal skins).[8]

Isidore dealt with skin disease in Book IV, which is divided into acute diseases, chronic diseases, and *Morbis qui in superficie corporis videntur*, "Diseases Seen on the Body's Surface." The dermatological terms from Book IV are listed in Table 5.1.

TABLE 5.1

Dermatological Terms in Isidore's *Etymologies*[9]

Alopecia	Loss of hair; from the Greek words ἀλώπηξ (fox) and ἀλωπεκία (fox-mange)
Parotidae	Swellings or tumors around the ears, which arise during a febrile illness; from the Greek παρωτιδες (around the ears)
Lentigo	Round freckles; from *lenticulae* (small lentils)
Erisipela	Erysipelas or *sacer igni* (holy fire); fiery red skin surface that spreads to nearby regions and causes fever
Serpedo	Red of the skin with pustules; from *serpendo* (creeping) spreads down the limbs
Impetigo	Dry, scaly, rough and round, on the surface of the skin; also called *sarna*
Prurigo	Itching; from *perurendo*, burning thoroughly, and *ardendo*, burning
Verrucae	Warts
Scabies	Rough, itchy skin
Lepra	Rough, scaly skin that turns black, then white, then red; from *lepidium* (pepperwort)
Elephantiasis	Similar to the hard, rough skin of an elephant or because it is a disease of great magnitude
Icteros	Jaundice; from the name of a yellow bird (the yellow-breasted marten); also known as *arcuatus morbus* (rainbow disease) and *regius morbus* (royal disease)
Cancer	Named from the maritime animal; not curable by medications, but can be cut away from the body, which might postpone inevitable death
Furunculus	Swelling rising to a point; from *fervunculus* and *fervet (*boils); also known in Greek as ανθραξ (anthrax)
Hordeolus	A small accumulation of pus by the eyelashes (stye); from *hordeum* (grain of barley)
Oscedo	Ulcerative disease of the mouths of children; from *oscitante*s (yawning)
Frenusculi	Ulcers near the opening of the mouth; from *frenum* (the harness used on beasts of burden)
Pustula	A swollen lesion on the surface of the body
Papula	Tiny, red protuberance of skin
Sanies	Ichorous matter discharged from the skin arising from blood, *sanguis;* differs from *tabes*, which is the same substance in the dead
Cicatrix	A wound covering that matches color of the surrounding skin; from *obducit* (cover) and, *obcaecat* (conceal)

Isidore described the major skin diseases using the same terminology that dates back to the time of Hippocrates and Galen, and while he offered little new information in his rather succinct summary, the concise overview is helpful because Isidore chose only the most pertinent information about the skin, and *Etymologies* focuses our attention on the dermatologic details most relevant to a sixth- or seventh-century nonphysician scholar.

Byzantine Medicine

Because the western part of Europe was increasingly controlled by various barbarian groups, scant documentation exists on medicine in the former Western Roman Empire in the early Middle Ages. The cultural and intellectual center of Europe shifted to the Greek-speaking East, and its two centers of medical learning—Alexandria and Ravenna (modern-day Italy). Located in Egypt, Alexandria had been for centuries the academic center of the known world. Medical education at that time focused on theory and philosophy more than practice. The students read a canon of Hippocratic and Galenic texts that were in Greek, but there were efforts to translate this literature into Latin in the sixth century.[10] The only other medical school of this period was located at Ravenna, the seat of the Ostrogothic kingdom, which ruled Italy until 540 when it was conquered by the Byzantines. For the next 200 years, Ravenna was a western outpost of the Byzantine Empire and an educational center. The medical school at Ravenna was unknown to historians until the nineteenth century, and it is now understood that efforts were undertaken there to Latinize medicine.[11] The quality and quantity of the medical knowledge disseminated at Alexandria and Ravenna should not be overestimated, however. The medical corpus available for consumption by Byzantine physicians in places such as Ravenna was a shadow of its former self, and as the writings of Galen morphed into Galenism, only Galenic treatises mattered from this point forward.[12]

The major theme of the early Middle Ages related to the history of medicine was the preservation of ancient medical information. This task was performed by several encyclopedic "compilers," all of whom were Greek. The majority of Galen's works, the Hippocratic corpus, and many of the other ancient medical texts were written only in Greek and never translated into Latin during ancient times because most of the Latin-speaking physicians of antiquity could also read Greek. But knowledge of the Greek language waned during the Middle Ages; only in the Byzantine Empire could the Greek language be spoken, written, and comprehended. The Byzantine writers copied the works of the ancients in Greek, limiting their value to Western Europe. These writers—"the medical refrigerators of antiquity"—were important to posterity for their preservative actions, but their works offer little excitement from original contributions to the body of knowledge.[13] Yet, the works reflect energy for acquiring and passing on medical knowledge and a flourishing of medical writing that should not be discounted.[14]

The first of the great Byzantine physician-compilers was Oribasius (320–403 CE). Like Galen, he was from Pergamon, studied medicine at Alexandria, and preferred the practical over the rhetorical. He was a friend and personal physician of the Emperor Julian the Apostate (r. 361–363), who commissioned Oribasius' two most significant works: a collection of excerpts from the writings of Galen, which has not survived, and *Medical Collections*, containing an encyclopedic array of writings from the ancient world. Oribasius preserved excerpts from many ancient authors that would have been otherwise lost, and, in the process, he prepared and packaged Galenism into the form that dominated for many hundreds of years.[15]

Oribasius did not include a descriptive section on the skin in his *Anatomica Galenica*, but he did write about pediatric skin diseases and was the first to discuss allergy to breast milk causing a skin rash. He believed that rashes presenting on a baby's skin (e.g., infantile eczema) were caused by the poor quality of the maternal milk or improper digestion of the milk or some "maleficence" of the skin beginning *in utero*.[16] Oribasius emphasized the following panacea for the management of sunburn, the prevention of wrinkles, and the brightening of the skin: cucumber and melon, the dung of the crocodile, dung of starlings, or chips of cypress and oakwood boiled into a concoction.[17] Oribasius preserved the seminal writings of Rufus of Ephesus (fl. first/second centuries CE) on plague (see Interlude 2). Perhaps Oribasius is more famous in the history of plastic surgery; for instance, he wrote about facial reconstruction and discussed the repair of the tip of the nose with an H-shaped flap of skin taken from the cheek.

Two chapters of his 70-chapter magnum opus are devoted to facial reconstruction. His writings also detailed how varicose vein surgery was performed in the Byzantine era.[18]

The next noteworthy Greek-writing physician of this period was Aetius (502–575) of Amida, a Mesopotamian town in modern-day southeastern Turkey. Known for being one of the earliest Christian physicians, Aetius, like Oribasius, compiled and preserved the writings of the ancient medical authorities. Aetius is credited with the first use of the term *eczema*, from ἐκζέματα, pronounced eczemata, meaning to bubble up or boil over. Aetius also described the use of table salts on the surface of the skin for the purpose of abrading a tattoo; the term for that procedure is called salabrasion. He classified genital warts, a malady equally prevalent in his time as now. He divided them into two types: (1) *condyloma*, which sometimes appear inflamed and (2) *thymi*: red, hard oblong protrusions appearing in the anogenital area, which sometimes bleed and have a benign and malignant form.[19]

THE ORIGINS OF THE WORD *ACNE*

Aetius also coined the word *acne*, a word with a controversial history.[20] The ancient Greeks referred to acne as *ionthi* and associated it with puberty—the word *ionthos* (singular) meaning "eruption with the first growth of the beard." Pliny, Celsus, and the Romans referred to acne by the term *varus* (plural *vari*). Prior to the second century CE, the Greek word ακμη, pronounced acme, meant apex, as in the height of a disease, but Julius Pollux (see Chapter 4) used the term in relation to puberty—the height of body's development or growth—and associated *acme* and *ionthoi*. Cassius, in the third century CE, stated that because the disease occurs during *acme* (puberty), the people call it ακμᾶς (*acmes*). So those patients who have mispronounced acne as acme all these years were not wrong! In the fifth century CE, Aetius called the pubertal rite of passage *acne* instead of *acme*, and it was commonly held by writers of the nineteenth and twentieth centuries that the word *acne* was a typographical corruption of the word *acme*. But five of the six original Latin publications of Aetius' works during the Renaissance contain the word *acne*. An alternative view is supported by the writings of Gorraeus (Jean de Gorris, 1505–1577) in 1564, who appeared to be in no doubt about the difference between acme and acne, as Gorraeus wrote that acne was so named because it did not itch and was a contraction of *a* (without) and *knesis* (scratching). Regardless, by the fifth century, *acme* converted to *acne* as the word for pubertal pimples. Both the terms acne and eczema disappeared from medical writings over the centuries, and in the interim, acne was referred to as *vari* (plural of *varus*, or pimple), and what we currently refer to as eczema was called many different things, including *scabies* and *prurigo*. Conrad Heinrich Fuchs (1802–1855) and Willan (see Chapter 12), respectively, reintroduced the terms in the nineteenth century. Fuchs divided acne into its various subtypes (*vulgaris*, *mentagra*, and *rosacea*).

The third Byzantine physician of dermatologic importance was Alexander of Tralles (525–605). Tralles was a city not far from the Aegean coast of Asia Minor. He came from a distinguished family—his brother Anthemius designed the Hagia Sophia. Alexander was a physician who practiced and wrote during the reign of the Byzantine Emperor Justinian (r. 527–565), but there is no evidence he was Justinian's personal physician. He likely learned medicine and surgery through apprenticeships. Rather than get involved with court life, Alexander became an itinerant physician before settling in Rome. He was an active, inquisitive, and kindly physician, gained enormous experience as he traveled around from province to province prescribing medications and performing various surgical procedures.[21]

Only three of Alexander's several works have survived, all in Greek: "Treatise on fevers," "Letter on worms," and his magnum opus, "Twelve Books on Medicine." There are no English translations of these works, nor known dates of publication. The 12 books are organized such that diseases of the head, starting with hair loss, are addressed first, then he worked his way down through the body: heart, lungs, stomach, kidneys, legs and feet, addressing angina, pneumonia, cholera, kidney stones, and gout along the way. Although the text is rife with references to Galen and Dioscorides, Alexander was not simply a compiler of information from the past. He demonstrated an original approach to his craft, with knowledge of equal parts pharmacology, surgery, diagnosis, and the art of medicine.[22] He believed in the efficacy of amulets and charms, long deemed to be outside the scope of medicine, because patients believed in them—and that belief could lead to clinical improvement. Alexander paid attention to traditional medicine and incorporated Far Eastern drugs, and he provided the reader with a listing of various ailments and the pharmacology of 600 medications. He was the first to treat gout with colchicine, a drug still used today. He promoted the humoral theory of medicine, believing the idea that melancholy resulted from an excess of black bile. Alexander of Tralles would be quoted and referenced by medical writers of the following centuries, and he was without a doubt the most outstanding physician of the sixth century.

Alexander wrote extensively about skin diseases, classifying them in the typical cephalocaudal fashion common in antiquity and the Middle Ages. The following topics relevant to dermatology are found in his *Twelve Books*: alopecia, loss of hair (male pattern baldness), nourishment of the hair, dandruff, pustules and exanthems of the scalp, purulent crusts and eruptions of the scalp, purulent ulcers and furuncles of the scalp, and ringworm of the scalp.[23] Two conclusions can be drawn from the list of chapter titles: the preservation of hair was as important in Alexander's time as it is today, and diseases of the scalp were a common problem in the Middle Ages. The prevalence of scalp disease is not unexpected since scalp hygiene is a crucial part of managing and/or preventing seborrheic dermatitis, psoriasis, and the numerous types of scalp infections that commonly arise without the regular washing away of scalp scales and sebum. Alexander recommended shaving, washing, and the application of tar and sulfur to the scalp to manage these conditions.[24] Alexander of Tralles was deemed an authoritative writer for several centuries and was referenced a millennium later in the important dermatological texts of Mercurialis in the sixteenth century and Turner in the eighteenth century.

The most exceptional physician of the seventh century was Paul of Aegina (ca. 625–690). Aegina is one of the Saronic islands in the Aegean Sea 17 miles southwest of Athens. While the exact dates of his life are not known, it is believed that he studied medicine and practiced in Alexandria. He is considered one of the last great physicians of that metropolis. More so than Alexander, Paul was a prolific compiler, and his *Epitomae medicae libri septem*, "Seven books of medicine," is considered the most complete overview of extant medical information available in the seventh century. Heavily influenced by Oribasius, Paul wrote about gynecology, poisons, pregnancy, diseases of childhood and old age, skin diseases, and pharmacology.[25] His sixth book on surgery is particularly noteworthy. Together with Alexander of Tralles, Paul of Aegina carried Galenic medical theory and practice into the Middle Ages, often referenced in texts for the next millennia. He was held in high regard by Muslim physicians of the next five centuries. Some have gone so far as to consider him the father of medical texts.[26]

In the history of dermatology, Paul of Aegina is the most important of the four great Byzantine physicians, and unlike the three previously discussed, we are very fortunate to have a revealing English translation with commentary by Francis Adams (1834).[27] Paul's third and fourth books contain information about skin diseases, and the fourth book, in particular, is nothing short of spectacular in its provision of information about seventh-century views of skin disease. The terse entries contain 10–20 percent diagnostic information and 80–90 percent therapy.

Paul started with *elephantiasis*, describing it as an incurable "a cancer of the whole body" because "it is impossible to find a medicine more powerful than it."[28] Adams pointed out that there has been much confusion over the centuries about the term *elephantiasis*; descriptions of it differ between the Greeks and Arabian doctors, and most of the medieval medical writers considered it a form of leprosy and note a change in facial appearance to that of a lion (leonine) or satyr.

Paul addressed *lepra* and *psora* in the next section; both are described as what a modern dermatologist would think of as psoriasis:

> Both of these affections consist of an asperity of the skin, with pruritus or wasting of the body, having their origin from a melancholic humor. But leprosy spreads over the skin more deeply in a circular fashion, throwing out scales which resemble those of fishes. But psora is more superficial and variously figured, and throws out furfuraceous bodies. In these cases, we must premise venesection when the body appears more than usually plethoric, but if not, we must by all means purge with those things which evacuate black bile.[29]

Paul's description of *lichen* reminds the dermatologist of a papulosquamous eruption such as guttate psoriasis, suggesting evolution in the meaning of that word away from its original impetigo-like meaning. In his section on *pruritus*, Paul clearly stated that itching of the elderly is incurable; the modern dermatologist would tend to agree with him.[30] Many of Paul's itchy patients likely had a scabies mite infestation. In the following section, the terms *leuce* and *alphos*, which repeatedly appear in the medical literature of the medieval period and Renaissance, refer to another incurable skin condition in which the skin loses its skin color; the two differ only in depth and severity. Ancient and medieval writers called them both "white forms of leprosy." It becomes quickly apparent when reading Paul that he and his predecessors considered vitiligo and psoriasis as types of *lepra*. His therapy for the white spots was intriguing—he recommended, among other things, that fig juice be applied to the patches and then the affected areas exposed to the sun. We know today that fig juice contains a phototoxic compound that can indeed darken the skin.

In the next few sections, Paul addressed *stigma*, which are marks on the skin caused by some injury to the skin (post-inflammatory pigmentation); *exanthemata*; *epinyctides* and *phylactaenae*, two extinct terms probably referring to vesicular forms of eczema; and *burns*, with emphasis on the use of Cimolian earth, a medicinal clay widely used in Aegean medicine. There is a section specifically describing the management of the wounds of "those beaten with scourges," which includes the following recommendation:

> For those who have been scourged, the skin of a sheep newly taken off, when applied yet warm, of all remedies cures the soonest, effecting this purpose in a day and a night.[31]

Perhaps it was the lanolin in the sheepskin that promoted the healing of these scourges. Also included are instructions for regrowing hairs on a part that has been burnt. Paul's subsequent four topics are as follows: *excoriation*; *myrmecia*, a type of wart that grows back when they are excised; *acrochordon*, a skin tag that does not grow back when cut out; and *ganglion*.

Paul had a typical understanding of skin infections for his time. What is known today as cellulitis, Paul reiterates Galen's definition of *phlegmon*, a red and painful swelling caused by an accumulation of good blood in the tissues. But "when yellow bile is seated in a part, it is called *herpes*," and "when blood and yellow bile together are collected in a part, *erysipelas* is formed."[32] Erysipelas was considered a very serious disease, "particularly about the head; so that if active treatment be not resorted to, it will sometimes prove fatal to the patient by suffocation."[33] When the inflammation generates pus, an abscess develops. When the inflammation does not form pus or resolve, *gangrene* and *sphacelus* manifest. The former refers to the early changes of "mortification;" the latter, a stage beyond gangrene when the affected area becomes "totally insensible."[34] Swollen glands are referred to as *phyma*, *bubo*, or *phygethlon*. A carbuncle occurs "when blood having become more melancholic than natural, ferments and fixes in a part."[35] Much of this information is simply a repeat of Galen's comments on the same terms.

Cancer, according to Paul, "occurs in every part of the body, but it is more particularly frequent in the breasts of women," formed "by black bile overheated; and if particularly acrid, it is attended with ulceration." He pointed out a difference of opinion regarding the way in which cancer got its name:

> The veins are filled and stretched around like the feet of the animal called cancer (crab), and hence the disease has got its appellation. But some say that it is so called because it adheres to any part which it seizes upon in an obstinate manner like the crab.[36]

He deemed cancer an incurable disease and advocated evacuating melancholic humors to keep it from increasing in size. Paul included sections on *oedema* (edema), which is caused by an accumulation of phlegm and is therefore cold and painless; *struma* (scrofula); three benign lumps: *steatoma* (lipoma), *atheroma* (epidermal cyst), and *meliceris* (hygroma); *favus* (a term still in use today); and sections on many types of ulcers, e.g., simple, unsuppurated, hollow, fungous [sic], spreading ulcers, putrid ulcers, sinuous, and malignant ones. Paul noted that malignant ulcers were called *chironian* or *telephian*: chironian ulcers were named after Chiron, the wise centaur whose ulcer was slow to scar over, and telephian ulcers were named after Telephus, who was wounded by Achilles and suffered for a long time with a nonhealing wound.[37]

In the last part of Book IV, Paul tackles several types of worms that he believed, in congruence with the Aristotelian doctrine, were generated from inside the body as "offspring of crude and thick pituitous matters with a suitable putrefaction."[38] He addressed the *dracunculus* (Guinea worm), offering a controversial approach to its removal without breakage by fixing "a piece of lead to the worm in order that its discharge may not take place at once, but gradually with the weight of the lead."[39]

The Byzantine physicians' contributions to the history of dermatology cannot be overstated. They were the direct heirs of the ancient physicians, and while there was little novel information in the treatises of Oribasius, Aetius, Alexander, and Paul, their efforts at preservation clearly benefited the generations of medical writers that followed them. They continued to be cited as authorities on skin diseases well into the nineteenth century. As the work of Celsus was for the ancient Romans, the work of Paul of Aegina stands out as the great dermatological authorship of the Byzantine Empire.

CONSTANTINE'S *LEPRA*

According to a hagiographic source entitled "The Life of St. Sylvester" (fifth century CE), the Roman emperor Constantine (272–337 CE) suffered from *lepra*. But as it was shown in Interlude 1, prior to the High Middle Ages, the word *lepra* had no relation to leprosy (Hansen's disease); therefore, it is highly unlikely that Constantine's condition was actually leprosy in the modern sense of the term.[40] Described as a scaly skin disease (our modern appreciation of leprosy is that it is typically *not* scaly), it is more likely that Constantine suffered from psoriasis, eczema, cutaneous T-cell lymphoma, or impetigo. Constantine's affliction was, by legend, cured by the baptism performed by the Pope, St. Sylvester, thus further validating Constantine's decision to convert to Christianity.

Constantine was not the only Roman Emperor to have reportedly experienced a chronic skin disease. The Roman historians Pliny the Younger and Suetonius both noted that Octavian (63 BCE–14 CE), better known as Augustus Caesar and the first Roman Emperor, had a chronic itchy skin disease. Since Octavian was also rumored to have asthma, it is very likely that Octavian suffered from atopic dermatitis.[41]

Anglo-Saxon Medicine

After the Romans withdrew from Britain in 410, the Roman and Celtic peoples (Britons) who were living there were forced to make room for migrations of both Angles and Saxons from modern-day northern Germany. By 600, the Angles had settled in the northern (Northumbria) and eastern portions of the main island, and the Saxons dominated the south, while the Britons maintained control of the western side. Soon, these peoples converted to Christianity and coexisted somewhat peacefully until Viking raiders destabilized the region starting in the late eighth century, with the Danes being the most successful.

The Venerable Bede (672–735), a Benedictine monk who lived and resided at the monastery of St. Peter in the Kingdom of Northumbria of the Angles, wrote in the relatively stable period preceding the Viking raids. Bede is most famous for his *Ecclesiastical History of the English People* (ca. 731), but he also collected and preserved works across many disciplines. His writings shed some light on Anglo-Saxon medicine, which combined medical theory and practice from classical antiquity with herbal remedies, charms, Christian amulets, superstition, folklore, and prayer. Bede's history also contains information about a smallpox epidemic in 545 CE and a bubonic plague epidemic in 664 CE (see Interlude 2).[42]

While the majority of Anglo-Saxon medical practitioners during this period were Christian monks and clerics, as they were in the rest of the Western medieval world, there was another type of healer who practiced a less-learned type of medicine. He was referred to as *lǣće* (pronounced "leech"). The word *lǣće* came into the English language with two separate meanings: medical practitioner and blood-sucking worm. The word *lǣće* was used to refer to medical practitioners in the Anglo-Saxon world up until 1200.[43]

In 878, Alfred, King of the West Saxons (Wessex)—later Alfred the Great, King of the Anglo-Saxons (r. 886–899)—conquered the Danes and forced their ruler to convert to Christianity. During his reign, Alfred was known to be a learned man who promoted education, scholarly pursuits, and other measures to improve the life of his people.

It was during this enlightened period that historians believe the *Leechbooks I* and *II* (copied together), *Leechbook III*, and *Lacnunga* were written. The Leechbooks—literally, book for the leech—are three of the oldest medical texts written in English and have been dated to circa 900. The books give us an excellent understanding of Anglo-Saxon medicine. The first two books are referred to as *Bald's and Cild's Leechbook* because of a colophon at the end of Book 2 that states, "*Bald habet hunc librum Cild quem conscribere iussit*," best translating as "Bald owns this book which he ordered Cild to compile."[44] Bald and Cild are otherwise unknown. Only one copy of this manuscript exists in the world; it is housed in the British Museum in London. Thomas Oswald Cockayne (1807–1873), a British philologist, translated these important works into modern English and published them for the first time in 1864–1866.

Bald's and Cild's Leechbook is essentially a list of recipes for remedies, most of which are plant-based and heavily influenced by Greek and Roman medicine. *Leechbook I* is devoted to external disorders; *Leechbook II* is devoted to internal ones. *Leechbook III* contains the oldest, most purely Northern information, consisting of recipes not seen in the other books. *Lacnunga*, which is old English for "remedies," is an authorless text associated with the Leechbooks that was likely compiled in the late tenth or early eleventh century. It not only contains several remedies from the Leechbooks but also includes charms and prayers for various ailments; it is the most superstitious and least rational of the texts.[45] The only writer mentioned by name in the whole series of Leechbooks is Pliny the Elder, but according to historians, portions of *Leechbook II* were taken directly from the writings of Alexander of Tralles.[46]

Anglo-Saxon medicine was on equal footing with the rest of Europe, and the *lǽce*, with his knowledge of plant remedies, was no less competent than the *medicus*.[47] The remedies in the Leechbooks were rational, observation-based, and intended to improve the well-being of the patient, sometimes with success.[48] The three Anglo-Saxon Leechbooks are filled with advice on how to treat various skin diseases. The remedies are herbal-botanical recipes for the most part, but prayers or incantations are often found as well. There is no theory or discussion about the skin itself or the nature of skin disease, or any disease for that matter. It is strictly practical medicine. All three Leechbooks incorporate magic in many of the remedies as the Anglo-Saxons believed in a disease-spirit that had to be driven out of the patient's body. There is also a strong Christian influence throughout the works with numerous Christian prayers and saints referenced, as the Anglo-Saxons were a culture at a crossroads between old pagan beliefs and a new Christian faith.

While the first and third Leechbooks have ample dermatologic information, there is no discussion on skin disease in *Leechbook II*, which focuses on internal diseases. The following are a few excerpts from *Leechbook I*:

> For worms of the eyes [lice of the eyelashes] take seed of henbane, shed it on gledes [live coal], add two saucers full of water, set them on two sides of the man, and let him sit there over them, jerk the head hither and thither over the fire and the saucers also, then the worms shed themselves into the water.[49]

> This shall be good for chilblain and in case that the skin of a man's feet come off by cold, let him take the netherward part of meadowwort and lustmock and oak rind, pound all to dust, mingle with honey, effect a cure with that.[50]

There is a discussion in *Leechbook I*, Section 32, concerning what Cockayne translated as "blotch" and what the Anglo-Saxons called *blaece*, from which we get the word "bleach." It is apparent that this could be vitiligo, but the ancients and medievals thought it was a form of leprosy characterized by hypopigmentation of the skin, and other sources refer to it as an itching disease.[51] Here is one of several treatments offered, which combines botanical medicines and a magical regimen to drive the spirit from the body:

> For blotch, take goose grease and the netherward part of helenium and vipers bugloss, bishopwort and hayrife, pound the four worts together well, wring them, add thereto of old soap a spoon full, if thou have it, mingle a little oil with them thoroughly, and at night lather on. Scarify the neck after the setting of the sun, pour in silence the blood into running water, and after that spit three times and then say, "Have thou this unheal, and depart away with it;" go again on a clean way to the house, and go either way in silence.[52]

Other conditions addressed in *Leechbook I* are shingles (which they called *haec circl adl*—the circle disease), wounds, "erysipelatous inflammations," and smallpox, which was called pock disease and was treated with this regimen:

> Against pocks, a man shall freely employ bloodletting and drink melted butter, a bowl full of it: if they break out one must delve away each one of them with a thorn, and then let him drip wine or alder drink within them, then they will not be seen or no traces will remain.[53]

Leechbook III addresses several dermatologic problems:

> For warts, take hound's mie (a wort) [an herb] and a mouse's blood, mingle together, smear the warts therewith, they will soon depart away.

> Against lice, give the man to eat sodden colewort at night, fasting, frequently: he will be guarded against lice.

> If a thorn or a reed prick a man in the foot, and will not be gone, let him take a fresh goose turd and green yarrow, let him pound them thoroughly together, paste them on the wound, soon it will be well.

> Against cancer, take goat's gall and honey, mingle together of both equal quantities, apply to the wound. For that ilk, burn a fresh hound's head to ashes, apply to the wound. If the wound will not give way to that, take a man's dung, dry it thoroughly, rub to dust, apply it. If with this thou art not able to cure him, thou mayst never do it by any means.[54]

DERMATOLOGIC MYSTERY IN THE LEECHBOOKS

The major dermatologic mystery of the Leechbooks involves the Water-Elf disease discussed in *Leechbook III*:

> If a person has the water-elf disease, his finger nails will be livid and his eyes tearful and he will look downwards. Do this for him by way of medical treatment: [take] carline, hassock, the netherward part of iris, yew-berry, lupine, elecampane, a head of marshmallow, dill, lily, betony, pennyroyal, horehound, dock, elder-wood, earthgall, wormwood, comfrey. Steep them in ale, add holy water, sing this charm:
>
> > Round the wounds I have wreathed the best of healing amulets,
> > That the wounds may neither burn nor burst,
> > Nor grow worse nor putrefy,
> > Nor throb, nor be filthy wounds,
> > Nor cut in deeply; but let him keep the sacred water for himself,
> > Then it will pain you no more than it pains the land by the sea.[55]

Although the Christian tradition was strong in Anglo-Saxon England by the time of the writing of the Leechbooks, the Anglo-Saxons could not erase an old pagan belief that held diabolical, disease-inflicting elves responsible for certain diseases. The works are replete with conditions such as "water-elf disease," caused by "elf-shot" or some other elf mischief. Elves were hard to see or invisible creatures who shot their victims with arrows that spurred diseases not known to have an apparent cause.[56] Victims would then need some sort of incantation (elf-charm) to exorcise from the body the spell or spirit introduced from the elf-shot. The excerpt from *Leechbook III* reveals that water-elf disease is treated with the combination of an herbal concoction and an elf-charm. The water-elf disease could refer to chickenpox, smallpox, or some other disease of the skin that affects the eyes and has a very "watery" or blistery appearance (ophthalmic zoster?).

Other dermatological complaints addressed include the "penetrating worm," jaundice, and burns by fire, liquids, or the sun, elephantiasis, and "dry disease" (inflammation), and "fig disease" (erysipelas). The Anglo-Saxon *lǽće* apparently trusted salves for a variety of concerns and prescribed them as often as drinkable concoctions. Many of these salves had a repellant effect. For example, *Leechbook III* contains formulas for protective salves for "nocturnal goblin visitors" and for "women with whom the devil hath carnal commerce."[57] In addition to herbal remedies, the *lǽće* prescribed saliva, blood, and excrements as treatments for various afflictions. Recipes frequently listed butter, milk, fat, oils, ale, wine, mead, vinegar, wax, and honey as ingredients.

In the *Lacnunga*, there is guidance on how to remedy carbuncles, lice (including a concoction applied thrice to the navel), itching, warty eruptions, black ulcers, erysipelas, and wens (infected follicle). For the latter,

> For a wen salve, take helenium and radish and chervil and ravens foot, English rape and fennel and sage, and southernwood, and pound them together, and take a good deal of garlic, pound and wring these through a cloth into spoilt honey: when it is thoroughly sodden, then add pepper and zedoary and galingale and ginger and cinnamon and laurel berries and pyrethrum, a good deal of each according to its efficacy: and when the juice of the worts and honey are so mingled, then seethe thou it twice as strongly as it was before sodden; then wilt thou have a good salve against wens.[58]

Incantations were an essential component of the therapeutic process of the *lǽće*. Swellings of the flesh were considered to be the dwellings of nine evil spirits, and the following charm was recited by the *lǽće* for furuncles, scrofula, and worms in an attempt to gradually reduce the spirits from the lesion:

> Nine were Noththe's sisters
> Then the nine came to be VIII
> and the eight to VII
> and the seven to VI
> and the six to V
> and the five to IV
> and the four to III
> and the three to II
> and the two to I
> and the I to none.[59]

Did any of these remedies work? For at least one of them, the answer is yes. Researchers in 2015 proved that the following leechdom for styes known as "Bald's Eyesalve" was repeatedly efficacious against methicillin-resistant *Staphylococcus aureus* (MRSA) infections:

> Work an eye salve for a wen, take cropleek and garlic, of both equal quantities, pound them well together, take wine and bullocks gall, of both equal quantities, mix with leek, put this then into a brazen vessel, let it stand nine days in the brass vessel, wring out through a cloth and clear it well, put it into a horn, and about night time apply it with a feather to the eye.[60]

The authors concluded that several ingredients are individually known to have antibacterial activity, but it was the combined action of several elements that made the concoction effective.[61] In 2018, it was shown that a substance known as allicin is the antibacterial ingredient found in the concoction, having bactericidal activity against resistant forms of both *S. aureus* and *Pseudomonas aeruginosa*.[62] However, in 2020, researchers proved that all ingredients of the eye salve were necessary to have an effect against bacterial biofilm on wounds.[63] This research into the so-called ancientbiotics of the Middle Ages is an exciting and promising field in the era of antimicrobial resistance that highlights the effectiveness of premodern medicine and the potential of ancient texts as a source of new antimicrobial agents.

Dermatology in the Eastern Medical Tradition

There is a paucity of translated source material for a history of skin disease in the East, and Eastern medicine followed a separate path from Western medicine until the mid-nineteenth and early twentieth centuries, when the Western brand of medicine was delivered to the East. A comprehensive survey of the history of skin disease in China, India, and other Eastern countries is beyond the scope of this book. Nonetheless, there is no space like the present to include a few comments about two of these nations—China and India—especially regarding any contributions that may have preceded developments in the West.

In traditional Chinese medicine, which is approximately 4000 years old, skin diseases are categorized under *wai ke*: external medicine (which includes disorders of the skin, hair, nails, muscles, bones, flesh, and sinews).[64] Skin diseases are manifestations of some internal imbalance and are characterized and organized by morphologic appearance, but not as named diseases. Traditional Chinese dermatology is holistic and reflects a view that skin disease in all cases signifies a problem with the health of the whole body. Sleep, emotions, diet, and digestion are just a few of the factors that can influence skin health. Disease was attributed to disturbances in the balance of internal wind, fire (hot blood), cold, summer heat, dampness, dryness, stasis (stagnant blood), or insect bites. Treatments of skin disease generally involved one or more of the following: dietary modification; the relief of internal blockages with acupuncture; herbal medications, in raw form, pills, baths, washes, pastes, powders, ointments, tinctures, oils, or wet compresses; fumigation, moxibustion (direct application of heat) or cupping. As in the West, skin disease was mastered and managed by the surgeon, after surgery (*yang yi*) separated from internal medicine, dietary medicine, and veterinary medicine in the eleventh century.[65]

The Chinese have a long history of writing about skin diseases, as summarized in Table 5.2.

Of these, the Chao Yuanfang title (610) is the most historically significant, as it contained descriptions of approximately 60 skin diseases. In that work can be found a discussion of the scabies mite and information on how to extract it from interdigital web spaces, proving that the Chinese knew about the scabies mite long before Western physicians.[67] Shen Dou-Yuan wrote "Profound insights on external diseases" (1604), considered China's first atlas of skin diseases. Dermatology as a distinct discipline for the Chinese had its beginnings during the Ming Dynasty (1368–1644) with the publication of various texts solely devoted to skin diseases.

The Chinese were among the first peoples to record information about history's most significant skin diseases: leprosy and smallpox. As was discussed in Interlude 1, leprosy was first written about in the *Feng zhen shi* 封診式, "Models for sealing and investigating" (266–246 BCE) under a generic term for skin disease called *li* 癘. The Chinese correctly recognized anesthesia as a feature of that disease. The earliest description of smallpox is from the fourth century CE in China, but there is evidence that it was in China some 600 years before that time.[68] The version of that virus faced by the Chinese in the first millennium must have been rather virulent and lethal. It is likely that trade between China and Japan led to the introduction of smallpox into Japan and the subsequent epidemic of 735–737 CE, killing a third of the Japanese people. Variolation, which the West learned about from the Ottoman Empire, first appears in Chinese in a text written in 1549, but less convincing reports suggest that the practice dates back to 1000 CE.[69] The Chinese method involved blowing smallpox material, kept at body temperature for one

TABLE 5.2

Classic Chinese Texts from the Common Era Containing Information on Skin Disease[66]

Prescriptions for Emergency	Ge Hong, 341
The General Treatise on the Cause and Symptoms of Disease	Chao Yuanfang, 610
A Thousand Golden Prescriptions	Sun Si-maio, 652
Essential Points of Wai Ke	Chen Zi-ming, 1263
The Main Points for Wai Ke	Qi Dezhi, 1335
Orthodox Manual of Wai Ke	Chen She-gong, 1617
The Golden Mirror of Ancestral Medicine	Wu Qian, 1742

month, up the nose.[70] There are no reports of a demography-altering pandemic of bubonic plague in the fourteenth century, and the first reports of syphilis did not occur in China until the sixteenth century. In addition to using mercury for various medical indications since 500 BCE, the Chinese wrote about scabies in ancient times and may have been the first to use sulfur to treat it.

In India, the ancient medical tradition that started in the Vedic period (1500–500 BCE), called Ayurvedic, placed both skin disease and skin health in focus. Disease was generally attributed to supernatural causes such as the curse of a god, or blamed on the machination of a demon or demons. But a humoral system of disease, involving three humors or *dosha* (*vata*, *pitta*, and *kapha*) and five elements (earth, air, fire, water, and ether), served as a more natural explanation. Traditional Indian medical texts discussed daily care of the skin with oil massage, trimming and care of the hair and nails, and the use of perfumes. In the *Sushruta Samhita* (unknown date, ca. 600 BCE–100 CE), an ancient Indian physician named Sushruta, who received the Ayurvedic medical knowledge of the god of medicine, Dhanvantari, dealt primarily with surgical management of disease and discussed such procedures as incision and drainage, cauterization, and dermabrasion.[71] Sushruta was a Hippocrates-like figure in that many different persons are believed to have contributed to the Sanskrit text under his name. The text contains a complete description of leprosy, including its highly specific diagnostic features of anesthesia. Chaulmoogra oil, which enjoyed a long run as a treatment for leprosy up until the twentieth century, was first mentioned as a treatment in this text. India can claim the first official writings on leprosy, which is not surprising since it appears the disease originated there.

In the medical counterpart to the *Sushruta Samhita*, the *Charaka Samhita* (unknown dates, ca. 400 BCE–200 CE), it is apparent that the ancient Indian physician knew the skin to have six layers and to be the residence of touch sensation.[72] The Sanskrit word *kustha*, which represented a number of skin ailments, including leprosy, was given 7 different subtypes in the *Charika* and 18 subtypes in the *Sushruta*. Among these subtypes can be identified several different skin diseases, including vitiligo, cellulitis, acne, melasma, and tinea.[73] A review of the Ayurvedic treatments offered in these works reveals a focus on herbal medicine, as well as an emphasis on special diets, meditation, yoga, laxatives, and enemas. Metals such as arsenic and mercury can also be found as common treatments, as alchemy held an important position in the Indian medical tradition.

The first writings on smallpox in India appeared around 400 CE, about the same time they did in China, but evidence suggests it existed in India before the birth of Christ, and Indian civilization was very likely inoculating with smallpox material as early as this period.[74] The Hindu people had a benevolent but dangerous goddess who personified smallpox named Sitala; she was revered and deemed responsible for smallpox epidemics in India. As in the case of China, there are no convincing reports that the Black Death ravaged India as it did the West or reports of syphilis in India before the sixteenth century. Indian medicine remained tradition-based until the mid-nineteenth century when the British imperial authorities imposed a modern Western approach to skin disease upon its Indian subjects.

Summary

The early Middle Ages (ca. 500–1000 CE) spanned a considerable period that deserves more appreciation for its intellectual achievement than historians, who previously referred to the era as the Dark Ages, have acknowledged. Early in that period, Isidore of Seville summarized the knowledge of his day, including all terms for skin disease that were in use at the time, making his *Etymologies* the single most influential encyclopedia of the Middle Ages. It has been shown that the Byzantine medical writers (sixth to eighth centuries) Oribasius of Pergamon, Aetius of Amida, Alexander of Tralles, and Paul of Aegina, compiled a great deal of classical medical knowledge in Greek in order to preserve it for the future generations of physicians. Within that corpus is documentation from these four writers about the skin and skin disease and the coinage of the words acne and eczema. As demonstrated in the Leechbooks, the Anglo-Saxons were writing and practicing a legitimate type of medicine in the ninth and tenth centuries. Their medicine was an amalgamation of Northern medicine, Greek and Latin medicine, and local superstitions with both pagan and Christian origins. Modern research into "ancientbiotics" has proven that at least one Anglo-Saxon remedy was effective against MRSA staphylococcal skin infection.

6

The Islamic Golden Age

After the seventh century, Greek and Latin medical erudition declined even in the Byzantine Empire. However, the torch of medical writing and compilation was not wholly extinguished; it was passed farther east. The Abbasid Caliphate was the Islamic state that ruled the Middle East and part of North Africa, including Alexandria, from 750 to 1258. During the era known as the Islamic Golden Age, Baghdad was founded in 762 and replaced Alexandria as the preeminent cultural center of the known world after it fell to the Muslims in 641. The Islamic Golden Age refers to the period of history when the economic flourishing of the Abbasid Caliphate allowed for an expansion of many aspects of Islamic society—including education, arts and culture, natural sciences, mathematics, and healthcare. The age began with the reign of Harun al-Rashid (r. 786–809) and ended with the siege of Baghdad by the Mongols in 1258. It was during these four-and-a-half centuries that the physicians of the Abbasid Caliphate managed to salvage classical medicine and preserve it for future eras.

The Greek-to-Arabic Translation Movement

Al-Rashid and his son al-Ma'mun (r. 813–833) sparked a period of scholarship known as the "Age of Translations." The task at hand was to translate as many of the available Greek texts as possible into Arabic in order to bring ancient medicine to the Muslim people. Established in 832, the Bayt al-Hikmah, "The House of Wisdom," was a library in Baghdad where scholars met to translate various works. The works of Galen were among the most revered. The most prolific of these early translators was an Arab Christian named Hunayn ibn Ishaq (809–873), known to the West as Johannitius. He translated 129 works of Galen from Greek into Arabic, and by the end of the ninth century, Arabic physicians had access to a wide range of ancient medical texts in up-to-date Arabic translations.[1] The collection of Hunayn's translations, known as the *Isagoge*, formed the basis of a medieval text called the *Articella* that later became the principal textbook used in Europe's medical schools (see Chapter 7). The Arabic translations of the Greek became a foundation of knowledge that would educate and inspire generations of learned Muslim medical men for the next 200–300 years.

The Arabs made outstanding contributions to the history of medicine, including the preservation of existing medical knowledge through translations, compilations, and commentaries on the writings of Galen and Hippocrates, as well as the Greek and Roman physicians of late antiquity and the early Middle Ages. The fruits of these labors formed the foundation of medical information that the Latin West used to educate its physicians for the next several centuries. But the Arabs also had original contributions of their own, particularly in the realms of pharmacology and alchemy, and they created the first pharmacies.[2] Some of their intellectuals made discoveries that were credited centuries later to Western physicians. For example, there is reason to believe that Ala al-Din ibn al-Nafis (1200–1288) discovered the pulmonary circuit of the blood. We may never know the full extent of the achievements of the Arabic doctors since many of the writings they produced were lost during the siege and sack of Baghdad in 1258 by the Mongols. Not only did the sack end the Islamic Golden Age, but the House of Wisdom was destroyed, and many of the manuscripts it held were thrown into the Tigris River. Fortunately, much of the knowledge preserved by the Arabic physicians of this age had been disseminated prior to the collapse of Baghdad through Western cities like Cordoba, Toledo, Salerno, and Palermo.

The Arabic-language medical writers of the Islamic Golden Age are owed a debt of gratitude for their contributions to the history of dermatology. Through their efforts in preservation and the translation

DOI: 10.1201/9781003273622-9

movement, the writings of the Greeks and Romans were safeguarded in the Arabic language so that future physicians and surgeons could benefit from the expertise of the ancients in the area of skin disease. Equally important were some examples of original input by the Arabic writers into our bank of knowledge about the skin and skin disease. While the contributions of many of these Arabic physicians are beyond the scope of this book, one in particular, Abu al-Qasim Khalaf ibn al-Abbas Al-Zahrawi, known as Albucasis, deserves at least a mention for several reasons: he was a founder of operative surgery, he authored a surgical compilation of the writings of Paul of Aegina, and he was the first to describe the neurological effects of leprosy. Our focus now turns to the contributions of the six most significant Arabic writers with following Latinized names: Rhazes, Haly Abbas, Avicenna, Averroes, Avenzoar, and Maimonides.

Rhazes (854–925 CE)

Muhammad ibn Zakariya al-Razi, better known as Rhazes (854–925), is considered by some the greatest physician and medical writer of the Middle Ages; he was also an influential alchemist and philosopher. Born outside of Tehran, in Persia, he spent much of his career in Baghdad. Although Rhazes practiced Galenic medicine, he was among the first physicians in history to question Galen; he wrote a treatise entitled "Doubts about Galen," and he believed that physician experience trumped book knowledge. He was not convinced of the concept of the four humors. Rhazes' doctoring was intertwined with his philosophizing; that is, he was a "physician of the body through medicine, and physician of the soul through philosophy."[3] Translated from Arabic and published in Latin in the thirteenth century, Rhazes' best original contribution is known in the Latin as *Liber continens*, "Comprehensive book on medicine," a diary of sorts containing case histories, notes, transcriptions, and observations. Another of his highly influential books was the "Book on Medicine for Mansur," a short medical textbook dedicated to al-Mansur, the governor of his hometown. Both books were familiar to medical students of the next half-millennium. His extraordinarily lengthy and diverse bibliography includes the seminal book on pediatrics, *Practica puerorum*, "Diseases of Children," and another for the poor, travelers, or anyone in need of a physician entitled "For one without a doctor," which suggested diets or drugs for self-treatment.

Rhazes was the most original and innovative of the six great Arabic-language writers on skin disease. In addition to his introduction of the concept of allergy as a cause of disease, description of the guinea worm, and work with mercurials, his most significant contribution to the history of the study of skin disease was his seminal treatise on smallpox and measles entitled *al-Judari wa al-Hasbah* (On Smallpox and Measles). He was the first to treat smallpox and measles as distinct diseases.[4] Prior to this publication, the two conditions were considered variants of the same illness, as both were exanthems that featured red macules. It is easy for us to distinguish the two today—smallpox is pustular, and measles is not. But the ancients did not separate febrile exanthems in this way; they lumped the two together based on their understanding of the underlying cause of the problem. Rhazes' discussion of the two exanthems demonstrates an in-depth knowledge of morphology; it is no wonder doctors used the book and its many translations until the eighteenth century, and it continues to impress even the modern dermatologist (see Interlude 4).

Haly Abbas (930–994 CE)

Ali ibn al-Abbas al-Majusi, known as Haly Abbas and widely regarded as the father of Arabic dermatology, authored a work entitled *Kitab Kamil as-Sina'aat-Tibbiyya*, "The Complete Art of Medicine." It was the first Arabic medical book translated into Latin.[5] Constantine Africanus brought a partial translation (1080) of the work to Monte Cassino, and it was one of the founding texts of the medical school at Salerno (see Chapter 7). In 1127, a complete translation of Haly Abbas' text by Stephen of Antioch (fl. early twelfth century) was published in Latin and became known as the *Liber regius* "The Royal Book" because Haly Abbas had dedicated the work to his king.

The Royal Book's section on dermatology contains superb information on skin disease, exhibiting both clarity and originality of thought. It addresses eczema, scabies, miliaria, favus, lice, seborrheic dermatitis, alopecia areata, lupus vulgaris, filariasis, leprosy, smallpox, chickenpox, measles, and erysipelas.[6] Haly Abbas was heavily cited later by Henri de Mondeville and Guy de Chauliac (see Chapter 7) and quoted heavily by Mercurialis in the sixteenth century (see Chapter 8). Seen as practical above all else, *The Royal Book* was very popular in the burgeoning medical schools of Europe, but enthusiasm for it waned with the arrival of Avicenna's *Canon*, which offered more detailed descriptions of skin diseases. The two works, however, shared the same explanations for causes, symptoms, and treatments of skin diseases.[7]

Avicenna (980–1037)

The next Muslim physician worthy of consideration is Abu Ali al-Husayn ibn Abdallah ibn Sina, better known as Avicenna. It could be argued that Avicenna was, instead of Rhazes, the greatest physician and medical writer of the Middle Ages in the East or West. There are no words to fully characterize the genius of this man; perhaps placing him next to Leonardo da Vinci will suffice. Avicenna was a Persian child prodigy and polymath born in Bukhara, in present-day Uzbekistan. He was a student of law, metaphysics, and science and wrote extensively on these topics (450 total works), but he is best known for his comprehensive accounts of human knowledge contained within the *Kita al-Shifa*, "The Book of Healing," and *al-Qanun*, "The Canon of Medicine." Contrary to what its title suggests, the former does not cover medicine but instead focuses on mathematics, logic, physics, and metaphysics and is famous for being the longest science book of its kind ever written.

The *Canon of Medicine* (1025) is a medical encyclopedia consisting of a million words arranged in five books, based on the works of Galen, Hippocrates, and Roman and Alexandrian physicians. He collected all the available medical information from classical antiquity and the early Middle Ages, arranging it in a clear, practical way. He addressed diseases of specific parts of the body, as well as diseases that spread over large areas of the body, such as fevers. He also described several hundred medications and therapeutic substances.[8] The eventual translation of Avicenna's magnum opus gave the medieval Western physician renewed access to Galenic medicine. Under the order of Frederick II, the Hohenstaufen emperor of the Holy Roman Empire, the *Canon* was translated into Latin in the thirteenth century by Gerard de Sabloneta, who is often confused with Gerard of Cremona. Its impact was lasting and profound, as the *Canon* was used as the standard medical school textbook in Europe until the seventeenth century, only falling out of favor when the Renaissance physicians chose the original Greek source material over the Arabic translations. But if longevity of influence is the criterion, then Avicenna's *Canon* is the single most important medical book ever written.

The fourth book of Avicenna's *Canon of Medicine* is one of the most important works in the history of dermatology. Avicenna became an oft-cited authority on skin disease for 700 years after his death. Avicenna did comment briefly on the skin in his masterful Book I of the *Canon*, which addresses anatomy, physiology, and the cause of disease, among many other general medical topics; however, there are only a few passages relevant to skin care. In addition to several pages of information about the beneficial effects of the water bath, he does caution the reader in regard to sunbathing, but not for the reason we would today be concerned. Avicenna believed that the sun causes the body to thicken and harden, and it "cauterizes" the pores of the skin, leading to obstruction of perspiration.[9] He also thought that the sun burns the skin more if one is motionless in the sun, as opposed to moving around.

Avicenna believed that the skin could function as a conduit whereby excessive humors could be expelled from the body, and obstruction of this process could promote disease. In Book IV, Avicenna revealed his rudimentary classification of disease. For the skin, he discusses swellings (aposthems), which are divided into hot swellings (phlegmon, erysipelas, and buboes), cold swellings (cancer, scrofula, and dropsy), and papular swellings (pustules, miliaria, scabies, warts, and vesiculobullous lesions). Disorders of the hair and color changes of the skin, such as alopecia and vitiligo, respectively, were not considered by him to be diseases; these were classified as disfigurements. (Sadly, even to this day, some health insurance plans do not consider vitiligo, a condition with significant, detrimental psychosocial effects, as anything more than a cosmetic concern.) Avicenna's comments on the transmission of disease from person to person were ahead of their time.[10] Lepra, scabies, variola, pestilential fever, septic inflammatory swellings, and ulcers could be spread from one house to the next or to a place in the direction of the wind. Avicenna espoused the belief that smallpox resulted when the blood boils but, unlike Rhazes, did comment on the contagiousness of that illness.

In Part 23, "On fevers," Part 25, "On Swellings and pimples," and Part 28, "On cosmetics," of Book IV, Avicenna left a legacy of knowledge about skin disease that would benefit future generations of physicians for several centuries. Pages and pages of diagnostic and therapeutic information are found within these parts. The information on smallpox and measles is complete, but it was obviously culled from Rhazes. After a lengthy and somewhat rambling introduction to "hot inflammatory swellings" in Part 25, Avicenna delineated the difference between erysipelas and other types of hot inflammatory swellings (cellulitis) in a concise, accurate manner: erysipelas is brighter, clearer, more blanchable, more superficial, more likely to blister, less indurated, associated with higher fever, less painful, and more likely to affect the face than cellulitis. All of this is correct information.[11] He described two types of pimples—ant-like and millet-type, both of which resemble forms of folliculitis. He later referred to urticarial lesions as scarlet pimples. Avicenna provided a plain definition of "Persian fire," a term for cutaneous anthrax: a pimple that emerges from the skin, blisters and burns the skin, forms a crust, and feels as if a hot object has been placed on the skin.[12]

Avicenna's descriptions of bullous eruptions may be an early description of pemphigus, a severe blistering disease now known to be autoimmune in nature. To Avicenna, there are two types of blistering: bubbles and blisters.[13] Bubbles are caused by the boiling of humors in the body which releases water and a thin part of the humor under the skin. These remain under the skin and do not contain pus. Blisters are caused by a thin blood substance released under the skin, which then putrifies, fills with pus, and inflates the skin.

Avicenna's definition of bubonic plague (see Interlude 2) still holds up today: a swelling that turns poisonous and putrefies the lymph node and changes the color of the surrounding area. He notes that such a lesion can have a negative effect on the heart through the arteries (sepsis) and lead to vomiting, abnormal pulse, and fainting.[14] The skin exam of a person with plague can prognosticate: if the swelling is red, there is hope for a cure; a yellow swelling is worse, but there is still a chance at a cure; a black swelling, however, means certain death.[15]

Avicenna stated that leprosy (see Interlude 1) is a "cancer" of the whole body, caused by the spread of black bile throughout the body, where it putrefies the organs and destroys their shape and condition.[16] He offers a very detailed description of leprosy's signs and symptoms.[17] Features of leprosy according to Avicenna are a blackened face, red eyes, asthma and breathing difficulties, constant sneezing, nasal sounds, thin hair, cracked nails, severe body odor, spiteful and stressed temperament, ugly and grim face, body lice, and skin ulcers. Late-stage features include destruction and loss of the nose, a malodorous discharge of bloody pus from all over the body, and the skin turning completely black.

The section entitled "On Cosmetics" has earned Avicenna the honor of "father of Arabic cosmetology."[18] It deals with problems that Avicenna deemed disfigurements of the skin rather than diseases, although the same medical treatments were used for both types of maladies. Avicenna devoted much time to the hair, which was believed at the time to derive from "smoky vapory matter coagulated in the tiny orifices of the skin." He included extensive recommendations for managing hair loss, protecting the hair from loss, protecting the eyebrows specifically, lengthening the hair, curling the hair, dyeing the hair, removing unwanted hair, and slowing the graying of hair. For something as simple as dandruff, which can sometimes cause purulence of the head and is produced from either pungent bilious humor or from black-bile-contaminated sanguine humor, Avicenna recommended bloodletting or purging, depending on the patient's needs, followed by cleansing topical medications and oils.[19]

Avicenna noted that skin beauty was tied to overall medical and mental health, and he believed that skin receiving more blood and vital energy was clearer and thicker. He urged protection of the skin from heat, cold, and wind. Chickpea, soft-boiled egg, meat soup, figs, unripe dates, and grape wine all promote beauty, as do radish, leek, onion, cabbage, and garlic. Other things promoting beauty of the face are getting angry, discussions, moderate exercise, wrestling, being happy, enjoying music, reading books, being friends with clean people, spending time with comedians, going horseback riding, and so forth.[20] If only it were that easy!

In this same section, Avicenna tackles vitiligo, tinea, impetigo, itching, scabies, warts, and corns. He attributed warts and corns to "thick black bile matter," and it is almost impossible to fathom that patients with warts and corns were treated with bloodletting and purging of black bile matter, but that is the case.[21] For single warts, Avicenna suggested a variety of topical medicaments and surgical options. Avicenna is recognized for using an alchemical substance termed cadmia (oxide of zinc) as a treatment for ulcerating skin cancer.

On hygiene, like the Romans, Avicenna promoted bathing; in the tenth century, Baghdad had more than 27,000 public baths with hot and cold water.[22] Finally, his set of rules for experimenting with and testing medications was groundbreaking in the path toward evidence-based medicine. There are numerous other innovations in the *Canon* that are beyond the scope of this book. Modern scholars tend to favor Avicenna as the greatest of all the Arabic writers because of his genius, attention to detail, and historical value, while others prefer Rhazes because of his inventiveness and accuracy of observation.[23]

Averroes (1126–1198) and Avenzoar (1094–1162)

Abu al-Walid Muhammad ibn Ahmad ibn Muhammad ibn Rushd, better known as Averroes (1126–1198), was a polymath who served as royal physician to the court of the ruling Almohad dynasty in Córdoba, in present-day Spain. Part of Spain (called al-Andalus) was ruled by the Muslims from 711 to 1492; Córdoba was the capital of Muslim rule in Spain for several centuries, and like Baghdad, an economically prosperous place as well as a center of learning. There were many libraries located there that contained countless Arabic translations of Greek texts. Averroes' most important medical work, published in Latin in 1482, was *al-Kulliyat*, "The Book of General Principles" (1162), also known as the *Colliget*, containing seven books based on Aristotelian as well as Galenic medicine. He is remembered more for his philosophy—his commentaries on Aristotle and the application of Aristotelianism to medicine—than for his dermatological writings. However, his *Colliget* did contain a substantial amount of dermatologic information, and he was the first to point out that a person could get smallpox only once in their lifetime.

Averroes was a collaborator with Abu-Marwan Abd al-Malik ibn Abi al-Ala ibn Zuhr, Latinized as Avenzoar (1094–1162), who was from Seville and was the most esteemed physician of his day. Averroes asked Avenzoar to write a compendium for the *Colliget*, and he complied. With the title *Kitab al-Taysir*, "Book of Simplification Concerning Therapeutics and Diet," their collaboration is the Andalusian counterpart to Avicenna's *Canon*.

MEDIEVAL KNOWLEDGE OF THE ITCH MITE

Avenzoar possibly knew of the scabies itch mite. He wrote in *Kitab al-Taysir*,

> Sometimes there arises on the body, under the external skin, little swellings which the vulgar call the scab, and if the skin is removed, there issues from various parts a very small beast, so small as to be hardly visible.[24]

However, another Arabic physician, Abu al-Hasan Ahmad ibn Muhammad al-Tabari (fl. tenth century), perhaps knew of the mite 200 years prior:

> this animalcule can be removed with the point of a needle … and it moves. If crushed between the fingers, one hears a crack.[25]

But there are questions concerning these observations: the mite, which is 0.4 mm in size, is generally too small for the naked eye to see or to crush with fingers, and it certainly would not make a cracking sound upon pressure. What he is describing sounds more like a flea or a louse.

There is much debate among historians of medicine as to who the first person in history was to "know about" the scabies mite. While there was no official publication about the microscopic organism until the seventeenth century, the abovementioned Arabic doctors (Avenzoar and Al-Tabari) are frequently discussed as being aware of the mite in the Middle Ages. Chao Yuanfang wrote about the mite in seventh-century China (see Chapter 5). Hildegard of Bingen and Trota of Salerno, both of whom will be discussed in the next chapter, are others who may have known of the mite. A final claim of early awareness of the mite centers around the 225th song of the *Cantigas de Santa Maria*, "Songs of St. Mary" by Alfonso X "The Wise" of Castile (1221–1284).[26] The peculiar story involves a priest who ate a spider that had fallen into his chalice during mass.[27] Rather than kill the priest with its poison, the eight-legged, hairy organism instead crawled about under his skin all over his body. Eventually, the spider made its way to his arm, and his arm began to tingle, which caused him to scratch. The spider emerged from under his fingernail, and he grabbed it, crushed it, and saved it for the next mass, at which time he ate the dead spider in front of his congregation. From that point on, the priest was more pious and not guilty of lustfulness. Perhaps knowledge of the scabies mite, which is like a tiny spider as it has eight legs, was the inspiration behind this bizarre religious tale.

Maimonides (1135–1204)

Moses ben Maimon, better known as Maimonides, was heavily influenced by his contemporary Averroes and is known today for his philosophy and Torah scholarship. Maimonides was a preeminent Jewish physician from Córdoba who wrote several medical works in Arabic, including "Extracts from Galen" and "Commentaries on the Hippocratic Aphorisms." His most important work, "Regimen of Health," contained advice on preventative medicine and was frequently copied and translated throughout the Middle Ages. Though he wrote extensively on the skin and skin disease in his book on medical aphorisms, a compilation of his random thoughts on medicine, he contributed little in the way of new discoveries.

In his aphorisms, Maimonides observed that acute inflammations occur in the spaces between skin and underlying muscle.[28] He understood and referenced Galen's knowledge on the sensory purpose of the skin.[29] Excessive sweat was abnormal and could be avoided by living a proper life and eating healthy, natural foods.[30] He believed that the epidermis is the layer of skin that retains liquids from the inside of the body, and the various eruptions of the skin were simply caused by retention and adherence of these liquids (humors).[31] Maimonides frequently mentioned excessive or defective chyme (El Qu-am) as a cause of disease, attributing pruritus and prurigo to irritating chymes.

Maimonides' surgical knowledge is most noteworthy for our study. He believed that black bile was the cause of both cancer (localized) and leprosy (generalized), two diseases commonly held to be on a spectrum with one another in medieval times.[32] Like Avicenna, he recommended cadmia to treat carcinomatous ulcers; he also discussed a general approach to treating skin cancer surgically, which reveals a rather forward-thinking approach for the Middle Ages:

> If one desires to treat a cancer through surgery, then one should commence by eliminating the black biles through purgation. Then one should excise the entire site of illness, until no residue therein remains. One should let the blood flow from the operative site, and not hasten to stop it. Then one compresses the surrounding vessels, and presses the thick blood out therefrom. After this one treats the wound.[33]

The modern dermatologist can appreciate his mindset toward surgery, except for the part about purging black bile. Other pertinent and reasonable surgical comments include his description of swellings that resemble "flour cooked in water" (epidermal cysts)—he recommended excision or to let them "putrify"—while for fatty tumors (lipomas), excision was the only option.[34] Ulcers, like cancer, needed internal treatment before external: phlebotomy daily for four days, then three purges of black "chymes," next, a diet promoting good chymes, and finally, wound care.[35] Maimonides would become a highly respected authority and reference source in the medical writings of the centuries that followed.

Summary

During the Golden Age of Islam, medical men such as Hunayn, Rhazes, and Avicenna translated, compiled, and/or commented on the classical medical writings of Galen, Hippocrates, and others, thus salvaging the knowledge of the ancients and preserving it in Arabic for future generations in both the East and West. Unlike their counterparts in the West, these writers delivered original work on skin disease. In particular, their work with the exanthems (smallpox, measles) and leprosy stands out, as do their seminal contributions regarding skin cancer, anthrax, cosmetology, and treatment of skin disease. Their understanding of the skin was in keeping with that of the ancients and the Western medieval physicians.

7

The Medieval West

Thus far, we have seen that the remarkable history of medicine in the Middle Ages began in the Greek-speaking East centered around Alexandria and moved into the Middle East and Muslim-dominated Spain. In addition, the Anglo-Saxons were continuing their own unique brand of medicine in what was formerly Roman Britain. What about medicine during the period in the rest of continental Europe—modern-day France, Germany, and Italy? We know of no famous medical writers or influential texts that survive from these regions. If there was such a thing as the Dark Ages, it was there and then—Western Europe from 500 to 1100, with its wars, corruption, superstitions, and "impenetrable mindlessness."[1] Missing was not only the medical theory but also the entire framework of intellect and education, which had fostered the ancient medical community.[2]

Carolingian Medicine

There was one significant bright spot of intellectual life during the early Middle Ages in Western Europe—at the court of Charles the Great, better known as Charlemagne. Western Europe was divided and controlled by various barbarian groups (Franks, Saxons, Visigoths, Ostrogoths, etc.) after the Roman Empire declined in the fifth century. These kingdoms were isolated, with the enduring Roman roads the only means by which information could travel between them. Charlemagne (742–814), the king of the Franks, unified Western Europe through conquest, forming what is called today the Carolingian Empire. In an attempt to revive the Roman Empire in the West, he was crowned emperor of the Romans by Pope Leo III on Christmas day in 800 CE. Over the next 150 years, the eastern part of the Carolingian Empire evolved into a principally central European entity called the Holy Roman Empire, beginning with the reign of Otto I (crowned emperor in 962). Thus, Charlemagne is considered by some historians to be the first Holy Roman Emperor. Charlemagne was not only great because of his unification efforts, but because he, like Alfred the Great whom he inspired, promoted literary and scholarly activity, the arts and architecture, and—most important to Charlemagne—education. This academic revival has been named the Carolingian Renaissance, the first of three medieval renaissances. The other two were the Ottonian Renaissance (936–1002) and the Renaissance of the twelfth century; the former had little influence in the history of medicine, the latter will be discussed shortly.

The Carolingian Renaissance was a period of increased cultural and intellectual activity that occurred during the ninth-century reigns of Charlemagne and his son Louis the Pious (r. 813–840). It was made possible by the peace and prosperity achieved by Carolingian rule, which stimulated a renewed enthusiasm for knowledge in an unenlightened people. Charlemagne's capital at Aachen, in modern-day western Germany, became a beacon for intellectuals all over Europe, most of whom were clerics. Charlemagne was able to lure the best and brightest across Europe to his court. The most famous of these was Alcuin of York (735–804), an Anglo-Saxon scholar and educator who founded the palace school at Aachen and was the most learned man at Charlemagne's court. Charlemagne issued an administrative order calling for the construction of monastic schools all over the empire in 787. The curriculum at the school contained the seven liberal arts divided into the *quadrivium* (music, arithmetic, geometry, and astronomy) and *trivium* (Medieval Latin grammar, logic, and rhetoric). Charlemagne and Alcuin believed that the production of copies of the works of classical Roman writers such as Cicero, Horace, and Julius Caesar would have practical benefits for Carolingian society. The main purpose was to reproduce a corpus of classical Latin texts from which to teach the students Latin at the schools across the Carolingian territory.

DOI: 10.1201/9781003273622-10

Latin had been the language of the Romans, i.e., those who lived in Rome—the emperors, the government, the military, the Roman people. But the elites of the Roman West were raised to be bilingual in both Greek and Latin, and for authors of literature, science, and medicine, Greek was the primary official language of the wider Roman Empire. When the Roman Empire split into two halves near the end of the third century CE, the Greek language yielded to Latin in the West. The Christian Church in the West converted from Greek to Latin; St. Jerome (347–420) translated the Greek Bible into Latin at the end of the fourth century. Greek writing dropped precipitously in the West during the period of late antiquity, but as we have seen already in the examples of the Byzantine medical writers, it thrived in the East.[3]

The Latin of Cicero and Vergil, known as Classical Latin, was a language taught primarily to children of the elite in a school setting during the time of the Roman Empire. It has been estimated that no more than 15 percent of the Roman people were literate; that is, they knew the grammar and could read and write the language.[4] The remaining majority, however, were dependent on learning an oral form of Latin from their mothers and, consequently, Classical Latin devolved in late antiquity into what has been termed Vulgar Latin, a crude version of spoken Latin that varied from region to region in Europe. These regionally distinct versions of Vulgar Latin ultimately spawned the Romance languages (French, Spanish, Italian, Portuguese, and Romanian). Classical Latin was on its deathbed as a language desperately in need of numbers, as the number of learned men proficient in the language had decreased dramatically prior to Charlemagne's time. There was a gap between the high form of the language that the educated knew and the lower form spoken by the masses. Although the exact numbers are unknown, scholars estimate that literacy dropped to 1–2 percent during the Middle Ages.[5] Rather than promote a new written Frankish language, Charlemagne chose to emphasize his inheritance of the Roman tradition, and he may have literally saved Latin. His educational reforms, termed the *Correctio* and written in the *Epistola de litteris colendis,* "Epistle on the Cultivation of Knowledge" (785), and the *Admonitio generalis,* "General Admonition" (789), mark a turning point in the history of Latin.[6] The reforms resulted in Latin not dying out; instead, it became the dominant language in Western Europe for the next thousand years.

Charlemagne and the Church ensured that Latin would continue as the language of the intellectual elite for centuries to come. Meanwhile, the Proto-Romance languages continued to develop among the masses in different regions of Europe. Europe as a whole, therefore, was becoming increasingly multilingual. In any particular region, however, the people were bilingual and spoke a burgeoning Romance language, while Latin was used for the written word by the few who had that ability. Latin proficiency among the clerics allowed them to produce corrected versions of the Bible and other liturgical works in order to deal with concerns that the everyday Carolingian cleric jeopardized the people's relationship to God by using corrupted Latin texts. God might not answer prayers that were accompanied by readings from error-filled texts. Thus, the terms Ecclesiastical Latin and Medieval Latin, considered interchangeable by some linguists, can be applied to the Latin written during the Middle Ages. It was different from Classical Latin in many ways and similar to it in others. The main differences in the Latin written after the Carolingian Renaissance were an overall simplification of the language brought about by the addition of punctuation and spaces between words, the addition of new words resultant from the intermingling with other cultures, and the formulation of the lower case, termed Carolingian minuscule.

A long-held view is that medicine was not given the same emphasis in the Carolingian educational reforms as grammar, rhetoric, and astronomy. Evidence to support this view includes the fact that Charlemagne refused to accept the advice of medical experts and that his principal biographer, Einhard (775–840), did not view medicine favorably in his biography of Charlemagne.[7] As a result, Carolingian historians and historians of medicine alike have considered the early Middle Ages as the nadir of Western medicine.[8]

Medical care in the Carolingian Empire was studied and delivered by monks and clerics; this medieval healthcare in Germany is referred to as *Mönchsmedizin.* The landscape of the West was dominated by castles and cathedrals, and anyone who knew how to read Latin likely lived in a monastery. Educated clerics were the only keepers of the knowledge of medicine and practical medical expertise.[9] Traditional physicians were few in number and typically associated with the courts of kings, but they were also active in some cities.[10] When the Rule of St. Benedict had called for the care of the poor and infirm in 516 CE, countless monasteries sprang up all over Europe as a result of this edict. Healing of the body was entrusted to the same person who could help to heal the soul: the monks.

We have details about the "health services area" of an ideal Carolingian monastery, albeit one that was never built. The Plan of St. Gall is the only set of architectural plans to survive the Middle Ages. It has been stored in the library of the Abbey of St. Gall, Switzerland, since 830. The plans reveal a large enclosed monastery containing a cloister for the sick, a separate chapel for the sick, bathhouse for the sick, bloodletting facility, herb garden for growing medicinal herbs, and a house for the physicians, which contained a pharmacy and an area for the critically ill.[11] The Plan of St. Gall sheds light on the emphasis placed on caring for the sick by the monks of the Carolingian Empire.

Medicine was indeed a concern of Carolingian intellectuals, according to some recent erudite scholarship, and Carolingian intellectuals left medical scholarship on a firmer footing than when they found it.[12] The evidence in support of this opposing view includes the fact that numerous medical works, translated from Greek to Latin, were produced in the Carolingian scriptoria, and that Alcuin held a favorable view of doctors according to a poem (796 CE) he wrote while at Charlemagne's court:

> The doctors hurry up at once, disciples of Hippocrates,
> one taking blood from veins, another mixing herbs in a pot,
> one brewing poultices, and another serving up potions.
> And yet, doctors tend to everyone without charge,
> so that Christ may bless and guide your hands:
> of all these things I approve,
> this is an order which I can praise.[13]

Having recognized that existing hospitals were in disrepair, Charlemagne requested that new ones be built at each cathedral in his realm.[14] There is also evidence in the *Lorscher Arzneibuch* (ca. 800) that Carolingian scholars were able to conciliate medicine and theology. Also known as the Lorsch Leechbook, this book of remedies in German produced by the Benedictine monastery at Lorsch is the most important original medical text to come out of the Carolingian Empire. In addition to its dietary recommendations and remedies for different diseases, the work is most famous for its defense of medicine from a Christian standpoint. Medicine had created a theological dilemma: should humans attempt to alter the state of their bodies and go against God's plan for them? In the Lorsch Leechbook, medical work was related to God's work, and the *medicus*, while subordinate to God, was God's agent, knowledgeable about the art of medicine as created by God, and equipped with "medicinal supplies of the Earth" provided by God.[15]

Thus, medicine and theology were integrated in the ninth century, and medieval views of disease intertwined the natural with the spiritual; if God controlled nature, disease could be both divine and natural.[16] This was an extremely important step in the history of medicine. Interpretation of disease as having a moral meaning resurfaced in this period, and conditions such as bubonic plague were often viewed as punishments. Prayer and penance for sin superseded natural remedies. Taking into account the fact that the relationship between religion and medicine was sorted out during this epoch, and that many medical texts were translated from the Greek into a more medieval type of Latin at this time, we can see that the Carolingian Renaissance had many lasting benefits.

Medieval Medicine and the Church

The pockets of scholarly activity in Western Europe during the early Middle Ages were Córdoba, Ravenna, Aachen, and Anglo-Saxon England, and there was significant activity in previously unmentioned medieval Ireland. The majority of the intellectual activity in these places was more preservative than innovative. What explains the paucity of scientific and medical innovations during the period stretching from ca. 500 to 1100 CE? In no particular order, it was the decline in literacy and the scarcity of learned men; economic stagnation; the de-urbanization of the population as the people fled to the countryside for subsistence; and the destabilization brought on by frequent war and unrest.

What about the long-held view that the medieval Church suppressed intellectual development in Europe during the Middle Ages? This stance was founded by myth-driving, nineteenth-century historians who popularized the idea that the Church stifled science and medicine during this period, citing examples from the writings of the apostle Paul (5–64 CE), Tertullian (160–240 CE), Basil of Caesarea (330–79 CE), and Augustine of Hippo (354–430 CE). Since that time, a widely held view is that scientific thinkers were subdued by the Catholic Church, both by the early Church fathers as well as by the medieval Church. Science historians today contend that this view has disappeared among scholars familiar with the Middle Ages.[17] Some of the most celebrated scientific achievements in the West were made by religious scholars, and there simply was no institution that promoted the investigation of nature more than did the Church.[18] The rise of the university, to be discussed shortly, is the most crushing blow to the myth, as the university enjoyed active support of the papacy, and 30 percent of the medieval university curriculum was concerned with the natural world.[19] From 1210 to 1277, the bishops of Paris did forbid the teaching of certain Aristotelian physics principles at the University of Paris; the Condemnation of 1277 was the most extensive. Some have interpreted this as evidence of a Church assault on science. On the contrary, a fresh look at the condemnations from modern historians results in the indictment of only a few local Parisian bishops, exonerates the Church as a whole, and notes that these condemnations might even have had the paradoxical result of elevating science.[20]

The idea that the Church condemned human cadaveric dissection was actually fabricated by the nineteenth-century historian Andrew Dickson White.[21] The Church did not oppose human dissection. Instead, dissection was not performed in the early and middle medieval periods simply because no one in any culture—pagan, Jewish, Christian, or Muslim—was interested in the ghastly endeavor.[22] It was a taboo that no one would challenge. Or maybe it was due to the general undeveloped state of medical learning in the Middle Ages.[23]

The practice of human dissection, becoming more common in the fourteenth century, was spurred by the development of universities and the efforts of the freethinking Holy Roman Emperor Frederick II (1194–1250), who in 1231 issued a decree mandating a human body be dissected at least once every five years.[24] Attendance was mandatory for anyone who was to practice medicine or surgery. Brewing intellectual fervor at the medieval universities caused the surge in dissections, not the Church getting out of the way of scientific advancement.

THE MEDIEVAL CHURCH AND THE SKIN

Indeed, there is a connection between the Church and the skin: the concept of "mortification of the flesh." This was the practice by penitent Christians, guilty of sins of the flesh, to hasten the death of the body with prolonged kneeling, fasting, or abstinence from some type of food or bodily need such as intercourse. Several examples of penance involve the skin. The *hair shirt*, also known as a *cilice* or sackcloth, was a shirt traditionally made of goat hair or other irritating fabric that was designed to bring discomfort and itching to the skin. A variant made of metal chain was worn around the legs. The *discipline* was a scourge (small whip) with seven tails (for each of the seven deadly sins) used to self-flagellate the back. A *spugna* was a spiked cord device used to strike one's chest. These instruments of dermatologic self-persecution have been used since biblical times and are still used today by a tiny minority of pious Christians in various parts of the world.

The Arabic-to-Latin Translation Movement

While Avicenna was leaving an unsurpassed legacy in the Middle East, the tenth and eleventh centuries were relatively quiet in Europe in the areas of science and medicine. After the Carolingian era, the Holy Roman Empire, modern-day Italy, and the Byzantine Empire experienced a decline in erudition. The quality of medical care in Western Europe was clearly lagging behind that of the Arabic world. There was, however, an intellectual reawakening in the 1100s, and the artistic and scholarly achievements of this century have been called the "Renaissance of the 12th century." Scholars attribute several causes for this awakening after the year 1000: the improvement of living conditions and social infrastructure coupled with the advancements in wheat production, the increase in population and trade, and the urbanization of Europe. By the twelfth century, there were more people with the leisure to pursue something beyond mere survival. In addition to a revival of interest in art, architecture, and literature, as well as the rise of paper as a replacement for parchment, the twelfth century saw two significant developments pertinent to our discussion: another translation movement and the rise of the universities and medical schools.

The Greek writings of Aristotle, Ptolemy, Hippocrates, Galen, and many others had all but disappeared from Western Europe. Latin copies of these works became a priority for the newly formed universities, thus spawning another translation movement. The source material for these translations, however, was not in the original Greek—copies in that language were exceedingly scarce or non-existent. It was the Arabic translations of the classical texts that would be translated into Latin. Consequently, it can be said that the Arabic compilers and translators of the ninth and tenth centuries preserved Aristotle and Galen for posterity. Without their efforts, these most influential works surely would have been lost for all time.

The Latin translation movement was concentrated in three places: the Italian city of Salerno, the Sicilian city of Palermo, and the reconquered Muslim city of Toledo, Spain. The movement began in the eleventh century with the career of a Muslim medical scholar named Constantine the African (ca. 1020–1099) who migrated to Salerno, lectured at the university there, and finished his career at the Monte Cassino monastery established by St. Benedict. Constantine translated a wealth of Arabic books into Latin, including the Arabic collection of writings of Hippocrates and Galen. Sicily, which had been under Muslim rule from 878 to 1060, was another site where translations were produced. In Palermo, an anonymous student translated Ptolemy's *Almagest* from Greek into Latin, and Euclid's *The Elements* was likely translated into Latin by the same anonymous student at that time.[25] Toledo was the most significant city of the translation movement of the twelfth century since there was a plethora of Arabic scientific, medical, and philosophical texts in the town's libraries and private collections. Gerard of Cremona (1114–1187) was among the city's most prolific translators of the Greek classics from Arabic to Latin. Originally from Italy, Gerard went to Toledo to find a copy of Ptolemy's *Almagest*, learn Arabic, and then translate it into Latin. Gerard's endeavors in Toledo elevated that city to the most important center for the transmission of scientific knowledge between Muslims and Christians.[26] Copies of these ancient works were then disseminated all over Europe to the monasteries, universities, and individual scholars.[27] Gerard translated 87 books in his lifetime, most of which were astronomical and mathematical manuscripts. Though he is often credited with the translation of Avicenna's *Canon,* it was another Gerard of Cremona who did that work. Also known as Gerard of Sabloneta, this other Gerard of Cremona focused on medicine and translated the *Canon* of Avicenna and *Liber Almansoris* of Rhazes.[28] The meandering geographic path of the knowledge in these texts was from Alexandria to Baghdad to Cordoba to Toledo. The universities of Western Europe were the final destination of these translations and the subject to which we now turn.

The Medical School

The medieval practitioner of healthcare was essentially a monk who had learned a basic medical curriculum at a monastic or cathedral school and had provided medical care to other monks and anyone who sought help at the monastic infirmary. This was the principal type of formal healthcare in the early and High Middle Ages. The most common treatment offered by these clerics was a concoction of plants and herbs. In addition, there were various other types of healers who provided a less formal type of care. These were persons who lacked the formal training but who had learned a sort of trade, based on secret knowledge and treatment protocols that were passed down verbally from generation to generation or learned through a master-apprentice program. These healers sought monetary gain, were often women and were referred to as the "empirics"—the surgeons, midwives, wise women, apothecaries, barbers, dentists, and many others. Latin illiteracy prevented these persons from achieving a certain level of education.[29] A sick person in the Middle Ages could make the journey to a monastic infirmary and see an educated cleric, or, more commonly, he or she could see a mostly illiterate, albeit practical-minded local healer. Or the infirm could simply take their chances with prayer, often to saints, or trust in the healing powers of an amulet.

Prior to 1088, schools attached to a monastery or cathedral were responsible for educating the clerical students of Europe. Monasteries were essentially the only repositories of medical knowledge in Western Europe. The Church administered the *trivium* and *quadrivium* to the students, who had access not only to a literate monastic instructor but also to a library containing varying numbers and qualities of texts. In 1079, Pope Gregory VII issued a decree calling for an educational expansion throughout Europe, and nine years later, the first university was founded at Bologna. The universities were open to all who wanted to attend, not just prospective monks. The University of Bologna began as a school with a focus on law. In 1134, a university in Salamanca, Leon (modern-day Spain), arose from the cathedral school there. Around 1150, the University of Paris evolved from the cathedral school attached to the Notre Dame de Paris; it quickly rose to an esteemed position as a center of excellence in theology and philosophy. In 1167, the University of Oxford was instituted, followed by the Universities of Cambridge, Padua, and Montpellier in 1209, 1222, and 1289, respectively. Each of these universities is still in existence today, and the university ranks as one of the most permanent legacies of the Middle Ages.[30]

Universities developed out of the renewed appetite for knowledge that characterized the twelfth century. Philosophy, logic, natural science, medicine, and law became disciplines of interest to eager students all over Europe. Increasingly available Greek and Arabic texts in Latin translation, especially that of Aristotle, provided new source material from which to discover, digest, and debate classical knowledge in the lecture halls with the *magister* (teacher) and fellow students. Since Aristotle wrote about a myriad of subjects, a basic university education consisted of lectures and disputations on Aristotelian material. Aristotelian scholasticism, the term for this method of learning, dominated the universities for the next 500 years.

The rise of the medieval university and the possibility of a medical curriculum for students interested in a career in medicine is undoubtedly one of the most significant developments in the history of medicine in the Middle Ages. The most influential medical school of the early medieval period, *Schola Medica Salernitana,* was founded ca. 850 in Salerno (modern-day Italy). It was not a university in the modern sense—rather, it was an informal group of medical educators around whom students gathered.[31] These teachers convened to debate one another, attracted students, regularized the debates and, thus, the university is born.[32] The nearby and unrivaled library of medical texts at the Abbey of Monte Cassino provided a regional invigoration for medical learning in the ninth and tenth centuries. But even in this advanced center for medical knowledge in Western Europe, the corpus of medical information paled in comparison to what the Arabs knew and practiced. Only when Arabic medicine permeated the universities in the twelfth and thirteenth centuries did the playing field even.[33]

The medical school at Salerno reached its zenith in the eleventh century when Constantine the African arrived with his translations of Greek and Arabic medicine, infusing the school with even greater knowledge to disseminate to its students. The early medical school there influenced other schools throughout Europe; the Salernitan corpus of medical texts—Dioscorides' *De materia medica*, Hippocrates' *Aphorisms*, and several of Galen's texts—became the nucleus of the medical educational material used throughout Europe. Salernitan medicine was initially more practical than theoretical.[34] Slowly, medicine transformed from a practical, monastic pursuit to an academic and professional one. And the result was an influx of laypersons into the universities pursuing a degree in medicine. With the rise of competing medical training programs in the twelfth and thirteenth centuries at Bologna, Padua, Paris, and Montpellier, Salerno's influence waned. The number of trained physicians did increase, but they were still too few to meet the needs of the entire community, and they were located mainly in urban centers. The majority of the population of medieval Europe lived in rural areas, with the result that there was no easy access to these urban, trained professionals.

Students were required to study three years of logic prior to embarking on a five-year program of medical education. The last step was a year of practical training with an attending physician, then an examination that the student had to pass before receiving a certificate to practice medicine.[35] The students studied Latin translations of Dioscorides, Galen, Hippocrates, Avicenna, and Paul of Aegina. In

TABLE 7.1

Contents of the *Articella*

Hunayn ibn Ishaq's *Isagoge*
Hippocrates' *Aphorisms*
Hippocrates' *Prognosis*
Theophilus' *On Urines* (seventh century)[a]
Philaretus' *On Pulses* (seventh century)[a]
Galen's *Ars Medicinae*

[a] Theophilus and Philaretus are the same person.[36]

the twelfth century, a collection of Arabic medical treatises called the *Articella* (see Table 7.1), which included Constantine the African's translation of Hunayn's *Isagoge,* was bound together and used as a textbook for several hundred years.

Medicine was influenced by Aristotelian scholasticism to the same degree as was natural philosophy, theology, and astronomy; as a result, medical knowledge of this period, known as *physica*, became more theoretical, i.e., scientific—it incorporated anatomy, physiology, and pathology.[37] Dissection of animals, particularly pigs, for the purposes of teaching anatomy was a mainstay of medical education in the twelfth and thirteenth centuries. Formal human dissection for educational purposes started in the fourteenth century at the University of Bologna with the career of the illustrious Mondino de Luzzi (1270–1326), an Italian physician and professor of medicine. De Luzzi assembled the first-known dissection manual since Galen entitled *Anathomia corporis humani*, "Anatomy of the Human Body" (1316), which was used in the medical schools of Europe for the next 200 years. By the turn of the fourteenth century, the University of Bologna had earned the reputation as the premier place to study medicine in Europe. This was in large part due to a Papal bull from Nicheolas II in 1292, singling out Bologna and certifying that any doctor who trained there could practice all over the world.[38] An additional purpose for human dissection at this time was to determine the cause of death for the sake of criminal justice or public health, but the local medical men capitalized on the opportunity for learning.[39] Human dissection took place next in France at Montpellier, then spread to the northern universities in the fifteenth and sixteenth centuries.

The Hospital

The rise of the hospital can be traced back to the Middle Ages and can be studied in terms of two different areas of development: Byzantine hospitals and Islamic hospitals. In the Byzantine world, the first hospital was known in Greek as a *nosokomeion* (from which comes the word "nosocomial," referring to an infection acquired while in the hospital). The *nosokomeion* emerged in Caesarea, Cappadocia (present-day Turkey), in 372 CE under the leadership of St. Basil and was eventually called *Basileias*. Later, similar hospitals originated in Alexandria, Thessalonica, Ephesus, and Constantinople.[40] At these early hospitals, Byzantine physicians provided care for weary travelers and the needy in the spirit of a Christian charitable institution. These facilities, like their Western European monastic counterparts, served more like hospices—in our modern sense—than hospitals, i.e., people were more likely to be "saved" in the spiritual sense than cured physically.

In 1136, Byzantine Empress Irene Komnenos founded the Pantocrator of Constantinople, a hospital representing the culmination of centuries of advancement in hospital medicine. The Pantocrator featured a more secularized type of healthcare that resulted in improved outcomes, and it had a more advanced organizational structure and layout than its primitive predecessors. It contained separate areas for surgery, the chronically ill, the mentally ill, the aged, and lepers, as well as a dormitory for hospital staff, a medical school, and several chapels, and it was run by a head physician, called an *archiatros*.[41]

The Muslims created the modern idea of the hospital by borrowing some of the institutional practices from the earlier Byzantine hospitals and then increasing the size of the structure and the number of services offered in their own version. The healthcare delivered in these Islamic hospitals was superior to their European counterparts: a disease could be diagnosed, a treatment for the disease administered, and a cure achieved. Islamic hospitals were secular institutions known as *bimaristans*. An early forerunner to the modern institution was the leprosarium founded in Damascus in the eighth century, but al-Rashid established the first documented hospital in Baghdad in 805.

Western Europe continued to deliver its healthcare at monastic infirmaries and Church-sponsored hospitals well into the sixteenth century. In England, for example, healthcare of the infirm took place under Church supervision until Henry VIII dissolved the monasteries in 1540, after which hospitals such as St. Bartholomew's in London came under secular control.

Medieval Medicine versus Ancient Medicine

The humoral theory of disease attributed to Galen and the ancient Greek physicians continued to serve as the principal means by which disease was explained throughout the Middle Ages and beyond. While occasional doubts about Galen surfaced in contemporary medical writings (see the writings of Rhazes in Chapter 6), there was surprisingly little-to-no questioning about the completely conjectured and unproven theory of the four humors set forth by the ancients. Therefore, medical treatments did not differ greatly from those offered in the ancient period. Bloodletting, purging with laxatives, emetics and enemas, cupping and blistering, application of leeches, herbal and botanical medicaments, and dietary changes continued to be the mainstays of treating most medical conditions. The purpose of all these treatments was to remove any excessive humor in order to achieve balance.

There are, however, five important distinctions about medieval medicine that differentiate it from ancient medicine. The first involves the rise of Christianity and the influence of religious belief on medical practice. Disease was often attributed to God's wrath as a punishment for sin or moral depravity, and prayer was a very powerful intervention in the healing process during this period, as it still is today. There were patron saints of diseases—hemorrhoids, headaches, etc.—to whom one could pray in addition to, or instead of, seeing a *medicus* or healer. The success rate of the available medical options could not have been high; prayer, in many cases, was simply a better option. A pilgrimage to a holy place or shrine in search of holy water or some relic was another option. In many cases, the medical professional supported and believed the idea that prayer and pilgrimage could lead to a cure. The Church had effectively taken over the medical care of Western Europe for the better part of the Middle Ages. Care of the sick was a mission of the Church; at a time when the expectation of success for a given treatment was undoubtedly low, saving the soul was every bit as important, if not more important, as saving the person's life. After all, the body was merely a container for the soul.[42]

THE PATRON SAINTS OF SKIN DISEASE

St. Bartholomew the Apostle is one of two patron saints of skin disease. The first-century legend about Bartholomew, an apostle of Jesus Christ, is that Bartholomew cured the daughter of an Armenian king, who subsequently converted to Christianity. Fearing retribution from the Romans, the king's brother had Bartholomew martyred with flaying followed by decapitation. Renaissance artists, including Michelangelo, depicted Bartholomew holding his own flayed skin in his hands. He was also revered as a protector against plague. The association of Bartholomew with skin is the basis for the claim that the saint is a patron of skin diseases and those who treat them. St. Anthony is the other patron saint of skin disease, and the veneration of St. Anthony by skin disease sufferers is described in Interlude 2.

The second major difference between medieval medicine and ancient medicine is the influence of astrology on medical practice. The astrological considerations in medicine that started in ancient times actually peaked late in the medieval period (fifteenth century) and thrived until the end of the seventeenth century. The medieval physician typically consulted astrological tables to predict whether a treatment administered at a certain time and to a specific part of the body was indicated or contraindicated. The "Zodiac Man" was a diagram that showed which zodiac symbol dominated which part of the body. For example, Aries dominated the head, and when the moon was in the "house" of Aries, it was potentially deadly to treat the head.[43] Phlebotomy could only be offered if the moon was in a particular constellation. Herbs and plants were offered if they were collected at times when certain affiliated planets were visible in the sky. The zodiac sign of a birth month could also predict which part of a person's body might be affected by disease and what type of humor dominated. These are just a few examples of the power of astrology to dictate the treatment plan. Tables containing this information were found in a handbook called a *vade mecum,* "go with me," which were carried by the physician for quick reference.[44]

Third, the Middle Ages saw greatly increased use of two diagnostic techniques that were founded by the ancients but became more commonplace in the medieval period: uroscopy and pulse checking. The former involved the close inspection of the urine to assess the patient for disease. Uroscopy became more widely used after the publication of *De urinis*, "On Urines," by the Byzantine physician Theophilus in the seventh century, a practice that Constantine the African resurrected in the eleventh century. The urine was placed in a urine flask called a *matula*, and the patient's diagnosis and prognosis were determined by comparing the specimen to a chart containing 20 different gradations of color. The medieval physician would also inspect the urine for sediment, pus, blood, and other substances. Uroscopy remained a mainstay of diagnostic procedure until the Renaissance, when its value was finally questioned. By the seventeenth century, uroscopy fell completely out of favor with physicians; those who continued to practice it were called charlatans, mountebanks, or quacks.

The medieval physician used the knowledge handed down from Galen to assess the patient by taking the pulse. While today the physician focuses on rate and strength of pulse, the medieval physician, without a yet-invented clock, cared less about quantity and more about quality. He characterized the quality of the pulse using animal analogies in order to infer the patient's temperament, humoral imbalance, and diagnosis. For example, a slithering, snake-like pulse indicated a melancholic temperament, while a phlegmatic person had a pulse that "will glide smoothly as a swan, slow, soft, and deep."[45] This type of discussion could be found in many of the major medical texts of the Middle Ages under the chapter heading *De pulsibus.*

The next major distinction is the increasing awareness of the contagiousness of disease. During the Middle Ages, laypersons and physicians alike believed that foul air emitted by a diseased person (breath) or object (e.g., stinky dung heap, carcass, or butcher's waste) was capable of causing disease in a person by breathing, contact with the skin pores, or simply gazing at the source. This theory of disease transmission is termed "miasma theory," from the Greek word for pollution. Miasma was considered to be the principal culprit for the Black Death. Lepers, by law, were supposed to stand upwind of a person so that their foul air could not emanate downwind on a person.[46] Medical writings of the period described several diseases, such as lepra, scabies, and smallpox, as contagious. While germ theory did not exist until the nineteenth century, medieval physicians deserve more credit than they have been given for at least recognizing that disease could be spread from person to person—something that was not emphasized by the ancients.

The last major development in medieval medicine that distinguishes it from ancient medicine is the rise of the barber-surgeon and the beginnings of scope-of-practice conflicts between physicians and surgeons and barbers. Surgical procedures were performed in ancient times, and the ancient medical writers wrote about surgery. But over the course of the first millennium, a delineation between physicians and surgeons developed to the point that physicians dealt with internal problems and surgeons dealt with external ones. Surgeons of the early Middle Ages underwent no formal training; instead, they learned their trade through a master-apprentice program. They were looked down upon by their physician brethren.

Around the turn of the first millennium, the barbers began encroaching on the surgeon's field of practice. The first barbers were men hired by monasteries to trim the hair of monks (tonsure). The barber's skill with sharp instruments, coupled with papal decrees against churchmen spilling blood, soon created opportunities for barbers to do other procedures traditionally performed by surgeons: paring of warts and calluses, application of leeches, cupping, draining of boils, and pulling of teeth. Bloodletting remained one of the principal therapeutic methods for treating skin diseases and was performed by both barbers and surgeons. They opened a vein or veins with instruments such as a lancet, a fleam, or a scarificator. The blood would run out into a small ceramic bowl, and the barber would taste and smell the blood as a means of determining the diagnosis. Later, both barbers and surgeons could be found on the battlefields of Europe, tending to the maimed and performing amputations.

In England, the barbers organized into the Worshipful Company of Barbers (founded in 1308, royal charter in 1462). The surgeons organized into the Guild of Surgeons in 1368. Eventually, the two groups merged into one in 1540 when Henry VIII, through royal charter, established the Company of Barber-Surgeons. The Barber-Surgeons placed a red, white, and blue pole outside of their establishments in order to advertise their trade. The red symbolized blood, the blue, the veins, and the white, the tourniquet. In an effort to gain control of the barbers and surgeons, the physicians organized in 1518 with the establishment of the Royal College of Physicians. The surgeons tried for 200 years to disconnect from the barbers, and they finally succeeded in 1745, during the reign of George II. Soon after the breakaway, John Hunter, the father of modern surgery, would elevate the discipline into a scientific specialty. In 1800, the Royal College of Surgeons was formed and still exists today.

There were regional differences in Europe between these groups. In France, at the College of St. Cosmas (a patron saint of physicians and surgeons), founded in 1210, there existed a complicated arrangement of the physicians, surgeons, and barbers, each struggling for turf. The confusion lasted until 1516, when the surgeons surrendered to the physicians so both could unite against the barbers.[47] In the German states, the barber-surgeons were unified, as they were in England, but not in Italy, Spain, and southern France.[48]

The barber-surgeon was second class to the physician throughout the Middle Ages everywhere in Europe, and every effort was made to ensure that the barber-surgeon could perform procedures only with a prescription from a physician. This arrangement would remain in place until the nineteenth century. In addition to these scope-of-practice issues, the Middle Ages saw the development of licensure and certification practices for these healthcare providers, with variable regulations throughout Europe. Regardless of these technical distinctions, the surgeons were the practical doers of medieval medicine; the physicians, the learned thinkers.

Skin Disease in the Middle Ages

Skin disease was "astonishingly prevalent" in the Middle Ages.[49] It is impossible to refute that claim, when one considers the single change of clothes, poor hygiene, extreme poverty, and abject filth in which the majority of Europeans found themselves. Scabies, herpes, tineas, head and body lice, staphylococcal and streptococcal infection (boils, cellulitis, erysipelas), and venereal diseases were just a few of the rampant skin problems faced in the medieval era. The extensive wardrobes often taken for granted today were indeed limited in this age. But lack of clean clothing was not the main problem that led to a prevalence of skin disease in the Middle Ages; in Western Europe at least, it is commonly believed that it was the non-prioritizing of a regular bath, rooted in the Christian tradition, that promoted skin disease:

> Jesus' indifference towards ritual purity accorded with what became a wider Christian distrust or neglect of the body. Somewhat paradoxically, the Jewish purity laws, especially at the time of Christ, emphasized the body's importance: the purity or impurity of the body at any given moment was a significant matter. Within a few hundred years of Christ's death, Christianity had gone in a different direction. It discounted the body as much as possible, devaluing the flesh so as to concentrate on the spirit.[50]

St. Jerome, in a letter on hermetic living, stressed that the baptismal bath was the only bath Christians needed when he wrote, "Is your skin rough and scaly because you no longer bathe? He that is once washed in Christ needs not to wash again."[51] Not only did the Christian Church ignore personal hygiene in its doctrine—unlike the Jewish and Muslim traditions which stressed it—the Church opposed bathing in public facilities because it often led to temptations of hedonism and generated concerns of both pride and sensuality.

There were also concerns about a weakening effect on the body from bathing at temperatures greater than that of the body itself.[52] In the wake of the Black Death, bathing fell under suspicion as a risky enterprise for acquiring disease.[53] Bathing in hot water in particular, which was believed to open the pores of the skin, could allow disease to enter the body through the skin. As a result of these issues, being clean was not at the top of the list of priorities of the medieval Western Christian. And with the constant exposure to filth and malodor—think of the chamber pot dumped onto the street as one passed by—you can almost imagine the average medieval person thinking, "what's the point of cleanliness?" Lastly, baths were not readily available. While the aristocracy may have had access to baths—in bathhouses or at home—the peasant class did not and had to resort to washing in natural sources of water such as streams and rivers. Bathing again fell under suspicion in the sixteenth century with the rise of syphilis and was not revived as a healthy habit until the nineteenth century (see Chapter 12).

Such are the commonly held beliefs about hygiene in the medieval period. However, recent scholarship has called into question this stereotype about medieval Christian peoples:

> Certainly, medieval Europeans did not bathe or launder their clothes as frequently as we do today. But that does not mean that they preferred being dirty or were oblivious to the benefits of good hygiene. Rather, the generally low level of personal hygiene, especially when compared to modern standards, can be attributed more to the limited facilities available for washing and the attendant inconvenience of using them than to any cultural bias against cleanliness or any ignorance of its benefits. This conclusion is supported by many surviving medieval tracts on health and numerous illustrations and records of everyday life.[54]

Yet, in a world without readily available soap, antiseptic cleansers, and laundry detergent, it was indeed commonplace for the people of the Middle Ages to suffer from a variety of skin conditions. Only healthcare workers who care for the homeless population of today can come close to appreciating the severity of the skin problems faced by a typical medieval person. In addition to skin diseases brought about by poor hygiene and resultant skin infection, such as impetigo and scabies, both benign and malignant ulcers were rampant problems. Cancer of the breast, for example, which presents today as a lump confirmed by mammography, presented in medieval times as an ulcerated lesion on the skin of the breast, due to the advancement of disease in a setting of no available means to diagnose and treat the problem in its early stages. Similarly, skin cancer likely presented in a very advanced state. Without vaccines, viral exanthems such as measles, varicella, and smallpox were commonly dealt with and frequently written about. Thus, the majority of conditions described in the skin disease sections of medieval medical texts were either infectious or neoplastic by nature.

The classical idea of the function of the skin as a protective covering for the structures underneath it thrived well into the Middle Ages. Discoveries during this period concerning the skin were few and far between. In the anatomical discussions throughout the period, there was a relative inattentiveness to the skin, and no texts were produced that focused primarily on the skin or skin disease. Before the thirteenth century, the skin was a structure not to be tampered with, as it was taboo to cut it open to investigate the interior structures of the human body. When human anatomic dissection became a more common practice, the skin was viewed as covering that was in the way, something to be passed through and pushed aside in order to get to the more important targets of the dissecting instruments.

In addition to its main function as a protective covering, later medieval writers eventually rediscovered the sensory functions and excretory functions of the skin—ridding the body of wastes, toxins, humors, and moisture—and the idea that the blockage of the excretory passages could lead to disease. To the late medieval physician, the skin was a patent membrane, which could be traversed in two directions, and it was responsible for health by means of the excretion of sweat and deleterious humors.[55] Moreover, the skin's color, temperature, and texture were viewed as guides to temperament (see Table 7.2).

A given temperament was considered a risk factor for certain types of diseases as well as an indicator of personality traits. Temperament ordinarily changed throughout life: infants were sanguine; youth, bilious; adults, melancholic; and the elderly, phlegmatic. Temperament could also change in certain disease

TABLE 7.2

Skin Temperature and Hydration as a Reflection of
Temperament and Humoral Imbalance

Temp/Hydration	Temperament	Imbalanced Humor
Warm/moist	Bilious	Yellow bile
Warm/dry	Sanguine	Blood
Cold/moist	Phlegmatic	Phlegm
Cold/dry	Melancholic	Black bile

states, and examination of the skin was one important way of determining a person's given diagnosis. For example, warm, moist skin signaled a sanguine temperament, which would lead the medieval physician to a differential diagnosis of conditions associated with excessive blood, which would, in turn, be managed with phlebotomy. Although it is obvious to modern physicians that bloodletting would be a huge mistake for a warm, moist patient in the throes of a fever, the above discussion of temperament was the sensible, rational approach in the mind of the medieval physician for this type of therapeutic action. However, in other cases, assumptions made about the appearance of the skin were more prejudicial than rational, as skin changes could also indicate defects in a person's moral or spiritual purity.[56]

Hildegard of Bingen (1098–1179)

Medieval Western medical writers did devote some energy to expositions on skin disease in their treatises. In the following sections, we will review the main contributors to the history of dermatology in the Middle Ages, starting with two medieval heroines. Although many women responded to the Rule of Benedict in caring for the sick at monasteries throughout Europe, while others served as secular healers and midwives, there was no opportunity afforded to women to get the medical education needed to reach the status of a learned *medicus* or *physicus*. As a result, female medical writers during the Middle Ages were rare. Women learned medicine by doing it, men by reading about it.[57] In the Renaissance of the twelfth century, however, two women demonstrated their knowledge and expertise in the medical field and left works for us to study and appreciate. Hildegard of Bingen and Trota of Salerno wrote engrossing medical compendiums that provide us with a fascinating inside look at medieval medicine at a monastery and a university, and they offer us a glimpse into the way in which several skin diseases were understood and managed in the Middle Ages.

Hildegard of Bingen is one of the most famous and extraordinary women of the Middle Ages. A German abbess who founded and served at monasteries in Rupertsberg and Eibingen, Hildegard is famous for having divine visions that she shared with her peers and incorporated into numerous Christian philosophical tracts. Interestingly, medical historians question whether these episodic "visions" could be epileptic fits or migraine auras.[58] She was also a prolific poet, playwright, and composer, and she wrote one text, *Lingua ignota*, "Unknown language," in an undecipherable code. Her renown inspired pilgrimages from all over Europe to Eibingen, where her counsel was sought in spiritual as well as medical matters. With her scientific mind and impressive knowledge of medicine, she recorded two major medical works between 1151 and 1158: the first was entitled *Physica*, a treatise on natural history containing the medicinal value of numerous plants, animals, and minerals; the other, *Causae et curae*, "Causes and Cures," a comprehensive overview of various diseases and treatments, "shown by God." The former is a work organized by treatment, the latter organized by ailment. English translations are available for both works.[59]

Physica contains chapters on plants, elements, trees, stones, fish, birds, animals, reptiles, and minerals. The book is therefore considered one of the first texts on natural history. The medicinal value of hundreds of items is described, and the ailment for which the item is most useful is discussed. In many cases, the target condition is a dermatological one, i.e., wheat is helpful for dog bites; rye is appropriate for scabies of the head; barley is for hard and rough skin; and lily is effective against both white leprosy and red leprosy. While there are doubts raised today about the efficacy of these concoctions, Hildegard's formula for essential oil of violet is still used in Germany today and has been shown to inhibit cyclooxy-genase, *NF-KB*, and other inflammatory mediators implicated in psoriasis.[60] Nightshade, which she sug-gested for ulcers, has been shown to have anti-inflammatory, proangiogenic, and collagen-remodeling effects.[61] Modern appraisals of medieval medicine are typically skeptical to the point of dismissal, but it is safe to say that at least some of Hildegard's concoctions actually worked.

Causae et curae is not just a medical treatise; Hildegard shared her worldview and cosmology in it and then incorporated disease into her larger understanding of the world around her. She attributed diseases to humoral imbalances and noted many of them to be more common in persons with certain personal-ity types or with moral and spiritual shortcomings. Her approach is one of an independent thinker. Her therapeutic armamentarium was principally composed of herbal and botanical ingredients used to cor-rect these imbalances, but she also included useful animals and minerals. Monastic medical providers cultivated herbs with medicinal value in the garden of the monastery, and Hildegard had an impressive knowledge of the healing power of these plants. She covered a wide variety of maladies, from the stench of the breath to swelling of the testicles to yawning, and she has a few topics of dermatologic interest, e.g., eczema, lice, and leprosy. Her entry on *scabies* reveals an extensive knowledge about skin disease:

> If bad humors have erupted in eczema over his entire body, a person should wait for them to fully develop and ooze out. When the skin between the sores begins to redden and to dry out, he should smear it with appropriate ointments lest, if he waited longer, the skin would develop greater distress from the ulcers and rotten matter.[62]

She recommended sulfur ointment applied for five days, which the modern dermatologist knows is an effective treatment for modern scabies.

Lice, according to Hildegard, commonly infested people with thin marrow and resulting thin fat, and because their skin was more porous, sweat passed more easily through the skin, giving rise to many lice.[63] Lice sometimes do not emerge from the skin and instead eat a person from within. Leprosy can result from three causes: gluttony and drunkenness, anger, or lust; the first leads to red swellings and red blisters, the second causes the skin to blacken and split down to the bones, the last type causes ulcers on red skin.[64] She treated hair loss in young men with bear fat mixed with ash from wheat. Tinea capitis resulted from gnawing worms.[65] For erysipelas, she prescribed crushed flies, which were to be spread around the affected area, then a crushed, shell-less red snail around the fly layer, and finally lily sap encircling the snail layer.[66] She also wrote about scrofula, ulcers, and worms. Finally, there is some sug-gestion that Hildegard correctly identified a burrowing organism as the cause of scabies; she used the term *gracillimi vermiculi*—which translates as "thinnest tiny worm"—in the *Physica* entry on horsemint and discusses similar parasites in other parts of the text.[67]

Hildegard's medical writings impress with the way in which her medical views fit snuggly into her cosmology, and she wrote with the same authoritative, matter-of-fact tone as any other medieval medi-cal writer. Hildegard of Bingen deserves to be honored for many diverse accomplishments; for our dis-cussion, she is to be remembered as the first woman to write about skin diseases. It was not until 2012 that Hildegard received official recognition from the Catholic Church when Benedict XVI declared her "Doctor of the Church." Though she was never officially canonized, she is often regarded as St. Hildegard.

Trota of Salerno (Eleventh to Twelfth Century) and *The Trotula*

Trota of Salerno is a mysterious, acclaimed person for whom there are few historical details concern-ing her life and career. She is important because she is deemed by many to be one of the first female physicians in history. Some scholars consider her to be the first female professor of medicine at Salerno and responsible for the most important text on women's medicine in the Middle Ages: the eponymous "Trotula." Other critics insist that this work was written by a man; still others believe that *Trotula* is simply the title of the book and does not refer to a person.[68] But there are records of a female physician who was active in Salerno around 1050 named Trocta de Ruggiero.[69] She was married to a physician and the mother of two sons, both physicians. She was an authority for her contemporaries and so famous in the two centuries that followed her life that Chaucer mentioned her in his prologue to the *Wife of Bath's* tale.[70] Exactly which of the manuscripts that are attributed to Trota were actually written by this person is a matter of scholarly debate. One of those manuscripts, *De curis mulierum,* "On Treatments for Women," has been attributed to someone named Trota, which was a commonly used woman's name in medieval Italy. Green, the preeminent expert on this puzzling work, wrote that Trota has as much claim to the authorship as her Salernitan contemporaries.[71] The other two, *Liber de sinthomatibus mulierum,* "Book on the Conditions of Women," and *De ornatu mulierum,* "On Women's Cosmetics," may have been written by a Salernitan colleague or colleagues.

The *Trotula* follows Greco-Roman humoral theory but is heavily influenced by Arabic medicine of the Islamic Golden Age.[72] The dermatology of the *Trotula* is focused entirely on skin diseases faced by women. Vaginal itching and excoriation of the pudenda are treated with specific unguents. Lice of the underarms and pubic area are managed with ashes and oil, while lice of the eyelids can be eradicated with aloe, white lead, frankincense, and bacon.[73] For scabies, an ointment composed of oil, vinegar, and quicksilver is described. The *Trotula* also has extensive information on whitening the face, reddening the face, freckles, fissures of the lips, and warts—all of which were apparently important cosmetic issues for women at this time. For wrinkles, a medieval version of a chemical peel is suggested: apply stinking iris to the face at bedtime and expect in the morning that the skin will swell; then apply an ointment of lily root, and the skin will peel and appear "delicate."[74] Unwanted redness of the face can be managed with leeches applied to the nose and ears bilaterally. Skin cancer is treated with an ointment consisting of frankincense, mastic, wax, oil, Greek pitch, galbanum, aloe, wormwood, mugwort, pellitory-of-the-wall, rue, and sage; however, the alternative application to the cancer of wild ivy leaves, cooked in wine, makes more sense to the modern dermatologist familiar with topical immunotherapy.[75] Cancer of the nose is managed with another specific powder. For feigning virginity, leeches can be applied inside the vagina the night before the marriage. In the brief section on cosmetics, there are recipes for depilatories, different agents for blackening/whitening/goldening/thickening/curling the hair, as well as remedies for thickness of the lips, roughness of the face from sun or wind, and sunburn. There is an ointment good for both covering the face blemished from mourning the dead and for the pustules of lepers.

The most peculiar dermatologic entry is entitled "On Itch-mites of the Hands and Feet," suggesting there was some knowledge about the scabies mite:

> For contracting the worm from the hands and feet, that is, the itch mite, which in English is called *degge*, take a heated brick and any kind of vessel full of water, and afterward let henbane seed be placed upon the burning brick. And let the patient hold her feet above the smoke, and you will see the worms falling into the water just like hairs.[76]

Scabies mites falling into water would not look like hairs, however. The mite is a pinpoint 0.4 mm in size and round. Trota's "worm" from the description sounds closer to cutaneous larva migrans, a condition in which a worm larva migrates through the epidermis. In the cosmetics section, itch mite is again the translation used in reference to itch mites eating the hairs. Medieval medical writers did not think a mite was responsible for tinea, but thought it was caused by little worms. Regardless of these translational difficulties, Trota and her colleagues appear to have been well versed in the idea of parasitic skin disease and may have known of the itch mite.

Skin Disease and the Medieval Surgeon

The careers of several important medieval surgeons in Italy, England, and France deserve special treatment for their minor or, in some cases, major contributions to the study of skin disease. Many medieval surgeons wrote extensively about skin diseases in their surgical treatises, but only a select few will be highlighted here. Roger of Palermo (ca. 1140–1195), also known as Rogerius or Roger of Salerno, was a twelfth-century Italian surgeon and a product of the medical school of Salerno. He authored an important medieval surgical text entitled *Practica chirurgia* (ca. 1180), the first major surgical text of the Middle Ages in the West. His main contributions were his recognition that some genital ulcers were sexually transmitted, his recommendation of topical mercurial salves for skin diseases, and for being the first to coin the term *lupus* (Latin, "wolf").[77]

THE ORIGIN OF THE WORD *LUPUS*

The Rogerian meaning of the word *lupus* thrived through the eighteenth century; it originally referred to ulcerated skin lesions of the lower limbs that resembled the bite of the wolf and that were differentiated from and often confused with what was referred to as *cancer*—similarly ulcerated lesions, but of the face.[78] In the Middle Ages, *noli me tangere* (touch me not) became an all-encompassing word for ulcerating lesions of the face, including what we today call skin cancer, lupus vulgaris, discoid lupus, and destructive lesions of syphilis. In 1851, the word *lupus* was revived by Cazenave, who first coined *lupus erythematosus* (see Chapter 13) for a non-ulcerating, scaly facial lesions (known today as discoid lupus); and by Willan, whose description of lupus Willani (lupus of Willan) matches the diagnosis later known as *lupus vulgaris*—the common type of lupus (see Interlude 1). In both of these latter cases, the author may have chosen lupus to reflect the sunken facial appearance of the patient resembling the face of a wolf, instead of the bite of the wolf.

The Italian Teodorico Borgognoni (1206–1296) was probably the most famous surgeon of the thirteenth century. A product of the medical school in Bologna, Borgognoni's greatest achievement in medicine was the four-volume *Cyrurgia* (1267), a revolutionary surgical text that challenged many of the prevailing beliefs of the time. In that work can be found this landmark quote:

> It is not necessary, as Roger (Frugardi of Salerno) and Roland (Capelluto of Parma) have written, as many of their disciples teach and as all modern surgeons profess, that pus should be generated in wounds. No error can be greater than this. Such a practice is indeed to hinder Nature, to prolong the disease and to prevent conglutination and consolidation of the wound.[79]

Borgognoni was the first to challenge the concept of "laudable pus," which refers to a misconception dating back to the time of Hippocrates that the presence of pus in a wound, especially yellow-white, thick pus, was a good sign and encouraged by the surgeon. While it is certainly better to have pus in a wound than the pus-less gangrenous changes of a severe necrotizing infection, the presence of pus, except in the case of inflamed sebaceous cysts or pyoderma gangrenosum, is generally a sign of infection and not something to "laud." Borgognoni opined that wounds should be kept dry and free of ointments and no effort is to be made to encourage pus accumulation. The fourteenth-century French surgeon Henri de Mondeville (see below) and the sixteenth-century French surgeon Ambroise Pare (see Chapter 8) also questioned the concept of laudable pus in their major surgical texts, but the medical community ignored their arguments, and pus continued to be "praiseworthy" until the nineteenth century when the work of Semmelweis, Pasteur, and Lister dispelled the myth forever (see Chapter 11).[80]

Gilbertus Anglicus (ca. 1180–1250) was an English physician about whom we have little biographical data, but he was a renowned physician both during his life and for several centuries afterward. Geoffrey Chaucer (ca. 1340–1400) included him in a list of famous physicians—many of whom are recognized in this present work—in the prologue to his *Canterbury Tales:*

> Wel knew he the olde Esculapius
> And Deyscorides and eek Rufus,
> Olde Ypocras, Haly and Galyen,
> Serapion, Razis and Avycen,
> Averrois, Damascien and Constantyn,
> Bernard and Gatesden and Gilbertyn.[81]

Gilbertus authored a comprehensive medieval medical overview called *Compendium Medicinae* (ca. 1240). This encyclopedic series consists of seven books and contains an important chapter on leprosy and measles, and he also discussed smallpox, a disease that he knew was contagious and for which he advocated steam baths and red coverings (see Interlude 4). The second book contains a discussion of skin diseases ordered *a capite ad pedes* (from head to toe).[82] Gilbertus noted that the hair is "a dry fume (fumus siccus), escaping from the body through the pores of the scalp and condensed by contact with the air into long, round cylinders."[83] Hair color is determined by humors: "red hair arises from unconsumed blood or bile; white hair, from an excess of phlegm; black hair, from the abundance of black-bile (melancholia), etc."[84] Gilbertus offered remedies for dyeing hair or removing it, and for the destruction of vermin on the hair. He delineated recipes for three different soaps with medicinal value. Among the skin conditions given attention in *Compendium Medicinae* were alopecia, dandruff (furfur), tinea, caries, favus and achor, rosacea, morphoea, and scabies.[85]

Gilbertus acknowledged that sometimes the physician is asked to advise the patient on cosmetic concerns. In a chapter entitled *De ornatu capillorum* "On the adornment of the hair," he wrote:

> The adornment of the hair affords to women the important advantages of beauty and convenience; and as women desire to please their husbands, they devote themselves to adornment and protect themselves from the charge of carelessness. In order, therefore, that our ministry may not be depreciated, and that we may not render ourselves liable to the accusation of ignorance, let us add a few words on the subject of the dressing of the hair and the general care of the person.[86]

Gilbertus advised ladies seeking a charming or youthful appearance to use steam baths to open the pores and soften the skin followed by drying the skin with a fine cloth; the cheeks could then be reddened with a lotion of brazilwood soaked in rose water, or if excessively red, blanched with the root of the cyclamen.[87] His text is complete with remedies for freckles, moles, warts, wrinkles, other blemishes, and for foul breath and body odor.[88] The text even contains a long chapter entitled *De sophisticatione vulvae* that contains detailed information on vulvar esthetics and techniques to feign virginity. Gilbertus apologized in advance of the chapter, not because of modesty, but because he was aware his information could be used for the purposes of deceit.

PETRARCH AND BOCCACCIO'S SCABIES

The father of humanism (see Chapter 8), Francesco Petrarch (1304–1374), then 61 years of age, once wrote a letter to his friend Giovanni Boccaccio (1313–1375), author of *The Decameron*, complaining about his scabies. At the time, this could have meant a scabby, itchy skin eruption, such as modern scabies, but could have also referred to dermatitis, eczema, impetigo, or many other dermatoses.[89] For five months, he could barely use his hands for any purpose other than to scratch.[90] Petrarch commented on the dangerousness of scabies, and it is correct, as we know that scratching unclean skin can lead to staphylococcal bacteria entering the body leading to sepsis and death.[91] In 1373, Boccaccio wrote to another friend about his own experience with the itchy disease, which caused him to scratch all day and to scratch himself to sleep every night.[92] One wonders if Boccaccio did not acquire the illness from Petrarch, or if the condition was just that rampant in fourteenth-century post–Black Death Italy and its still-crowded, unsanitary cities.

Henri de Mondeville (1260–1320)

Two French surgeons from the fourteenth century deserve some attention as they were the last of the important figures from the Middle Ages who contributed in part to the history of dermatology. Together their work is a sort of final summary of medieval medical knowledge, especially as it relates to skin disease. The first was Henri de Mondeville. He was born in Normandy and received medical training at both Montpellier and Paris, later spending some time under Theodoric Borgognoni. Mondeville's credentials were unusual for the time period. While he was a true physician surgeon, he later served as professor of anatomy and surgery at Montpellier, where he conducted the university's first unsanctioned human dissection in 1315. He was eventually employed as a royal surgeon for the Capetian monarchy. Henry started—but never finished—a landmark treatise on surgery in Latin called *La Chirurgie* in 1306. Mondeville earned recognition for using *Chirurgie* to elevate the field of surgery, and it was the book's groundbreaking illustrations that did so more than the text itself. Thirteen high-quality illustrations, typical in this era only for religious texts and intellectual treatises, simultaneously complemented the text and enlightened its surgeon readers.[93]

Mondeville had antithetical views that were rejected by his colleagues, but his views proved to be ahead of their time. While in the service of the king's army, Mondeville first cleaned wounds with wine and then applied bandages soaked with wine, but a few days later, applied an antiseptic plaster made of plantain, betony, ache [celery], resin, wax, and turpentine along with a large dry compress over the dressing as a whole.[94] It would take 600 years for his efforts to finally be appreciated with the advent of modern antiseptic techniques.

Mondeville's section on leeches gives us an inside look into this peculiar practice. Leeches were used for the same reason as cupping and phlebotomy: to reset humoral balance by removing blood from the body. He points out that leeches remove blood from deeper in the body than cupping, but not as deep as phlebotomy. Their application is useful not only in the treatment of several skin diseases, but also in cancer, delirium, and depression. Mondeville noted that one should select leeches as slender as a rat's tail and avoid feeding the leeches for 24 hours prior to their use.[95]

La Chirurgie extensively addresses skin disease, as there was an agreement between physicians and surgeons in the Middle Ages that the surgeon was restricted to dealing with external problems, and, therefore, a medieval surgical textbook needed to have a lengthy section on skin disease. Mondeville grudgingly included two chapters on cosmetics, as he believed that cosmetics were fraudulent in that they hid something and had nothing to do with God, justice, or illness.[96] For men, the cosmetic issues Mondeville covered are excessive redness (treated with leeches and cupping), pale areas, sunburn and windburn, dark and unsightly blemishes, unwanted hair, and lack of facial hair (except in the case of eunuchs). He did note playfully that a surgeon who develops good skills in the cosmetic field could become very popular with women, noting that a woman's favor "is more desirable than the good favor of the Pope or of the Lord."[97]

With a misogynist stance and tone typical for his epoch, Mondeville, on the embellishment of women, discussed sweat boxes, massages, baths, and a few ointments and lotions.[98] He advised against using camphor in contrast to his contemporaries who recommended it, because it could thwart the libido in men. After a brief discussion of vaginal rejuvenation and depilatory methods, Mondeville described the way women could prevent enlargement of the breasts—at the time an embarrassing thing—and the eradication of lice from the armpits. He explained how women could clean, color, and scent the hair, stating that strawberry-blonde is the most popular and desirable color. He cautions surgeons who might take on the task of dealing with a woman's face, noting that even the most beautiful women are not content with their beauty. He offered guidance on blemishes, wrinkles, foul odors in the woman's nose, and bad breath.

Mondeville addressed scabies and itch, which to him were two different conditions. Although he was unaware of the itch mite, he did appreciate scabies as a contagious illness, and he also noted the toxic effects of mercury used to treat it. His understanding of miasma theory as an explanation for contagious disease is fascinating: morbid matter under the skin is expelled through the skin into the air, which is contaminated with "malignant fumes."[99]

Mondeville then exhibited disdain toward the chaos in the nomenclature for skin diseases among the Greek, Roman, and Arabic medical writers:

> In respect of these lesions and many others, the authorities contradict each other as to the definitions, the treatments, etc. First came the Greeks, including Hippocrates, Galen, and Constantine, followed by the Arabs, including Avicenna, Rhazes, Serapion, et al., and then the Latin writers of Salerno and all the others who until the present have dealt with the questions. I have not to find

two of them in complete agreement about these infections [skin disorders]. It is almost as if they agree to disagree. One cannot take from them a single 'true fact' because what one calls serpigo, another calls impetigo, and a third says pannus. A fourth names one as a subset of another and insists on the same treatment for both. A fifth says that there are three categories of impetigo, each requiring a different treatment. They deal with morphea and its ilk in the same way, or with even more vague arguments. So it is that we must be skeptical about what any single author or a single practitioner says, something that may contradict or give incomplete information.[100]

In an attempt to clear up some of the confusion, Mondeville offered his own classification of skin diseases of the face—which he called infections but could also have been translated as blemishes or alterations: infections within the skin only, within the subcutaneous layer, involving both the skin and subcutaneous layer, involving the bone as well as overlying skin and subcutaneous layers, and infections between the skin and subcutaneous layer.[101] While Mondeville's primitive classification system has largely been ignored, it was possibly the first system from a dermatopathological point of view.

Other notable observations from Mondeville's skin disease section include his comment that comedos are called *verbles* in French, which is the word for maggot, because of the appearance of the emitted material upon squeezing them. This analogy of worms or maggots for comedones will return again in the seventeenth-century discussion of *Morgellons* (see Chapter 9). He added further to the confusion in his discussion on morphea, which was either modern-day vitiligo, tuberculoid leprosy, or, in some cases, what we think of today as the condition known as morphea (which was named after the Greek shape-shifting god, Morpheus). He called leprosy a shameful disease that is more of a medical than a surgical disease. His description of the face of the leper was, according to Pusey, unequaled before or since.[102]

Mondeville clearly had a unique interest in skin disease compared to his peers. He refers to winter itch as *salt-phlegm* and miliaria as *night-sweats*. He echoes Aristotle in that lice are spontaneously generated from the skin, explaining that the two outer layers of the skin give rise to the carapace of the organism. He describes the differences between warts and *porreaux* (seborrheic keratosis). He wrapped up the section with another brilliant exposition on the confusion of the disease names and a philosophical point about the unnecessity of knowing the names of diseases:

> How important is it to know that *dartre* and *impetigo* are not the same things, especially when we treat both of them with the same ointments? Does it annoy you that certain infections of the skin and subcutaneous tissues are alike or different, since you usually treat all of them with the same corrosive ointments and a few other things?[103]

He repeated his frustration again later in the text when he talks about aposthems (see below) and the lack of agreement on how they should be managed.[104] It is easy to see how confused Mondeville and other medieval surgeons might have felt with all the conflicting information in the medical books of the last millennia. The exasperation of the medical writer with the dermatologic nomenclature was a recurring theme over the centuries. Mondeville had the loudest voice of the medieval period in calling for clarity of the dermatological nomenclature. For this reason, Mondeville's *Chirurgie*—a glorious text, truly the first of its kind, and completely readable and lasting in its value to historians of medicine and surgery—is also a crucial and underappreciated work in the history of dermatology.

Guy de Chauliac (1300–1368)

The other surgeon whose work is of major historical significance to our study is Guy de Chauliac, the author of *Chirurgia Magna* (1363). Chauliac was born in Chaulhac in south-central France. The exact nature of his training and occupation has baffled historians over the centuries, but it is generally agreed that he was educated as a cleric and became a master of medicine at Montpellier, and although he was never a barber-surgeon, he practiced surgery. Thus, like Mondeville, Guy de Chauliac's career was a blend of surgery and medicine. He served no kings, but he did serve as papal physician to several of the Avignon Popes.

Chauliac's *Chirurgia Magna* was very well received and became the most influential and well-read surgical text for the next several centuries, at least until Richard Wiseman's surgical treatise in the seventeenth century. It has been praised by many historians and biographers over the years as being on par with the works of Galen, Hippocrates, and Avicenna. While not as innovative as the work of the great sixteenth-century French surgeon, Ambroise Pare, Chauliac has been noted as taking "a middle of the road position between timidity and recklessness" that raises his book's value above all other works as the seminal achievement in the history of surgery.[105] It was the first complete work for surgical education in the history of the world, representing a comprehensive collection of all the known information about surgery during the Middle Ages. We are fortunate to have Nicaise's tally of referenced authors by Chauliac: Galen was referenced 890 times, Avicenna 660, Rhazes 161, Haly Abbas 149, and Hippocrates 120 times.[106] The text consists of seven treatises: I—Anatomy; II—The Aposthems; III—On Wounds; IV—On Ulcers; V—On Fractures and Dislocations; VI—Miscellaneous Maladies; and VII—The Antidotary. The last treatise is an invaluable section summarizing all medieval procedural and pharmaceutical treatments.

Chirurgia Magna contains an abundance of dermatological information. In treatise I, Chauliac refers to the skin as a tissue containing a network of nerves, veins, and arteries that was designed to act like leather and protect the body and provide sensation.[107] In lieu of any more comment on the skin, he referred his reader to Galen's *On the Usefulness of the Parts*. That is the entirety of the space he devoted to the anatomy of the skin. However, the skin was important to Chauliac, as evidenced by his numerous sections on skin disease.

In treatise II, Chauliac defines the medieval word, aposthem, as any tumor, inflation, enlargement, bulge, elevation, or excrescence of the body. A simplified version of his classification scheme for aposthems is seen in Table 7.3. To Chauliac, humors were either natural (pure) or non-natural (corrupted/diseased), and an aposthem was a collection of humor that varied by its temperature and whether the humor was natural or non-natural.

Several of these terms are still used today. The best modern word for a true phlegmon is inflammation, but cellulitis comes to mind from his description. Esthiomene, according to Chauliac, denotes the corruption spreading by undermining and liquifying the surrounding tissue. The "non-natural" sanguine diseases consist of several different names and synonyms for a host of infectious cutaneous lesions. Erysipelas and herpes apparently meant something different to Chauliac than what they mean to the modern dermatologist. Notice that cancerous tumors developed from a corrupted melancholic humor.

Treatise VI also contains dermatologic information. Like Mondeville, Chauliac included a brilliant chapter on leprosy, noting the six unique signs (rounded eyes and earlobes; hairless brows; dilated nostrils; deformed lips; hoarse nasal voice with foul breath and body odor; and an "ugly Satyr-like stare") and 17 shared (or equivocal) signs.[109] The lengthy historical and diagnostic information about leprosy must have been extraordinarily informative to the medieval surgeon or physician. He urges caution when making the diagnosis, as the stakes were so high for the patient and the populace. Get it wrong, and the world will abhor an "innocent" person, or a leper might go free and expose the healthy population.[110]

TABLE 7.3

Chauliac's Classification System of Aposthems[108]

Warm, sanguine, natural	True phlegmon
Warm, sanguine, non-natural	Carbuncle, furuncle, braise, Persian fire, malignant pustule, anthrax, malignant carbuncle, esthiomene or gangrene, St. Anthony's fire, or St. Martial
Warm, choleric, natural	Erysipelas
Warm, choleric, non-natural	Herpes
Cold, phlegmatic, natural	Edema
Cold, phlegmatic, non-natural	Tissue emphysema, aqueous aposthems, phlegmatic excrescences, glands, scrofulas, loupes (cyst), turtles, goiters, hernias, melicerides (of horses), steatomas, lipomas
Cold, melancholic, natural	Sclerosis, true phlegmons
Cold, melancholic, non-natural	Sclerosis, true induration, cancerous aposthems

Chauliac addressed skin diseases typically found in a medieval medical text: white-and-black morphea, impetigo and serpigo, scabies and itching, and lice, nits, and the like, and leeks, warts, and horns.[111] Interestingly, his description of "nits" is the closest we have seen to that of the scabies mite: nits are "tiny animals who tunnel between the skin and underlying flesh."[112] Nits today refer to the eggs of the louse. He ignored variola because it is a problem belonging to the realm of the physician, not the surgeon (the physicians often dealt with exanthems). But he otherwise offered little new information and was less negative than Mondeville about the conflicts among medical writers concerning the names and descriptions of cutaneous diseases. Under "Maladies of the Head," he discussed tinea and disorders involving hair loss; the latter is a basic reiteration of Galen's definitions and causation. After a discussion of the confusing nomenclature for tineas, he offered a simplified description of tinea: an ashen-gray, malodorous, scabies-like malady of the head, with scales and crusts that moistens, depilates, and disfigures the scalp.[113] This is a perfect example of Guy de Chauliac's impressive ability to break down into simplistic terms what he knows about a condition.

The part of *Chirurgia Magna* that is dedicated to skin disease concludes with several pages on cosmetics, in which Chauliac points out for surgeons the disclaimer that the desired result cannot be guaranteed to the patient.[114] True surgical embellishment was worthy of a medieval surgeon's time and attention, but the application of cosmetic preparations was not. He reminded his reader with a quote from Galen about cosmetic medicine and the female patient: it is not a surgeon's purpose to know what makes a face beautiful, but he can manage the aging face with honor and "eliminate what offends her husband."[115]

Summary

Skin disease in the medieval West fell under the dominion of the surgeon, as demonstrated by the career and writings of Gilbertus Anglicus, Theodoric Borgognoni, Henri de Mondeville, and Guy de Chauliac. The skin remained largely an envelope, but there was a revival of the ancient acknowledgment of the skin's excretory and sensory functions. As both skin disease and epidemic viral disease were rampant due to poor hygiene and filthy conditions in most of Western Europe, there was special emphasis on skin disease in the writings of many medieval surgeons. Numerous medical writers of the Middle Ages devoted countless pages to the diagnosis and treatment of many different skin diseases, including leprosy, scabies, erysipelas, and scrofula. The detailed and accurate descriptions of leprosy found in the works of Mondeville and Chauliac represent the highest level of dermatology in the Middle Ages and signify the value of dermatology at a time when diagnostic accuracy became crucial to securing the livelihood and freedom of persons affected with skin disease, which may or may not have been leprosy. The contributions of two heroines in our story—Hildegard of Bingen and Trota of Salerno—to the history of dermatology should not be forgotten.

8

The Renaissance

The Renaissance was the period of European history that lasted from approximately the beginning of the fourteenth century until the end of the seventeenth century. The word *renaissance* means "rebirth" and refers to the revival of European artistic and intellectual life after the Middle Ages. Its onset was marked by the production of some of the first Italian Renaissance art (such as Giotto's Scrovegni Chapel frescoes in Padua, 1305) or the publication of Dante's *Divine Comedy* (ca. 1320) or the discovery of the lost letters of the ancient Roman writer and orator, Cicero, in 1345 by Francesco Petrarch (1304–1374). The Renaissance can be divided into two thematic periods: the backward-looking early period characterized by humanism and the forward-thinking later period of change, which included the Protestant Reformation (beginning in 1517) and the Scientific Revolution (starting in 1543). In the early days of the movement, Renaissance writers, thinkers, artists, scientists, and physicians rediscovered the writings and world views of the ancients and assigned them supreme value. This stance toward Greek and Roman writers is a key feature of the period known as humanism, led by Petrarch (1304–1374), the "Father of Humanism," who resurrected the works Cicero and Vergil, and Desiderius Erasmus (1466–1533), the most famous scholar of the Northern Renaissance. It is to this early period that the story now turns. The Scientific Revolution will be considered in the next chapter.

The Renaissance began in Italy because of unique social and political factors in places such as Florence that stimulated cultural revitalization. It is widely held that the Black Death (see Interlude 2) contributed to the onset of the Renaissance. The Black Death devastated the European population, especially in Italy, which caused an increase in wages for the working class because there were fewer people to do the work. There were also fewer people to pay rent, resulting in severe financial hardship for the land-owning nobility. Merchants and opportunists lacking any birthright found themselves financially able to compete with the nobility. To compensate for their humble backgrounds, they patronized the arts, prompting an explosion in demand for artistic works. Due to a thriving sophisticated economy in Italy, the individual, with a newfound dignity and intellectual freedom, could now rise to realize his potential. It was this increase in freedom to express one's self—exemplified in the following quote by the illustrious Florentine philosopher Giovanni Pico Della Mirandola (1463–1494) from his *Oration on the Dignity of Man* (1487)—that initiated the artistic and scientific achievements in the centuries that followed the Black Death:

> Oh unsurpassed generosity of God the Father, Oh wondrous and unsurpassable felicity of man, to whom it is granted to have what he chooses, to be what he wills to be!

The preoccupation with death in the fourteenth century undercut the religious orthodoxy and caused the fifteenth- and sixteenth-century intellectuals to question the world around them. Learned men of the period first turned to classical antiquity for answers. Renaissance medicine in the humanistic period experienced a revival of the works of Galen and Hippocrates in their original Greek language, as well as new Latin translations of the works.[1] The motto was *ad fontes*, "back to the sources." There was concern among these pro-Hellenic learned men, such as Niccolò Leoniceno (1428–1524), that the existing translations of these ancient works were full of errors, spurring the desire to study the texts in their unaltered, original format without the nearly 1500 years of scholastic modification.[2] The humanists sought to clarify what was "lost in translation" as the texts had journeyed across the medieval world—first in Greek, then in Arabic, and finally in Latin. The controversy concerning the practice of bloodletting was an example of a conflict between the source material and the medieval versions that needed clarification: the Greek texts suggested that the patient be bled on the same side as the original source of the illness,

DOI: 10.1201/9781003273622-11

whereas the medieval version stated it should occur on the opposite side.[3] Ancient medical practices were deemed superior to any practices developed in late antiquity and the medieval period, and the association of ancient authority with church orthodoxy further cemented this worldview. Leoniceno was also convinced that careful examination of the original Greek of Hippocrates and Galen could reveal that syphilis existed in ancient times (see Interlude 3). Leoniceno never lived to see his dream realized for an authoritative publication of Galen's complete works in the original Greek, but it came to fruition a year after his death. This landmark humanistic medical publication of the Renaissance, the culmination of over a hundred years of scholarship, was printed by the Aldine Press in Venice in 1525.

PARACELSUS (1493–1541)

Not every physician in this period supported a revival of the original form of Galenic medicine. The most famous anti-Hellenic practitioner was Theophrastus Philippus Aureolus Bombastus von Hohenheim, known today as Paracelsus, a self-imposed nickname meaning "better than Celsus." He was an eccentric Swiss physician who, while lecturing, donned an alchemist's apron rather than the customary robe. He lacked any official university-based education, stating that "the universities do not teach all things, so the doctor must seek out old wives, gypsies, sorcerers, wandering tribes, robbers and such outlaws, and take lessons from them."[4] To some, his unprecedented efforts to reject Galen indicate that he was a founder of modern medicine; others consider him an insignificant mystic and quack.

To Paracelsus, medicine needed a complete overhaul in its understanding of disease. His passion was so strong that he publicly burned Avicenna's *Canon* and several Galenic texts during a professorship in Basel in 1527, stating they were no longer relevant to the study of medicine. He developed his own disease system involving three chemicals—salt, sulfur, and mercury—instead of humors. He is also known as the father of toxicology, having famously claimed that "all things are poison, and nothing is without poison, the dosage alone makes it, so a thing is not a poison." The iatrochemists (chemical doctors) followed in his footsteps, and his chemical basis for disease would compete with humoral theory in the centuries to follow. He was one of the first describers of syphilis and the first to propose mercury as an effective treatment for that disease; he also popularized the use of sulfur, antimony, iron, and arsenic.[5] He is considered the first to recognize the value of laudanum as an analgesic, and he was a forerunner of the antisepsis movement. While Paracelsus' system of disease would not take hold in mainstream medicine in Europe, this controversial figure deserves a place in the pantheon of medical history for his groundbreaking discoveries and forward-thinking scientific stances.[6]

The Discovery of Human Anatomy

The most significant milestone of Renaissance medicine was the discovery of human anatomy. A basic understanding of normal human anatomy and physiology was first necessary for medicine to modernize. It is difficult to imagine that physicians before the fifteenth century had little-to-no specific knowledge of human anatomy, but that is indeed the case. This discovery was only possible because of the promotion of human dissection as a scientific endeavor in the fourteenth through sixteenth centuries. In ancient and medieval times, human dissections were rarely performed as it was either taboo or outlawed; instead, Galen and others believed that human anatomy could be inferred from the dissection of animals, such as monkeys and pigs. Consequently, no knowledge of anatomy inherited from Galen was based on human dissections.

As the practice of human dissection grew in the fourteenth century, the anatomist ordinarily dissected the corpse of an executed criminal, performed during the winter since formaldehyde was not yet discovered and the corpse decomposed more slowly in the cold. At the University of Padua (est. 1222), a frontrunner of medical education, the anatomy department became world-famous. Over the next few centuries, its famous dissection amphitheater drew several giants in the field of anatomy. As the thirst for knowledge that characterized the Renaissance accelerated in Italy, more and more individuals participated in human dissection, and interest in the procedure spread all over Europe. With the Church's hands-off policy for the practice of dissection, the only limit to the endeavor by the fifteenth and sixteenth centuries was the unavailability of corpses to dissect. A black market for dead bodies, especially in England, arose to meet anatomical scientists' demands. After the heyday of the bodysnatchers, Britain passed the Anatomy Act in 1832, which allowed for the dissection of non-criminals in medical schools.

The fascination with human anatomy first arose outside the medical world, in the realm of the Renaissance artists.[7] To paint or sculpt more naturalistic works, the artist became a student of human anatomy. One famous artist's fascination grew into an obsession. That artist, Leonardo da Vinci (1452–1519), wrote in 1508:

> And this old man, a few hours before his death, told me that he was over a hundred years old and that he felt nothing wrong with his body other than weakness. And thus, while sitting on a bed in the hospital of Santa Maria Nuova in Florence, without any movement or sign of any mishap, he passed from this life. And I dissected him to see the cause of so sweet a death.[8]

Da Vinci painted only 15–20 paintings in his 50-year career, which left him with time for other pursuits—namely scientific ones. With his legendary appetite for knowledge, he focused on human anatomy at two different times in his career; the most important period was 1506–1513. Throughout his life, he had a desire to publish a treatise on his anatomical findings. He acquired a vast knowledge of human anatomy during the later years of his life, largely through the dissection of almost thirty cadavers.[9] He drew 750 depictions of his discoveries with detailed annotations in the margins. Unfortunately, the work was never published, and Da Vinci's investigations would have no influence on the developments toward modern medicine. His drawings disappeared for two and a half centuries, only to be found again in 1760 in a chest in Windsor Castle. Only his famous "Vitruvian Man" drawing is remembered, but that work was more a demonstration of Da Vinci's obsession with proportions and symmetry than with anatomy, i.e., the order and design of the human body in harmony with the order and design of the natural world.

Andreas Vesalius (1514–1564)

Da Vinci did not get credit for his "discovery" of human anatomy; that credit went to the Flemish physician, Andreas Vesalius. Born in Brussels with the name Andries van Wesel, Vesalius was the son of an apothecary to Charles V, Holy Roman Emperor. Vesalius's father inspired him to enter a career in medicine. He went to medical school in Paris under the mentorship of Jacobus Sylvius (1478–1555), a leading Galenic physician of the sixteenth century and a proponent of anatomic dissection. Sylvius inspired young Vesalius to explore the human body, but Vesalius soon became exasperated with his teacher's blind trust in the ancients when he realized that the knowledge of anatomy imparted by Galen was often incorrect. Sylvius believed that everything Galen and Hippocrates had ever written was entirely true.[10] Vesalius learned for himself that this assessment was inaccurate, and in so doing, risked the ire and persecution of religious authorities as well as his colleagues. He studied the intricacies of the human skeleton during his excursions through the Cimetière des Innocents, "Holy Innocents Cemetery," in Paris. Vesalius' interest in human anatomy became an overt obsession, the intensity of which "hints at pathological impulses."[11]

Vesalius left Paris for the University of Padua, where at 23 years of age, he received an appointment as a professor of anatomy. Vesalius desired to explore the human body and was willing to go to any length to secure a cadaver for his pursuits. He famously stole the hanging remains of a condemned criminal and publicly lectured on anatomy while dissecting the corpse. With dissection after dissection, Vesalius ultimately gained the knowledge to correct many anatomical mistakes that Galen had made, and he systematically dismantled Galen's version of the human body. For example, Vesalius disproved Galen's claim that blood passes between the right and left sides of the heart through the tiny pores in the heart's wall. To Vesalius, the reason for Galen's errors was an easy one: he relied on animal carcasses and inferred human anatomy from these dissections.

While at Padua, the 29-year-old Vesalius set out to publish what he had hoped would be the greatest book on anatomy ever published. It is widely believed—but not definite—that he hired illustrator Jan van Calcar (1499–1546) to draw the anatomical depictions; van Calcar was a pupil of the artist Titian, the grandmaster from nearby Venice. After five long years of production, *De humani corporis fabrica libri septem*, "On the Fabric of the Human Body in Seven Books" was published in 1543. Vesalius' challenge of Galenic dogma resulted in a somewhat expected denigration from his detractors whose orientation was Galenic. His own former professor, Sylvius, went so far as to write in his *Vaesani cuiusdam calumniarum in Hippocratis Galenique rem anatomicam depulsio*, "A Refutation of the Slanders of a Certain Madman against the Anatomical Topic in Hippocrates and Galen" (1551):

> I implore his imperial Majesty to punish severely, as he deserves, this monster born and bred in his own house, this worst example of ignorance, ingratitude, arrogance, and impiety, to suppress him so that he may not poison the rest of Europe with his pestilential breath.[12]

But all of these efforts to suppress Vesalius failed, and he soon became the personal physician to Charles V. He later served Charles' son, Philip II, who moved the court of the Empire to Madrid in 1559. Vesalius' *Fabrica* would go on to become a sensation and possibly the single most important text in the history of medicine. Sylvius, desperate to save face and salvage his own life's work that defended Galen's anatomy, claimed that the anatomy of the human body must have changed since the time of Galen.

The story of Vesalius' death is one of legend. Vesalius' life ended at 50 years of age when he became ill after being shipwrecked on an Ionian island during a return voyage from a pilgrimage to Jerusalem. The pilgrimage was a penance demanded of him by Philip II, who pardoned him after a conviction by the Spanish Inquisition for vivisection. Vesalius had performed an autopsy on a Spanish nobleman, only to find his heart still beating during the procedure. Scholars contend that the story is a myth and that Vesalius was on a pilgrimage in order to escape hostile colleagues at the Spanish court.[13]

The publication of the *Fabrica* was a milestone as it was the first time the medical world had been updated with new information in almost 1500 years. Its release signaled the onset of the anatomic revolution—the fervor of this revolution driven by the desire to see for oneself instead of trusting the ancients.[14] From then on, medicine would direct its focus toward the inside of the body to better understand the source of disease.

The *Fabrica*, containing over 200 folio illustrations and 700 pages of text, is composed of seven books: (1) bones and cartilages, (2) ligaments and muscles, (3) veins and arteries, (4) nerves, (5) organs of nutrition and generation, (6) the heart and associated organs, and (7) the brain. A second edition was released in 1555. Only 700 original copies are known to exist in the world today, but the *Fabrica* was translated into an extraordinary English reconstruction for modern readers in 2014.[15]

Vesalius devoted an entire chapter to the skin—Chapter 5 of the second book—and his description of the skin, though short, is valuable to this history.[16] He noted that like other substances of the body, the skin is subject to generation and corruption and its quality falls somewhere in the middle of hardness and softness. It is also in the middle of sinew and flesh, neither bloodless like sinew nor full of blood like the flesh. The skin of different parts of the body vary in their concentration of nerves as well as thickness, with facial skin soft and thin and the skin of the scalp and soles thicker. Vesalius made an interesting comment that the skin is the largest continuous structure of the body, but it does have tiny openings that allow for the release of "sooty wastes." He noted that the epidermis is bloodless and thin and transparent like the outer layer of an onion, except in places where it is thicker, like on the palms and soles. Vesalius addressed a debate among Renaissance anatomists as to whether the sense of touch came from the skin or from deeper structures within the body. Small nerve fibers, which course through the skin after branching off of larger, deeper nerves and which give us our cutaneous sensation, were not yet discovered. Vesalius urged his reader to disregard Aristotle's contention that the skin has no sensation, noting the bellies of muscles such as those of the thigh have much less feeling than the skin of the face and hands.[17] Also included in Chapter VI of Book 2 are details as to how to observe the skin and its layers during dissection. Unlike previous dissectors, who saw the skin as in the way of the more important structures targeted in the task at hand, Vesalius gave the skin the attention it deserved.

Ambroise Pare (1510–1590)

There was another major publication in the sixteenth century that would change medicine forever. Its source material was not found in a dissection theater but on the battlefields of war-ravaged Europe, where its author, Ambroise Pare, served as a French army surgeon. A quote commonly attributed to Hippocrates states, "He who wishes to be a surgeon should go to war," and it proved true in Pare's case that the "learn as you go" training on the battlefield was without equal.[18] It was during his time in the army that Pare discerned the way to reduce traumatic bleeding, as well as bleeding caused by surgical intervention, by tying off vessels with ligatures. His groundbreaking work in the surgical field was first published in 1545 in French rather than the expected Latin; in 1617, his battlefield discoveries would finally be published in English under the title *The Method of Curing Wounds Made by Gun Shot (Also by Arrows and Darts)*.[19] Pare contributed the most significant advancements in Renaissance surgery, a field that required four major milestones in order to enter the modern era.[20] After the publication of Vesalius' *Fabrica*, Pare's discovery of ligatures was the second of these milestones. Only the nineteenth-century inventions of anesthesia and antisepsis remained.

Pare's pupil, Jacques Guillemeau (1550–1613), translated Pare's other writings into Latin, which were subsequently translated into English by Thomas Johnson (ca. 1600–1644) as *The Complete Works of Ambroise Pare* in 1634. Pare referred to the skin as having an epidermis or "bastard skin," and a dermis or "true skin"; he viewed the epidermis as having a strictly ornamental purpose and believed that it formed as an excrement of the dermis, while the dermis he viewed as having the following use:

> …to keep safe and sound the continuity of the whole body, and all the parts thereof, from the violent assault of all external dangers, for which cause it is everywhere indewed with sense, in some parts more exact, in others more dull, according to the dignitie and necessitie of the parts which it ingirts, that they might all be admonished of their safetie and preservation. Lastly, it is penetrated with many pores, as breathing places, as we may see by the flowing of the sweate….[21]

These texts reveal the sixteenth-century surgeon-anatomist views of the skin and its diseases. The reader is referred to the excellent English translation of Pare's masterpiece of Renaissance-era surgery and, in particular, his discussions of cancer and the plague.[22]

Jean Fernel (1497–1558)

Paracelsus, Vesalius, and Pare. These are the figures who get the most attention in any trustworthy overview of the history of medicine during the Renaissance. A lesser known genius of the period was the French physician Jean Fernel. While Vesalius was laboring to discover and document the entire human anatomy, Fernel attempted to do the same for physiology: explain the function of every part of the human body. He returned to Galen, Aristotle, and Hippocrates for assistance with this ambitious endeavor but introduced medieval and Renaissance ideas into his synthesis. Fernel is considered "one of the great restorers of medicine, and the first after Galen who wrote ably on the nature and cause of diseases."[23] Credited with introducing the terms *physiology* and *pathology*, he masterfully stated, "Anatomy is to physiology as geography is to history; it describes the theatre of events."[24] He was not interested in the "what" of the human body; he preferred the "how." Fernel complained that the study of anatomy lacked intellectual depth and the "holistic principles of causation and function."[25] Fernel was one of the foremost medical writers of his day, and if he is less well known today than Vesalius or Pare or Paracelsus, the preoccupations of medical historians with these figures are to blame.[26]

Physiologia was the first part of a trilogy, along with *Pathologia* and *Therapeutice*, that constituted Fernel's greatest work, *Universa medicina* (1567). As a staunch Galenist, the content of his *Physiologia* reads like a Renaissance update of Galen's *De usu partium corporis humani*, "On the usefulness of the parts of the human body." His logical system of belief about the practice of medicine is entirely correct and modern in its main conclusion: first, learn physiology, and then you can truly understand pathology, which can then lead to an understanding of therapeutics. He warned that the more typical path of contemporary physician training—philosophy then human anatomy then the study and treatment of individual diseases—effectively "covers their eyes in thick darkness."[27]

Among all the works examined in preparation for this book, the *Physiologia* is one of the most extraordinary in its comprehensiveness, detail, and brilliance. While it contains no new discoveries, the work incorporated Galenic medicine in "wider Renaissance visions" and was enormously popular (97 complete editions or translations between 1554 and 1680) among the physicians, anatomists, and surgeons of the sixteenth and seventeenth centuries.[28] In *Pathologia*, Fernel devoted Book VII, entitled *De externis corporis affectibus*, "On the external affections of the body," to skin "affections." Fernel's succinct descriptions are unusual for this period. Fernel is credited with the first use of the term, *lues venerea*.

Jean Fernel's comments about the skin in his *Physiologia* complement nicely the same in Vesalius's anatomic treatise and reveal an even more advanced understanding than shown in the latter treatise from 24 years earlier.[29] To Fernel, the skin is a membrane that covers the whole body, thicker than membranes within the body because of the mass of the whole body is greater. It has small "vents" for exhalation from the inside and contains equal parts flesh and nerve. It gets nourishment and *pneuma* (spirit) from the ends of veins and arteries that can be found within it and its sense of touch from the "lengthy ramification of nerves" underneath it. What the Greeks called the epidermis is made from the "dried refuse" of the true skin, and a thermal blister arises when the epidermis is separated from the dermis. The skin covers the entire body except in the openings in the body (the ears, the nose, eyes, mouth, genitalia, and anus). Most impressively, Fernel was aware that the muscles of facial expression are embedded within the skin: he noted that the skin of the forehead and the rest of the face, and especially the lips, is "intimately combined" with these muscles. The skin of the hands and feet allows these regions to bend and grasp in every direction and have a more precise sense of touch.

Now that we have reviewed the understanding of the skin in the mind of an anatomist, a surgeon, and a physiologist of the Renaissance, some general comments are in order about the knowledge of the skin and its diseases during this period. The skin, in keeping with the Galenic theory, was most often described by Renaissance writers as a porous outer covering, and Plato's idea of the fisherman's net (see Chapter 3) was revived. It had two layers—*cuticula* (epidermis) and *cutis* (dermis), with the former excreted by the latter. Its only function was waste removal, but it was appreciated for the beautification of the body it provided. A major difference between Renaissance thinking on skin and traditional Aristotelian views is that the Renaissance physician knew that the skin was the organ of touch and rejected Aristotle's view that the source of the sense of touch was in the flesh underlying the skin.

The skin did not yet have its own diseases, but the "affections" of the skin (what skin diseases were called at this time) instead reflected an expulsion of morbid material from inside the body, and he divided skin diseases by the humoral source of the lesion. An eruption on the skin after several days of fever would be welcomed in relief by the family and the physician at the bedside, and efforts to suppress the eruptions were considered dangerous because the morbid material needed to come out of the body. Knowledge about the meaning of the different skin conditions was important to the Renaissance physician or surgeon, as it could dictate the underlying diagnosis, prognosis, and treatment given to the patient. Cosmetic concerns had no place within the Galenic framework in which the average Renaissance physician worked, but these physicians were frequently tasked with handling cosmetic complaints and expected by their patients to deal with them.[30] Hence, an increasing number of chapters or treatises on cosmetic concerns is found throughout the period. Finally, during the Renaissance, the skin became increasingly a concern of the physicians or surgeons who found themselves at the frontlines against the greatest scourge of the period—a dermatologic one—namely, syphilis (see Interlude 3).

Minor Renaissance Contributors

In the fifteenth and sixteenth centuries, numerous Italian, French, Dutch, and German physicians—some famous, some not—made minor contributions to the history of dermatology. The following medical writers covered skin disease in their writings. Note that none of the figures discussed in this chapter were

English; English medicine lagged behind the rest of Europe and did not make significant advances until the seventeenth century.

Gabriel Fallopius (1523–1562), an Italian professor of anatomy and medicine at the University of Padua, was one of the most important anatomists of the sixteenth century. He was a pupil of Vesalius and discoverer of countless anatomical entities, most famously, the tube bearing his name. He wrote extensively about topics commonly found in the skin chapters of medical texts of the Renaissance: venous ulcers, tumors, psora, lepra, itching, pediculi, erysipelas, etc. He was also known for his writings on syphilis and invented a Renaissance version of the condom (see Interlude 3).

Filippo Ingrassia (1510–1580) was a Sicilian professor of medicine at Naples and a former student of Vesalius and Fallopius. He is considered the "Sicilian Hippocrates." In addition to his work with the study of bones, he promoted hygiene and disease prevention, understanding that disease could be transmitted from one person to another. For dermatology, he was among the first to describe scarlet fever clearly and distinguish it from measles.[31] He may have been the first to describe chickenpox (or it was Guidi—see below).[32] Chickenpox, also known as varicella ("little variola"), was not distinguished from smallpox until the nineteenth century.

Guido Guidi (1509–1569), also known by the Latinized name Vidus Vidius, was a Florentine surgeon and anatomist. He authored a surgical textbook beautifully illustrated by Renaissance artists entitled *Chirurgia e greco in latinam conversa*, "Surgery, translated from Greek into Latin" (1544). He devoted many pages to skin diseases in his *De curatione generatim*, "On Medical Care, in General" (1587), and he may have been the first to describe chickenpox.[33]

Giovanni Manardo (1462–1536) was an Italian physician from Ferrara who authored an important work entitled *Epistolae medicinales*, "Medical letters" (1521), a compendium of 103 letters based on case histories, professional discussions, and personal observations. Like his mentor Niccolò Leoniceno, Manardo studied ancient Greek medicine in the original Greek tongue. He was among the first to separate astrology from medicine and venereal from non-venereal diseases.[34] Among the letters is one on external diseases addressed to the Ferrarese surgeon Michael Santanna, a work that is one of the first devoted entirely to skin disease.[35] He described milk crust (cradle cap), eczema, psoriasis, and syphilis. He supported the use of guiacum for syphilis (see Interlude 3).

Michelangelo Biondo (1497–1565), better known as Blondus, was an Italian surgeon who penned a short treatise in 1544 on the determination of a person's character from the form and color of their hair, skin, and nails.[36] His comments on nevi (moles) reveal superstitions that were retained in this progressive period. For example, moles arising on a part of the body of a child could predict attributes of a person or prognosticate the type of person they would become.[37]

Ludovico Settala (1552–1633) wrote an entire book on moles entitled *De Naevis Liber*, "Book about Moles" (1606), and discussed the relationship between the skin of the face and the rest of the body.[38] The position of a nevus on the body could predict a person's qualities and deficiencies.[39]

Marco Antonio Montagnana (d. 1572) penned *De herpete, phagedaena, gangraena, sphacelo, & cancro*; "On herpes, phagadena, sphacelsus, and cancer" (published posthumously in 1589). A professor of surgery at Padua for 25 years, Montagnana's work on ulcers and carcinoma is detailed, comprehensive, and ahead of its time.

Laurent Joubert (1529–1583), a dynamic figure in sixteenth-century French medicine and a graduate of Montpellier, questioned old wives' tales and superstitions of his era in an important work entitled *Erreurs populaires*, "Popular Errors" (1578). He studied laughter, as scientifically as any Renaissance writer, and reported his findings in "Treatise on Laughter" (1579), and he translated Guy de Chauliac's *Chirurgia Magna* into French in 1578 (see Chapter 7). He wrote 130 pages on skin diseases in a section of *De affectionibus pilorum et cutis praesertim capitis et de cephalalgia tractatus unus*, "One treatise on the diseases of the hair and skin especially of the scalp and on headache" (1582). In that work, Joubert mentioned syphilitic alopecia and a primitive description of trichorrhexis nodosa; his emphasis on scalp disorders is typical for the Renaissance.

Pieter van Foreest (1521–1597), also known as Petrus Forestus and "the Dutch Hippocrates," was a Dutch physician who studied medicine at the Universities of Leuven, Padua, and Bologna and then settled in Delft, where he practiced medicine for nearly 40 years. His most significant contribution to the history of medicine was an enormous, 32-book collection of his case histories entitled *Observationum et Curationum Medicinalium sive Medicinae Theoricae & Practicae.* The first volume was published in 1588; most of the work was published posthumously in the century after his death. He detailed approximately 1350 patients, identified by name and location, whom he diagnosed and treated during his career. *Observationum* contains a short volume, *De Fucis* (Volume XXXI, 1606), containing 11 cases related to cosmetic medicine, including recipes for cosmetic remedies. Topics covered include skin blemishes, pallor and redness of the face, pustules and impetigo of the face, removing and lightening scars, removing vestiges of measles and smallpox, restoring the hair, teeth whitening, burns from fire and water, lightening the hands and the skin, obesity and how to avoid getting thin, and thinness and how to avoid becoming obese.[40]

Hieronymus Mercurialis (1530–1606) and *De Morbis Cutaneis* (1572)

In 1572, Hieronymus Mercurialis (Girolamo Mercuriale) wrote the most significant dermatological publication of the Renaissance, *De morbis cutaneis et omnibus corporis humani excrementis tractatus*, "Treatise on diseases of the skin and all excrements of the human body," a compilation of all information accumulated about skin diseases dating back to ancient times. Its value rests not in that it contained any new developments, but that it was the first work in which skin disease was placed front and center.

Born in Forli, Italy, the son of a physician, Mercurialis was an extraordinarily learned man who migrated throughout his career when opportunities presented themselves, making him one of the most famous physicians of his time. After being educated in Bologna, Padua, and Venice, he went to Rome where he caught the attention of Cardinal Alessandro Farnese, a major patron of the arts. Mercurialis entered the Farnese household, where he lived and wrote for seven years while surrounded by some of the most eminent men of letters in Rome. In 1569, at 39 years of age, he accepted the position of Chair of Medicine at the premiere medical university in Italy, the University of Padua. Two years later, he married Francesca Bici and the couple had five children. It was during his time in Padua that he published *De morbis cutaneis*. In 1573, he went to Vienna to care for an ailing Emperor Maximilian II, before returning to Padua for another professorship, where he remained until 1587. After six years at the University of Bologna, he finished his career at the University of Pisa upon the request of Ferdinando de Medici, the Grand Duke of Tuscany. He retired to his hometown of Forli in 1606, the year of his death.

For a better characterization of Mercurialis, we turn to his eighteenth-century biographer, the German physician Friedrich Boerner (1723–1761).[41] In 1755, he portrayed Mercurialis as having a kind disposition and an industrious work ethic. He was celebrated with many honors and the high esteem of everyone who knew him. With his broad brow, handsome features, and impeccable manners, he stood out among his peers for his remarkable skill, gentle nature, and teaching ability. He lived a pure and pious life, preferring writing and academia over money and fame.

Mercurialis should be remembered for several reasons beyond his seminal work in dermatology (which will be discussed shortly). First and foremost, he was a prototypical humanist physician, with not only a philological interest in the texts of Galen and Hippocrates, but also antiquarian leanings.[42] He translated the classical works himself and supported with material evidence from the past, he critically assessed and questioned them. Siraisi considered Mercurialis superior to the rest of the humanist physicians for the historical evidence outside of medical texts he sought and employed.[43] Mercurialis took the appraisal of the past to a whole new level. Among Renaissance physicians, there were not many equals who could apply philological, antiquarian, and historical methodology.

As one of the most prolific medical writers of the period, *De morbis cutaneis* was not his most famous work, nor was it the only book he produced on the subject of the skin. His most famous work was his first publication, *De arte gymnastica*, "On the art of gymnastics" (1569), the first complete work to address the relationship among exercise, health, and wellness, in which he reintroduced ancient exercises to his contemporary readers. Written during his time with Cardinal Farnese, this first work on sports medicine made Mercurialis a star in the medical world of Renaissance Italy. In addition to *De morbis cutaneis*, his other dermatological text was *De decoration*, "Book about adornment" (1585), in which he expounded on cosmetic issues of the skin: beauty, blemishes, wrinkles, scars, skin care, hair care, warts, corns, boils, body odor, and nail diseases, to name a few. His second professorship at Padua marked Mercurialis' most prolific period when he authored the following works: "On plague" (1577), "On diseases of women" (1582), "On disease of children" (1583), and "Censure of the works of Hippocrates" (1583). As a generalist, he did not specialize in any one field. He also wrote on the feeding of infants, on diseases of the eyes and ears, on poisons, epidemics, medicines, and the practice of medicine.[44]

MERCURIALIS AND THE PLAGUE OF VENICE (1576–1577)

Mercurialis is also remembered for a brief fall from grace, and later, redemption. In 1575 and early 1576 in Venice, a few deaths from a plague-like illness got the attention of the *Provveditori Alla Sanita*, the local health department.[45] The *Provveditori*, convinced that the cause of death was plague due to an outbreak in nearby Padua and Mantua in 1575, began isolating the sick by establishing quarantine hospitals called lazarettos. Mercurialis had returned recently from Vienna and led a group of Paduan physicians to Venice to assist the *Provveditori* with the outbreak. He determined that the illness affecting the city was not plague but some other less serious pestilential fever. His rationale was the predilection for illness among the poor (historically, plague did not show a preference toward any particular demographic) and the low number of deaths up until that time. Mercurialis and the Paduans felt that the quarantine efforts should be stopped because they were causing widespread panic, with large numbers of Venetians fleeing the city. After much debate, the Doge sided with the Paduan advisors, and the plague preparations ended. This proved to be one of the worst misdiagnoses of all time, and during the next few months, the bodies began to pile up. In fact, the Venetian plague of 1576–1577 would claim the lives of 50,000 people.[46] With his reputation significantly—but only temporarily—damaged, Mercurialis offered no apologies and quickly rehabilitated himself in the eyes of the medical community with lectures on the plague at Padua, as well as a publication, *De pestilentia*, "On plague" (1577).[47] The debacle in Venice was soon forgotten, swept under a rug made of erudite writings and lectures.

First published in Venice in 1572, *De morbis cutaneis* contains a series of lectures given by Mercurialis at Padua that were transcribed by his medical student, Paulus Aicardius. A second edition was released in 1585, followed by reprints of that edition produced in 1601 and 1625 (the version used in the research for this book was the 1601 edition). The book is dedicated by Aicardius to Cardinal Guglielmo Sirleto (1514–1585), the son of a physician himself and a great linguist who served as custodian of the Vatican Library, which he augmented with the addition of many classical texts. In the introduction, Aicardius depicts Mercurialis as a humble genius, reluctant to have his words published, fearing an unpolished final product.[48] Aicardius eventually persuaded Mercurialis to allow publication for the sake of preserving his words for his students, using the argument that Aicardius could eliminate any errors found in circulating unofficial copies of his lecture material that could discredit him.

The work contains 210 pages, divided into two parts: the first focusing on skin disease (94 pages) and the other on excrements (*De excrementis*, 115 pages), such as urine and feces. The 94-page section on diseases of the skin is itself divided into two parts: at 60 pages long, "Liber 1" discusses all the known diseases of the skin confined to the scalp, whereas the 34-page "Liber 2" discusses all of the known diseases of the skin that can occur anywhere on the body. Almost two-thirds of *De morbis cutaneis* focuses on the scalp (including hair loss). A dermatologist and student of the Latin language, Richard L. Sutton (1908–1990), accomplished the painstaking feat of deciphering difficult medieval Latin to provide the only English translation of *De morbis cutaneis* for the modern reader.[49]

Mercurialis referenced more than 70 authorities in *De morbus cutaneis*, 19 of whom were before the Common Era and another 33 from the first 700 years of the Common Era. Thus, two-thirds of Mercurialis' sources were from the period stretching from early ancient times to late antiquity.[50] This quintessential Renaissance text reveals the author's reverence for Hippocrates and Galen, whose names and opinions are prominent throughout. Like other Renaissance humanist physicians, Mercurialis promoted the Galenic understanding of disease that the balance of the four humors—blood, yellow bile, black bile, and phlegm—determines one's health. Mercurialis collated what was handed down by the Greek and Arab physicians, and for the many conflicts of viewpoint between the ancient and medieval authorities, he mediated the debate with a judgment of whose opinion was preferable.[51]

According to Mercurialis, the skin serves as a protective covering for the flesh, binds the body parts together, and acts as a receptacle for waste materials, whereas the hair purifies the head of excrement and provides for the dignity of appearance and adornment. He recalled that Hippocrates saw the skin as a binding for the body parts, while Plato correctly likened the skin to a fisherman's net.[52] Mercurialis offered a unique classification of skin disease: diseases of color (e.g., leuce, vitiligo, alphos, and exanthemata); diseases of roughness or smoothness (pruritus, scabies or psora, impetigo, and lepra); and diseases of bulk (papules and all skin tumors).[53] He addressed the idea that skin diseases, such as *scabies* or *lepra*, are not really diseases in the opinion of Galen and Hippocrates because they do not impede function in any way; instead, they are disfigurements. In contrast, Mercurialis pointed out that while the skin does not have many functions in common with the rest of the body, it does have its own individual actions, and diseases such as *scabies* or *lepra* interfere with the skin's own actions. The skin's main action, according to Mercurialis, is the reception of nourishments from the veins, which the skin must then process; hence, the disruption of an action equates to disease.[54] Mercurialis foreshadowed a major break from the ancient authorities: the skin had its own diseases. Jan Jessen (see below) would formally argue this new way of thinking about the skin at the end of the sixteenth century.

Mercurialis' understanding of the origin of hair was in line with a typical Renaissance conception of hair—a waste product expelled through the skin that forms into shape by the straight passageway from which it is discharged.[55] He addressed five disorders of hair: *defluvium, calvities, canities, alopecia*, and *ophiasis*. *Defluvium* is today what is called telogen effluvium, the shedding that occurs a few months after surgery, birth of a child, major illness, or infections such as the Covid-19 virus. It is distinguished from *alopecia*, according to Mercurialis, as hair falling out not due to abnormality of humors but due to other causes. It is most likely to occur after a prolonged illness, and the root cause is the thinness of the scalp pores, a thickening of the scalp, or a scarcity of nutrients to build the hairs. Other causes of *defluvium*, as identified by Mercurialis, are the ingestion of poisons, touching salamanders, starvation, and prolonged fatigue. The presence of *defluvium* can sometimes denote a poor prognosis, as in the case of diarrhea: if the diarrhea is so severe that your hair falls out, death is imminent. The treatment of *defluvium* entails a diet rich in "astringent" foods (i.e., foods with a dry flavor), baths, and topicals. No internal treatments are necessary, but he advocated shaving the head followed by the application of labdanum, an essential oil. An example of Mercurialis' blind acceptance is noted; he recommended shaving the head so that the medicament could be used properly and because Cornelius Celsus wrote that shaving the head is beneficial.[56] This "because—_____—said so" type of evidence is ubiquitous in the book. Fill in the blank with Galen, Celsus, or Hippocrates, or countless other writers of the ancient world.

Concerning the way in which hair continues to grow after a person dies, Mercurialis remarked that Aristotle and others believed that the hair and nails continue to grow after death because much excrement is produced in death, and this ample supply feeds the hair and nails. Mercurialis rejected this idea and instead favored the correct reason, proposed by Alexander of Tralles (525–605): when we die, the skin retracts as it decays and dehydrates, and the hair roots become exposed, giving the hair a longer appearance.

Regarding *alopecia* and *ophiasis*, the former involves loss of almost the entire head of hair, whereas *ophiasis* is a loss in only certain areas and resembles the pattern of a snake (*ophis*, Greek for snake). When decayed, blood, phlegm, yellow bile, and black bile can each give rise to these types of hair loss. Management of both conditions depends on first determining the causative corrupt humor, then purging the patient of that humor, maintaining a healthy diet that promotes good juices and easy digestion, and avoiding sexual indulgence and other exertions. When blood is the causative humor, the patient is bled from the side of the body more heavily affected by the hair loss; if phlegm is the cause, bleeding is to be avoided, but a separate purging medicament is suggested. For bile, purging using rhubarb pills is appropriate. He described the proper linament (topical agent) to treat the affected areas of the scalp, with the best are ones able to penetrate deep into the scalp and "break up, evacuate, and dissipate heavy humors."[57] His concluding comments that the cantharides enhance penetration of other medications through the blistered skin are still relevant and used in modern dermatology practices.

Calvities is Mercurialis' term for male pattern baldness. True *calvities* for him was hair loss that occurs at a certain time of life, does not affect women, and primarily involves the anterior part of the scalp. He preferred Galen's explanation for the cause of *calvities*: age-related withdrawal of the brain from the cranium, so that the bone cannot nourish the hair, and the hair falls out.[58] Insomnia, worry, late study, and too much coitus are causes of *calvities*, and true *calvities* is not curable. Women do not experience *calvities* because of their cold temperament and extremely wet brains.[59] *Calvities* occurs mainly in the front of the scalp because, according to Aristotle, the part contained there is the "most vigorous part of the brain."[60] Mercurialis unknowingly got that right. *Calvities*, therefore, is detrimental to a person's health because drafts of air could penetrate more easily in this region and damage the brain.[61] It is best prevented with a diet rich in fat and low in fruits and wines, both of which accelerate *calvities*. Cool air is preferred to warm, and the person should sleep more and worry less. Cutting the hair regularly down to the scalp helps prevent *calvities*. That, of course, is not accurate.

For graying of the hair (*canities*), Mercurialis reviewed all the classical opinions on cause—dryness, phlegmatic moisture, or inadequacy of innate heat relative to external heat—and settled on the last of these causes, held by Aristotle and then Galen, as being the most convincing. Essentially, hairs succumb to decay because external heat damages the humors of the scalp, which lack their own innate heat. *Canities* starts at the temples because the bones are thinner there, and the humors are therefore more susceptible to external heat factors. Women, according to Mercurialis, gray with age more quickly than men because of their cold and moist nature and are thus more susceptible to this type of corruption.[62] He distinguished *canities* of old age and *canities* related to disease and then offered advice on how to manage patients with this complaint: eat healthy food; avoid warm, thick air; exercise moderately; massage the head and the whole body; never cover the head; keep the bowels loose and regular; and dispel all perturbations of the mind, especially anxiety and grief. He urged his reader to not neglect to learn about this problem, as "vain white-haired women, anxious not to displease their husbands" will seek treatment.[63]

Mercurialis classified diseases of the scalp as either ulcerative or non-ulcerative. The non-ulcerative conditions are *pediculation* (lousy scalp) and *furfuration* (scurfy scalp), and the ulcerative ones include *achors*, *favus*, *sycosis*, and *psydracium*. Lice are spontaneously generated by the human body, excreted from the body as decayed byproducts of digestion.[64] Those at most risk for lice, according to Mercurialis, are children and women, sailors and prisoners, and people who fail to care for their bodies with exercise and bathing. Eating papaya or snake meat promotes the growth of lice.[65] Mercurialis knew of several types of lice: *hexapods* (head lice), *plactulas* (pubic lice), *pedicelli* (body lice), and *lendines* (nits). Having head lice causes no detriment to one's health; if anything, it is beneficial because the animals consume much excrement in feeding and reproduction.[66] Lice leaving the body is a sign of imminent death because the lice know to seek a better home.[67] Mercurialis suggested a proper diet and meticulous hygiene as means of prevention, while purging, bloodletting, and a variety of oral and topical medicaments were methods of treatment.

What Mercurialis called *porrigo* is seborrheic dermatitis or atopic dermatitis—the formation of scales and flakes upon scratching the head.[68] Mercurialis settled on the following cause of *porrigo*: healthy humors rise from the body into the head and are corrupted and thickened by a distemper of the head. Removing the scale and examining the underlying skin color can reveal the humoral material there: red, sanguine; yellow, bile, etc. Risk factors for porrigo include a diet rich in salty and acrid foods, such as onions and garlic, excessive coitus, doing the wrong exercises before or after meals, taking baths after a meal, and anger—all which cause the humors to boil.[69] Treatment is largely the same as that for lice, being mindful that efforts to strengthen the skin too much can be detrimental because, according to Celsus, interfering with the reception of corrupted humors into the skin can lead to dangerous retention of these humors in the body.[70]

Mercurialis addressed what he considered to be common diseases, *achor* and *favus*, described as two types of ulcerative scalp diseases that he classified as moist types, as opposed to the dry type of scalp ulcers that he terms *tinea*.[71] *Achor* and *favus* are characterized by an exudation of sticky humors. *Achor* has small openings from which a thin exudate oozes, while *favus* has larger openings and a thicker, honey-like exudate (*favus*, Latin for honeycomb). The former term is no longer used today but probably represented an infected form of scalp dermatitis, whereas *favus* now refers to a rare type of tinea capitis (scalp ringworm). According to Mercurialis, both conditions begin with itching, then swelling in response to scratching, and subsequent oozing. He preferred Galen's opinion that the cause of these scalp diseases was an "acrid, serous, erosive humor mixed with a thick one" and that tasting and touching the humor could aid in the diagnosis. If the humor tastes slightly bitter, the source is bile; if acid, phlegm or melancholy. If the ulcer feels warm, the disease is bilious, and if cold, phlegmatic.[72] *Achor* and *favus* of the child are treated primarily with topical remedies; for adults, bloodletting followed by purging and then the application of topical liniments (lotion) is the treatment protocol. For bloodletting, he recommended venesection of the frontal or postauricular veins if the condition is extensive as opposed to the more traditional use of the common ulnar vein.

The discussion on *tinea* reveals that Mercurialis recognized the various forms familiar to the modern dermatologist: black-dot, gray patch, kerion, favus, etc., but in Mercurialis' time, the terminology was poorly defined and quite confusing to the modern reader. Mercurialis likely sourced information regarding tinea from Avicenna because he noted he could not find a clear description from any Greek author.[73] Listed as tinea's causes include bad foods, contagion, heredity, other diseases of the scalp, and the failure to adequately treat *achor* and *favus*.[74] Sufferers were encouraged to consume a diet lacking in sweets and rich in vinegar, but Mercurialis cautioned, per Hippocrates, that vinegar taken alone without ingesting certain foods can draw melancholic humor into the scalp and worsen the condition.[75] Treatment included bloodletting followed by purging, as well as one unique recommendation for tinea that is not seen in other chapters: the removal of infected hairs with tweezers or chemical depilatories. Recognizing the value of mercury's use as well as its danger, particularly if the "poisonous medicine" reaches the brain, Mercurialis mentioned it for the first time but only considered it a last resort.[76]

Leuce and *alphos* are two related diseases of skin color that are similar to vitiligo in that they involve whitening of the skin. In fact, Mercurialis used the terms *leuce* and *alphos* interchangeably with *vitiligo*. The terms are defined by each of his various sources, but there is little agreement among these sources on the nomenclature. Mercurialis saw the two conditions as distinct from one another. *Leuce* was more widespread than *alphos* and more likely to whiten the hairs in affected areas; *leuce* spreads throughout the body with continuity and was thought to be incurable. The prognosis could be made by puncturing the skin and if, instead of blood, a white humor oozes out, the case is hopeless.[77] This test is obsolete and contradicts our modern experience with vitiligo. Mercurialis contended that *leuce* and *alphos* occur when the skin is nourished by viscid and thick phlegm for a very long time; it is not contagious because the viscid and thick phlegm cannot easily be transmitted from one person's skin to another.[78] If phlegm accumulates inside the skull, epilepsy occurs, whereas if it accumulates outside the skull, *leuce* and *alphos* occur. Men and older women are more susceptible to these conditions than children and younger women; it is prevented in the latter by the cleansing effect of menstruation, while old women are like old buildings and more susceptible to cracks.[79]

Treatment of *leuce* and *alphos* entailed a regimen that not only drew phlegm from the body but also prohibited the development of phlegmatic humors. An environment with warm, dry air was most desired, and adequate sleep was promoted as sleep is the superior state for digestion.[80] Exercise was encouraged, and depression, grief, and sexual activity were discouraged, as was drinking water, which was considered harmful. Instead, "old, strong, good wine," as well as meats that promoted a dry warmth, were best for the phlegmatic patient. Purgatives were controversial because they were thought to be unable to pull humors out of the superficial layers of the skin, where leuce and alphos occurred. Mercurialis opposed the idea of using fire to darken the white areas as he thought that the risk of worsening the appearance of the skin was too great.[81]

Regarding *pruritus*, which remains in place as the modern term for itch, Mercurialis defined two forms: a milder form relieved by scratching and a more severe form not so easily quelled. In both forms, the skin appears unaltered without edema, ulceration, and excoriation, as opposed to other skin conditions which have itching as a feature.[82] Mercurialis delved into the idea of itch, and he was very modern in his thinking that *pruritus* was a type of pain.[83] We now know that itch and pain are closely related neurologically as both are transmitted by unmyelinated C fibers.

As it turns out, according to Mercurialis, scratching causes the itch to intensify in *pruritus* because new humors are brought to the site, and the ones left are more inflamed by the rubbing and scratching. *Pruritus* is said to be rarely chronic because continued scratching can cause the situation to devolve into *scabies*, which is characterized as a pruritic condition with sores, papules, and pustules on the skin brought about by scratching. The itch of *scabies* is even more intense and persistent.[84] This idea of the "itch that rashes," familiar to modern dermatologists, convinces the present author that Mercurialis' continuum of *pruritus* and *scabies* includes all the different types of eczema, as well as modern scabies. The cause of *pruritus*, again in accordance with Galen, is due to a thin, salty, phlegmatic humor building up in the skin that is not released completely from the skin as it is in scabies, which has a thicker liquid that emanates from the skin. Risk factors for *pruritus* include a hot, dry body, young or old age, and an unclean lifestyle.

Treatment of *pruritus* involved removing the salty and bitter humors from the body, avoidance of extremes of temperature, refraining from exercise, sexual activity, rubbing and scratching, and any perturbations of the mind.[85] Good sleep is important with this condition as well. Keeping the bowels regular was emphasized, using enemas or broths if need be. In regard to a controversy over whether salt water or freshwater baths were preferable, Mercurialis interestingly favored freshwater because of a reference to Homer, who had Nausicaa wash her clothing in a river rather than a sea.[86] A diet rich in lettuce, vinegar, goat's meat, and chicken was promoted, with the meats preferentially boiled instead of baked or fried. The bowels should be loosened, the blood let out, and the humors purged with various purgation recipes, repeated until relief is noted.

Concerning the confusing disagreement in his available literature as to the correct term for what he identified as scabies, Mercurialis remarked that the Greeks were referring to *scabies* when they used the term *psora*. He determined that *scabies* was a pruritic condition characterized by dry or moist exudates; with the dry caused by an abundance of melancholic juices and the moist by a salty phlegm, a sanguineous humor, a bilious ichor, or all of the above.[87] Mercurialis quoted Galen's understanding of *scabies*; it results from defective humors arriving at the surface of the skin but they cannot escape and thus decay.[88]

Risk factors include poor hygiene and poor diet, with men more likely to contract scabies than women. Interestingly, like *pruritus* degenerating into *scabies*, *scabies*, if untreated, can transform into *lepra*. Treatment entails a diet similar to that for *pruritus*, as well as and the traditional stepwise plan of evacuation of the bowels, bloodletting, purgation, and finally, topically applied remedies, including sulfur baths. Mercurialis settled another debate: if melancholic humors are the cause, the bloodletting should occur on the right side because the liver (the generator of black bile) is situated on this side. Mercurialis condemns mercurial medicine peddled by quacks for scabies, his main argument against this "poisonous" agent underpinned by the fact that Greeks did not mention it.[89] To Mercurialis, only in chronic and severe forms of the disease should it even be considered an option.

INFERNAL ITCHING

In the *Inferno* portion of Dante's Divine Comedy (1320), Dante is guided through the nine circles of Hell by the Roman poet Virgil, descending into each circle designated for progressively more wicked crimes and where one is destined to agonize for all eternity. In the eighth circle, called *Malebolge* and where fraud and crooks (including alchemists and counterfeiters) were doomed, Dante recounted what he saw:

> We step by step went onward without speech,
> Gazing upon and listening to the sick
> Who had not strength enough to lift their bodies.
> I saw two sitting leaned against each other,
> As leans in heating platter against platter,
> From head to foot bespotted o'er with scabs;
> And never saw I plied a currycomb
> By stable-boy for whom his master waits,
> Or him who keeps awake unwillingly,
> As every one was plying fast the bite
> Of nails upon himself, for the great rage
> Of itching which no other succour had.

And the nails downward with them dragged the scab,
In fashion as a knife the scales of bream,
Or any other fish that has them largest.
"O thou, that with thy fingers dost dismail thee,"
Began my Leader unto one of them,
"And makest of them pincers now and then,
Tell me if any Latian is with those
Who are herein; so may thy nails suffice thee
To all eternity unto this work."[90]

Longfellow's "scab" was the translation of Dante's "la scabbia"—scabies, which we have seen in previous chapters refer at this time to any itchy, scabby eruption. Dante had medical knowledge as he had once enrolled in the guild of physicians and apothecaries in Florence. Dante's choice of itching as the second-worst-type of punishment a human can experience in Hell reflects the degree of unpleasantness with which medievals viewed itching and skin disease. The only fate worse than eternal itching is to be perpetually trapped in ice. Virgil's wish—that scratching with fingernails "suffice thee to all eternity"—is a haunting reminder that in a world without ineffective dermatological treatments, the only remedy is to give in to the impulse brought about by the sensation, i.e., scabere, "to scratch."

On *lepra*, Mercurialis notes that according to Galen, Oribasius, Paulus, and the others, the materia is the same as in *scabies*.[91] From the descriptions, there is no doubt that Mercurialis's *lepra* is modern-day psoriasis. In *lepra*, as in psoriasis, the skin is noted to be thickened and scaly. He referenced Julius Pollux (fl. second century CE), who noted the nail involvement that is distinctly and correctly a feature of *lepra*, and he referenced Nicander (fl. second century BCE), who said the word *lepra* means "to be made scabby and white."[92] This type of *lepra* is the "Lepra of the Greeks," so named by Avicenna and the Arabian physicians. According to Mercurialis, there was also a lepra known to the Arabs that was the same disease the Greeks called *elephantiasis*, a kind of swelling of the whole body. This clarification supports the contention that the "elephantiasis of the Greeks" and the "Lepra of the Arabs" are the same disease as our modern understanding of leprosy (see Interlude 1). *Lepra* is caused by an imbalance of the liver, spleen, or both, which leads to an abundance of melancholic humor. Risk factors include heredity, intercourse with a menstruating woman, old age, and walking in woods heavy with dew.[93] If untreated, *lepra* can evolve into elephantiasis (essentially, the entire body is affected and swollen), and interestingly, elephantiasis can evolve into lepra. The treatment of lepra is the same regimen as for scabies, but according to Mercurialis, it required stronger medication.

Mercurialis addressed *lichen*, known today as impetigo, a disease that can affect the whole body, but particularly arose on the face and chin. *Lichen*, per Mercurialis, was dangerous because it can spread over the entire face, and involve the eyes, or it may cause disfigurement; it was identified by its numerous round sores and broad plaques with itching, burning, and roughness.[94] Mercurialis stirred up a controversy involving *lichen* and another ancient skin disease, *mentagra* (see Chapter 4), and he claimed that they two conditions were not the same as Pliny had suggested.[95] His reasons: *lichen* was an old disease described by Hippocrates, and Pliny's *mentagra* was new; *lichen* of the chin, according to Galen, was painful and itchy, and dangerous, while Pliny's *mentagra* was not painful or dangerous; and finally, Pliny's *mentagra* affected the eminent men of Roman society, while *lichen* affected anyone.[96] Such was the type of discourse that can be found throughout Mercurialis' work. Treatment for *lichen* includes the same administered for pruritus, scabies, and lepra. Mercurialis pointed out that *lichen* can evolve into *scabies* and *lepra*, thus completing a continuum of disease in which the main dermatologic diseases are all connected to one another.

In sum, Mercurialis' milestone work is a comprehensive review of the writings of ancient and medieval authorities dating back to the time of Hippocrates (460–370 BCE). As the first volume devoted primarily to dermatology, it can be appreciated as a complete overview of all the available information regarding skin diseases up until the mid-sixteenth century. He excelled at giving readers different viewpoints on authorities; then, acting as an assured mediator, he interjected his opinion to correct the view when he thought it necessary. In some cases, his viewpoint was original, but in others, Mercurialis showed a heavy bias toward the Greeks, especially Galen and Aristotle, and often twisted their words so that they fell in line with Renaissance thinking. Although the modern physician is more likely to respect the results of a current research article than one from the early twentieth century, in Mercurialis' mind, the opposite is true: the Greek ancients could do no wrong. Later authors had the bravery and confidence to challenge the Greeks with a different way of thinking about these diseases. Mercurialis, for the most part, did not. While he himself offered little to no new contributions, he deserves credit for his erudite survey of diseases of the skin—a milestone of humanism and the elevation of old knowledge.

De Decoratione Liber (1585)

Briefly, a few comments about *De decoratione liber*, "Book on Adornment," a collection of notes from Mercurialis' lectures compiled in 1585 by Giulio Mancini (1559–1630). The 44-page text (each numbered page with an unnumbered reverse side) is significant because its topics represent the skin issues that a Renaissance physician would typically ignore, though Mercurialis is hopeful, per the subtitle, that doctors, philosophers, and students of all disciplines would find the book useful.[97]

The table of contents of *De decoratione* reveals that the principal cosmetic concerns of a Renaissance-era patient involved the face and hands: the cosmetic art or adornment, and a discussion of beauty and ugliness; the origin and authors of the cosmetic art; the usefulness of the cosmetic art; under which part of medicine it should be placed; how the beauty is spoiled by many blemishes and what things should be done from the beginning; obesity of the whole body or part of it; being slender; blemishes of the skin, and with discoloration defiled from its original color; in which many things are discussed related to skin color; sun spots on the face and hands; the skill of the adorner, and how the defects may be lessened; hair care; skin care; spots on the face; scars; bruises or livid spots; how the substance of the skin is disturbed by these blemishes and why an odor might even emanate; fissures; blemishes that render the skin uneven chiefly about warts; calluses; acne; boils; miliaria; wrinkles; nail diseases, primarily of their falling off; thickened and deformed nails; nails in leprosy; dirty nails and color change of nails; paronychia; and body odor.

In the first few chapters, Mercurialis reveals that Galen accepted "cosmetic art" as a discipline of medicine, with Mercurialis himself echoing that it was a discipline worthy of a physician's attention. As in the case of most of the skin diseases discussed in *De morbis cutaneis*, cosmetic defects, such as pimples, result from humoral imbalance and are managed with a combination of internal (e.g., bloodletting and purging) and external remedies, and in the case of acne, extraction. No secret from Mercurialis' text can be found to the age-old problem of wrinkles since he believed "they are able to be disguised, or even hidden at times; however, but they are never able to be healed."[98]

GASPARE TAGLIACOZZI AND THE "ITALIAN METHOD"

De decoratione is also famous for having the first reference to the nasal reconstruction techniques pioneered by the Italian surgeon Gaspare Tagliacozzi (1545–1599), a contemporary of Mercurialis, who did not officially publish his method until 12 years later in a work entitled *De Curtorum Chirurgia per Insitionem,* "On the Surgery of Defects by Grafting" (1597). Dueling with rapiers, a popular method among men dealing with conflict during the sixteenth century, not infrequently resulted in someone losing his nose, if not his life. The forehead method, in which forehead skin is donated and flapped down to cover the nasal defect, originated in India some 2000 years ago and is still used today.[99] Tagliacozzi is considered one of the founding fathers of plastic surgery for devising the "Italian method," a type of skin flap in which the arm was fixed in position for several weeks in close proximity to the nose, while a flap of skin from the biceps was partially excised and placed on the nose. Once the flap "took" on the nose, it could be severed from the arm, and the person could finally lower his arm.

Jan Jessen (1566–1601)

Mercurialis was unquestionably the prototypical representative of the Renaissance for the history of dermatology, and his two texts will forever be considered among the most important works in the history of the specialty. But there is one last figure whose contributions may represent more of a turning point toward the modern era.

Jan Jessen, also known as Johannes Jessenius or Jan Jesensky, was a Bohemian polymath who delved into medicine, philosophy, politics, and poetry. Born in Breslau (present-day Wrócław), he studied medicine in Wittenberg and Leipzig, and then Padua, where he overlapped with Mercurialis and the esteemed anatomical educator, Hieronymus Fabricius (1533–1610). Jessen is most famously associated with Prague and for working as a physician, rubbing elbows with the astronomer, Tycho Brahe, and performing that city's first public cadaveric dissection. He also served as a politician on behalf of the Protestant cause, which resulted in his execution in Prague in 1601 during the Thirty Years' War.

In addition to a description of his public dissection named *The Prague Anatomy* and an important surgical text called *Institutiones chirurgices*, both of which appeared in 1601, Jessen authored in that same fateful year a short treatise on the skin entitled *De cute, et cutaneis affectibus*, "On the Skin, and the Affections of the Skin." *De cute* is a brief, 12-page disputation that contains Jessen's 21 arguments that he himself made at a disputation at the University of Wittenberg in the year prior to its publication (1600). Only three copies of the work are known to exist.

Jessen was among the first to identify skin affections as diseases "of the skin," not merely disruptions on the surface of the body as an indication of disease inside the body. According to Galenic theory, the skin could not have its own diseases because disease was defined by Galen as a disruption of function, and since the skin had no function, it could not have diseases. Jessen viewed the skin differently, seeing much more purpose and function than a simple covering. For him, the skin was a defensive barrier that regulated the body's emissions, temperature, and beauty.[100] It was also a window into the internal organs; therefore, if you studied a patient's skin, you could learn a lot about the condition of the whole body.[101] Like Mercurialis, Jessen organized skin diseases by roughness or hardness, or by color or blemish.[102] He saw some skin diseases as caused by external forces, while others were caused by an imbalance of internal forces.[103] To Jensen, any an attack on the attractiveness of the skin was every bit a disease as an attack on its porosity.[104] He advanced itch as an abnormal sensation, but not a disease.[105]

How Jessen viewed the skin is strikingly similar to the modern view, and his short work on the skin— as opposed to Mercurialis' longer, decidedly Galenic work—is the first great dermatologic text of the modern era. Mercurialis' text, though significant for being the first of its kind to focus solely on the skin, did not herald the modern era of dermatology that would follow. But Jessen's work did offer the first whispers of modern dermatology. According to Murphy, *De Cute* arose out of necessity; the practical-minded surgeons and physicians of the era needed to better understand the skin as they were faced with public health crises that involved the skin: the Black Death (see Interlude 2) and the rise of syphilis (see Interlude 3).[106] Jessen's contribution was finally writing down what medical men for the last hundred years had begun to conclude, i.e., the skin was a structure that could indeed have its own diseases, even if Galen did not say so. In spite of Jessen's modern view, however, it will be seen in the chapters that follow that Galenism survived the sixteenth century.

Summary

Renaissance physicians carried on the long tradition of relying heavily on the terms, classification, and treatments of skin disease proposed by Galen. The physicians and surgeons of the period continued to promote purging and bloodletting in order to correct the humoral imbalances that were considered the cause of skin diseases. At this time, skin disease was classified into only two categories of disease: of the head and of the rest of the body. Most writers of the period considered the skin a sort of membrane or envelope surrounding the body, with its main function the excretion of waste products from the body. The skin was excluded from the "anatomical revolution" of the rest of the body. Still, the Renaissance was not lacking in advances in knowledge related to the skin and its diseases, as it was the era in which the first textbook of dermatology was written: *De morbis cutaneis* by Mercurialis (1572). Mercurialis further organized skin diseases on the basis of roughness, color, or bulk (thickness). We also see the first indications of the idea that the skin could be diseased itself, that it was not always an innocent bystander, affected only by the process of evacuating morbid material from the body through its layers. Because of the repercussions of epidemic diseases involving the skin (such as bubonic plague and especially syphilis), the skin entered the consciousness of practitioners, such as physicians, surgeons, and quacks, as well as the layperson, in a way unequaled in the past. Evidence from this period suggests there was no scarcity of medical writings about skin disease. Although these documents contained information that did not differ greatly from that of the ancient Greek and Roman physicians or the compilers and preservers of the Middle Ages, the very fact that there was so much talk about skin disease underpins the premise that modern dermatology's subtle beginnings originated during this period.

Interlude 2

The Black Death and Other Pandemics

Throughout history, deadly pandemics of highly infectious diseases have ravaged large populations of people, often altering the course of history for the affected societies as a result of colossal mortality. Except in the case of the cholera and influenza epidemics of the nineteenth through twenty-first centuries, virtually every historically significant epidemic disease had major manifestations on the skin. In this section, it is our task to deal with the great plagues of history, particularly as they relate to the skin. The ultimate epidemic disease affecting the skin, i.e., smallpox, will be dealt with in a later section.

The Plague of Athens

The earliest recorded pandemic in human history was the Plague of Athens (430–426 BCE), an epidemic that inflicted a devastating blow to the Athenian people at a time when war with Sparta had just broken out again. As much as a quarter of the population of Athens, including its famous leader Pericles, died during this outbreak.[1] The following is a description of the disease by the classical Greek historian Thucydides (460–400 BCE), who survived the disease himself and whose name was attached to the syndrome (Thucydides syndrome):

> Persons in full health were seized suddenly, without any ostensible cause, with hot flushes about the head, redness and turgescence of the eyes, while the parts within, both the pharynx and the tongue, became, at once, blood red, and the breath was extremely fetid; and in succession to these symptoms, followed sneezing and hoarseness. Shortly afterwards the disorder descended into the chest, occasioning a violent cough, and, settling on the heart, it caused both a reversion of the heart and every kind of bilious evacuation which has ever been designated by physicians; and these were accompanied by great distress, that is, to use medical terms, were accompanied by tormina and tenesmus. A hollow hiccup came on in most cases, giving rise to a violent spasm, which, in some instances, ceased soon, and in others only after a considerable interval. The surface of the body was neither very hot to the touch nor was it pale, but reddish, livid, and covered with small vesicles and sores; while inwardly it was so burnt up that the sufferers were impatient of garments of the lightest tissue or covering of the finest linen; their only desire, in fact, was to lie naked, Thus, they longed for nothing so much as to cast themselves into cold water; and many, who were not well attended to, urged by an unquenchable thirst, actually did so, by plunging into the cisterns; and yet whether they drank much or little, it was all the same…Very many, however, of those who survived those critical days, were eventually carried off by the debility and exhaustion which ensued from the disease passing down into the abdomen, and there causing extensive ulceration together with profuse diarrhea. For the disease, which had its first seat in the head, beginning from above, passed through the whole body, and, if any one did get safely through its most dangerous stages, he had yet to endure a seizure of the extremities, which left traces of its virulence behind. The malady, in fact, lighted upon, or rather, to speak medically, it was by a process of metastasis, resumed in the pudenda, the fingers, and toes, with such violence, that many of those who recovered were not only deprived of those parts, but some of them also lost their eyes; while others, at the commencement of their recovery, had so completely lost their memory as to have no recollection either of their friends or themselves.[2]

The disease that caused this epidemic is, to this day, one of the great medical mysteries of all time. The condition appeared to start in the head and neck with "hot flushes about the head" (headache),

DOI: 10.1201/9781003273622-12

red eyes (conjunctivitis), and a sore throat. Then the afflicted suffered from cough, chest pain, and laryngitis, implying that the infection had descended down the airway. Next is vomiting, diarrhea, and weakness. The red, burning rash sounds like a cephalocaudal vesicular exanthem. All of these complaints suggest that the Athenians were dealing with a viral illness. We can infer from the loss of fingers and toes that some of the Athenian victims experienced disseminated intravascular coagulation (DIC). To the present author, the specifics of insatiable thirst (due to either dehydration or diabetes insipidus) along with vision loss (due to either corneal scarring or optic nerve damage) and memory loss are the crucial symptoms. Smallpox can cause corneal scarring and dehydration. These features also bring up encephalitis as a possible diagnosis; it can cause diabetes insipidus, memory loss, and damage to the ophthalmic system. In sum, we are looking for an epidemic viral syndrome that causes a cephalocaudal vesicular rash and DIC, and if the mechanism of vision loss and thirst is corneal scarring and simple dehydration, then smallpox is the best retroactive diagnosis. But if the mechanism of the vision loss and thirst is cerebral inflammation, some type of viral encephalitis is the most likely cause.

Measles has been reported to cause both encephalitis and DIC. Cunha noted that the internal sensation of heat, relieved with immersion in cold wells, is specific for measles, noting that in the Fiji Islands outbreak of 1875, many of the outbreak's 40,000 measles victims ran into rivers and streams to relieve the sensation of heat.[3] However, blisters and ulcers are not seen in measles. In that case, smallpox fits better, but scholars have argued that smallpox did not arrive in the classical world until several centuries later (see Interlude 4).

Numerous other infectious diseases have been postulated as the cause of the Athenian plague. In 2005, researchers claimed to have extracted *Salmonella typhi* DNA from the teeth of the ancient remains in a mass grave, leading to the conclusion that typhoid fever was the cause of the plague. However, convincing arguments have come forth that the research was flawed.[4] And the constellation of mucosal and skin findings described by Thucydides are not seen in typhoid fever, which has "rose spots" (small red flat spots on the torso), as its only skin finding. Other candidates for the Athenian plague are bubonic plague, epidemic typhus, and meningococcemia. Thucydides neglected to mention glandular swellings (buboes) as a feature of the disease, effectively ruling out bubonic plague. Another interesting hypothesis is that the Athenian plague was caused by Ebola hemorrhagic fever.[5] Olson et al. point out that the plague was believed by the Greeks to come from Africa. Ebola is also associated with a sudden onset of fever, headache, and pharyngitis, followed by cough, vomiting, diarrhea, severe weakness, a red rash, and hemorrhage from various orifices. Arboviral (mosquito-borne) diseases, which can lead to encephalitis, should also be considered.

Not long after the Plague of Athens, in 396 BCE, an unknown infectious disease struck a Carthaginian army while it besieged the Greeks of Syracuse, a city in Sicily, allowing the Greeks to break the siege and crush the Carthaginians. The only source of information about this so-called Carthaginian Plague comes from Diodorus Siculus (fl. first century BCE). Diodorus described the syndrome as having the following symptoms: sore throat, burning pain all over the body, fatigue, diarrhea, delirium, and a pustular skin rash (*phlyctenae*).[6] Smallpox is the most likely candidate for the cause of those findings, and if you consider the proximity in time of this scourge to the Plague of Athens, it can be suggested that the Carthaginian Plague was simply a continuation of the Plague of Athens, which was therefore caused by smallpox. Perhaps smallpox arrived in the classical world much earlier than previously acknowledged.

The Antonine Plague

The Antonine Plague (165–180 CE) was a devastating epidemic that occurred during the reign of Roman Emperor Marcus Aurelius Antoninus; it was also known as the Plague of Galen since the greatest eyewitness to this plague was none other than the physician Galen. Although Galen never devoted an entire treatise to the epidemic, he did leave scattered accounts. A skin rash was a major feature of the Antonine Plague; Galen described it as black pustules which erupted all over the body, dried up and scabbing over, leaving behind scars.[7] His description perfectly coincides with the evolution of the smallpox exanthem, and scholars generally believe that the smallpox virus caused the Antonine Plague.

Approximately 10 percent of Rome's population died in this epidemic, including the emperor Marcus Aurelius, making it the worst pandemic in human history up to that time.[8] The Antonine Plague coincided with the last years of the *Pax Romana*, but it is unclear how significant this plague was for the empire's eventual decline. While Edward Gibbon did not consider the Antonine Plague particularly problematic in his famous book, *The Decline and Fall of the Roman Empire*, modern scholarship considers the Antonine Plague a significant turning point, one that changed the trajectory of Rome, but it was not a coup de grace.[9]

The Plague of Cyprian

The Plague of Cyprian (249–262 CE) was the second major plague to strike the Roman Empire; this plague was even more devastating than the Antonine Plague because it further heightened the instability of an already politically and economically unstable time known as the Crisis of the Third Century. It was named after St. Cyprian of Carthage (ca. 200–258 CE), an important figure in the history of the Western church in the third century who left an eyewitness account of the plague entitled *De mortalitate*, "On the plague."[10] Only from the Christian record can we draw conclusions about this obscure event; there was no historian like Thucydides or physician like Galen, leaving us a detailed account.[11] The magnitude of the loss of life is unclear. We do know from Cyprian that the plague was empire-wide in its scope, with approximately 62 percent of the population of Alexandria succumbing to the disease, and as many as 5000 persons per day dying in Rome at one point.[12] A major social effect of the plague was the strengthening of Christianity, as people looked to the new religion and its promise of a rewarding afterlife.[13]

The infectious disease that caused the Plague of Cyprian is unknown, but the skin does not appear to have been involved in this plague as in others. Still, historians have argued that smallpox or measles was the cause.[14] Smallpox is a natural candidate for the Plague of Cyprian, but in no place is a diffuse pustular rash mentioned in descriptions of the syndrome. The first definitive descriptions of measles did not appear in the medical literature until Rhazes' works of the tenth century CE. It is hard to believe that a condition as distinct and impressive as measles would exist for seven centuries and receive no attention in the medical literature of Late Antiquity. Perhaps, the measles rash was lost inside a body of literature fraught with diagnostic confusion. A process known as selection-aware molecular clock modeling places the origin of the measles virus in the sixth century BCE, confirming that the measles virus, a paramyxovirus, diverged from a devastating cattle plague known as rinderpest as humans intermingled with cattle in antiquity.[15] Incidentally, rinderpest is the only other viral disease besides smallpox to be completely eradicated from the world. If smallpox and measles are excluded as candidates for the Plague of Cyprian on the basis of no evidence for skin involvement in the syndrome, with the major features of this syndrome being fever, diarrhea, vomiting, and hemorrhage, diseases that deserve stronger consideration include typhoid fever, pandemic influenza, Ebola, and other hemorrhagic fevers.[16]

MEASLES

A highly effective vaccine for measles eliminated this potentially devastating illness from the United States by 2000, but both the influx of unvaccinated travelers and immigrants and the anti-vaccination movement have caused a resurgence of measles in the United States starting in 2015. Worldwide, measles continues to affect millions each year, and with approximately 100,000 people dying from the disease annually, measles is one of the leading causes of vaccine-preventable death.[17] It is presently the most contagious disease on earth, with a basic reproduction number (R_0) of 16–18, meaning that a person infected with measles will transmit the virus to 16–18 people.

The Plague of Justinian

The Plague of Justinian (541–750 CE) was the first of three historical pandemics of bubonic plague. The Second Pandemic of Plague began with the Black Death in the fourteenth century, and the Third Pandemic occurred in the nineteenth century in China. The Justinianic Plague was named after the Byzantine emperor Justinian (r. 527–565), who was famous for attempting to restore the empire by reconquering Italy and nearly succeeding. Much of what we know about this Plague comes from the writings of the two principal eyewitnesses of the Justinianic Plague: Procopius of Caesarea (ca. 500–560) and John of Ephesus (ca. 507–588).

The initial wave of the Plague of Justinian (541–544) was the most devastating, especially to Constantinople, but repeated waves struck Europe and the Near East for the next 200 years. While some scholars contend, based on the literary evidence, that the Justinianic Plague was responsible for the death of half of the population of Europe, others argue that this high mortality rate is not supported by the demographic and economic trends gleaned from the archeological evidence (papyri, coinage, inscriptions, land use, and ancient DNA).[18] Still others contend that the Justinianic Plague was devastating enough economically and militarily to squelch Justinian's ambitions for recapturing the Western Roman Empire.[19]

Scientists have supporting evidence—DNA studies of plague victims' teeth—that the Justinianic Plague was caused by the *Yersinia pestis* bacterium.[20] This organism is transmitted by a vector, the Oriental rat flea (*Xenopsylla cheopis*), which introduces the disease to humans through its bite; although its natural reservoir is the rat, other mammals, such as prairie dogs, are suspects for hosting this bacterium. In humans, infection with *Y. pestis* presents in three major forms: bubonic, septicemic, and pneumonic. All three forms are typically seen in a pandemic. A victim has the best chance of surviving bubonic plague, which occurs after a bite and is characterized by the presence of buboes—large, painful lymph node swellings that eventually suppurate. If the infection spreads from the buboes to the bloodstream, septicemic plague ensues, and dark purpuric lesions develop all over the body. If the infection spreads to the lungs, the patient is said to have pneumonic plague, which can spread from person to person by respiratory droplets. Both septicemic and pneumonic plague are uniformly deadly without antibiotics. However, because persons with these more serious forms of plague were likely to die before having a chance to spread the disease, it is widely held that the bubonic form was most responsible for the transmission of the infection throughout the pandemic.

Y. pestis was first isolated in 1894 by Swiss-French physician Alexandre Yersin (1863–1943) during his research of the Third Pandemic of Plague (1850–1960) in Hong Kong. Though Yersin named the organism after his mentor, Louis Pasteur, it was later renamed *Yersinia* to honor its discoverer. While it is generally accepted that *Y. pestis* is the cause of bubonic, pneumonic, and septicemic plague, it remains controversial among some scientific circles whether *Yersinia* was indeed the cause of the Justinianic Plague and the Black Death (see below).

Little was known about pre-Justinianic bubonic plague until 2010, when phylogenetic studies indicated that bubonic plague originated in China some 2600 years ago. This conclusion was questioned in 2015 after *Y. pestis* DNA dating up to 5000 years ago was found in Eurasian remains.[21] In 2018, *Y. pestis* DNA was discovered in skeletal remains in Sweden, placing the bacterium in Europe some 4900 years ago, which could explain population declines that occurred in Neolithic Europe (7000–1700 BCE).[22] It has also been suggested that the presence of the Greek word βουβών (*boubōn*) in the Hippocratic corpus is evidence that the Hippocratics knew about plague. But the word in ancient Greek refers simply to the area below the abdomen (the groin area). The term *boubōn* was used in many instances in regard to medical conditions unrelated to plague, and of the 12 occurrences of the term in the entire corpus, none meets the criteria for a description of bubonic plague.[23]

The first legitimate literary evidence of bubonic plague is attributed to Rufus of Ephesus, writing in the first century CE. Most of the writings of Rufus do not survive, but the Byzantine compiler Oribasius (320–400 CE) included in his *Medical Collections* a passage entitled, "From the works of Rufus. On *boubōn*." In that passage, Oribasius wrote, quoting Rufus,

> Then there are the *boubónes* called pestilential, which are especially seen around Libya and Egypt and Syria, and are most deadly and highly acute.... And they said that a sharp fever

followed closely and terrible pain, disturbance of the entire body, and delirium and the swelling of *boubónes* that are large, hard, and not suppurating, not only in the accustomed places, but also on the part behind the knee and at the bend of the arm although such inflammations do not happen there at all.[24]

There is no doubt from the description that Rufus was talking about bubonic plague; it can, therefore, be inferred that it was an active disease in the regions he mentioned, but not particularly common in Rome. The only other author to discuss "pestilential *boubónes*" was Aretaeus of Cappadocia, who described them in his "On the Causes and Signs of Acute Diseases" as arising from the liver and being "especially malignant."[25] In contrast, Galen, in his more than 20 volumes and thousands of pages, does not once mention them.[26] It is likely that for someone as learned and prolific as Galen to omit bubonic plague from his writings speaks to the fact that the condition was not common in the Greek-speaking world and certainly argues that a pandemic of the disease never took place in antiquity.

The challenge of explaining so much death was unimaginably difficult for the Byzantines. The principal sixth-century historian Procopius characterized this dilemma when he wrote of the Justinianic Plague:

> During these times there was a pestilence, by which the whole human race came near to being annihilated. Now in the case of all other scourges sent from heaven some explanation of a cause might be given by daring men, such as the many theories propounded by those clever in these matters, for they love to conjure up causes which are utterly incomprehensible to man.... But for this calamity, it is quite impossible either to express in words or to conceive in thought any explanation, except indeed to refer it to God.[27]

The best description of the effects on the body of the Justinianic Plague, also from Procopius, is in keeping with our modern understanding. He noted that first, the victims had a sudden fever but without any change in color or feeling of warmth. Then, on the next day or in the next few days, a bubonic swelling "took place not only in the particular part of the body which is called *boubon*, that is, 'below the abdomen,' but also inside the armpit, and in some cases also beside the ears, and at different points on the thighs."[28] Then some of the sufferers entered into a "deep coma," while others a "violent delirium," while many others "died straightaway"; in those cases "where neither coma nor delirium came on, the bubonic swelling became mortified and the sufferer, no longer able to endure the pain, died."[29] Procopius then commented,

> Now some of the physicians who were at a loss because the symptoms were not understood, supposing that the disease centered in the bubonic swellings, decided to investigate the bodies of the dead. And upon opening some of the swellings, they found a strange sort of carbuncle that had grown inside them. Death came in some cases immediately, in others after many days; and with some the body broke out with black pustules about as large as a lentil and these did not survive even one day, but all succumbed immediately. With many also a vomiting of blood ensued without visible cause and straightway brought death...
>
> Now in those cases where the swelling rose to an unusual size and a discharge of pus had set in, it came about that they escaped from the disease and survived, for clearly the acute condition of the carbuncle had found relief in this direction, and this proved to be in general an indication of returning health; but in cases where the swelling preserved its former appearance there ensued those troubles which I have just mentioned. And with some of them it came about that the thigh was withered, in which case, though the swelling was there, it did not develop the least suppuration. With others who survived the tongue did not remain unaffected, and they lived on either lisping or speaking incoherently and with difficulty.[30]

Note that the discharge of pus (suppuration) from the buboes was viewed as a favorable prognostic finding. Procopius' comment about the difficulty with speech in survivors of the plague correctly points out that stroke was a possible complication of this infection due to its tendency to trigger hypercoagulability.

The term for this increase in the thickness of the blood is DIC; the phenomenon is not unique to plague but a feature of several blood-borne infectious diseases. One cannot mistake the Justinianic Plague for something other than the bubonic plague.

The Black Death

The Black Death (1347–1351) was the deadliest pandemic in recorded human history, taking the lives of a staggering 30–60 percent of the population of Europe, or tens of millions of people. This particular outbreak was part of a larger so-called Second Pandemic of Plague, which started in 1331 in either China or the steppes of central Asia, then spread westward toward the Middle East and Europe by the Mongols and Far Eastern traders on the Silk Road. This Second Pandemic lasted for several centuries. Contemporary European accounts, as well as recent scholarship by historians of the Black Death, have long assumed that the pandemic originated in Asia and devastated China and India before spreading to Europe. But a review of contemporary written evidence in both regions reveals no substantive proof that the pandemic ravaged either China or India as it did in the West.[31]

According to the famous account by Gabriele de Mussi (ca. 1280–1356), the plague was first introduced in Eastern Europe during the siege of Kaffa (Crimea) in one of the earliest examples of biological warfare. In 1346, the city was under attack by the Mongols, who flung their plague-infected dead by trebuchets over the walls and into the city. The plague then migrated westward to the ports of Constantinople, Messina (Sicily), and Marseilles in 1347–1348, presumably carried by rat-infested cargo ships. The widening pandemic expanded in a clockwise fashion to England by 1348, central Europe by 1349, Scandinavia by 1350, and Russia by 1351, leaving in its path a trail of dead bodies never seen before or since.

The plague returned again and again in various places all over Europe until the eighteenth century; the most famous of these recurrences was the Great Plague of London (1665–1666). Fourteenth-century writers called this pandemic the "Great Mortality" (*mortalitas magna*) or the "Great Pestilence" or *atra mors*, meaning "terrible (or dreadful) death." When Johannes Isacius Pontanus (1571–1639) referred to the Plague of 1347 as *atra mors* in a work entitled *Rerum danicarum historia*, "History of the Danish People" (1631), it was translated for the first time as the "Black Death."[32] *Atra* was the Latin word for the color black, but it was also used emotively to mean "dark" or "ill-omened." It could also mean "terrible" or "grisly," and it was a word associated with funerals and mourning. Regardless, starting in the seventeenth century, the Great Mortality became known as the Black Death. Traditional beliefs for the use of the color black to describe this plague are as a reference to either the black skin lesions that erupted in the hours before death; a black comet seen before the arrival of the plague; the color of the widespread mourning due to the high mortality rate; or the plague symbolized as a man on a black horse or as a black giant.[33]

While the majority of researchers believe that the Black Death was caused by *Y. pestis*, support for this claim among scholars of the subject is not unanimous.[34] Refuters of *Y. pestis* as its cause have brought forth some very compelling arguments, such as the conditions being too cold in places such as Iceland for flea activity or that rats were simply not present in certain areas where the plague was rampant.[35] The incubation period for the Black Death has been established to be too long for what is necessary to control the spread of bubonic plague. The medievals used a 40-day-long quarantine—the word "quarantine" derives from the Italian word for 40 days (*quaranta giorni*), a duration which has biblical roots—to mitigate the transmission of the disease, whereas the incubation period of modern bubonic plague is only a few days.[36] And the Black Death was too deadly, too rapidly spreading, too contagious, and too relentless to blame bubonic plague, a condition which is historically less lethal than the Black Death, and typically slow moving through populations, remitting with reductions in flea-activity during the winter; reductions in the incidence of the Black Death were not seen in the winter.[37] The differential diagnosis of bubonic plague includes viral hemorrhagic fever, including Ebola, or other infectious diseases such as anthrax, typhus, typhoid, and relapsing fever; perhaps these diseases deserve at least some consideration. Or perhaps medieval bubonic plague was very different from modern plague in terms of its virulence, transmission, and epidemiology. The present author's opinion is that it is very unlikely that contact with draining buboes was the means by which widespread transmission occurred.

The contemporary descriptions of the Black Death shed some light on the controversy. The most famous non-medical literary voice of the Black Death was Giovanni Boccaccio (1313–1375), the Florentine writer who authored a collection of 100 short stories called the *Decameron* (1353). His description of the signs of the plague is the most illuminating:

> Yet not as it had done in the East, where, if any bled at the nose, it was a manifest sign of inevitable death; nay, but in men and women alike there appeared, at the beginning of the malady, certain swellings, either on the groin or under the armpits, whereof some waxed of the bigness of a common apple, others like unto an egg, some more and some less, and these the vulgar named plague-boils.

> From these two parts the aforesaid death-bearing plague-boils proceeded, in brief space, to appear and come indifferently in every part of the body; wherefrom after awhile, the fashion of the contagion began to change into black or livid blotches, which showed themselves in many [first] on the arms and about the thighs and [after spread to] every other part of the person, in some large and sparse and in others small and thick-sown; and like as the plague-boils had been first (and yet were) a very certain token of coming death, even so were these for every one to whom they came.[38]

Guy de Chauliac, the medieval surgeon who witnessed the Black Death in Avignon in 1348 and never left his post, wrote the most widely read contemporary medical description of a seven-month-long epidemic of plague.[39] The first form of plague, which only occurred in the first two months of the epidemic, caused fevers and coughing of blood (pneumonic plague) and led to death within three days. The second type occurred for the duration of seven months and was characterized by "carbuncles" in the axillae and groin and death within five days. Guy noted that those who were coughing were particularly contagious, and the afflicted generally died alone, without servants, priests, or family members at the bedside. Guy himself contracted the Black Death but survived it.

In addition to his famous exposition of the beginning of the Black Death, Gabriele de Mussi vividly described the stages of plague experienced by the victims in Piacenza, his hometown.[40] The first feature was chills and stiffness and a general tingly or prickly sensation. Then a very hard and solid bubo erupted in the armpit or groin. Next were the fever and headaches, along with an insufferable odor for some; for others, it was vomiting of blood or "swellings" on the back, chest, or thigh, the latter signifying imminent death. The majority of the afflicted died between days three and five. Raymond Chalin de Vinario, a late fourteenth-century French contemporary of Chauliac and physician to three popes, left another significant account of the Black Death from a medical standpoint.[41] Besides commenting on the black spots on the skin, he described an additional feature of the plague: carbuncular inflammation of the throat with difficulty swallowing, to the point of suffocation. John VI Kantakouzenos (1293–1383), a Byzantine emperor and historian, also wrote about the plague, but the description of what he witnessed, in even his own son, is in some places a word-for-word copy of Thucydides' description of the plague of Athens, which was a totally different disease and experience than the Black Death.[42] Dozens, if not hundreds, of plague accounts exist as wave after wave of the plague struck Europe well into the modern era.

A few thousand cases of bubonic plague occur each year in the world today; these cases provide us with a modern look at the medieval disease. A comparison of the medieval accounts to a summary of modern accounts of bubonic plague in Arizona and Madagascar supports the diagnosis of plague as the cause of the Black Death.[43] Modern plague starts with fever, chills, weakness, and headache a few days after a flea bite. Then, the patient develops a bubo, which is a markedly enlarged, exquisitely tender infected lymph node in the region of the flea bite. Flea bites, which occur most commonly on the lower extremities, are most likely to cause buboes in the groin region. Children, who typically play low to the ground, are susceptible to flea bites on the upper extremities. In these cases, and in cases associated with a cat bite or scratch, the buboes are more common in the underarm or neck. Untreated bubonic plague can lead to sepsis with DIC, pneumonia, or meningitis. Septicemic and pneumonic forms of plague can both occur with or without a preceding bubo; pneumonic plague can result from inhalation of infected aerosolized respiratory secretions. Plague patients can uncommonly experience severe tonsillitis (pharyngeal plague) or prominent gastrointestinal symptoms, confusing the picture. The most atypical reported route of acquiring plague was a case of pharyngeal plague after the ingestion of camel meat from camels infected with plague by flea bites.[44] Indeed, in modern plague, the flea appears to play a crucial role in the transmission of the infection.

The dermatologic features of the Black Death, as described by its contemporary writers, serve as evidence for some scholars that the cause was something other than bubonic plague. In addition to the buboes, numerous accounts from the fourteenth through the sixteenth centuries contain references to black or livid spots, carbuncles, blisters, and pustules found all over the body in plague victims. Samuel Cohn, a most persuasive voice against *Y. pestis* as the cause of the Black Death, argued that the absence of widespread pustules and other skin lesions in the Third Pandemic data from India, suggests that something other than bubonic plague was the cause of the Black Death.[45] In the fourteenth-century plague treatises, pustules were an important feature of the disease and relevant for prognosis, and the presence of widespread pustules and carbuncles was associated with a worse prognosis.[46] From the modern descriptions of the plague, we know that the vast majority of patients with modern plague do not have skin lesions other than the draining buboes. But if left untreated, plague can lead to several dermatologic findings that have been reported in the modern literature: purpura, ecthyma gangrenosum, carbuncles, blisters, eschars, and pustules.[47] Butler pointed out that pustular rashes were uncommonly, but not rarely, identified in plague patients in Vietnam in the 1960s.[48] Again, these findings are not a major feature of the disease, but it is incorrect to say that pustules or "carbuncles" do not or cannot occur in bubonic plague.

The most classic skin lesions of plague are livid or black spots which we would today call purpura; they form as a result of DIC and can evolve into necrosis and subsequent gangrene of the distal extremities. The presence of black spots on the skin in the pre-antibiotic era signaled a death sentence. Another potential mechanism of skin lesions in the setting of plague is the development of vasculitis in the skin, a consequence of the immune response to the infection as one's immune system generates antibodies that bind to the bacterial proteins and accumulate in vessels of the skin, leading to inflammation of the vessel wall and hemorrhage. Vasculitic skin lesions appear not uncommonly as hemorrhagic pustules.

Perhaps this debate can be finally put to rest. In 2010, *Yersinia* DNA was discovered in the tooth sockets of the remains of fourteenth-century plague victims from mass graves all over Europe; they offered this as proof that *Y. pestis* was indeed the cause of the Black Death.[49] Perhaps the rat and its flea played a limited role in the transmission of the Black Death. Perhaps other vectors like the human flea (*Pulex irritans*) or the body louse (*Pediculus humanus*) actually transmitted the disease.[50] Perhaps *Y. pestis* was more virulent and deadlier in the fourteenth century. Perhaps comparing the Second and Third Pandemics is misguided when considering the contextual differences of individual and public health, hygiene, nutrition, medicine, and living conditions of periods that are 500 years apart in time.

The medieval writers who described the Black Death were aware that the bubonic form and the pneumonic form were two different presentations of the same disease, but they struggled to explain such an utterly devastating illness with Galenic humoralism. Instead, even their most scientific explanations involved either astrological or religious influences (or both). The general consensus for the time, as summarized by Guy de Chauliac, was that the Black Death had its origins in the heavenly bodies, specifically "from the conjunction of the three superior planets, Saturn, Jupiter and Mars that had been preceded by another conjunction on March 24, 1345, in the 14th degree of Aquarius."[51] It was widely held that conjunctions (when two or more planets line up exactly) could bring about major changes: new kings, the appearance of prophets, or great plagues. Conjunctions between Jupiter and Saturn occur every 20 years: the last was December 21, 2020, the first year of the Covid-19 pandemic.

Another prevailing interpretation of the cause of the Black Death had religious underpinnings. God was angry at man for his sins—especially his sensuality—or testing man's patience, but ultimately God's plan was not to be understood; it was to be feared.[52] Even the skin lesions were placed in a religious context. The black or livid patches, noted frequently on the chest and back and which occurred when the infection spread into the bloodstream, were referred to in popular contemporary literature, such as that of Daniel Defoe and William Shakespeare, as "God's tokens," since death soon followed after their appearance.

As miasma theory was the dominant theory to explain infectious diseases at the time, it was believed that the source of infection lay in the stench of the axillary and inguinal boils. Strong perfumes were developed at this time to mask the offensive odors, and the sweet-smelling essences—cinnamon, cloves, musk, saffron, rose oil, and camphor—were applied to clothing to protect a person from the miasma emitted from the diseased person. Doctors wore long robes and beaked masks filled with fragrant herbs to protect themselves on the job. For medieval medical and surgical management of the plague, Guy de Chauliac offered the most comprehensive advice. He instructed his readers to flee the regions where the plague is flourishing, but if plague is omnipresent, use purgative pills and get phlebotomized while keeping the air in one's surroundings pure by burning a fire in the hearth. He recommended theriac to help the heart and sweet-smelling items to rectify the humors. He treated active cases with phlebotomy, laxatives, electuaries (herbals mixed with honey), and sweet cordials, and advanced the buboes with ground figs, boiled onions, yeast, and butter, while gas-filled carbuncles were scarified and cauterized.[53]

We are fortunate to have numerous accounts of the plague to study for the purposes of learning the human experience of the Black Death.[54] But even in the era of Covid-19, it is impossible to fully comprehend the fear, the dread, and the despair that the Europeans must have felt from the Great Mortality all around them. Since *Yersinia* continues to "plague" the human race to this day, we must continue to study the Black Death in order to learn about the disease, its transmission, how to identify it, and how to react to it.

St. Anthony's Fire and *Ignis Sacer*

The historical record shows that on numerous occasions during the Middle Ages, the peoples of Europe faced local epidemics of a pestilential disease known as St. Anthony's Fire or *ignis sacer*, "holy fire." These terms cause some confusion because *ignis sacer* had been used since ancient times by several medical writers, including Celsus and Cassius Felix, to describe a variety of painful skin conditions, which we today could refer to as erysipelas, shingles, or some ulcerative disease such as pyoderma gangrenosum. Furthermore, St. Anthony's Fire can today refer to either the medieval pestilence presently discussed or the streptococcal skin infection known as erysipelas. The reason for the confusion is that the term *ignis sacer* was borrowed—either mistakenly or intentionally—from the ancients by medieval medical writers to designate a new epidemic disease characterized by burning pain in the legs and feet, followed by swelling, red blistery areas, peeling of the skin, and ultimately, loss of sensation, gangrene, and autoamputation of the fingers and the toes.

The first mention of this pestilence occurred in the *Annales Xantenses*, "The Annals of Xanten." Xanten had an abbey along the Rhine in modern-day Germany. The entry for the year 857 reads, "A great plague of swollen blisters consumed the people by a loathsome rot so that limbs were loosened and fell off before death."[55] Forty-thousand people died in and around Aquitaine (France) in 994 in one of the worst outbreaks of the Middle Ages. Barger, a twentieth-century scholar of this disease, placed it in the context of the end of the millennium, and he offered a description of the horror:

> And when a plague of invisible fire broke out, cutting off limbs from the body and consuming many in a single night, the sufferers thronged to the churches and invoked the help of the Saints. The cries of those in pain and the shedding of burned-up limbs alike excited pity; the stench of rotten flesh was unbearable; many were however cooled by the sprinkling of holy water and snatched from mortal peril.[56]

Initial accounts of this pestilence referred to it as *ignis ocultus*, "hidden fire," but by the tenth century, it was consistently referred to as *ignis sacer.*[57] Other accounts referred to it as a type of erysipelas. Epidemics of this disease struck the French regions of Metz in 1001 and Lorraine in 1089; the latter was described by chronicler Sigebert of Gembloux (1030–1112): "a great number of people were afflicted by a gruesome disease which caused their limbs to become as black as coal, and from which the patients died miserably, or were reduced to an unhappy life, having lost hands and feet."[58] Six outbreaks of *ignis sacer* were recorded in the tenth century, seven in the eleventh, ten in the twelfth, and three in the thirteenth; the majority of these occurred in France.[59] Other epidemics occurred at various times in Germany, Denmark, Burgundy, and less so in England.[60] *Ignis sacer* sickened parts of Europe again and again until the nineteenth century, when it became very uncommon.

The medievals attributed the cause of *ignis sacer* to divine wrath, and thus two saints became associated with this plague. The first of these was St. Martial (third century CE), whose aid was invoked by the people in the region of Limousin (Limoges, France) during the tenth century. The local bishop there led public prayer and carried relics of St. Martial in a processional in order to attenuate the outbreak.[61] The other was St. Anthony (251–356 CE), whose name became associated with this pestilence in the eleventh century. In the 1090s, a church was built in Vienne, France, to honor St. Anthony and house his relics. Those afflicted with the pestilence made pilgrimages to this revered place, and an order known as the Hospital Brothers of St. Anthony was established in 1095 to care for the pilgrims, giving hope to persons suffering from this plague all over Europe. It was widely recognized that just a week-long stay at the Abbey of St. Anthony could result in a cure.[62]

In addition to the expected adoration of St. Anthony, afflicted pilgrims could anticipate in Vienne good nutrition and treatments from the Brothers, who would apply plant-derived poultices for the purpose of pain relief and healing. The order's reputation for success with the treatment of St. Anthony's fire and other skin diseases grew; their monastic order expanded to several cities in France, Germany, and Scandinavia. They later cared for victims of the Black Death in the fourteenth century. By the fifteenth century, there were 370 Antonine hospitals, with their characteristic red paint, across central Europe.[63] Visits to these hospitals became so popular that "beggars, impostors, and simulators" feigned St. Anthony's Fire by applying dressings, falsifying bleeding with fake blood made from blackberries, creating ulcers with caustic juices, using a broken egg on a bandage to make what looks like pus; they could even recreate a convincing case of gangrene.[64]

The most famous of these Antonine hospitals was at Isenheim near Colmar, France, where today can be found the spectacular altarpiece by Nikolaus of Haguenau and Matthias Grünewald (created 1512–1516), who depicted St. Anthony in several portions of the massive work along with a person suffering from St. Anthony's fire and Christ studded with plague spots. The attention to skin disease in the Isenheim altarpiece is distinctive.

St. Anthony's Fire was almost exclusively a disease of the peasantry, and children were more susceptible than adults. It began with intense pain in the legs or feet, with the surface of the extremities feeling cold to the touch. The skin typically then turned livid or black; sometimes, it was studded with blisters and red, as seen in erysipelas. Gangrene ensued, and limbs eventually autoamputated; this was considered a good prognostic sign.[65] In areas east of the Rhine, the gangrenous features of this syndrome were less common; instead, after the initial sensory symptoms, nausea, vomiting, and diarrhea ensued, followed by fits of convulsions, mania, and/or hallucinations. Such was the natural history of this illness, so what exactly was the cause of it?

In the sixteenth and seventeenth centuries, physician investigators in Germany and France, such as the Frenchman Denis Dodart (1634–1707), started to suspect that the cause of these mysterious epidemics was the ingestion of bread made from spurred rye. Spurred rye, or cockspur rye, results from contamination of the ergot fungus, *Claviceps purpurea*, when there is a harsh winter followed by a rainy spring. Rye bread made from spurred rye turns a red color. Ergot fungi contain ergotamine, an alkaloid and potent vasoconstrictor; ergotamine, a serotonin agonist, also effects the brain and is a precursor to lysergic acid diethylamide (LSD). It promotes uterine contractions, reduces postpartum bleeding, and alleviates migraine headaches. For these purposes, ergot alkaloid derivatives are still available today, although they are much less commonly prescribed than in the past.

Toxicity from consumption of substantial amounts of ergotamine can manifest as severe limb pain and peripheral vasoconstriction (gangrenous ergotism), or seizures, muscle spasms, delusion, confusion, and hallucinations (convulsive ergotism). The prevalence of ergotism among the poor is explained by the tendency of the poor to consume spurred rye. The dissimilarity in the manifestations of ergotism east and west of the Rhine remains somewhat of a mystery. Modern researchers suggest that it was variability in the concentration of ergot alkaloids in the grain due to various reasons: regional differences in the strains of *C. purpurea*, differences in the soil or habitat where the grain was grown and stored, and degradation of the ergot over time after prolonged storage.[66] Less rye was grown in Italy in the Middle Ages; hence, St. Anthony's Fire was not mentioned in medieval Italian chronicles.[67]

Scholars have counted at least 83 epidemics of ergotism dating back to the ninth century.[68] One of the earliest outbreaks of ergotism occurred in Paris ca. 945. Numerous people in Paris developed the painful skin sores and went to St. Mary's Church in Paris in search of relief. They were taken in by the church, but after a quick recovery, the ill returned home, only to develop the sores again. The nourishment at St. Mary's Church was from the duke Hugh the Great's uncontaminated grain stores, and simply a break from the dangerous grain at home led to resolution of the skin lesions.[69]

It is difficult to quantify the morbidity and mortality caused by ergotism throughout history, but it is likely in the millions. While gangrenous ergotism is yet another fascinating example of pestilential disease involving the skin, the most intriguing aspect of this phenomenon concerns the circumstantial evidence for the role ergot may have played at various times throughout history. Scholarly research has shown that in the eighteenth century, rye consumption in parts of Europe stunted population growth by its interference with fertility; wheat-eating England saw its population grow at times when rye-eating France did not, and even in England, when wheat prices were high, rye consumption increased, because rye is much cheaper, and fertility rates decreased.[70] In 1722, Russia's Peter the Great was campaigning with his army in the Caucasus and had to abandon his ambitions for Persian lands because of ergotism, which decimated his army by an estimated 20,000 deaths.[71] The Great Fear (July 22–August 6, 1789) was a period of panic, mass hysteria, and revolt within the peasant class at the beginning of the French Revolution that has been attributed, with rather compelling data, to ergotism; "1789 was an 'ergot year' in Northern France."[72] Convulsive ergotism may explain the bizarre behavior of the young women accused at the Salem witch trials (1692–1693). The soil near the affected households was ideal for the growth of rye; the climatic conditions in Salem were suitable for ergot to prosper; and there is evidence of red-colored bread being used in religious services in Salem at the time.[73] Historians have postulated that convulsive ergotism was responsible for unusual behaviors of persons throughout history, but in most cases, there is no proof. Examples of these conjectural instances include the behavior of the Viking berserkers, the hallucinations of Hildegard of Bingen and other Christian mystics, and the Eleusinian Mysteries of Ancient Greece.

Whether ergotism was a strictly medieval phenomenon or also prevalent in the ancient world is one of the great unanswered questions about this topic; however, there is no reason to think that the *C. purpurea* was not present in ancient times since several textual references exist to ergot in ancient documents. A Babylonian tablet dated to 2500 BCE mentions in an inscription that "the women who gather noxious grasses" were "expelled from the city with the exorcists and mutterers of charms," while a Sumerian tablet of the same period describes reddening of damp grain.[74] An Assyrian tablet (660 BCE) alludes to a "noxious pustule in the ear of grain," and the sacred book of the Parsees (Zoroastrian Persians) dating to 400 BCE references "noxious grasses that cause pregnant women to drop the womb and die in childbed."[75] The Chinese were using ergot as early as 1100 BCE in obstetrics, and Hippocrates' *melanthion* may have been ergot as he knew of its benefits with postpartum hemorrhage.[76] The *ignis sacer* of the Greeks and Romans, however, appears to refer to several different skin diseases that involve fiery pain or the spread of the condition like fire, but not the specific syndrome of ergotism that involves gangrenous necrosis of the extremities.

Ergotism ravaged European societies throughout the Middle Ages and the early modern period. Yet, it remains a relevant condition for public health authorities today. There was an outbreak of what may have been ergotism as recently as 1951 in Pont-Saint-Esprit, France, which affected 250 persons with an acute psychiatric illness after ingesting poisoned bread. Interestingly, a compelling argument exists, supported by declassified documents, that the actual cause of the illness was CIA experiments with LSD on this population.[77] In 2011–2012, 14 high school students in LeRoy, New York, began to collectively exhibit Tourette's syndrome-like behaviors with vocal and motor tics. Ergotism and other environmental poisonings were considered but ultimately ruled out; authorities concluded that conversion syndrome and/or mass hysteria were the cause.[78] Ergotism is a fascinating phenomenon and a reminder that what we ingest can have major implications for us as individuals as well as for societies as a whole. The reader is referred to some extraordinary scholarship by Foscati on the entire subject of St. Anthony's Fire.[79]

Tarantism and the Dancing Plagues

Tarantism is a disorder characterized by dancing to music following the bite of a spider. It was first reported in the eleventh century but was most commonly recorded in the fifteenth through eighteenth centuries. The spider of concern at the time was the Apulian tarantula of southern Italy; now known as *Lycosa tarantula*, this spider is not a tarantula but a type of wolf spider, whose bite is as harmful as a bee sting. It is more likely that it was the Mediterranean black widow (*Latrodectus tredecimguttatus*) that caused cases with an organic neurologic syndrome arising after the bite.[80] Both of these spiders were more active in the summer when tarantism was more prevalent. A person who was bitten by one of these arachnids would then engage in fast tempo, upbeat dancing to music called a *tarantella* in order to avoid death from the bite. Stephen Storace (1762–1796), an English composer of the eighteenth century, witnessed an outbreak and documented the music in a letter, giving us one of the best eyewitness accounts of this bizarre phenomenon:

> It happened one day that a poor man was taken ill in the street, and it was soon known to be the effect of the tarantula, because the country people have some undoubted signs to know it and particularly (they say) that the tarantula bites on the tip or under lip of one's ear, because the tarantula bites one when sleeping on the ground: and the wounded part becomes black, which happens three days after one is bit.... The people at the sight of me cried out—play—play the tarantella: (which is a tune made use of on such occasions). It happen'd that I had never heard that tune, consequently, cou'd not play it.... I told them I could not play it but if any would sing it, I would learn it immediately; [a] woman came, and helped me to learn it; which I did in about ten minutes time ... the man began to move accordingly, and got up as quick as lightning, and seem'd as if he had been awaken'd by some frightful vision, and wildly star'd about still moving every joint of his body; but as I had not as yet learn'd the whole tune, I left off playing, not thinking that it would have any effect on the man. But the instant I left off playing the man fell down and cried out very loud, and distorted his face, legs, arms, and every other part of his body, scraped the earth with his hands and was in such contortions, that clearly indicated him to be in miserable agonies ... and then the people cried out faster-faster; meaning that I should give a quicker motion to the tune, which I did so quick, that I could hardly keep up playing and the man danced in time.... I suffered a long patience to keep up such a long time, for I played (without exaggeration) about two hours, without the least interval.... The people took him up and carried him into a house, and put him into a large tub of tepid water, and a surgeon bled him.... He sweated a great deal and fell asleep, which he did for five or six hours, when he awakened, was perfectly well, only weak for the great loss of blood he had sustained and four days after he was entirely recover'd.[81]

Tarantism appears to have been a phenomenon that primarily affected persons who were hysterical, melancholic, depressed, frustrated, neurotic, or otherwise mentally ill.[82] It has been associated with lycanthropy, fanaticism, prejudice, superstition, religion, misery, and poverty.[83] Attempts to explain the bizarre phenomenon have linked it to rabies, ergotism, financial hardship, the consumption of enormous quantities of wine, as well as sun and heatstroke.[84] Scholars today generally agree that tarantism had little to do with the effects of the bite itself and more to do with a type of epidemic (or mass) hysteria that grew out of psychological distress in the context of local cultural influences, superstitions, and folklore.[85]

In the case of tarantism, the dancing and music were seen as therapeutic for the effects of the bite of the spider. Literally, dance or die. These facts differ from other dancing plagues that occurred in different parts of Europe, which appeared spontaneously and seemed to have no association with spider bites. The first of these occurred in 1021 in Kölbigk (Germany), but the most famous of the dancing plagues occurred in Aachen in 1374 and Strasbourg in 1518. In 1374, thousands of people in western Germany, the Low Countries, and northeastern France danced in agony for days or even weeks, begging for priests or anyone to save their souls, while in Strasbourg in the hot summer of 1518, as many as 400 people succumbed to the outbreak, which claimed the lives of about 15 men, women and children every day.[86]

Scholars such as Kohn link the dancing manias to the flagellant (self-scourging) movement and place the manias in the context of religious self-chastisement.[87] Ergotism has been proposed as a cause for this phenomenon, but scholars such as Waller cannot link rye ingestion to each of the outbreak locations, which occurred in various places throughout Europe.[88] It is more likely that dancing plagues, like tarantism, represent a type of mass psychogenic illness, or epidemic hysteria.

ST. VITUS' DANCE

Contemporaries of these plagues first believed the episodes to be conjured by saints, such as St. Vitus, who had been venerated with dancing parties over the centuries, to cleanse the body of demonic possession. Perhaps more and more people would join into these "plagues" in order to be a part of the religious cleansing, wanting others to think that they too were touched by a saint. The dancing plagues became known as St. Vitus' dance (coined by Paracelsus) when a group of dancers in Strasbourg touched the nearby church containing the relics of that saint.[89] Note that these dancing manias are to be distinguished from the other types of chorea (a neurologic disorder characterized by rhythmic dance-like jerking motions), such as the chorea that accompanies rheumatic fever and that was named Sydenham's chorea after Thomas Sydenham (see Chapter 9).

The English Sweating Sickness and the Picardy Sweat

The next epidemic with dermatologic implications was the Sweating Sickness, also known as the "English sweat" or *sudor anglicus*, that struck England and other parts of Europe in five epidemics between 1485 and 1551.[90] The first outbreak occurred not long after the Battle of Bosworth Field, when Henry Tudor (the future Henry VII) and his French mercenary soldiers—who possibly brought the sickness to England—crushed the House of York and took the throne of England.[91]

These were terrifying times. An English physician named John Caius (1510–1573) penned the main eyewitness account of the Sweating Sickness called *A Boke or Counseill against the Disease Commonly Called the Sweate or the Sweating Sickness* (1552). Review of Caius' text reveals no mention of a rash or respiratory symptoms occurring at any point in the syndrome. The illness was quick, deadly, and came out of nowhere, characterized by a sudden onset of fever, weakness, and sweating. Tens of thousands died, often within 24 hours of the onset of the illness. Unlike other epidemics which affected the poor, the Sweating Sickness preferentially affected middle-aged, wealthy, professional-class males.[92]

The etiology of these epidemics remains among the most baffling medical mysteries in the history of medicine; relapsing fever, influenza, typhus, plague, arboviruses, botulism, and ergotism have all been both argued for and rejected as causes. The current prevailing theory places the blame on an unknown hantavirus that may or may not have gone extinct. Hantaviruses are rodent-borne viruses that cause a similar syndrome, but the Sweating Sickness appeared to spread from human to human without a rodent vector.[93] Other candidates include anthrax, meningococcal disease, dengue fever, and a tick-borne hemorrhagic fever known as Crimean-Congo hemorrhagic fever (CCHF).[94] Research into the cause of this epidemic disease will hopefully continue, as this devastating illness could potentially return again.

A less deadly version of the English Sweat, known as the Picardy Sweat, appeared in Picardy, France, in 1718 and occurred again and again in small epidemics for almost 200 years. In addition to having a lower mortality rate and the presence of neurological symptoms, the Picardy Sweat differed from the English Sweat in that affected persons experienced itching within 12–24 hours of the illness and a reddish rash within the first 48 hours.[95] The rash, according to a vivid report written in 1833 by Dr. Prosper Ménière, of Ménière's disease, represents miliaria (also known as prickly heat) which sometimes occurs in the setting of high fever and perspiration and is caused by obstruction of sweat ducts; sadly, the rash offers no clue to the etiology of this disease:

> The sweating is often prodigiously great, patients being obliged to change their shirts 20 to 30 times in the course of one night, and this "flux" continuing to the like extent for two or three days. Its odor was that of rotten straw, or of a weak solution of chlorine, or of the evacuations

of the cholera morbus. The water halitus from the skin is kept rarified by the heat of the bed-clothes; when these are removed, it is condensed, and forms a thick cloud, which speedily resolves itself into a sort of rain. The bowels are usually constipated, and the urine is scanty. The sweating lasts sometimes for four, five and six days, and it ceases gradually without the substitution of any other critical evacuation, or the occurrence of other symptoms; but in the majority of cases, a vesicular eruption on the chest, neck, back, and successively over all the body, appears on the second, third, or fourth day. It varies exceedingly in different patients: the vesicles are usually of the size of millet seeds—here and there a few larger ones are scattered. In the early stage, the rash appears papular; when it dies away, the part is found covered with furfuraceous scale.[96]

The description of this so-called miliary fever rules out diseases such as scarlet fever or measles. Considering the neurologic symptoms, Kohn noted stronger evidence for acute meningococcal disease as the cause of the Picardy sweat, while Heyman contends that a hantavirus is most likely responsible for this illness.[97]

Plica Polonica

The next topic of this section was not actually a plague but a cultural phenomenon. The term *plica polonica* (*plica* from Latin, "to knit" or "to fold together," as in "complicate") is translated as "Polish plait" and refers to hair that is so matted and entangled that it becomes an impregnable mass of keratin, resembling a bird's nest. Another term for it was *trichoma*, a tumor or mass of hair. It was a condition associated with the people of Eastern Europe, particularly Poland, traditionally considered brought there by the Mongol invasion in 1287.

Plica was first described by the German physician Johannes Schenck von Grafenberg (1530–1598), also known by the Latin moniker, Schenckius. In 1584, he described plica as "an irreversible plaiting of the hair accompanied by lice, headache, mutilating arthritis, scoliosis, and onychog-ryphosis."[98] Referred to as *trica incubarus* (devil's hair), *weichselzopf*, and *plica polonica*, early descriptions of this entity focused as much on its perceived spiritual roots as its medical origins. A variety of causes was attributed to plica, originating in Eastern European folklore and superstition: a witch's curse, the work of wicked elves (termed elflock), or a punishment from God. It was generally accepted by the learned physicians of Europe as a medical condition resulting from internal disease until the mid-nineteenth century. It was believed that morbid material left the body and resided in the scalp; both laypersons and physicians of the seventeenth and eighteenth centuries maintained that cutting the matted mass could lead to death, and that further entanglement of the hair could mean relief from existing internal disease. Villagers, beggars, and the elderly were deemed more susceptible to this disease; other risk factors included feelings of sadness, anger, resentment, and horror, and living in swampy or unhealthy conditions.[99] But, in general, a person of any age, gender, or social status could suffer from plica. Some authors held that it was contagious, while others believed it was congenital.[100]

By the mid-nineteenth century, physicians finally came around to the idea that plica was not a disease, nor should its formation be considered a treatment for disease; rather, it was a symptom of poor hygiene and caused by the neglect of brushing and cutting the hair in a population controlled by superstition. Cazenave considered it a complication of seborrheic dermatitis, and Kaposi viewed it as end-stage neglect (see Chapters 13 and 14).[101] Additional contributing factors to the formation of the mass of hair were the entanglement promoted by lice nits and infection of the underlying scalp. The leading academic nineteenth-century physicians engaged in an uphill battle to convince the naive peasantry that their beliefs, promoted by local priests and physicians, were erroneous and that the treatment for plica—cutting the plait away—would not lead to death. In 1884, the condition became known as plica neuropathica, in reference to the association of neglected, matted hair with psychological disturbance.[102]

Anthrax

Anthrax is an infection with the Gram-positive, rod-shaped bacterium, *Bacillus anthracis*, that more commonly attacks livestock than humans. Humans who tend to infected cattle, such as wool handlers, are at high risk for the disease by either skin contact, inhalation, or ingestion of *Bacillus* spores. Anthrax most commonly presents first on the skin; this form is known as cutaneous anthrax and is characterized by a solitary, painless black nodule with a peripheral red halo. Fortunately, cutaneous anthrax is not particularly deadly, unlike the pulmonary and gastrointestinal forms of the disease, but all forms can be successfully cured with antibiotics.

Anthrax is an ancient illness, believed to have existed in pharaonic Egypt and possibly even responsible for the cattle-killing (fifth) and the boil-riddling (sixth) plagues of Egypt in the Book of Exodus. The word anthrax derives from the Greek word for coal, in reference to the black center of the skin lesions, and according to the Bible, the Sixth Plague occurred after "soot from a kiln" was thrown by Moses, dusting all of Egypt.[103] Virgil (70–19 BCE) wrote extensively about anthrax in his *Georgics*.[104] It is widely believed that Avicenna's "Persian fire" was cutaneous anthrax. Throughout history, the impact of *B. anthracis* has largely been felt through devastating epizootics, especially in the seventeenth through nineteenth centuries. It was first officially described as a human disease—and called the malignant pustule—in the mid-eighteenth century. The bacterium was first identified by Davaine and Rayer in the blood of sheep in 1850 (see Chapter 13). Robert Koch (1843–1910) was a founder of the germ theory of disease, and his "Koch's postulates" (see Chapter 11) were developed directly from his work with anthrax, proven to be caused by *B. anthracis* in 1867. Anthrax remains relevant today, in reference to the October 2001 US anthrax scare and the 1972 Sverdlovsk (Yekaterinburg) anthrax outbreak that occurred after an accidental leak of anthrax spores from a military research facility that resulted in the death of dozens of Russian citizens. Anthrax is endemic in Russia, and there are concerns that melting of the permafrost due to climate change in East Siberia might expose millions of frozen livestock carcasses and their immortal and deadly anthrax spores.[105]

Yellow Fever

The next epidemic disease to discuss as it relates to the skin is yellow fever, but the only cutaneous symptom of this disease is jaundice, the yellowing of the skin caused by liver damage that occurs in 15 percent of cases. Yellow fever is a typically short-lived viral disease that is transmitted by the bite of a mosquito (*Aedes aegypti*) infected with an RNA flavivirus. The classic symptoms of yellow fever are fever, nausea, back pain, and headache, all of which improve in just a few days. For the unlucky ones who get liver damage, the yellowing of the skin (jaundice) typically starts at the end of the first week, when the fever breaks and the patient starts to improve symptomatically. Around 30 percent of persons with jaundice die from liver failure.[106] It is a gruesome way to go, as the liver failure causes impaired coagulation, and the infected vomit blood and bleed from every orifice.

The history of yellow fever is a relatively short one compared to other epidemic viral diseases; it is believed to have originated as an endemic disease in Africa which was brought to the New World by the shipping industry and the African slave trade starting in the seventeenth century. While there were outbreaks in southern Europe in the nineteenth century, yellow fever devastated cities of North and South America from the seventeenth through twentieth centuries. The deadliest period in US history was from 1793 to 1905; the 1793 outbreak in Philadelphia ended the lives of 10 percent of that city's population. The coastal towns of the US eastern seaboard and Gulf Coast such as New York, Charleston, Baltimore, Norfolk, and New Orleans were particularly susceptible to outbreaks, having imported the mosquitos along with commercial goods from places like Havana and Santo Domingo. No city suffered more with yellow fever in the nineteenth century than the present author's hometown of New Orleans, where 40,000-plus persons died in repeated outbreaks from 1817 to 1905; the deadliest year was 1853 when the "Yellow Jack" took the lives of 8000 residents. New Orleans—with its mosquito-laden surrounding swamps, necropolis-like cemeteries, haunted French Quarter locales, and voodoo traditions—wasn't always "The Big Easy"; it was once the "City of the Dead." The last US outbreak occurred in New Orleans in 1905. Yellow fever remains a significant problem today in Africa and South America; 78,000 persons died of the disease in Africa in 2013.[107]

The major breakthrough in medical science that led to the ultimate eradication of yellow fever from the United States was the recognition that the disease was transmitted by mosquitos. Cuban epidemiologist Carlos Finlay (1833–1915) is credited with the theory (1881), and a team led by Walter Reed (1851–1902) confirmed Finlay's theory in 1900. The elimination of infected mosquitos in places like Havana (by 1901) and Panama (by 1906) secured the eradication of the virus in the United States. The Panama Canal was being constructed around this time, and the United States was only able to take over the construction of the Panama Canal from France—and achieve significant economic and geopolitical strength—because yellow fever (and malaria) had decimated the French engineers.[108] The advancement of medical theory by Finlay and the Reed Commission allowed the construction to proceed without the casualties brought about by yellow fever in the past. In 1927, the yellow fever virus was the first human virus isolated, and a highly effective vaccine was developed the following decade. Unlike other viral illnesses, however, the only way to eradicate this virus from the world is to eradicate the mosquito that transmits it.

THE YELLOW PLAGUE OF 664 CE

Yellow fever is not to be confused with the Yellow Plague. The Yellow Plague of 664 CE was the first major epidemic recorded in English history.[109] The only source of information about this plague comes from the Venerable Bede's (672–735) *Ecclesiastical History of the English People* (731), which noted that the plague erupted soon after a total eclipse of the sun. Because of the widespread mortality noted by Bede, both smallpox and bubonic plague have been speculated as to the cause of this historical mystery, but there is no description of the symptoms of this plague or explanation why it and a similar Irish plague in the 540s were called yellow. Perhaps it was in reference to the yellow pustules of smallpox. Also worth considering are epidemic diseases besides yellow fever that are associated with jaundice, including viral hepatitis (especially hepatitis A), malaria, CCHF, and dengue fever.

Epidemic Typhus

Epidemic typhus is an infection with a bacterium called *Rickettsia prowazekii* that is transmitted from person to person by the human body louse; the bacterium resides in the feces of the louse. This louse is slightly different from the lice that infest the hair of schoolchildren. Instead, it infests the body and garments of persons of poor health and hygiene living in unclean conditions. Scratching the louse bites causes the person to rub the louse feces into the wound, thus inoculating the body with the bacterium. The signs and symptoms of typhus include fever, chills, headache, rapid breathing, body aches, cough, nausea, vomiting, confusion, and a rash. The red, petechial rash starts on the torso and spreads outward to the arms and legs. The mortality rate of untreated epidemic typhus is anywhere from 10 to 60 percent; with antibiotics, the condition is uniformly survivable. Epidemic typhus should be distinguished from endemic (murine) typhus, which occurs worldwide and is spread by the rat flea, and typhoid, a febrile condition with red spots on the skin caused by *S. typhi*, made famous in the twentieth century by the life and career of "Typhoid Mary."

The origins of typhus are unknown. While typhus is occasionally promoted as the cause of the Athenian and Antonine Plagues, the first definitive typhus epidemic in Europe occurred in Spain during the reconquest of Grenada in 1492, and the first episode of typhus in the New World (Mexico) was clearly described in 1545.[110] Typhus was first described—and distinguished from plague—by Girolamo Fracastoro in his 1546 work *De contagione*, "On contagion." It is not clear whether typhus was brought from the Old World to the New World, or vice versa.

Typhus became a major problem in two principal settings: jails and wars. In the filthy European prisons of the early modern period, typhus, better known at the time as "jail fever," spread like wildfire, killing off inmates before they could even be executed, and the nidus of infection that was the jail became of a public health liability in places like London. Repeated wartime epidemics occurred in Europe during the seventeenth through twentieth centuries; the most famous of these claimed lives of many of the half-million soldiers Napoleon lost as his Grand Army retreated from Russia in that particularly brutal winter of 1812–1813.[111] Among many other wars, typhus figured prominently in the Thirty Years' War (1618–1648), the American Revolution, the Bolshevik Revolution, and both World Wars, and in the Nazi concentration camps.[112] Hans Zinsser, an American bacteriologist and writer noted for his work with typhus, argued in his masterpiece *Rats, Lice, and History* (1935), that throughout history, typhus caused more deaths in war than the warfare itself.[113]

Typhus was thought to be the same disease as typhoid until the eighteenth century. The role of lice in the transmission of typhus was discovered in 1909, and in 1916, Henrique da Rocha Lima (1879–1956) isolated the organism responsible for typhus and named it after Howard Ricketts (1871–1910) and Stanislaus von Prowazek (1875–1915), both of whom died of typhus while investigating the disease. Today, epidemic typhus is a rare disease; the last outbreaks occurred in 1995 in Burundi and in 2012 in Rwanda. Persons impacted by poverty, poor hygiene, and unsanitary living conditions are at the highest risk for contracting typhus. Typhus has a wild animal host (the flying squirrel), and, therefore, *R. prowazekii* could reemerge during a future time of war, famine, or other human catastrophes. Minor outbreaks of the disease have occurred in homeless camps in various parts of the world, including the United States.

Human Immunodeficiency Virus/Acquired Immunodeficiency Syndrome

The first case of human immunodeficiency virus (HIV) infection occurred in 1959 in the Congo, but it is believed that the virus had been transmitted from chimpanzees to humans as early as the 1920s. The first person to die from HIV infection in the United States did so in 1969. The HIV epidemic did not ignite, however, until the late 1970s, and it reached its zenith in the 1980s and 1990s. Since the beginning of the epidemic, 79 million people have been infected with HIV, and 36 million people have died from it as of 2020.[114]

The skin figures prominently in the HIV/AIDS epidemic. The most classic of the myriad cutaneous manifestations of AIDS—the syndrome of depressed immunity caused by the virus—is a type of skin lesion called Kaposi's sarcoma (KS), first described by Moriz Kaposi in the nineteenth century (see Chapter 14). It is caused by human herpesvirus-8; a weakened immune system allows this virus to form tumors in the lymphatic system, and restoration of the immune system often causes the tumors to disappear. The purple-red papules and plaques of KS soon became a dermatologic stigma of possible HIV infection in the 1980s. Countless other dermatoses were also seen, including severe seborrheic dermatitis and psoriasis; molluscum-like cutaneous lesions of opportunistic fungal infections (e.g., cryptococcosis); a generalized itchy, papular eruption; and more severe presentations of cutaneous viral, bacterial and fungal infections. Knowledge of all the possibilities of skin diseases in this unique patient population was essential in the 1980s through 2000s. Today, there are highly effective treatments for HIV and prophylactic medications that are able to limit the transmission of the disease both sexually and transplacentally. Thus, the severity of cutaneous disease observed in HIV positive patients in Western medical clinics has been greatly reduced starting in the 2010s, but in parts of the world where access to these medications is poor, the many dermatologic manifestations of HIV disease remain problematic.

Coronavirus Disease-2019 (Covid-19)

In December 2019, the first cases of a novel coronavirus infection were documented in Wuhan, China. The cause was SARS-CoV-2, a highly contagious virus that attacks the respiratory system and causes death (most commonly due to respiratory failure) in <1 percent of all persons infected with the virus, but with a higher risk of death according to age and comorbidities. Within a few months, the virus had spread all over the world, and the death toll rapidly mounted. As of May 2022, 521 million people have been infected with SARS-CoV-2, and 6.2 million people have died worldwide. Four different types of vaccines (RNA, viral vector, whole virus, and protein subunit) have been released all over the world to bolster immunity against this virus.

Infection with SARS-CoV-2 can lead to various types of cutaneous manifestations. The most famous of these is called "Covid toes"—a condition which dermatologists refer to as perniosis. Perniosis is theorized to be caused by hypercoagulability or hyperviscosity of the blood, and in cold-sensitive parts of the skin surface, such as the toes, the skin experiences small thromboses (clots) and inflammation. The most common sequela of Covid-19 is a classic viral (morbilliform) exanthem, but it can also cause hives (urticaria), a papulovesicular rash (blisters), livedo reticularis, vasculitis, petechiae, erythema multiforme-like lesions, and acral-ischemic lesions.[115] The diversity of these skin lesions reflects the virus' ability to induce variable immune responses in the host. Three months after infection, diffuse shedding of the scalp can occur in what is termed telogen effluvium. As of the publication of this text, our understanding of this novel virus' effect on the human body—and the skin—is evolving.

Summary

The skin has played a role in almost all of the significant pandemics of history. The first major recorded pandemic is known as the Athenian Plague (430–426 BCE), and the cause of that pandemic remains one of the great medical mysteries of all time. It is likely that either smallpox or measles was the cause, but many researchers believe that both of those diseases arrived in the classical world several centuries later. The Antonine Plague (165–180 CE) was almost certainly caused by smallpox and may have been the first major epidemic caused by that disease. The Plague of Cyprian (249–262 CE), which may or may not have been the beginning of the end for the Roman Empire, had little to do with the skin, but scholars have argued for measles or smallpox as a cause of that plague also. The Plague of Justinian (541–750 CE) was the first major pandemic of bubonic plague, while the second started in the fourteenth century and was known as the Black Death. The Black Death was the first dermatologic nightmare of all nightmares, and there is ample literature left behind about the dermatologic implications of that pandemic. Other important illnesses in the history of dermatology were St. Anthony's fire, tarantism, the English Sweating Sickness, the Picardy Sweat, anthrax, typhus, yellow fever, plica polonica, HIV/AIDS, and Covid-19.

Part II

Order

I do not know what I may appear to the world, but to myself I seem to have been only like a boy playing on the sea-shore, and diverting myself in now and then finding a smoother pebble or a prettier shell than ordinary, whilst the great ocean of truth lay all undiscovered before me.[1]

Isaac Newton

Our century is called ... the century of philosophy par excellence ... The discovery and application of a new method of philosophizing, the kind of enthusiasm which accompanies discoveries, a certain exaltation of ideas, which the spectacle of the universe produces in us – all these causes have brought about a lively fermentation of minds, spreading through nature in all directions like a river which has burst its dams.[2]

Jean le Rond d'Alembert

For the recognition of a disease of the skin, no other assistance is required than a knowledge of the objective symptoms, which are visible on the surface of the body in each particular case. We do not attach any value whatever, either to the history or to the subjective phenomena in investigating a cutaneous affection; for we ought to be guided in this matter only by those symptoms which are appreciable by the sight, the touch, or (sometimes) by the smell. These afford certain and infallible grounds for the establishment of a diagnosis, for they have their origins in the malady itself. They are, so to speak, the alphabet, of which the letters are traced on the skin, and our task is but that of deciphering the writing.[3]

Ferdinand von Hebra

It is remarkable that in the journalistic paeans in which the triumphs of medicine in the glorious reign of Queen Victoria have been lately recounted, dermatology has had no part. Why should this branch of our art be thus unhonoured and unsung? It is a form of specialism, no doubt; but specialism is no longer looked upon as an unclean thing—except by some survivor of an antique world here and there. Dermatology, although its victories have perhaps been less showy than those won in some other special departments, has not lagged behind in the onward march of medicine.[4]

Malcolm Morris

DOI: 10.1201/9781003273622-13

9

The Scientific Revolution

The brilliant minds of the seventeenth century recognized that the scientific knowledge of the world around them had stood alone on the word of the great thinkers of the ancient past. It was now time to develop a new "system of the world," one based on empirical data and observation, not on old texts from millennia ago. The scholars of this era developed a natural philosophy (i.e., science) from new hypotheses, experiments, results, and conclusions. This scientific spirit also began to reform in medicine, with observation and empiricism eventually challenging the authority of the ancients. This fascinating period of intellectual development is known as the Scientific Revolution.

The roots of the Scientific Revolution arose in 1543, a year that should be remembered for the publication of two of the most important works in the history of the world. The first was Vesalius' *De humani corporis fabrica*, discussed in the previous chapter. The other was *De revolutionibus orbium coelestium*, "On the Revolutions of the Heavenly Bodies," by the mathematician and astronomer Nicolaus Copernicus (1473–1543).[5] In the tenth chapter of the first book, Copernicus controversially wrote:

> At rest, however, in the middle of everything is the sun. For in this most beautiful temple, who would place this lamp in another or better position than that from which it can light up the whole thing at the same time? For, the sun is not inappropriately called by some people the lantern of the universe, its mind by others, and its ruler by still others …. Thus indeed, as though seated on a royal throne, the sun governs the family of planets revolving around it.[6]

His bold statement and supporting evidence contradicted the system described by the ancient Greco-Roman astronomer Claudius Ptolemy (100–170), which placed the earth at the center of the universe, with the planets, sun, and stars revolving it in a perfect circular motion. Copernicus was not the first to propose this heliocentric theory; Aristarchus of Samos (310–230 BCE) had done so previously, but his theory was overshadowed by that of Ptolemy, and the Ptolemaic system dominated for 1500 years. Ptolemy was to astronomy what Galen was to medicine. The discoveries of Copernicus signified the first major revolt against the authority of the ancients, but it would take another 125 years until the Copernican system was generally accepted.

What followed were the efforts to prove the Copernican system in spite of attempts by the Catholic Church to reject the ludicrous concept. The Danish astronomer Tycho Brahe (1546–1601) combined the Copernican system and the Ptolemaic systems, resulting in the theory that the moon orbits the earth, the planets orbit the sun, but the sun still orbits the earth. Unlike the Copernican system, however, the Catholic Church did not denounce the geocentric Tychonic system. The extraordinary German mathematician/astronomer Johannes Kepler (1571–1630) worked for a time under Brahe, then inherited his astronomical data, which he tried to rectify with the heliocentric theory of Copernicus. In the process, Kepler discovered his laws of planetary motion, including the hypotheses that the earth does orbit around the sun and that its orbit was elliptical rather than circular; he published the laws in *Harmonices Mundi*, "The Harmony of the World" (1619).

Galileo Galilei (1564–1642) was an Italian astronomer known for being a defender of the Copernican system and for extensive writings on the subject, which earned him the wrath of the Catholic Church. While he disagreed with Kepler's planetary laws, he formulated his own laws, chiefly in regard to falling bodies. He was the first to state that mathematics could be used to delineate the laws of nature. Galileo's general idea can be found in the following quote commonly attributed to him, but which is actually a paraphrasing of his words: "Mathematics was the language in which God has written the universe." Galileo's writings enraged the Church—the defenders of a scripture-based, Aristotelian worldview—and

DOI: 10.1201/9781003273622-14

Galileo was put under house arrest. These battles—coupled with his writings promoting observation and experimentation, his dealings with gravity, and his crushing blows to Aristotelian scholasticism—give Galileo, according to Albert Einstein, the designation of "the father of modern physics—indeed, of modern science altogether."

The other founder of modern science was Francis Bacon (1561–1626). In his book *Instauratio magna*, "The Great Instauration," Bacon wrote:

> Men have sought to make a world from their own conception and to draw from their own minds all the material which they employed, but if, instead of doing so, they had consulted experience and observation, they would have the facts and not opinions to reason about, and might have ultimately arrived at the knowledge of the laws which govern the material world.[7]

And with these words, Bacon heralded the Scientific Revolution in 1620s England. He had called for the development of a natural philosophy that is based on experience as well as observational data and its testing and interpretation: the scientific method. Among the themes in Bacon's writings was the idea that knowledge equaled power and that scientific knowledge should be separated from theology. He promoted inductive reasoning, in which one makes observations and, from them, hypotheses, which are then tested by experiments in nature, as opposed to deductive reasoning, which applied opinions of the past. He called for a cooperative effort in what he termed a "House of Solomon" (an institute or society for scientific pursuits), and he argued that there was no limit to what could be learned, as there never could be a point where all was known. Bacon believed that the systems instituted by the Greeks did not benefit mankind and that any prior knowledge that did not improve the lives of humans should be ignored. He wrote that knowledge should be acquired "for the glory of the Creator and the relief of man's estate," meaning the relief of the human condition or human suffering.[8]

After a royal charter was granted by Charles II in 1660, the scholarly giants of England established the Royal Society. As the intellectual center of seventeenth-century Europe, the Royal Society was devoted to the improvement of natural knowledge and divided into subgroups focused on the following disciplines: physics, astronomy, optics, anatomy, chemistry, agriculture, the unknown, and correspondence. It was the realization of Bacon's wish for a "House of Solomon," where hypotheses were formulated, experiments tested the hypotheses, and the results were communicated to one another. Its main publication, *Philosophical Transactions of the Royal Society*, is the world's oldest continuously running scientific journal, dating from 1665. Its motto has always been *Nullius in verba*, "on the word of no one," meaning trust only that which can be proven with observation and experience, not because it was said once by someone or written down somewhere, no matter how weighty the voice or pen.

FIRST FELLOWS OF THE ROYAL SOCIETY

England was home to several revolutionaries of science in the seventeenth century: Robert Boyle (1627–1691), the founder of modern chemistry; John Locke (1632–1704), a philosopher whose writings focused on empiricism and epistemology; Robert Hooke (1635–1703), a polymath (elasticity, microscopy, coiner of "the cell," architecture); Christopher Wren (1632–1723), another polymath (architecture, physics, astronomy, mathematics); Edmond Halley (1656–1742), astronomer, mathematician, and physicist; and Isaac Barrow (1630–1677), professor of mathematics and optics.

Two Fellows of the Royal Society merit more attention here. The first is Irish-born chemist Robert Boyle, a natural philosopher and founding member of the Royal Society. He inherited the principles of Bacon and performed scientific investigations, particularly in the realm of chemistry, with the idea that no past knowledge was fact unless it could be proven by experiment. These experiments could produce positive or negative results, and both were equally worthy of publication. Boyle answered Bacon's call for each scientific discipline to have a "natural history"—a collection of observations and experimental results. If Bacon was the "thinker" behind this movement, then Boyle was the first and most significant "doer."

The other Fellow deserving further discourse here is John Locke. Locke, both a philosopher and a physician, is known for his philosophical letters and treatises on epistemology, the study of knowledge. He subscribed to the belief that both knowledge and ideas are acquired through experience, as opposed to René Descartes (1595–1650), who had proposed that they were innate. In his "Essay on Human Understanding" (1689), Locke wrote, "no man's knowledge here can go beyond his experience."[9] Expressed another way, knowledge was acquired only from sensation (observation) and reflection of what was observed. Locke, like Boyle, appreciated Bacon's guidelines for the new philosophy and promoted the formulation of new knowledge founded on empirical data and experience. Locke and Boyle are significant contributors to the history of medicine in that they both supported the idea that experimental philosophy could be applied to medical knowledge.

While this new Baconian, anti-Aristotelian natural philosophy was being promoted by the fellows of the Royal Society, the curriculum taught in Latin at the universities such as Oxford and Cambridge in the seventeenth and part of the eighteenth centuries remained one based on Aristotelian scholasticism, as if they had never heard of Copernicus and Galileo or the great figures in anatomy and physiology outlined in the last chapter.[10] The official college charter of Cambridge's Trinity College requested that their students ignore other authors and only study Aristotle and his followers.[11] The universities were not at the vanguard of intellectual discovery; it was the genius thinkers of the Royal Society that advanced Bacon's vision while the universities were stuck in the past. It took another hundred years and yet another genius for this to change.

There are no words to adequately describe the genius of Isaac Newton (1623–1727) or the magnitude of his contributions to the Scientific Revolution, but all disciplines of the intellectual world were never the same after the publication of his greatest work—the single most influential scientific book ever written—*Philosophiae naturalis principia mathematica*, "Mathematical Principles of Natural Philosophy" (1687). In the *Principia*, Newton explained "The System of the World" with his laws of motion, his law of universal gravitation (the attractive force between two objects is equal to the product of their masses divided by the square of the distance between them), and his confirmation of Kepler's laws of planetary motion, thereby proving the heliocentric theory and closing the door forever on the Aristotelian and Ptolemaic models of astronomy. Embedding in the work his foundations of what he called the "infinitesimal calculus," Newton provided mathematical proof of the orderly natural forces of the world. The Baconian vision had been fully realized.[12]

The publication of the *Principia* in 1687 marked the end of the Scientific Revolution, but it would take several decades for Newton's labors to be digested and its fruits to take hold. This era also marked an end of the adherence to old ways of thinking, and it had become evident that with the scientific application modeled by Bacon, new ways of thinking could be formulated and either proven or rejected.

The Medical Revolution

Medical science also experienced its own revolution in the sixteenth and seventeenth centuries, as represented by a series of important discoveries and advancements. While Galen continued to have a strong influence on medicine into the nineteenth century, it was during the 1600s that new theories about human physiology, as well as the origins of disease, would emerge. This was the result of medicine becoming a discipline commandeered increasingly by curious scientists rather than dogmatic traditionalists.

The most significant medical advancement of this period was the discovery of the circulation of the blood by the Englishman William Harvey (1578–1657). The account of his findings was published in *Exercitatio anatomica de motu cordis et sanguinis in animalibus*, "An Anatomical Essay Concerning the Movement of the Heart and Blood in Animals" (1628). In his dedication of the book to King Charles, Harvey wrote:

> The heart of animals is the foundation of their life, the sovereign of everything within them, the sun of their microcosm, that upon which all growth depends, from which all power proceeds.[13]

Building on the work of Michael Servetus (1511–1553), the discoverer of the pulmonary circulation, and Hieronymus Fabricius (1537–1619), the describer of venous valves, Harvey proved that blood flowed in a circle: from the heart to the lungs, from the lungs back to the heart, from the heart to the tissues through the arteries, and from the tissues through the venous circulation, back to the heart. The last step was the most revolutionary of all his claims. After the work of Vesalius, Harvey's publication would be the second major crushing blow to Galen, this time to his physiology. Galen had viewed a blood system of two independent pathways—a venous conduit that moved nutrition from the liver to the tissues, and an arterial one that moved *pneuma,* coming from the lungs, from the heart to the tissues.[14] Harvey was guided by Aristotelian principles throughout his career, but after seeing for himself the human body in the Paduan anatomical theater, he became convinced of this new way of thinking about the heart and blood. Harvey confirmed what Vesalius had suggested when he said, "I profess to learn and teach anatomy not from books but from dissections, not from the tenets of philosophers but from the fabric of nature."[15]

The work of Harvey would enthrall the succeeding generation of physician-scientists, none more so than Thomas Willis (1621–1675). Willis was a founding member of the Royal Society and a physician, as well as an anatomist and a chemist. With his publication of *Cerebri anatome* (1664), Willis "did for the brain and nerves what William Harvey did for the heart and blood."[16] He added the word "mellitus" (honey-like) to diabetes, noting the sweet taste of the diabetic's urine. Chemistry was a burgeoning field at this time, and Willis combined Aristotelian and Paracelsian chemical theory into a system that proposed that all bodies consisted of five elements or principles—spirit, sulfur, salt, earth, and water. Over time, Willis's dissections and chemical experiments would eventually lead to his discounting the theories from Aristotle and Galen.

Willis was not alone in his pursuit to rectify chemistry with physiology; Franciscus Sylvius (1614–1672) was a Dutch iatrochemist whose theory of acid and alkali balance in the body competed with humoral medicine and the Paracelsian chemical theory. It was also during the seventeenth century that Anton Leeuwenhoek (1632–1723) developed his microscope, Robert Hooke (1635–1702) coined the term "cell," and Marcello Malpighi (1628–1694) completed Harvey's circulatory pathway with the discovery of the capillary.

Thomas Sydenham (1624–1689)

But one seventeenth-century physician undoubtedly heralded the modern era of the actual practice of medicine. Celebrated as the "Father of English Medicine" and the "English Hippocrates," Thomas Sydenham (1624–1689) was a one-of-a-kind physician who rejected it all: the academia, the dissections, the speculation, and the theories. Having renounced the entire extant body of work in medicine, he instead set about to create a new science of medicine. When asked what medical textbook he recommended, he famously quipped, "Read Don Quixote, it is a very good book. I still read it frequently." Sydenham was heavily influenced by Bacon. In his writings can be found the employment of many of Bacon's methodologies: forming a natural history, studying abnormalities, repeating experiments, etc.[17] Both Robert Boyle and John Locke influenced and supported Sydenham's independent reasoning. In a letter to fellow philosopher William Molyneux (1656–1698), Locke described the value of Sydenham's independence:

> You cannot imagine how far a little observation carefully made by a man not tied up to the four humours, or salt, sulphur, and mercury, or to acid and alkali which had of late prevailed, will carry a man in the curing of diseases though very stubborn and dangerous; and that with very little and common things, and almost no medicine at all.[18]

Sydenham respected Robert Boyle for his empiricism, and Boyle encouraged Sydenham in his epidemiological research. It is apparent that others could not deal with his rejection of their new ideas or his disapproval of old dogmatic ones. Sydenham was not well regarded by his colleagues, if not plainly derided by them, so he was never a Fellow of the Royal Society, a member of the Royal College of

Physicians (only a licentiate), or appointed university chair. On one end of the spectrum were the Galenic physicians, and on the other end, there was Sydenham, and in the middle were the scientists of the new philosophy, among whom only Boyle and Locke supported Sydenham. There was no place yet for a Sydenham, a quintessential man "ahead of his time."

Sydenham repeatedly wrote about the physician studying "with his own eyes, not through the medium of books."[19] He very famously stated his opinion about the burgeoning scientific disciplines,

> All this is mighty fine! but it won't do. Anatomy—botany—nonsense! Sir, I know an old woman in Covent Garden who understands botany better; and as for anatomy, my butcher can dissect a joint full as well; no, young man, all this is stuff; you must go to the bedside, it is there alone you can learn disease![20]

Sydenham ushered in a new era of medical ethics, always trying to follow the best course for his patient. He was one of the first to understand and profess that sometimes the treatment was worse than the disease. The idea of *Primum non nocere,* "first do no harm," was attributed to Sydenham, who often opted to let nature take its course. He was less apt to offer traditional treatments of disease and more likely to "consult my patients' safety and my own reputation most effectually by doing nothing at all."[21] He was skeptical of traditional theories of physiology and the treatments based on these untrustworthy theories. His extreme Puritanism did, in part, impede a truly modern approach to medicine; he found the microscope neither useful nor necessary in studying disease processes, nor did he venture into the realm of anatomical pathology. He believed that only through the senses did God intend for man to perceive the nature of things.

The Sydenham chorea of rheumatic fever is named after him. He described scarlatina (scarlet fever) and how it differed from measles, and he wrote extensively on syphilis and controversially on smallpox. Other noteworthy contributions of Sydenham include his antithetical cooling therapy for smallpox and other fevers, the naming of pertussis for whooping cough, the prescription of Peruvian bark (quinine) for malaria, the distinction between gout and rheumatism, and the promotion of the use of a new preparation of laudanum for a variety of conditions. On the latter, he famously opined, "Among the remedies which it has pleased almighty God to give man to relieve his sufferings, none is so universal and so efficacious as opium."[22]

He was given credit as the first to call for classification of diseases when he wrote in *Observationes medicae* (1676):

> It is advantageous that all diseases be re-organized into definite and certain species, with precisely the same diligence and accuracy which has been done by botanical writers in their own phytology.[23]

Sydenham's idea of "species" of diseases—that diseases were distinct entities—was a novel one, which would be greatly expanded upon in the next century. Within his writings could be found natural histories of diseases that he attempted to get exactly right from his experience at the bedside. To Sydenham, the correct diagnosis leads to the correct treatment. He was a firm believer that a specific disease would generally present with similar symptomatology in different individuals, noting that "nature, in the production of disease, is uniform and consistent."[24]

He was the author of numerous medical treatises including *Observationes medicae,* "Observations of Medicine" (1676), which became a widely used textbook for 200 years, and *Processus integri,* "The Process of Healing" (1692), but his masterpiece was his "Treatise on Gout" (1683), himself a sufferer of that disease. Sydenham, like Hippocrates, published his own informal "oath" in the preface to *Observationes medicae,* which effectively summed up his ethics, spirituality, and conscience:

> Whoever takes up medicine should seriously consider the following points: firstly, that he must one day render to the Supreme Judge an account of the lives of those sick men who have been entrusted to his care. Secondly, that such skill and science as, by the blessing of Almighty God, he has attained, are to be specially directed towards the honour of his Maker, and the welfare of

his fellow-creatures, since it is a base thing for the great gifts of Heaven to become the servants of avarice or ambition. Thirdly, he must remember that it is no mean or ignoble animal that he deals with. We may ascertain the worth of the human race, since for its sake God's Only-begotten Son became man, and thereby ennobled the nature that he took upon him. Lastly, he must remember that he himself hath no exemption from the common lot, but that he is bound by the same laws of mortality, and liable to the same ailments and afflictions with his fellows. For these and like reasons let him strive to render aid to the distressed with the greater care, with the kindlier spirit, and with the stronger fellow-feeling.[25]

Other than his work on the rashes of scarlet fever, measles, smallpox, and syphilis, Thomas Sydenham did little to advance the development of the field of dermatology per se. This is understandable since he was a physician, not a surgeon, and it was the surgeons of the seventeenth and eighteenth centuries who promoted the study of skin disease more than their physician counterparts. Still, Sydenham's writings would inspire future generations of physicians and surgeons, including one of the true heroes of the history of dermatology in the seventeenth and eighteenth centuries: Daniel Turner (see below).

Dermatology of the Seventeenth Century: Samuel Hafenreffer (1587–1660)

Four important developments in the seventeenth century deserve our attention as they represent important steps toward the development of dermatology as a specialty of medicine. The first of these developments was a publication in Latin in 1630 by Samuel Hafenreffer (1587–1660) with the Greek title Πανδοχειον Ἀιολοδερμον, transliterated as "Pandocheion aiolodermon." A difficult title to unravel, the present author loosely translated it as "Complete Compendium of Skin Affections."[26] A second edition was released in 1660 with the title *Nosodochium*, "Compendium of Disease." The complete title of both editions continues with:

> In which all of the afflictions of the skin and of parts adhering to it, are very faithfully handed down with particular treatment for both knowledge and healing. Which in addition has been illustrated with various Galenic, chemical, cosmetic and other chosen established remedies. The work is agreeable and useful for doctors as well as surgeons: and where the adjacent supporting footnotes succinctly inform the reader for the sake of exploring Arabic, Greek, Latin, and German content.[27]

Hafenreffer has received little attention in histories of dermatology, perhaps because there is no English translation of his work, and little has been recorded about his life. It is known that he was born in Herrenberg, Germany, and died a professor of medicine at the university in Tubingen. He is occasionally recognized in some dermatology textbooks—in the chapter on pruritus—for being the first to define pruritus (itch) as the unpleasant sensation that invokes the desire to scratch. We know he was highly revered by Thomas Browne (see below).

An in-depth analysis of the obscure *Pandocheion aiolodermon* (*Nosodochium*) is beyond the scope of this book, but the front matter reveals something about Hafenreffer and his contribution. The book was dedicated to a Count Paul Andreas von Wolkenstein (1595–1635), "the most serene and powerful of the Bavarian electorate." In the *Amicorum ad autorem votiva*, "Friends' Offerings to the Author" found in the front matter of the book, Gregorius Horstius (1578–1636) wrote:

> Samuel, you work with all variations of human skin when you teach, and you restore [the skin] with a healing hand. What do you hope to get for yourself from this? Or should the thanks you receive from the skin alone be your reward for your services? That's what many people, lacking true virtue, conclude, who pay a small pittance for your healing power. However, may you not be downcast. Indeed, that type of person does exist which sincerely loves you inside and out. Meanwhile, let scabies, verruca, phlogosis, attack anyone who has rejected your treatment of the skin.[28]

Perhaps this mysterious man deserves a little more recognition for his early interest in skin disease than posterity has given him. His book was significant because he gave the names of skin diseases in various languages, allowing us to cross-reference the different names for the same condition.[29] The work reveals in parts bizarre teachings about disease. For example, it was believed that gonorrhea could be cured through coitus with a virgin.[30] Hafenreffer was representative of the merging of academic and public medicine; his section on *examen leprosum*, "exam of the leper," and certificates of medical examination reflect involvement in public affairs (see Interlude 1).[31] Hafenreffer encouraged completely stripping the patient of clothes for the examination and focusing principally on dermatologic findings to support or refute a diagnosis of leprosy.[32] The nearly 600-page book impresses with its comprehensiveness, far surpassing the Mercurialis book (see Table 9.1). A much-needed English translation would shed light on this obscure character and his contribution.

Richard Wiseman (1621–1676) and the King's Evil

The second major development in the history of dermatology during the seventeenth century was the promotion of surgery as a respectable discipline by the Englishman Richard Wiseman (1621–1676). While dermatology today is a field that aligns equally with medicine and surgery, that was not always the case. In fact, dermatology grew out of the surgical field. Skin diseases and ailments were primarily managed by surgeons and barbers (the barber surgeons) in the sixteenth through eighteenth centuries. The medical physicians of this era were more focused on internal diseases such as pneumonia, fevers, gout, and rheumatism. In order for dermatology to become a specialty in its own right, surgery had to attain some credibility as a modern discipline. Wiseman took the first steps forward in this regard.

TABLE 9.1

Chapter Titles of Samuel Hafenreffer's *Pandocheion Aiolodermon*

Book 1	Book 2	Book 3	Book 4
The skin	Ulcers and their general division	Wounds in general	Tumors troublesome to the skin in general
Alphus	General treatment of ulcers	Symptoms and treatments of wounds	Enumeration and treatment of tumors
Leuce	Symptoms of ulcers	Wounds from stabbing or gunshot	Cosmetics
Pallor	Smallpox	Human bites	
Lentigines	Fistulas	Wild animal bites	
Remaining species of macules	Treatment of fistulas	Bite of the rabid dog	
The hair	Cancer	Treatment of the bite from a dog inflicted with rabies	
Affections of the hair	Gangrene	Reptile bites	
Acridones	Carbuncles	Other kinds of lesions from reptiles	
Sweat	Pestilential ulcers	Puncture from insects	
Papules	Syphilis	Treatment of wounds inflicted by reptiles and insects	
Pruritus	Enumeration of remaining ulcers		
Scabies and its species	Division and signs of named ulcers		
Signs and treatment of scabies	General treatment and types of ulcers		
Wet scabies			
Excoriation of the skin			

Wiseman had a varied and exciting life; in spite of his illegitimate birth, and without having a university education, he rose to the level of personal surgeon of King Charles II and later became the first consultant surgeon in London. He served in the Royalist Army during the English Civil War and after in the Spanish/Dutch Navy. He survived military and civil imprisonment, the Great Plague of London (1665–1666), which killed 68,000+ persons, and the Great Fire of London (1666), which destroyed seven out of eight homes in London. He wrote two important works: *A Treatise on wounds* (1672) and *Severall chirurgical treatises* (1676). The latter was published in six editions and became a very influential surgical text for the next century, with evidence of its use by medical students until 1778.[33] The surgical treatises demonstrate the influence of his military and naval background, and the work was advertised as being particularly useful for ships' doctors.[34] The case histories (popularly known as "Wiseman's Book of Martyrs") are not for the squeamish. Someone like Sydenham, with his "do no harm" approach, might have found the treatises particularly appalling, though we have no record of Sydenham ever commenting on them.

The division between physician and surgeon was so vast that it is not likely the two great Englishmen ever met.[35] Sydenham and Wiseman, coincidentally, were only ever in the presence of one another on the battlefields during the English Civil War (1645) between the Crown and the Parliament. At the Battle of Weymouth, Sydenham, then a cavalry officer, led raids while Wiseman, surgeon to a Royalist foot regiment, treated casualties.[36] Wiseman narrowly escaped capture in a battle his side ultimately won, but he was later captured in 1651 at the decisive battle of Worcester, which the Royalists lost and after which Cromwell and his parliamentarians took control of the government. Wiseman remained a Royalist for his entire career, though he ironically married the granddaughter of Sir Thomas Mauleverer, a signatory of Charles I's death warrant.[37]

Even with his traditional support for the humoral theory of disease, in effect, Wiseman did for surgery what Thomas Sydenham did for medicine. Dedicated to King Charles II, *Severall chirurgical treatises* (1676) is composed of eight treatises (see Table 9.2) containing 650 case histories of Wiseman's own observations, which, according to the author in his Epistle to the Reader, "was more conformed to my own judgement and experience than other men's authority." This sounds very Sydenham-like, and the treatises are a model of practicality and common sense, as well as a scientific spirit. His target audience, the young Chirurgeon—and his disdain for academia—are clearly stated in the epistle.[38] Wiseman was quite proud of his profession, describing it as 'noble' in his epistle to the reader:

> The nobility and dignity of Chirurgery [from the Greek, "handwork," the origin of the word surgery] are too well known to want the Help of an Oratour to set them forth. If a Panegyrick were necessary, it were best made by running through the Particulars of the Art, and the History of the Diseases cured thereby. He that shall duly consider the deplorable Misery of Mankind, and how much it wanteth relief in such a Multitude of Instances, must needs acknowledge us to be, what Antiquity hath long since call'd us, (viz). The Hands of God.[39]

Of the eight treatises, the lengthy fourth, "Of the King's Evill [sic]," is historically the most important. "The King's Evill" refers to the condition we know today as scrofula, a complication of tuberculosis that primarily affects children, in which infected lymph nodes, especially of the neck, enlarge slowly and later form sinus tracts with the overlying skin surface, leading to ulcerations. As it was the most discussed dermatologic ailment of his time, Wiseman was obliged to deliberate about it in great detail. He provided ample anecdotal evidence of his experience with the disease that he treated with a combination

TABLE 9.2

Wiseman's Severall Chirurgical Treatises

Treatise I: Of tumors	Treatise V: Of wounds
Treatise II: Of ulcer	Treatise VI: Of gunshot wounds
Treatise III: Of the diseases of the anus	Treatise VII: Of fracture and luxations
Treatise IV: Of the king's evill [sic]	Treatise VIII: Of lues venerea

of cathartics, purgatives, incision and ligature, and application of caustic medications to the ulcerations. The first to address this condition, Wiseman did so in an erudite and comprehensive manner.

The chapter reveals that one of the fathers of English surgery was not above promoting miraculous types of cures along with his many pharmacological and surgical interventions. He believed in the "King's touch" as a cure for scrofula. Dating back to the reigns of Edward the Confessor (1042–1066) of England and Philip I of France (1059–1108), there was a ceremonial custom in which the monarchs of England and France touched directly with bare hands the draining skin lesions of scrofulous persons, often thousands at a time, in order to heal them from this particular malady. Elizabeth I was particularly devoted to this custom.[40] The practice peaked with the Stuart dynasty, especially during the reign of Charles II. Richard Wiseman did not dispute the efficacy of the practice. In the first chapter of the fourth treatise, entitled "Of the cure of the Evill by the King's Touch," Wiseman stated,

> I my self have been a frequent Eye-witness of many hundreds of Cures performed by his Majesties Touch alone, without any assistance of Chirurgery, and those, many of them, such as had tired out the endeavors of able Chirurgeons, before they came thither …[41]

We will never know if Wiseman truly believed what he wrote or whether his opportunism under the Stuart Crown influenced this chapter of the treatise, keeping in mind that his writings were dedicated to Charles II himself. We do have evidence that even more scientific minds than Wiseman, such as Robert Boyle, believed in this type of faith healing.[42]

THE KING'S EVIL IN SHAKESPEARE (MACBETH)

MACDUFF:
What's the Disease He Means?

MALCOLM:
'Tis call'd the evil:
A most miraculous work in this good king;
Which often, since my here-remain in England, I have seen him do.
How he solicits heaven,
Himself best knows: but strangely visited people,
All swoln and ulcerous, pitiful to the eye,
The mere despair of surgery, he cures;
Hanging a golden stamp about their necks,
Put on with holy prayers: and 'tis spoken,
To the succeeding royalty he leaves the healing benediction.
With this strange virtue,
He hath a heavenly gift of prophecy;
And sundry blessings hang about his throne,
That speak him full of grace.[43]

Historians have examined this practice in many different contexts, from religion to magic to the "divine right of kings," to mass hysteria.[44] Regardless of his shortcomings for touting the efficacy of what Thomas Macaulay (1800–1859) called "an absurd superstition of a pre-enlightened age," Richard Wiseman should be remembered for his surgical treatises and their guidance of several generations of surgeons that followed him.[45] Like Sydenham, Wiseman would later profoundly influence Daniel Turner, the first British dermatologist. Sir Thomas Longmore, one of Wiseman's principal biographers, once remarked that the advances in surgery in the century after Wiseman's death were "traceable to the fact of his writings having been so widely diffused."[46]

The Scientific Revolution Reaches the Skin:
The Discovery of the Skin's Microanatomy

The third important development in the history of dermatology in the seventeenth century was the discovery of the microanatomical structures of the skin. The invention of the microscope gave the anatomists of this period the opportunity to look at the skin from a new perspective. Marcello Malpighi (1628–1694), an Italian biologist and physician, was among the first to apply this technology to the study of the human body, and he would eventually become the first person admitted to the Royal Society as a foreign member in 1669. In addition to his recognition for the discovery of the capillary and renal glomerulus, Malpighi is known for applying the microscope to examine the skin and for identifying a layer of the epidermis—which he saw as one unit—consisting of the stratum basale and the stratum spinosum (now termed the Malpighian layer). In a work entitled *De externo tactus organo anatomica observatio*, "An anatomical observation of the external organ of touch" (1665), he reported on the presence in the skin of the sebaceous glands and the pores from which sweat emanates, the latter believed to exist since the time of the ancient Greek physicians. The Danish scientist Nicholas Steno (1638–1686) is often credited with being the first to argue for the existence of sweat glands in 1664, but they were not actually discovered until 1833 when Johann Purkinje (1787–1869) reported on them. Malpighi's work also contains descriptions of the pigmentation seen in darker skin types, and he was the first to document in Western texts the presence of ridges and furrows in the fingers (fingerprints). In Europe, Johann Mayer (1747–1801) was the first to prove that fingerprints could be used to identify a person based on their uniqueness to the individual.

William Cowper (1666–1709) was a barber-surgeon and an anatomist who published the seminal work *The Anatomy of the Humane Bodies* in 1698. It became one of the most authoritative surgical and anatomical texts of the eighteenth century and brought much fame to Cowper, who was granted Fellowship of the Royal Society in 1699 and would be known in the history of medicine as one of the first surgeon-scientists. The work was enormous in physical size, weighing almost 20 lb (9 kg) and containing 114 illustrations from copperplate engravings. The majority of the illustrations (105) were drawn by Dutch artist Gerard de Lairesse (1641–1711) and were far superior to anything preceding them.

COWPER'S COPPERPLATES

The illustrations, however, mired Cowper in controversy as he was accused of one the most famous acts of plagiarism in the history of letters. The problem was that the copperplates originally appeared in a Dutch anatomical text entitled *Anatomia humani corporis*, "Anatomy of the Human Body" (1685), by Govard Bidloo (1649–1713), the personal physician of William III (William of Orange). That particular work sold poorly, and the plates were eventually acquired by Cowper. It is unclear whether Bidloo's publisher sold the plates to Cowper's publisher in order for Cowper to write an English translation of Bidloo's work, or whether Cowper was more complicit in their acquisition for his own aggrandizement. But he did purchase them, and since there were no copyright laws until the Statute of Anne in 1710, Cowper broke no laws in publishing the plates. They were incorporated into Cowper's own "The Anatomy of the Humane Bodies," and the written text was Cowper's alone, though Bidloo and Lairesse were not given proper credit for the plates. Cowper even used the same frontispiece, replacing Bidloo's name and title with his own. Bidloo was furious and complained in 1700 to the Royal Society, to no avail. The tension never abated between the two, with a spat documented between them while they were both present at the autopsy of William III in 1702. Cowper's reputation was tarnished somewhat by this affair, but it is important to recognize that the content written by Cowper to accompany the plates was as influential as the glorious anatomical illustrations the work contained.

Like Malpighi and Bidloo before him, Cowper applied the microscope to the study of the skin. He wrote in the legend to the Fourth Plate, which addresses the skin:

> With the Assistance of the Microscope, the *Cuticula* [epidermis] appears composed of divers *Strata* or Beds of Scales, fastened to the Papillary Surface of the Skin; and are so intangled with each other, as that they appear a continued Pellicle or Membrane when rais'd from the True Skin [dermis], whether by the Application of Blister-Plasters in Living People, or Scalding Water, Hot Irons, or the like, in Dead Bodies: According to the Number of these *Strata* or Beds of Scales, the Skin appears to be more, or less fair, and the Person is commonly said to have a thicker or thinner Skin, tho very frequently, the Jaundice and other Diseases give it an ill Tincture. The *Cuticula*, like the True Skin is not Uniform, in divers parts of it the Number of its Scales and their *Strata* exceed those of others ...[47]

The microanatomy of the skin is described, and Cowper's work demonstrates how anatomy was becoming even more scientific than it had been since the time of Vesalius. Cowper was not only an anatomist but also a surgeon, and he was responsible, even more so than Wiseman before him, for introducing the surgeon to science. As the history of medicine's first "enlightened" surgeon, Cowper led other surgeons to take the surgical art more seriously as an intellectual discipline.[48]

The Discovery of the Scabies Mite

The last of the major dermatological advancements of the seventeenth century was the discovery of the scabies mite by Giovanni Cosimo Bonomo (1666–1696) and Giacinto Cestoni (1637–1718), although Cestoni's contribution is undocumented.[49] This discovery was the direct consequence of the fervor of scientific investigation heralded by Bacon in the early part of the century that thrived in Italy as much as it did in England. Bonomo was an Italian physician and disciple of the great Italian biologist and physician Francesco Redi (1626–1697), a major figure in the history of biology. Redi, for example, was the first to prove rather controversially, through experimentation with rotting meat, that maggots did not arise spontaneously, as previously believed, but from the eggs of flies. Cestoni was an Italian naturalist, apothecary, and collaborator of Redi who hosted men of letters at his pharmacy in Livorno.

Sometime between 1685 and 1687, while collaborating with Cestoni and using a microscope to inspect the fluid of an infested person's skin lesions, Bonomo discovered the itch mite. Bonomo wrote a letter to Redi describing his discovery, and Redi published the research in a work entitled "Observations about the "pellicelli" of the human body, made by Gio. Cosimo Bonomo and written by him with other observations in a letter to Francesco Redi, Florence, 1687." In the letter to Redi, Bonomo wrote,

> I quickly found an itchy person, and asking him where he felt the greatest and most acute itching, he pointed to a great many little pustules not yet scabbed over, of which picking out one with a very fine needle, and squeezing from it a thin water, I took out a very small white globule scarcely discernible: observing this with a microscope, I found it to be a very minute living creature, in shape resembling a tortoise of whitish color, a little dark upon the back, with some thin and long hairs, of nimble motion, with six feet, a sharp head, with two little horns at the end of the snout. Not satisfied with the first discovery, I repeated the search in several itchy persons, of different age, complexion and sex, and at different seasons of the year, and in all found the same animals; and that in most of the watery pustules, for now and then in some few, I could not see any.[50]

Whereas mites are arachnids, all of which have eight legs, Bonomo's description of six-legged organism suggests he may have been looking at the larval stage of the mite.

This discovery should have had an immediate impact on the medical world. It was a landmark breakthrough, proving that itching, long-held to have a humoral origin, could be caused by an ectoparasite. It was actually the first time in medical history a microorganism was claimed to be the cause of any disease. The term *scabies* did not specifically refer to an itchy rash caused by the itch mite until the nineteenth century; *scabies* was a word dating back to ancient times that was used to refer to any itchy, scabby skin eruption.

Yet, in the immediate aftermath of the publication of Bonomo's letter, the personal physician of three popes of this period, Giovanni Lancisi (1654–1720), with the pope's power and influence behind him, disputed Bonomo's claims, effectively silencing him.[51] The revelation of Bonomo and Cestoni was largely forgotten, even with the research being published by Richard Mead of the Royal Society in 1703; the skepticism about the claim within that organization probably contributed to its ignomi. And the letter would be lost, only to be rediscovered in 1924. In 1710, 23 years after Redi published Bonomo's letter— and well after Bonomo's death—Cestoni came out with a claim that it was he alone who discovered the mite.[52] Many historians refute this assertion because only Bonomo's name is associated with the letter and the publication. Another controversy stemmed from the allegation in 1689 by Giovanni Calvoli (1625– 1706) that he had discovered the scabies mite ten years prior to Bonomo and Cestoni's announcement. He claimed that these two had been introduced to the idea of the mite's existence when they were given some drawings by Calvoli of the mite rendered by an artist named Salvetti, whom Calvoli had employed. Neither of these claims has gained any support from researchers on the subject, and history will continue to remember both Bonomo and Cestoni as the discoverers of the itch mite as the cause of scabies.[53]

The dermatologic writers of the seventeenth and eighteenth centuries did not accept a causal link between itching and the mite. Thomas Willis and Richard Wiseman both considered itching to have in all cases an iatrochemical root cause, while Boerhaave (see Chapter 10) attributed it to purulent matter in the blood.[54] Daniel Turner (see below) and Thomas Spooner (see Chapter 10), who both authored chapters or treatises on itch, missed the opportunity to distinguish the mite as *the* cause of *the itch*. A few attempts were made throughout the eighteenth century to confirm the theory of this disease, but no one could find the mites for himself. The problem was due to the fact that the mite is scarcer than the eruption would suggest, i.e., the average infested patient has a few dozen or so burrowing mites on him or her. Modern dermatologists are familiar with the diagnostic challenge of scabies; the mite is not easily found with microscopic preps. Thanks to the advent of dermoscopy, however, scabies can be diagnosed instantaneously and microscopic tests are now obsolete (see Chapter 16). In addition, they looked for the mites in the wrong place, with Bonomo erroneously claiming the mite was within the blisters of the eruption, when actually the leading edge of the burrowing track is the hot spot for finding the mite.[55] It was not until 1834 that an undergraduate student in Paris named Simon-Francois Renucci proved that *Sarcoptes scabiei* was the etiologic agent in scabies. He used knowledge imparted to him by peasant women of his home island of Corsica, who long held the know-how to extract the mite with a needle from the tip of a burrow (see Chapter 13).[56]

Thomas Browne (1605–1682) and the *Morgellons*

The history of dermatology in the seventeenth century cannot be completed without a few ancillary notes about happenings in this period. The first of these is a rather bizarre and mysterious story that has baffled historians for several centuries and one that was revived in the early part of the twenty-first century. It involves Thomas Browne (1605–1682), the English physician and polymath—and the original "know-it-all"—who wrote about many subjects and is considered one of the true geniuses of English letters. He was probably the most well-read person of his time, having an extensive library containing virtually every major publication of and before his time.[57] Browne was quite interested in the skin and its diseases.[58] Not only did he write of "a gruesome, vermiculate disease marring children in southern France," he wrote his Leiden dissertation on smallpox and once recommended that his son read Mercurialis and Hafenreffer.[59]

The mystery begins with a vague reference in his "Letter to a Friend" (1656) concerning this vermiculate disease affecting infants and children in Languedoc, a historical region in southern France of which Toulouse is the largest city. Browne wrote,

> Hairs which have most amused me have not been in the face or head, but on the Back, and not in Men but Children, as I long ago observed in that endemial Distemper of little Children in Languedock, called the Morgellons, wherein they critically break out with harsh Hairs on their Backs, which takes off the unquiet symptoms of the Disease, and delivers them from Coughs and Convulsions.[60]

The *morgellons*, a term coined by Browne, was also known as *crinones* and *masquelons*, and a topic of debate for the learned physicians of the era. The term refers to a condition that affected primarily infants exhibiting hair-like or worm-like material in the skin of the back, arms, and calves. The first reference to this affliction occurred in a 1544 posthumous publication by Leonello Vittori (1450–1520), also known as Faventinus, but the first treatise on the matter was not written until 1674, entitled *De vermiculis capillaribus infantium,* "On the worm hairs of infants," by the German physician and scholar, Georg Hieronymus Welsch (1624–1677).[61] Several medical writers of the intervening years would attempt to describe this disease, all agreeing this was a disease unknown to the ancients, as there was no medical literature about the affliction from the ancient writers. The first writers on this topic often confused it with dracunculiasis, a legitimate parasitic disease caused by the burrowing Guinea worm. Ambroise Pare, our battlefield surgeon hero of the sixteenth century, was able to distinguish the two, with the skin finding in question being hairs rather than worms:

> The mention of the Dracunculi, calls to my memory another kind of Abscess, altogether as rare. This our Frenchmen name Cridones, I think *a Crinibus*, i.e., from hairs: it chiefly troubles children and pricks their back like thorns. They toss up and down being not able to take any rest. This disease ariseth from small hairs which are scarce of a pin's length, but those thick and strong. It is cured by a fomentation of water more than warm, after which you must presently apply an ointment made of honey and wheaten flower; for so these hairs lying under the skin are allured and drawn forth; and being thus drawn, they must be plucked out with small mullets. I imagine this kind of disease was not known to the ancient physician.[62]

Pare's surgical student, Jacques Guillemeau (1550–1613) provided an excellent summary of the peculiar "hairs," including the link with epilepsy, and how the old wives managed them:

> As soone as little Children are taken with this disease they crie and take on extreamely and yet one cannot perceive any cause, why they should do so, which brings them oftentimes even to their grave, for that this disease drawes along with it Epylepticall convulsions; because the sinewes which come foorth of the backebone and are scattred on each side are over burdened and filled with some fuliginous vapour, of which Haires are bred, and they by their great length and continuity are carried directlie to the braine, whither when they are come, they cause this disease. The Women of the countrie of Languedocke, because it is a common disease with them, make no great reckoning of it and doe help it in this manner. With the palme of their hand they do rub the bottome of the childs backe and reines downe to the crupper-bone so long till they feele through the pores of the skinne the tops of very stiffe and pricking haires to come forth like unto hoggs bristles, which as soone as they see that they are come foorth, they pull them away by and by with their nayles, or else with such little Pincers as women use to pull the haire from off their eyebrowes. The same Montanus counselleth the woman to rub her hand first with some new milke; which being done and the haires pulled away, the child presently recovers his health and leaveth his ordinarie cries and laments.[63]

Johannes Schenkius (1530–1598) gave us a very detailed description of his understanding of *crinones/morgellons* that he believed was caused by "intercutaneous worms."[64] These worms infest children between the ages of six months and two years and are born in the muscles of the arms, legs, and back from humors that are trapped in the pores of the body, and the humor subsequently "undergoes putrefactive changes and becomes alive and ... is converted into worms." Schenkius' worms do not leave the pores but do stick out their heads, which appear as black dots on the skin. The infestation causes warmth, itching, insomnia, and restlessness, as the worms "plunder away the living flesh" of the infant child.

The debate as to whether the structures seen extruding from the surface of the skin were hairs or worms would go on for at least another century, with the majority of the writers of the seventeenth century voting for worms rather than hairs. In 1682, Michael Ettmuller (1644–1683) was the first to publish drawings of what he believed to be a living organism.[65] By the eighteenth century, however, the tide would turn against these structures being worms or any other type of living organisms, as demonstrated in the writings of Daniel Le Clerc (1652–1728):

> Ettmuller indeed challenges us to the Test of Experience, and affirms by the Assistance of the Microscope he had seen those Crinous, that is, true Worms; but since Leuvenhoeck by using the same Instrument did not discern them to be little Worms, but Hairs or Bundles of Hairs, and in an inanimate Matter, it remains that we make a Judgment to ourselves which of the two we will believe, and which not. But if we enquire whether of them understood the Art of managing the Microscope best, or used it most frequently, no Body, I am of Opinion, will prefer Ettmuller to Leuvenhoeck, who was the most eminent that Way of his Age; so that if either err'd, it is most probable 'twas Ettmuller.[66]

Writing in the 1770s, Plenck (see Chapter 10) called the condition *crinones* and referred to the lesions as *setae* (Latin for bristles), noting that they sometimes resembled worms or comedones (blackheads and whiteheads). Other writers discussed the excessive swaddling of the infants as contributing to the eruption of the lesions. We know today that such swaddling can lead to "prickly heat" (miliaria). The above descriptions indicate to the present author that the spots Browne and others claimed were worms or hairs were either a form of keratosis pilaris, infantile acne (blackheads, when expressed, can have a vermiculate appearance), heat bumps (miliaria), trichostasis spinulosa, or folliculitis. The primitive microscopists of the seventeenth century may also have been looking at clothing fibers that are commonly seen under the microscope along with skin scrapings. The physicians and surgeons, influenced by both superstitions as well as valid reports of helminthic disease in a growing medical literature, could have fostered misinterpretation of the *morgellons* as a parasitic disease.

MORGELLONS DISEASE

Fast forward to the beginning of the twenty-first century for the conclusion of the story—when persons unwilling to accept a diagnosis of delusional parasitosis in themselves or their loved ones discovered Browne's *morgellons*, coined the term "Morgellons disease," and attributed their condition to this disorder. Morgellons disease is a self-diagnosed, unofficial skin condition characterized by a crawling sensation on the skin and skin lesions that contain some sort of fibers. Morgellons disease has been a controversial topic, with skepticism outweighing support by the medical community. Believers in this disease reference the above seventeenth-century medical literature as support for their diagnosis. Skeptics consider it just another version of delusional parasitosis, an uncommon, but not rare, monosymptomatic hypochondriasis disorder in which the afflicted person experiences a fixed delusion that their skin is infested with bugs, worms, fibers, or other organisms. Delusional parasitosis is one of the most challenging forms of mental illness to treat, and because patients with the disease often refuse to see a psychiatrist, whom they desperately need, dermatologists are at the front lines managing this condition. While many cases represent a primary psychiatric illness, others are secondary to the use of illicit amphetamines, prescribed stimulants for attention-deficit hyperactivity disorder (ADHD), and/or narcotic pain medications, all of which in the author's experience contribute to a variety of skin problems, including hyperfixation on the skin.

Jean Riolan the Younger (1580–1657) and Nicholas Culpeper (1616–1654)

Several additional figures from this time period should be acknowledged for their significant contributions to dermatology. French anatomist and physician Jean Riolan the Younger (1580–1657), also called Riolanus, was a known vehement supporter of Galen and opponent of Harvey. Riolan's magnum opus, originally written in Latin and translated into English by English physician/botanist/herbalist

Nicholas Culpeper (1616–1654), was published in several editions with the title "A sure guide, or, The Best and Nearest Way to Physick and Chyrurgery" (1657).

Riolan was the first to study the difference between dark skin and light skin types.[67] Using a blistering agent to blister the skin of an African man, Riolan then analyzed the specimen and correctly determined that the pigment was found in the thin outer layer of the skin known then as the cuticula (today termed the epidermis) and that underneath this layer, black skin was exactly the same as white skin. Malpighi later independently confirmed Riolan's observation and pointed out that the pigment was specifically found in his so-called Malpighian layer of the cuticula.

Riolan considered the skin to be a reflection of the overall health of the human body, similar to our modern sense of the skin "as a window into the internal organs." He believed that the skin of the face, in particular, "is the looking-glass wherein are seen the diseases of the body, especially of the liver, spleen and lungs."[68] According to Riolan, the skin can undergo a variety of changes: experience shifts in temperature; be "gnawn through" or completely lost; lose its smoothness and become rougher; be disfigured by pustules; its passages can be stopped up or more open than they should be, or lose its connection as in wounds and ulcers. He concluded that

> The Skin, seeing it is the breathing place of the whole body, is subject to an infinite number of Diseases; and if the pores be shut, the Body suffers great discommodities, by reason transpiration is hindered.[69]

The nineteenth-century physician Erasmus Wilson (see Chapter 12) credited Riolan with constructing a primitive classification system that influenced the morphology-based systems of the late-eighteenth and early-nineteenth centuries, noting that Riolan divided them into three groups—Pustules, Deformities, and Tubercles.[70] As someone who thought about the skin more scientifically than any of his predecessors, Jean Riolan the Younger was an important figure at the crossroads between the Renaissance and the early modern period.

The aforementioned translator of Riolan, Nicholas Culpeper, was an interesting astrologer-physician who penned an influential text entitled "The English Physitian, or an Astrologo-physical Discourse of the Vulgar Herbs of This Nation" (1652). Later known as "Culpeper's Complete Herbal," it was a popular and lengthy compendium of medicinal herbs. Although not formally trained in medicine and having failed to complete his apprenticeship to be an apothecary, the maverick Culpeper nonetheless practiced medicine among the poor of London, as perhaps that city's "first general practitioner."[71]

In the introduction to his excellent book, Culpeper lamented the realities of seventeenth-century medicine, and by writing his text in English, he delivered medical knowledge to the masses. His purpose was to protect the layperson from quacks and pretenders:

> Hence it becomes evident that the study of Physic ought to form a part of the education of every private gentleman, and should become the amusement of every individual whose occupation in life affords an opportunity of investigating this valuable branch of literature. No science presents to our contemplations a more extensive field of important knowledge, or affords more ample entertainment to an inquisitive philanthropic mind …

> It is a melancholy reflection, daily confirmed by observation and experience, that one half of the human species, labouring under bodily infirmity, perish by improper treatment, or mistaken notions of their disease. What greater inducement then can be offered to mankind, to acquire a competent knowledge of the science of physic, than the preservation of their own lives, or that of their offspring?

> Not that it is necessary for every man to become a physician; for such an attempt would be absurd and ridiculous. All I plead for is, that men of sense, of probity and discernment, should be so far acquainted with the theory of physic, as to guard their families against the destructive influence of ignorant or avaricious retailers of medicine.[72]

After a description of the nature and use of nearly 400 herbs, Culpeper included a "Medical Part" which contained an "Anatomical Analysis of the Human Frame." In that section, Culpeper offered to his common reader the following eloquent description of the skin, drawn heavily from the writings of Riolan, as well as a summary of seventeenth-century views of the skin:

> The skin is a membranous covering of the body, similar, spermatic, having blood mixed with it, reddish, white, loose, and the instrument of feeling. It hath cutaneous veins and arteries, as also nerves; from the last of which, it receives its quickness of sense. From the capillary veins and arteries it receives blood for nourishment and vital spirit for quickening. Its temperature is cold and dry, or rather exquisitely temperate, yet so that it may be the judge of feeling. The skin on the top of the head is thickest, that on the sides thin, that on the face and palms of the hands thinner, that on the lips thinnest of all; that on the tops of the fingers is mean, so that the sense of touching may be the more perfect: its texture is slight, and very full of small holes or pores, for the insensible transpiration of fumes, vapours, and sweat. It takes its colour from the predominant humour, unless it be such from the birth, as in Ethiopia. It has a double substance: the one is external, called *cuticula*, or the scarf-skin, because it is placed upon the skin, as a cover or defence, every where perforated with pores, without blood and without feeling; its connexion is to the true skin, from whence it has its figure and colour; but, in blackmoors, the *cuticula* being pulled off, the skin itself is white. It has no action, only use, which is to shut the pores of the skin, that icho[r]ous substance may not issue from the veins and arteries; to defend the skin from immoderate heat or cold; and to make it smooth, beautiful, polished, and even. It is generated of a viscous and oleaginous vapour of the blood. The other is the true skin, of which we have first spoken, which is six times thicker that the scarf-skin; its pores will appear in winter-time, if it be made bare and exposed to the cold: for, where they are, the *cuticula* will appear like goose-skin. The skin receives two cutaneous veins, through the head and neck, from the jugulars: two through the arms, breast and back, from the axillaries: two through the lower belly, loins, and legs, from the groins, which are conspicuous in women after hard labour, and in such as have the *varices* in many branches. It has a few arteries, and those very small, in the temples and forehead, fingers, scrotum, and yard.[73]

The last section of the work, "Of Diseases in General, their Prevention, and Cure," contains diagnostic and treatment information for virtually every complaint, including numerous skin conditions, e.g., the "malignant, putrid, or spotted fever" [typhus], miliary fever, smallpox, measles, scarlet fever, erysipelas, "the King's evil," the itch, abscesses, wounds, burns, bruises, ulcers, venereal disease, buboes, and chancres.

Culpeper challenged the idea that medical knowledge was owned solely by the medical profession and truly succeeded in his task of demystifying and translating medicine so that the masses could benefit from it. Popular among the poor, whom he often treated *pro bono*, he was nevertheless disdained by the medical community—for practicing without a license, for giving away the secrets of the trade to the masses, and for his antiquated, astrology-based medical worldview. Culpeper, conversely, loathed physicians and apothecaries, whom he saw as greedy and untrustworthy. The book was enormously successful and was brought to the New World by the pilgrims, where it heavily influenced colonial medicine in the decades that followed. Considered one of the founders of alternative medicine, Culpeper wrote the most successful book on herbals of all time, as the book is still in print to this day.

POISON IVY DERMATITIS DESCRIBED

Captain John Smith (ca. 1580–1631), the explorer who helped settle the first British colony in the New World at Jamestown, Virginia, actually contributed to the history of dermatology, with the first account of poison ivy dermatitis, which he published in 1624 while back in London. The plant, which is not native to Europe, was described in the following manner:

> The poisoned weed, being in shape but little different from our English yvie; but being touched causeth redness, itchinge, and lastly blysters, the which howsoever, after a while

they passe away of themselves without further harme; yet because for the time they are somewhat painefull, and in aspect dangerous, it hath gotten itself an ill name, although questionless of noe very ill nature.[74]

By the middle of the seventeenth century, the plant was carefully gathered up by travelers to the New World and imported into England and France, where it was planted in the estate gardens because of its beauty, studied by physician-botanists for its medicinal value, or used by craftsman for its shine-producing sap on furniture.

The First Dermatologist: Daniel Turner (1667–1740)

Finally, the seventeenth century saw the first surgeon, Daniel Turner (1667–1740), dedicate much of his time to the treatment of skin disease and write a book about the topic. Often referred to as the "first English dermatologist," one could argue that Turner was the first dermatologist of any country. That is, unless details about the obscure career of Samuel Hafenreffer, discussed above, someday emerge to dissuade us. Daniel Turner was born on September 18, 1667, in Holborn, London, the third son of John and Rebecca Turner. While he did not receive any formal university education, he did learn Latin and Greek in his grade school years. His upbringing was Anglican, and he was taught to revere the Bible. This strict moral rearing would later influence his professional life and his worldview as a physician. At seventeen, he became an apprentice to a London surgeon, Charles Bateman of the famous Bateman lineage (see Chapter 12), until 1684, when he came under the tutelage of Thomas Lichfield in 1686, under whom he served as an apprentice until he completed his requisite seven years of training in 1691. With his diploma in hand, he began his career as a surgeon in London, but it took him an additional eight years before he was granted membership in the Company of Barber-Surgeons.

Turner was closer to a modern surgeon in actual practice than many of the barber surgeons around him and before him. He was very well read; all throughout his surgical writings, he quotes the works of many of his contemporaries and predecessors who inspired him. It is apparent from the referencing that on Turner's bookshelves were the writings of esteemed men such as Richard Wiseman, Lazarus Riverius, Daniel Sennert, Wilhelm Fabry, Theodore Turquet de Mayerne, and, without equal in his mind, Thomas Sydenham. Riverius (1589–1655) was a French chemist and physician whose *Institutiones medicae* (1656) and *Praxis medica* (1640) were influential texts, each noted for their emphasis on observation and for detailed pharmacological information. Riverius was a professor of medicine at the renowned medical school in Montpellier. Daniel Sennert (1572–1637) was a German chemist, physician, and prolific writer at the University of Wittenberg. He penned an important series of six medical volumes entitled *Practicae medicinae,* completed in 1636 and available in an English translation, in which he sought to rectify Galenic medicine with Paracelsianism. His fifth volume (on surgery) contains a lengthy section on the skin, hair, and nails.[75] That great work contains extensive information about the removal of various undesired spots on the skin, an erudite section on plica polonica expressing decidedly unmodern views of the basis of that condition, and the first description of rubella (German measles). Wilhelm Fabry (1560–1634), referred to as Fabricius Hildanus in Turner's works, was the first learned German surgeon. Turquet de Mayerne (1573–1655) was a fellow of the RCP who was knighted by James I and very much respected by Turner.[76]

From his case histories, we can understand the type of surgeon Turner was and the type of practice he had. He treated patients from all social classes—both gentlemen and gentlewomen, as well as tradesmen and artisans, and the less fortunate. He saw patients in the study of his residence, or at their homes, or in local hostels, and it was often in the evening or in the middle of the night when Turner would make his calls.[77] Early in his surgical career, accidents were the most common things he addressed, with fractures being the most common accident for which he was called. He also managed external ulcers, tumors, lesions, boils, and swellings and performed amputations, extracted bladder stones, and repaired ruptures and fistulas.[78]

Turner used bloodletting, purging, and relieving of blocked pores with diaphoretics, baths, and brushes to relieve fever. In his view, fever was caused by obstruction of insensible perspiration, due to certain blockages in the pores of the body, and he believed the skin pores were conduits between the inside and outside of the body that could be controlled to promote humoral equilibrium. He cautioned that bloodletting was not meant for every patient, only those who could endure the loss of blood. Purging was also a standard treatment and was believed to save a person's life; it should be administered pre- and postoperatively. He was also emphatic about diet as a way of managing skin disease—he had a different type of diet to recommend for each type of problem.

Turner deserves credit for being a forerunner in promoting patient autonomy and informed consent. Throughout his works, it is evident that Turner's focus was not on diagnosis but on therapy. He would have lengthy discussions about the treatment course, being respectful of a patient's right to refuse treatment or need for time to decide whether he or she would proceed with the treatment.[79] These procedures were somewhat ghastly and painful, and Turner's compassionate side came out in his writings about the decisions he and his patients made together about how to proceed.

It was during Turner's career as a surgeon that he gained much experience in treating skin disease. The skin served as the dividing line between the jurisdiction of the surgeon and the physician in the seventeenth and eighteenth centuries. Physicians managed internal disease, while the surgeons managed external diseases and were expected to limit their practice to prescribing externally applied medications, applying caustics to the skin, or draining corruptive material through the surface of the skin. Physicians were trained and knowledgeable about skin diseases and would manage them, particularly in cases where skin involvement arose from an internal source of disease, as in the case of the exanthems. But the lofty physicians of Turner's day were in general uninterested in skin diseases and instead focused on diseases such as consumption, fevers, gout, wheezing, rheumatism, and palsies.

After an 11-year run as a surgeon, Turner grew tired of his career choice, instead preferring to be a physician. Perhaps he desired to improve his standing in the world, to achieve the respect of his peers, and to be better recognized for his knowledge and accomplishments. He was released, after paying a fine of 50£, from the Company of Barber-Surgeons. In 1711, he sought a fellowship in the RCP, but without the requisite doctorate diploma from Cambridge or Oxford, it was not allowed. Instead, Turner obtained a license that officially allowed him to practice medicine, but he could no longer practice surgery. In his greatest work, *De Morbis Cutaneis, A Treatise of Diseases Incident to the Skin in Two Parts* (1714), Turner dedicated the book to the president and censors of the RCP, considering it his duty to offer the first publication to the president and censors to "convince them that they had given that Privilege to no idle, and I hope, to a useful Person."[80] Becoming a physician was a significant step up in Georgian society, one that ultimately enabled him, at 45 years of age, to marry a woman of the landed gentry, Elizabeth Altham.

In 1723, Yale University awarded Turner an honorary doctorate, even prior to the establishment of a medical school there. Just how he achieved a medical degree from Yale from across the ocean is an interesting anecdote. Established in 1701 and the third oldest college in the American colonies, Yale needed more books in its library and was soliciting gifts of books from London donors. Turner sent 25 books from his personal library to Yale, along with a letter stating that he would greatly appreciate a doctoral degree in return. Yale was happy to comply, and Turner became the first-ever honorary degree recipient from that university.[81] A contemporary critic of Turner insinuated that the letters MD on his diploma stood for *multum donavit*, "he donated much."[82]

Daniel Turner was a prolific writer during his years as a physician, and he wrote significantly more texts than his contemporaries. Without any formal education, Turner had something to prove, and he would strive to be known as an authority his whole career. Yet, Turner was never admitted into the ranks of the Royal Society. He was not born a gentleman, nor a Freemason, as many members were, and he was not connected enough to existing members who could have sponsored him.[83] Even without an acceptance into the society, Turner had the nerve to steal the Society's motto for his portrait, *Nullius in Verba*—"on the word of no one."

Besides Turner's writings on skin disease, his areas of intellectual focus included the elevation of surgery, instruction on venereal disease, and the attack of quackery. His first publication, *Apologia Chyrurgica* (1695), was simultaneously a defense of surgery and a condemnation of the "gross abuses offer'd thereunto by Mountebanks, Quacks, Barbers, Pretending Bone-setters, with other Ignorant Undertakers."[84] His writings about venereal disease in *Syphilis, A practical dissertation on the venereal disease* (1724) describe in detail how syphilis was experienced in eighteenth-century London, and how it was recognized and treated (see Interlude 3). His massive two-volume text, *The Art of Surgery*, written 11 years into his career as a physician, summarized the known surgical information of his day and included dozens of personal cases from his surgical career. It was the most successful of his books during his life. Nevertheless, even with its size and completeness, *The Art of Surgery* did not replace Robert Wiseman's *Severall Chirurgical Treatises* as the preeminent surgical text in Britain, and Turner's book eventually fell into obscurity. Only *De Morbis Cutaneis* would survive the test of time to be remembered today.

Turner tried to elevate his surgical brethren by trying to dispel some myths about them, i.e., that they were cruel, barbaric, hasty, and uninformed. In Turner's mind, surgeons should be given the same level of respect as physicians, and they should be allowed to dispense internal medications to their patients. Surgical patients often needed internal treatment, Turner argued, and many of the external treatments applied by surgeons had internal effects, so why are surgeons disallowed from prescribing internal medications? The physicians, however, wanting to protect their professional domain had the position of power in this turf war, and it would take another half-century for surgeons to get the prescriptive authority for internally administered medications. In Turner's time, the line would remain drawn at the level of the skin, with the surgeons outside it and the physicians underneath it.

In addition to his role as surgical apologist, Turner spent a lot of time and energy writing about quacks, their methods, and how to spot them. Turner deserves credit for shedding light on this issue, and in many ways, he was a forerunner of evidence-based medicine. To Turner, a quack was an intruder in the surgical and medical professions who practiced surgery or medicine with no diploma, training, or certificate and who proclaimed grandiose promises of healing through false advertisement. Uroscopy had become obsolete by Turner's time, but the soothsayer types and the quacks kept it in their bag of tricks. Turner loathed these "dangerous" people and spent his career attacking them in his writings. Turner was accused of quackery by his critics, especially when mercurial salivation for syphilis had generally fallen out of favor by his peers, and he continued to promote it for many years thereafter. In his defense, Turner did make several pleas for more testing of reportedly effective remedies.

Published in 1714, Turner's *De Morbis Cutaneis* had five English editions and was released in French in 1743 and in German in 1766. Turner's decision to write and publish it in English—instead of Latin— was highly unusual for this period and even more unusual considering the book's Latin title. *De Morbis Cutaneis* is 524 pages, divided into two parts in a single volume. Book One, "Of Diseases of the Skin in General," functions as an overview of the known diseases of the skin at that time that were believed to arise from inside the body. Book Two is an overview of diseases arising from external factors, entitled "Of Diseases of the Skin, Incident to some particular Parts of the Body." Turner used the following format: introduce the disease; discuss the diagnosis, cause, and prognosis; review the known treatments of the time for the disease, giving credit to the authors; and conclude with a lengthy selection of cases from his practice or that of his colleagues. Turner listed in the beginning of his work the 155 authors he consulted. The overwhelming majority of names are Greco-Roman, along with a few recognizable contemporaries such as Cowper, Willis, Drake, Harvey, and Fuller. Turner's complete textbook on skin disease contains all the knowledge available in his day, dating back to ancient times. His numerous cases are the most valuable part, as they reveal the step-by-step practicalities of treating skin disease in late seventeenth and early eighteenth-century London, and lay bare for the first time in history, the humanity, the vulnerability, and the suffering of persons with skin disease.

Turner started off with an introduction to the known anatomy and physiology of the skin. It is a summary based on the work of his countryman and "excellent anatomist" William Cowper. Turner divided the skin into two layers: the cuticula (scarf-skin) and the true skin. The cuticula (the epidermis) is a white, fine membrane that covers the whole body. The color of one's skin is determined according to the humors underneath this cuticula: jaundiced—yellow bile, red—sanguine, aethiopian—black bile, pale—phlegmatic. Its functions include touch, protection of the true skin from injury, the release of humors from its pores and perforations "to ventilate the Flame," and for "Ornament and Comeliness" for the person.[85] The true skin (the dermis) is also a membrane layer encompassing the entire body, serving the same functions as the cuticula, with the addition that the true skin also serves as the root of the hairs and indicates the overall temperament or constitution of the body.

Focusing primarily on treatment, Turner shared numerous anecdotes about cases with which he was involved and the surgical interventions he delivered while contrasting his work with that of the so-called "Pretenders," persons posing as surgeons without the licensure or fellowship of the College of Surgeons. The following case is an example of the type challenges that Turner undertook:

> An elderly Person, a Brewer's Servant, came to me late one Even, the Winter that I quitted the Practice of Surgery, and before he made his Complaint, stank so horribly that I car'd not much to tarry the hearing of his Story; but upon his great Importunity, and telling me he was undone if I would not assist him, I ask'd him his Case, when taking on in pitiful Manner, he drew forth his *Penis*, wrap'd round with some Sort of Plaister, with which he had been dress'd by a licensed Physician (so calling himself) of twenty Years Experience, but with much more Truth a Quack, who after so long trying Experiments upon unwary and deluded Persons, is yet to seek which Way to go about the Cure of a *Periphymosis*. When the Plaister was taken off, I discover'd a Sight not very usual, the *Glans Penis* of a monstrous Size, as big as a double Fist, black as the Chimney, and mortify'd a great Way through, over which the *Prepuce* (turn'd back of the same colour) lay in several thick and rumpled Folds … which had strangled the *Glans*, was not to be come at …[86]

> It had been this Fellow's Misfortune, being drunk, to engage with a foul Slut, who had not only clapt him, but he unmindful to return the *Prepuce*, the next Morning in vain attempted it; and thereupon meeting with this Pretender's Bills, or seeing them upon some Pissing-Post, applies for Relief; when after a Fortnight's Pain, well drain'd of his ready Money, with his dripping rotten *Penis*, came to me; on whom, when I had thus taken off the Symptoms, and not able by the common Mercurials both inwardly and outwardly to obtain my Ends, I hasten'd a Salivation, and thereby heal'd his Sores: the *Glans* incarn'd, and looks tolerably handsome … by Reason of the Cicatrix, having a small Knob which hinders it from playing freely over the *Glans*; but which he may at any Time, if so minded, be freed by Circumcision. As a Martyr in the Cause of *Venus* and unbridled Lust, he thinks he has shed Blood enough already; and if it now suffice to carry off his Water, he talks (at least at present) that he has no other Occasion.[87]

Another case discusses a more mundane problem for the modern dermatologist, i.e., shingles:

> A Merchant's Man after freer drinking over Night than usual, complain'd next Day of a Smart and Tingling upon one of his Shoulders, which neglecting for a Day or two, and going to shift himself, he found his Linen to stick in some Places, and having got it off, perceiv'd it stain'd with a certain Humour, and wetted also with the same. The Itching, Smart and Burning increasing, and beginning to stretch it self to other Parts of the Back, I was sent for, and perceiv'd a large Cluster of Pustules, some of them already burst and drying up with Scab; whilst in others the Skin was thick set with Pimples of the same Kind, arising near unto: I clipped off the Heads of those that were full of Matter, and whilst a Servant went to his Apothecary for a Gally-pot of *Diapomphol*, I let him Blood, and after dressed the Parts with some of the same spread on a Rag and apply'd plaister-wise: Next Day I purged him with the common Potion of *Rhubarb, Sena, Tamarinds, Sal. Tart*, &c. other Days he took 3ij [2 drams] of *Crem. Tart.* in his Water-gruel: After the second Purge, they ceased to come out in any new Places, in those which were first out, began to dry away; the others I order'd to be snipt in like Manner as they arose, and gave him a Box of my *Unguent Lap. de Cal.* with which he was drest daily, 'till they were all healed.[88]

Turner wrote about what is considered the first randomized, controlled clinical trial in medicine, between Turner's topical therapy and the "chymist's" Spirit of Wine. He described a patient "having been making merry with his Friends, getting out of the Boat, mist his footing, and bruised both his Shins against the Stairs."[89] Turner was called to see the patient, and when he arrived at the bedside, there was a chemist (apothecary) already there.[90] The drunk man wished that each of the two men treat a leg, and it was quickly apparent to Turner that this would be a golden opportunity to prove that his treatment was more effective than that of the chemist, so Turner let the chemist choose which leg he wanted to treat. Turner gave us day-by-day assessments of the legs' response, and it was soon obvious that Turner's leg was improving, and the chemist's leg was not. Consequently, an abscess formed in the leg treated by the chemist, and Turner, forced to intervene surgically on behalf of the patient, saved the patient from a serious outcome. The trial ends with a merry conclusion:

> About a Month after my Patient was got Abroad, he sent for me to the Tavern, being in Company with his Chymist, where he paid me his Acknowledgment for my Attendance and Service done him: and over a Glass of Wine the Chymist ask'd me if I would be so free as to tell him the Composition of my Plaister.[91]

The most famous, fascinating, and controversial chapter in Turner's *De Morbus Cutaneis* is Chapter XII, entitled:

> Of *Spots and Marks* of a diverse Resemblance, imprest upon the Skin of the *Foetus*, by the force of the Mother's *Fancy*: with some things premis'd of the strange and almost incredible Power of *Imagination*, more especially in *pregnant Women*

While there are a plethora of obvious fallacies in the first 11 chapters, those fallacies were par for Turner's time, built by contemporary understanding of disease. But in Chapter XII, Turner stained his legacy by affirming his imaginationist viewpoint that one's "Fancy" could produce in that person any disease, or in the case of a pregnant woman, her fetus could be affected by birthmarks. Turner, quoting Thomas Fienus (1567–1631), explained the phenomenon this way:

> The *Fancy* … by causing a Motion of the Humours and Spirits in the Bodies of Men, is capable of producing almost every Disease therein; for as the same [the Fancy] is of sufficient Power to determine the said Humours to any Part thereof, it is able therein to produce the Indisposition incident thereunto … we shall take Notice of some monstrous Births, or otherways deform'd and blemish'd by Marks from the strong Imagination or disappointed Longings of the Mother …[92]

He then recounted numerous examples of this phenomenon from the available literature and from his own experience, e.g.,

- a noble woman with a white husband gives birth to a child of "Ethiopic complexion" which was caused by the woman intently viewing a picture hanging in her bed chamber of an infant exactly resembling the infant.[93]
- a girl was born with hair all over the body as a result of the mother's unhappy ruminating and often beholding the picture of St. John the Baptist, hanging at her bedside, drawn in his typical hairy clothing.[94]
- a woman "of the meaner Sort" was delivered of a child "well-shaped in every respect, but had the head of a cat" because she lived in fright of a cat that had "gotten into her bed."[95]
- the niece of Pope Nicholas III had a monstrous birth "all over hairy … with Bear Claws, instead of Toes and Fingers" which was ascribed to her looking at a picture of a bear and which resulted in the pope giving an order to destroy all pictures of bears in the city of Rome.[96]
- A boy was born with his liver, intestines, stomach, and spleen outside the body below the navel; after his death his mother revealed that she had witnessed some soldiers killing a calf and she saw "how the bowels came tumbling from the belly."[97]
- a woman gave birth to a child already circumcised at birth because she, while pregnant, had overheard a conversation of a guest at her house detailing the manner in which the Jewish circumcision was performed.[98]

- an actor dressed in a devil's costume returned home to his wife and she being frightened at the time of conception, after "brought forth a Child of the same diabolical Figure the Man was dress'd in."[99]
- a woman, while quarreling with another woman, "put herself into such a Passion, that she was unable to contain her self" and was then delivered of a daughter, "of a couragious and heroik Mind, but her Feet and Hands contracted as if ready to fight ... in a trembling posture, after the Manner of angry People unable to govern their Passion."[100]
- several cases of pregnant women frightened by seeing beggars with defects, such as missing arms or hands, giving birth to children with the same defect.[101]
- a pregnant woman, "longing to bite the naked Shoulder of a Baker passing by her," gets her "good natur'd husband" to hire him "at a certain Price" for this purpose, and after "the big-belly'd Woman had taken two Morsels," getting only two of the three bites she desired because the baker would not suffer it again, she gives birth to two live children and one dead one.[102]

The listing goes on for pages and pages (with examples of Siamese twinning, a child that looked like a frog and one who looked like an ape, a child with speckled skin akin to a pebbled ground the mother would fix her eyes upon during her devotion, and most commonly, examples of birthmarks said to look like fruit, such as cherries or strawberries, because the mother longed for that fruit during the pregnancy). This section of the book leaves the impression that Turner was naive and hypocritical; he denigrated quacks for their promises and snake oil treatment but could not question the validity of a story about an infant with a lizard for a head. Furthermore, Turner cannot explain how these strange altera-tions, as he put it, appeared on the fetus, other than merely by the force of the mother's imagination, noting that the exact mechanism for these defects was *supra captum*—"beyond his understanding."[103]

The more forward-thinking critics of his day vilified Turner for the chapter, with James Blondel (1665–1734) as the most outspoken of these. Blondel was a physician who trained in Leiden and was made a licentiate of the RCP in 1711. Some 13 years after the publication of *De Morbus Cutaneis*, Blondel, without singling out Turner in any way, published anonymously a treatise entitled *The Strength of Imagination in Pregnant Women Examin'd and the Opinion that Marks and Deformities in Children arise from thence demonstrated to be a Vulgar Error* (1727). Daniel Turner considered the work to be an attack on his Chapter XII, which Blondel denied repeatedly. In September 1729, Turner countered with the pamphlet vociferously addressing Blondel's work, *A Defense of the 12th Chapter of the First Part of a Treatise, De Morbis Cutaneis*. Later that year, Blondel issued a second work, *The Power of the Mother's Imagination over the Foetus Examin'd*. He confronted Turner directly in his introductory chapter, describing his cases as "fictitious ... insufficient and frivolous" and "wretchedly weak, and shallow—silly—ridiculous—insipid—best answered with Contempt," while lamenting Turner's stance and approach:

> Oh! what a pity, that a Gentleman, who has a good share of Reputation, should, out of Compliance to his Friends, engage himself in a Cause which can never be fairly defended by sound and close Arguments, but only by Quibbles and Puns, Suppositions and *Canterbury* stories ...

> The great Misfortune is, that by repeating so often, that the Effects of *Imagination* are incom-prehensible, Persons are apt to make a Merit of Ignorance, and for Truth to worship Falsehood, because 'tis intricate and contrary to Reason ...

> [continuing in the PREFACE] *My Opinion implies no Absurdity. 'Tis clear and intelligible, and easily deduced from the Laws of Motion, which God has established amongst Bodies ...*

> *The other Opinion is precarious, and depending upon Hear-says, and false Stories: 'Tis unphi-losophical and grounded upon occult Qualities ...*

> *'Tis sawcy and scandalous, in supposing that those, whom God Almighty has endowed, not only with so many Charms, but also, with an extraordinary Love and Tenderness for their Children, instead of Answering the End they are made for, do breed* Monsters *by the Wantoness of their Imagination.*[104]

Blondel went on to refute the beliefs of the "imaginationists" by employing a rational, deductive approach that involved hypothesis testing and anatomic concerns.[105] By invoking Newton's laws of motion, Blondel stood for the Enlightenment, the scientific method, and the modern era, while Turner trusted in the ancients and looked to the Creator to explain these natural skin lesions. In this war of pamphlets, the controversial topic was placed in the consciousness of eighteenth-century scientific thought, and though Turner was on the losing side of this argument, the engagement on issues that resulted from his pamphleteering advanced the understanding of the pathogenesis of disease through scientific discourse. It would take another 50 years for the imaginationist dogma to fall away in the writings of physicians and scientists of the era. Turner would have the last word in 1730 with yet another pro-imaginationist pamphlet. And the fourth edition of *De Morbis Cutaneis*, released in 1731, retained an unedited original twelfth chapter.[106]

Daniel Turner was a proud man who desired, more so than anything else in his life, to be recognized as an authority in medicine by his peers with an admission to the RCP. Unfortunately, he never achieved this lifelong goal. He was exceptionally hardworking, eventually sought by patients for his service over other practitioners, and extremely prolific in his writings compared to his contemporaries. He was significantly more religious than his Enlightenment peers, and he tried to live a virtuous life, guided by the Bible, while considering himself a handservant to God, delivering treatments that would only be successful if God willed it.[107] From his writings, it is obvious that Turner was a compassionate physician, and somewhat unusual in his ethic for patient autonomy in regard to decision-making. He was more a master of therapeutics than diagnosis, with an overwhelming majority of the pages in *De Morbis Cutaneis* devoted to prescription recommendations and case studies of his treatment courses. He was very direct and did not hesitate to express his opinions in his writings. He became irritated by incompetent practitioners who caused or risked significant harm to patients. He used very strong unprofessional language, calling out those whom he deemed quacks. He was coarse, as one might expect from his not being born with a gentleman's status or brought into the professional world through the university system. From his writings, we can see that Turner was proud of his career, but not to the point of conceit, as he was equally likely to divulge his treatment failures to his reader as he was his successes. His pride got in the way only when it came to admitting defeat, as when astute Enlightenment colleagues, such as Blondel, so eloquently pointed out his mistakes and his failure to humbly rid himself of his imaginationist beliefs.

Posterity has not been kind to Daniel Turner, as he has certainly had more critics than fans. It is possible that during the very competitive milieu in which he found himself, there was some spite and envy from his contemporaries. Their disdain for Turner, a non-Fellow, clouded an honest assessment of his work that was carried out in large part in isolation. In a 1730 Grub Street Journal, John Martyn (1699–1768) called Turner's work digressive, meaning full of passages designed to amuse and distract from the melancholy nature of the cases.[108] Thomas Bateman (1778–1821) referred to Turner as "our credulous countryman," in reference to Turner's willingness to believe anything he had heard from colleagues or read in texts.[109] In his *Epitaphian Mementos* (1827), William Wadd referred to Turner as "dirty old Daniel."[110] Norman Moore's 1899 entry in the *Oxford Dictionary of National Biography* stated that Turner's "medical attainments were small, and the records of cases are the only parts of his works of any permanent value."[111] Even the rare modern scholarship on Turner has not been favorable. Cock had a compelling and critical take on Turner as one who put his own aggrandizement above all else.[112] Citing numerous examples throughout his work, she pointed out that Turner committed significant shaming of not only his patients but also competing practitioners in order build himself up as an authority.[113] Turner's infamous twelfth chapter made him a total laughingstock, overshadowed the rest of the work, and tarnished his reputation irreversibly among the physician-scientists of his day, almost canceling out his better qualities. Moreover, he continued to promote topical remedies, especially mercurial ones, and salivation for syphilis at a time when it had fallen out of favor because internal treatment of external disease was deemed most appropriate; consequently, Turner was seen by some as antiquated at best, or at worst, a quack.

The minority view holds Turner in high regard. If judged by its circulation and number of editions (five) and languages (three), *De Morbis Cutaneis* was a success, and the most important text on cutaneous medicine to circulate in the first half of the eighteenth century.[114] Turner's text on syphilis had a long run, and had Astruc not arrived on the scene, it may have dominated his era.[115]

Fordyce (1858–1925) bracketed Turner's name with Sydenham and Boerhaave.[116] Rayer (see Chapter 13) valued the practical nature of Turner's book.[117] Hare argued in 1967 that Turner lacked both a formal education and "the advice of a good editor and perhaps even more of a good wife," either of whom could have mollified his "intransigent attitude."[118] Turner's *Ceratum de Lapide Calaminari*, "ointment of calamine ore (zinc)," was mentioned frequently in his works as a treatment for many different skin diseases, including burns, ulcers, boils, and shingles. A mixture of butter, yellow wax, olive oil, and calamine, the simple compound would become celebrated as "Turner's Cerate," and it could be found in dispensaries in the United States as late as 1955.[119] His advocacy for the use of the condom should not be overlooked.

One of the most important British dermatologists of the twentieth century, Alan Lyell (1917–2007), wrote the greatest defense of Daniel Turner, claiming that Turner was the true founder of British dermatology with the following supporting statements.[120] At the time of Turner's writing, the ignorance about the diseases of the skin was so great that very few, if any, could adequately judge the value of what he had written. Jealousy and suspicious, not complimentary remarks, was the norm for his era. His colleagues were likely very perturbed by his writing in English, dropping the "air of mystery" that typically cloaked the work of doctors. Most interestingly, Lyell pointed out that "a curtain was drawn deliberately across the memory of Daniel Turner by the cult of Robert Willan, before whom, people were led to believe, all had been chaos."[121]

Daniel Turner's career represents a fascinating transition point in the history of dermatology, an enigmatic man with views arising from two contrasting eras. On the one hand, he held in high regard the authority of his predecessors with their archaic understanding of disease and untested therapeutics (i.e., it is effective because Galen or Riverius said it is effective), and he frequently referenced the "old wives." On the other hand, Turner saw himself as a protector of the public from quackery and its ineffective or dangerous treatments. Turner's pleas later in his career for clinical trials, as well as his choice of publication in English rather than Latin (which could introduce the specialty to the masses), were very forward thinking. He is positioned at the crossroads between the Renaissance and the Enlightenment, and the conflicts within his writings—anecdotal versus evidence-based—confuse us in how to assess his career. While he will likely always be a difficult figure for us to pin down, Turner should be remembered as a pioneer in the field of dermatology as he was the first practitioner to demonstrate clearly an immense interest in skin disease. Most of all, he was the first to document and adequately characterize the suffering that skin disease could cause and to offer compassionate treatment suggestions, with patient autonomy in mind, which resulted from his obsessive research into the known information of his day.

Summary

The seventeenth century can be characterized as a period of intellectual upheaval stemming from the conception of the scientific method. The promotion of observation and the application of the principles of empiricism began to replace the tired approach of looking to the ancients for answers to scientific or medical questions. While Newton's *Principia* was the culmination of nearly 125 years of work in mathematics and physics to prove Ptolemy's system was incorrect, Harvey's *De motu cordis* was the major breakthrough that led the anatomists, physicians, and surgeons of the period to realize that Galen's system was also incorrect. Medicine and surgery, led by Thomas Sydenham and Richard Wiseman, respectively, would continue on separate paths during this time, but each would become increasingly more scientific and more modern in their approaches, and skin disease remained under the jurisdiction of surgeons more so than physicians. There was nothing groundbreaking in Hafenreffer's major dermatologic publication of the period in regard to the nomenclature, diagnosis, or treatment of skin disease, but it did demonstrate a fervor for skin disease in at least one major thinker of the period. Once the newly-invented microscope was in the hands of Marcello Malpighi and William Cowper, proof existed that the skin was not just a protective covering of the internal anatomy, but that it had its own anatomy. Modern dermatology was not yet born in the seventeenth century, but in many ways, modern medicine and surgery were—if by modern, we mean stripped of antiquated beliefs and ancient texts and backed by the observations of the naked eye at the bedside and the aided eye at the microscope. Now that physicians and natural philosophers could study the skin microscopically and visualize each of its minuscule components, it was only a matter of time before the skin and its diseases could be studied scientifically with this extraordinary invention.

10

The Enlightenment

The intellectual developments that dominated eighteenth-century Europe are collectively known as the Enlightenment. Some scholars, with a focus on France, define the era as the period beginning after the reign of Louis XIV; he died in 1715. Others look at the Enlightenment more broadly since the movement occurred in many parts of Europe and the United States, and they consider it a second phase of the scientific revolution, marking its beginning with the publication of Bacon's *The Great Instauration* (1620). Still others see the Enlightenment beginning sometime in the late 1680s with the revocation of the Edict of Nantes (1685), the publication of Newton's *Principia* (1687) and John Locke's works (1689–1690), and the overthrow of the Stuart monarchy by William of Orange in the Glorious Revolution (1688).[1] For our purposes, this last definition is most suitable. All scholars agree that the Enlightenment ended with the events leading up to the American (1776) and French Revolutions (1789).

As for the causes of the Enlightenment, historians generally frame this period of intellectual history as a reaction to one or more of the following: the incessant warfare of the preceding centuries, especially the apocalyptic Thirty Years' War (1618–1648); as a natural progression from the Scientific Revolution; as a breaking point after centuries of poor treatment of the lower and middle classes by the monarchies of Europe; or simply as the natural order of things after the introduction of that ever-wonderful and greatest of brain fuels, coffee. Coffee was introduced into Europe after the siege of Vienna in 1683 when the victorious Austrians acquired the spoils of coffee from their defeated besiegers, the Turks. Coffee was being consumed in the Arabic world for at least 200 years prior, having arrived there at some point in the late Middle Ages from Ethiopia, the legendary birthplace of the beverage.

The *Philosophes*

The Enlightenment started in France, where a community of thinkers and writers emerged at the crossroads among "human superstition, despotism, ignorance, and suffering" with the possibility that human suffering could be reduced and well-being increased after applying the principles of empiricism and observation to societies.[2] The philosophy of these eighteenth-century thinkers was heavily influenced by the empiricists Frances Bacon (1561–1626) and John Locke (1632–1704) and the rationalists René Descartes (1596–1650) and Baruch Spinoza (1632–1677). Empiricism—the idea that one's experience is the most important source of knowledge—and rationalism—the idea that reason is the most direct route to knowledge—were two competing philosophical stances that emerged out of the seventeenth century. Empiricism refers to inductive learning based on sensory input acquired through experience and experiment. Rationalism refers to deductive learning through intellect without the need for experiment. One was not better than the other, and Bacon hoped for an alliance between the two faculties, the men of experiment and the men of dogmas (the reasoners):

> The men of experiment are like the ant, they only collect and use; the reasoners resemble spiders, who make cobwebs out of their own substance. But the bee takes a middle course: it gathers its material from the flowers of the garden and of the field, but transforms and digests it by a power of its own.[3]

The best methods of the experimental and rational faculties were applied by the Enlightenment thinkers—in France, called *philosophes*—in their assault on the institutions of their day. Their targets were religious faith, superstition, despotic government, intolerance, social immobility, and human suffering.

DOI: 10.1201/9781003273622-15

The themes of the Enlightenment—now known as liberal ideals—were individual freedom, the right to happiness, the right to property, sensual pleasure, religious tolerance, and equal opportunity. Both the American and French Revolutions were products of the Enlightenment; the Conservatism and Romanticism movements of the early nineteenth century were reactions to the Enlightenment.

WHO WERE THE *PHILOSOPHES*?

So, who were these so-called *philosophes* and other important figures of the Enlightenment? In no particular order, they included Denis Diderot (1713–1784), co-founder of the *Encyclopédie*, the most defining publication of the Enlightenment; David Hume (1711–1776), the empiricist heir to Bacon and Locke; Cesare Beccaria (1738–1794), who advocated revision of the penal codes and opposed the death penalty; Immanuel Kant (1724–1804), the quintessential rectifier of both empiricism and rationalism; Montesquieu (1689–1755), who believed in the separation of state powers; Jean-Jacques Rousseau (1712–1778), who proposed the social contract and popular sovereignty; and Voltaire (1694–1778), author of *Candide* and especially known for his criticism of the Catholic Church and his defense of the freedom of speech; Adam Smith (1723–1790), whose *The Wealth of Nations* laid the foundation for free market economic theory; and Catherine II of Russia (1729–1796), Joseph II of Austria (1741–1790), and Frederick II of Prussia (1740–1786), considered enlightened despots of the period. Benjamin Franklin (1706–1790) and Thomas Jefferson (1743–1826) were Founding Fathers of America, heavily influenced by Bacon, Locke, and Newton and proponents of the same Enlightenment ideals as their European counterparts.

In addition to the political, religious, and social impact of the Enlightenment, there was obviously an impact felt in the realm of natural philosophy (science), and later, in medicine. Bacon, Descartes, Galileo, Newton, Locke, and other intellectual giants of the preceding century were the awe-inspiring idols of Diderot, Voltaire, Franklin, and the others. The founders of the new philosophy had ushered in enthusiasm among the *philosophes* for the idea that the application of scientific knowledge and principles had the potential to improve the human condition. And these eighteenth-century natural philosophers learned from Bacon and Galileo to study nature for oneself rather than trust the received authority of the past; from Descartes, to doubt everything; from Locke, that experience matters most; and from Newton, that the world was orderly, designed, and governed by laws.[4] The enthusiasm in the *philosophes* for the application of scientific principles was reinforced by the fact that they had already seen the fruits of this new philosophy: Kepler's planetary motion, Galileo's mechanics and motion, Harvey's circulation of the blood, Gilbert's magnetism, Hooke's elasticity, Torricelli's air pressure and the vacuum, Boyle's pneumatics, Huygens' pendulum and centripetal force, and Newton's motion, optics, and universal gravitation.[5]

The *philosophe* admired inductive reasoning, rational analysis, and experimental confirmation.[6] There was an emphasis on mathematics and mechanics. He shunned superstition and old wives' tales and rejected the authority of the ancients. Because the universities continued to teach Aristotelian scholasticism, he avoided these places and instead sought to meet for discourse at cafes, salons, and burgeoning Academies; many of the important philosophes lacked a university education. They were opposed more to religious intolerance than religion per se. Above all, utility reigned supreme in the philosophy of this era, meaning the highest value was placed on whether a particular nugget of scientific knowledge could increase human happiness or decrease human suffering.[7]

The *philosophes* not only defended their viewpoints in academies, cafes, and salons, but they also wrote about these arguments in lengthy treatises, books, and pamphlets. In addition, writers in this period attempted to popularize the natural philosophy of the preceding century in terms that the lay public could understand; Newton's *Principia* was just too convoluted for the average person, or even the *philosophe*, to comprehend.[8] Like disciples, the generations after Newton and Bacon delivered a message to the masses that contained both a more easily digested version of natural philosophy and a plethora of Enlightenment ideals.

Iatromechanics (Iatrophysics)

During the Enlightenment, there was the advancement of theories that were in opposition to Galenic humoral physiology, although Galenism would continue to dominate the teachings at the major medical institutions of Europe until the nineteenth century. We have seen in previous chapters that the first competing theory—iatrochemistry (chemical medicine)—was founded by Paracelsus and promoted by Thomas Willis and Franciscus Sylvius. After a century of digesting Harvey's *De motu cordis* (1628) and Newton's *Principia* (1687), the scientific minds of the generations that followed those great works advanced another school of thought in which physics and mathematics, proven to be so powerful by Newton, could be applied to human physiology and medicine. It was a school of medicine in which terms such as static and dynamic, contraction and expansion, motion and friction were utilized in its discussions. The foundation of this school can be traced back to the careers of Santorio Santorio (1561–1636), Giovanni Borelli (1608–1678), and Giorgio Baglivi (1668–1707). Santorio was among the first to use instruments such as thermometers to try to quantify vital aspects of the human body. His major publication was *De statica medicina,* "On medical measurement" (1614). Borelli, the father of biomechanics, applied physics to both animal and human musculoskeletal systems and published his findings in *De motu animalium,* "On the movement of animals" (1680). Baglivi performed physiologic experiments and calculations to demonstrate that the human body was essentially a machine and that the fibrous solids of the organs were more important than the body's fluids.

Termed iatromechanics (mechanical medicine), iatrophysics, or iatromathematics, this school of thought explained the human body not as varying ratios of four humors or three chemicals, but as a clockwork machine composed of microscopic particles, capable of mechanical functions like muscle contraction and the movement of fluids through vessels. Although the iatrophysics movement originated in the early seventeenth century, it did not reach its heyday until after the publication of the *Principia* in 1687. Around that time, several English and Scottish physicians, either close to or within Newton's inner circle, put forth an effort to bring about the "Newtonianization" of medicine.[9] Their focus was the hydraulics and velocities of circulating fluids calculated based on the dimensions of vessels or their obstruction, which, when altered, led to different types of diseases. Their writings incorporated complicated mathematical calculations, geometrical diagrams, experimentation, and observational data. Newtonianism was ultimately deemed a flawed system. It has been argued that hydraulic iatromechanism was in large part meant to win favor with Newton, who had presided over the Royal Society during this period, but it did not survive for very long after Newton's death in 1727. It became increasingly clear that careful attention to details at the bedside, not mathematical experiments, was the route to discovering the answer to medicine's many questions and that Bacon, not Newton, was the best source of inspiration for physicians wishing to make scientific advances in medicine.[10]

The *Encyclopédie*

Dictionaries and encyclopedias in the modern sense arrived during the Enlightenment. The *philosophe* found the authoritative nature of these types of books the perfect format for the comprehensive exercise of explaining everything in terms of the new philosophy. The best examples of this endeavor were the *Encyclopédie ou Dictionnaire Raisonné de Sciences, des Arts et des Métiers,* "Encyclopedia, or a Systematic Dictionary of the Sciences, Arts, and Crafts" (published from 1751 to 1772), edited by Denis Diderot and Jean le Rond d'Alembert (1717–1783). In the preface to the *Encyclopédie,* Diderot stated the objective:

> To collect all knowledge scattered over the face of the earth, to present its general outlines and structures to the men with whom we live, and to transmit this to those who will come after us, so that the work of the past centuries may be useful to the following centuries, that our children, by becoming more educated, may at the same time become more virtuous and happier, and that we may not die without having deserved well of the human race.[11]

As a project that extended from 1751 to 1772 in which savants such as Voltaire, Montesquieu, and Rousseau were able to communicate their ideas to the masses by contributing an article, the *Encyclopédie* was the most influential publication of the Enlightenment. Featuring a broad range of topics including the arts, technology, and history, the final product contained 28 volumes, in excess of 70,000 articles and 3000 illustrations from more than 160 contributors. The entire corpus of these contributions represents the consummate accomplishment of the Enlightenment. Diderot, recognizing the value of this magnum opus to civilization, wrote:

> A revolution may even now be burgeoning in some remote region of the world, or be smouldering at the very center of a civilized country; should it break out, destroy the cities, scatter the nations anew, and bring back ignorance and darkness, all will not be lost, if a single copy of this work survives.[12]

The *Dictionnaire philosophique* (1764) Voltaire's own smaller scale version of the *Encyclopédie*, containing over 100 articles of various topics on religion, freedom, and morality, with the following entry on medicine illustrating the characteristic flavor of his work:

> Regimen is superior to medicine, especially as, from time immemorial, out of every hundred physicians, ninety-eight are charlatans. It is not, however, the less true that an able physician may preserve life on a hundred occasions, and restore to us the use of our limbs...I distinguish not between physicians and surgeons, these professions being so intimately connected...Men who are occupied in the restoration of health to other men, by the joint exertion of skill and humanity, are above all the great of the earth.[13]

How were the skin and skin disease viewed by the Enlightenment *philosophes*? There is no better way to find the answer to that question than to consult the defining and most inspired work of the entire age: Diderot and d'Alembert's *Encyclopédie*. A search using the keyword *peau* is a logical place to start, and it yields enlightening declarations about the skin and its ailments in three entries that pertain to our discussion. The first entry, on the skin itself, reads:

> *Peau* (skin): A reticular plexus or a body of vessels is situated immediately under the cuticle or the epidermis. The vesicles of the skin contain a mucous liquid: Malpighi and others think that the color of the skin comes from the dyeing of this liquid; they test themselves on the fact that Black skin is white, and their blood red, etc. and that the only thing that is particular to them in this part is the color of this liquid. The skin is composed of fibers of its own, or according to Steno, it is formed of tendon productions of the subjacent parts, which end in an infinity of pyramidal nipples, intertwined with innumerable numbers of nerve fibers & other vesicles which form what is called parenchyma; it is by means of these nipples that the skin becomes the organ of touch. The skin is generally bound to the subjacent parts by the adipose membrane, and by the vessels which are proper to it, the veins, arteries, nerves, etc. Its purpose is to cover and envelop the whole body, to be a general emunctory for the matter of perspiration, and to be the organ of touch. The diseases of the skin are scabies, leprosy, smallpox, measles, purpura, and erysipelatous inflammations.[14]

The second entry, "Pores de la Peau," was written by Chevalier Louis de Jaucourt (1704–1779), the most prolific writer of the whole *Encyclopédie*, if not the most industrious scholar of all time. He studied medicine at Leiden with Boerhaave and was an iatromechanist. He wrote more than 17,000 articles from 1759 to 1765 on virtually every topic including biology and medicine, with his contributions totaling approximately 24 percent of the entire encyclopedia.[15] An entry dedicated to the pores of the skin reflects a fascination with the skin's excretory functions that was common in this period, as Jaucourt noted, "each part of human skin is filled with excretory conduits or pores that continually expel superfluous humors of the fluid that circulates."[16]

The third entry, on *Maladies de la peau*, "Diseases of the skin," was written by Menuret de Chambaud (1739–1815) and provides an invaluable source of information about the status of skin disease in the eighteenth century. Chambaud was a Montpellier-trained physician who contributed countless articles on medicine for the *Encyclopédie*. He wrote:

> Diseases of the skin are all characterized by some eruption more or less sensitive, more or less elevated, which changes the color, destroys the suppleness, disturbs the polish and the uniformity; these eruptions are sometimes pimples or small tumors raised above the surface of the skin; at other times they are mere spots which offer to the eyes only an alteration in color, without any sensible elevation; in some cases there are scales covering the skin, etc. The diseases of the skin can be distinguished into chronic and acute; this distinction is very well founded and very important. In the first class, lepra, scabies, scabs, ringworm, elephantiasis, etc. Among the acute diseases are chiefly smallpox, measles, scarlet fever, miliary, purpura, erysipelas, etc...[17]

He divided skin diseases into acute and chronic, noting that acute diseases are generally left to nature, while chronic diseases do not resolve without treatment.

Chambaud questioned the prevailing iatromechanical Boerhaavist (see below) notion of his time that skin disease was caused by the acrimony of the humor which gets arrested in the skin and its stagnation, leading to the various eruptions, and resultant pain, itching, or excitation of the skin. He called Boerhaave's acrimonies "imaginary" and his principles "false," "vague," "arbitrary," and "ridiculous." He noted:

> But what is most unfortunate is that these erroneous principles have given rise to pernicious consequences; a false theory has established bad practice, especially in the treatment of chronic skin diseases. If all the humors are acrid, it has been said, if their acrimony is the basis, the foundation, and the root cause of these diseases, it will only be necessary to destroy it in order to put an end to its effects. Let us, then, put in the blood watery, sweet, mucilaginous medicines, we will drown the salts, soften their pungency, envelop and entangle, so to speak, their point; at the same time the vessels smeared by these fatty, unctuous juices will be less susceptible to irritation; defended by this shield, they will be safe from the stinging of these pointed globules, they will resist their action, to the weaker efforts they make to penetrate into their tissue, then also the quantity of aqueous liquid which will serve as a vehicle for these medicines, will dissolve the lymph, and the blood will diminish its cohesion, the neighborhood of the globules; by this means these two fundamental vices of the blood will be effectively corrected; the humors will be watered down and made more flowable, hence more stagnation, more engorgement & more tumor, at the same time more irritation, more tingling, & thus, complete cessation of the itching & pain; and by a subsequent necessary consequence, the most perfect calm, harmony, and uniformity are re-established in the animal economy. This is how these doctors heal in their surgeries and consultations: the indications are very natural, the remedies exactly correspond to the indications; but unfortunately success is not achieved by them: it is a very pretty novel; but there is nothing real; situations are well managed, well brought in; but they are imagined: the characters are well supported; but they are false, they do not exist in nature...[18]

Chambaud is clearly challenging the prevailing notions of the Leiden iatromechanists, and to some extent, the whole of humoral theory, concluding that their approach may sound good but never actually succeeds. Instead, he promoted the enlightened physician with empiricism, reason, and the scientific method as his best tools. He also disparaged "imprudent surgeons" with their "murderous hands" for applying topical remedies to the skin. To Chambaud and other physicians, topical therapies could drive back the disease into the body, leading to serious or fatal consequences:

> It is very essential to warn the sick to carefully remove the murderous hand of the imprudent surgeon, to avoid with the last circumspection any external application, any remedy which might act in some way on the skin; there is no medium, if the remedy is not useless, it will be pernicious, it cannot do good; the greatest evil that may result from fear is the action of these topicals, which the charlatan, with brazen promise, distributes without knowledge, and which the ignorant and credulous people buy and employ with confidence; the bad effects of these remedies are

terrible and quick. They dissipate the affection of the skin quite well; they make the pustules, the exanthemas disappear, and it is from this too prompt cessation that all the danger comes. How many sudden deaths have followed these kinds of inconsiderations; all the books are full of the fatal accidents which this kind of credulity attracts; there is no one who has not seen or heard any similar event; and yet one is always the dupe of those subaltern physicians, fertile in promise, the hope of healing prevails over the fear of danger. It is easy to hope for what one desires with ardor, and there is no business in which one seeks less to base one's hopes than in regard to health, so there is none where one is most often deceived.[19]

According to the physicians of this era, skin disease was best treated from within. Recall that the surgeon Turner, in the appendix of his magnum opus, *De Morbis Cutaneis,* promoted topical therapies, and Turner and surgeons like him were the targets of this attack. Chambaud concluded with the comment that the promotion of perspiration was the safest and most effective therapeutic option in the treatment of chronic skin diseases.

Carl Linnaeus (1708–1778) and the Classification of Living Things

In addition to the exhaustive drive to define everything, there was an equally powerful drive to classify all things, and no individual of the Enlightenment better demonstrated that drive than Carl Linnaeus, the most influential naturalist of the eighteenth century. He was a Swedish botanist, zoologist, and physician who developed the binomial taxonomical system used to classify all living things. Newton's proof that the "system of the world" was one of order and law influenced every aspect of knowledge during the Enlightenment. In the realm of biology, the classification system of Linnaeus was an attempt to order all natural things. To Linnaeus, every animal, including man, every plant, and every mineral had a neat place in the world. From Aristotle's writings and the work of Neoplatonists such as Plotinus (205–270 CE), the idea of *scala naturae,* "the ladder of nature," later, "The Great Chain of Being," had existed since ancient times. It would be modified over the centuries by Saint Augustine and Thomas Aquinas. At the top of this ladder sat God, and underneath God were the angels, then man, then the animals, the plants, and finally rocks and minerals. Various political and social versions of this concept surfaced during the course of human history. The rationalists—Descartes, Spinoza, and, especially Gottfried Wilhelm von Leibniz (1646–1716)—modified the Great Chain of Being, describing it in terms of a degree of perfection in relation to God, with God the perfect being, and each rung on the ladder down (man, animals, etc.) increasingly less perfect compared to God.

The Linnaean system broke away from this idea of a vertical, descending order of being and instead placed all living things in different kingdoms with no category above any other. Linnaeus organized expeditions and sent his students, later known as his "apostles," all over the world to catalog species of plants, animals, and insects. At 28 years of age, he published the fruits of his ongoing research in 1735, with the title *Systema naturae,* "The System of Nature." He wrote:

> The first step in wisdom is to know the things themselves. This consists in having a true idea of the objects; objects are distinguished and known by classifying them methodically and giving them appropriate names. Therefore classification and name-giving will be the foundation of our science.[20]

Systema naturae underwent ten editions, with the most definitive being the markedly expanded, two-volume tenth edition (1758). He drew criticism from fellow scientists and theologians by classifying humans as animals and placing them next to apes. Interestingly, Linnaeus was not the first to introduce a binomial taxonomy. He credited Gaspard and Jean Bauhin, two Swiss brothers and students of our Mercurialis (see Chapter 8), for their introduction of the idea in 1596. Even so, Linnaeus was quite proud, if not vainglorious, of his accomplishment and his place in history; the quote *Deus creavit, Linnaeus disposuit,* "God created, Linnaeus organized," though probably incorrectly attributed to him, exemplifies his pride. Linnaeus did not lack critics. His toughest contemporary critic, Comte Georges-Louis Leclerc de Buffon (1707–1788), found his system artificial and wrote in his *Histoire naturelle* (1749–1804) that the "Genera, Orders, and Classes exist only in our imagination."[21]

More recently, science historians have also criticized Linnaeus' work as decidedly unscientific and Eurocentric in its assessment of differing human races; it failed to discover evolution where it must have been glaringly obvious with such research.[22] But Linnaeus was a religious man and, in his mind, his work supported the existence of God and God's plan. Furthermore, he was cognizant of angering the ecclesiastics with controversial statements. And though he was not an evolutionist, his work did lay the groundwork that would ultimately lead to the theories of evolution promoted over the next century. With *Systema naturae*, Linnaeus became the hero of eighteenth-century natural philosophy. Rousseau was known to have said in a message to Linnaeus, "Tell him I know of no man on earth who is greater than he."[23] Only time will tell if the Linnaean taxonomical system can survive the recent efforts to replace it with a phylogenetic (evolution-based) nomenclature.

LINNAEUS' HELLISH FURY WORM

The story would not be complete without a mention of Linnaeus' *Furia infernalis*, the "Hellish fury worm." Linnaeus himself had once been attacked by an unidentified organism, and his affected arm eventually required surgical intervention in order to rid him of a consequential serious illness. Years later, Linnaeus decided that the culprit was a tiny, threadlike worm discovered by one of his students, which Linnaeus, in his *Systema naturae*, named after the vengeful Furies of Greek mythology. It was described by Linnaeus as having the thickness of human hair, with a gray body and black legs.[24] The organism fell from the air and landed on the skin, which it pierced and entered, causing unbearable pain. The fury worm captured the imagination of both laypeople and naturalists for the next century. Many medical treatises from the late eighteenth and early nineteenth centuries, including that of Plenck, contained descriptions of this illness. Others doubted the worm's existence, and the Academy of Sciences in Stockholm offered a reward if someone could come forward with the worm, but no one did. Later in life, Linnaeus himself became skeptical about the existence of *Furia infernalis*, and scholars have concluded that Linnaeus was likely bitten by a horsefly.[25]

Nosology: The Classification of Diseases

While Linnaeus was defining and classifying living things, Enlightenment physicians attempted to define and classify diseases, a discipline termed nosology. Recall that Thomas Sydenham, in the seventeenth century, had originally called for the classification of diseases based on his novel idea of "species" of disease. Nosology developed from the desire to bring order to a large body of disorganized facts, to encourage more satisfactory explanations of therapeutics in the iatrochemical and iatromechanical framework, and to make a stand against rising radical skepticism.[26] Several important physicians in the eighteenth century attempted to answer Sydenham's call. Interestingly, many of these physicians, like Linnaeus, were also botanists, and the approach taken to classify disease followed the approach to classify plants. Plants at this time were classified based on directly observable external structures, and diseases were classified by directly observable signs and symptoms.

The most significant of these physician-botanists was François Boissier de Sauvages de Lacroix (1706–1767), a professor of medicine at Montpellier and very close friend of Linnaeus. They frequently corresponded to discuss their research and writings, influencing one another equally. Sauvages' first attempt at a classification system was published under the title *Nouvelle classes de maladies*, "New Classes of Diseases" (1731), and like Linnaeus, Sauvages spent his whole career expanding and fine-tuning his classification system. The culmination of his life's work was entitled *Nosologia methodica sistens morborum classes genera et species juxta Sydenhami mentem et botanicorum ordinem,*

"Methodical nosology placing classes, genera, and species of diseases according to the reasoning of Sydenham and the arrangement of plants" (1763). Sauvages had delineated 10 classes, 44 orders, 315 genera, and 2400 species of diseases. The system was based only on the constant symptoms of a disease but suffered from "endless subdivision;" for example, Sauvages listed 17 varieties of cough and 29 types of hiccups.[27] Previous less scientific approaches to listing diseases dating back to ancient times organized them either alphabetically, regionally (location in the body), or etiologically.

Linnaeus, a physician as well as a biologist, published his own classification of disease in a work entitled *Genera morborum,* "The Types of Disease" in 1763, the same year *Nosologia methodica* was published. Unlike the work of Sauvages, it had little impact on contemporary medicine because Linnaeus could not properly distinguish between symptoms and diseases.[28]

Next was William Cullen (1710–1790). First a surgeon, then a physician, and then a professor of medicine at Edinburgh, William Cullen was the most influential English-speaking medical educator of the eighteenth century. Students and practicing physicians alike from all over Europe traveled to Edinburgh to hear him lecture. He was also a botanist and chemist, and he was an acquaintance of the Enlightenment giants David Hume and Adam Smith. Cullen's understanding of disease was different from the mainstream; he was an early rejecter of humoralism. Because he instead believed that all pathology resulted from disordered action ("spasm") of the nervous system, he earned the nickname "Old Spasm."[29]

Cullen published several highly authoritative texts, the most important of which were *Synopsis nosologiae methodicae,* "Synopsis of methodical nosology" (1769) and "First Lines of the Practice of Physic," (1777), with the former containing his nosology, the latter a textbook of medicine in English that is widely considered his magnum opus. Cullen's nosology, far simpler than that of Sauvages, contained only four classes of disease instead of ten: pyrexias (fevers), cachexias, neuroses, and local diseases. The work is of tremendous value to medical historians because it contains in its first volume all of the major published nosologies for the purpose of convenience and comparison.

LESSER KNOWN NOSOLOGISTS

In addition to Sauvages' and Linnaeus' systems, Cullen included in his publication the nosologies of Vogel, Sagar, and Macbride. Rudolf Augustin Vogel (1724–1774) was a German professor of medicine at the University of Gottingen, and later, the personal physician of George III of England; he published several important works, including a nosology entitled, *Definitiones generum morborum,* "Definitions of the Kinds of Diseases" (1764). Johann Baptiste Michael Sagar (1702–1778) was a Viennese physician to whom a great debt is owed for his *Systema morborum symptomaticum,* "System of symptomatic diseases" (1771). David Macbride (1726–1778), an Irish physician and nosologist, wrote *A methodological introduction to the theory and practice of physic* (1772). In every corner of Europe, physician-writers were producing their own unique classification of diseases, a fervor that peaked in the 1760s and 1770s.

A formal classification system organized solely for skin disease was not published until the last quarter of the eighteenth century, but it is important to note that the great physician classifiers of this age— Sauvages, Linnaeus, Cullen, Vogel, Sagar, and Mcbride—all included skin diseases in their classification systems. In the present day, the vast majority of the known skin diseases are understood to be localized to the skin and arise from the skin. But the eighteenth-century physician carried on the age-old belief that changes in the skin reflected the internal health of a person, believing that it was a humoral imbalance or an "acrimony" of the humors inside the body that caused the skin changes. This understanding of skin disease, still referred to in this period as "affections," is reflected in the classification systems of the Enlightenment.

The categories used to organize the known diseases were ones based on a contemporary understanding of symptomatology, pathogenesis, and pathology. Headings used for classes and orders included *febres* (fevers), *spasmi* (spasms), and *fluxus* (flux, flowing out, as in diarrhea). Sauvages (1731 and 1763, see above) was first; he categorized skin diseases under two of his ten classes: *Vitiae,* "defects," and *Phlegmasiae,* "inflammation." Linnaeus (1763) put all of the skin diseases in his class XI, *Vitiae,* and divided them into two orders, *Scabies* (Latin for roughness or scaliness) and *Maculae.* Cullen (1769), with the longest, most detailed, and yet most simplistic system, had skin affections divided among three of his four classes: *Pyrexia* (fever), *Cachexia,* and *Locales.* Vogel, with one of the more sensible systems (1764), placed them in his tenth class, *Vitia,* categorizing them into six different orders: *Inflammationes, Tumores, Extuberantiae* (swelling), *Pustulae et Papulae, Maculae, and Dissolutiones.* Sagar (1771) had skin affections spread throughout in his 13-class system: distributed among four classes called *Vitiae, Plagae* (wounds), *Cachexiae* (chronic wasting), and *Exanthemata* (eruptions). McBride (1772) paid the least attention to skin diseases and mentioned only a few under an order called *Inflammationes.* In each of the above instances, skin diseases were not given their own category, and little detail was given about the nuances that distinguished one from another.

Herman Boerhaave (1668–1738) and Albrecht von Haller (1708–1777)

Excluding the work of Bernhard Albinus (1697–1770) and Giovanni Morgagni (1682–1771), considered the most important anatomists of the eighteenth century, the major contributions in the theory of medicine occurred in the realm of human physiology. The University of Leiden was home to two of the giants in this field, and the University rose to prominence during the career of Herman Boerhaave (1668–1738), who succeeded Govard Bidloo (see Chapter 9). Because of Boerhaave, Leiden became the premier center for medical education in Europe in the first half of the eighteenth century, and Boerhaave, referred to often as the Dutch Hippocrates (recall that Pieter van Foreest of Chapter 8 also given this nickname), was the most famous physician in the world during its apogee. Like many of his esteemed colleagues, he was a chemist as well as a botanist, and he made his mark in those fields. His medical writings were inspired by Newton, Descartes, and Borelli; therefore, he was a quintessential iatromechanist, someone who viewed the circulation of the blood in terms of mechanics, pressures, and hydraulics.[30] Boerhaave compiled the theories of Willis, Borelli, and Baglivi into a comprehensive iatromechanical system that attempted to reduce the conflict that arose in the early eighteenth century among Galenic medicine, iatrochemistry, and iatromechanism.

In addition to his iatromechanistic leanings, Boerhaave's legacy includes his reintroduction and popularization of bedside teaching, which had fallen out of favor since the end of the 1500s.[31] At Padua, Giovanni Battista da Monte (1498–1591) was the first to promote teaching in the hospital at the bedside. Any physician practicing today could tell you about his or her memorable days in the hospital wards where the attending physician used the patient in the bed as the reference to embark on an educational discussion. With his 12 teaching beds at St. Cecilia Hospital, Boerhaave popularized this practice and ensured it would remain a fixture of medical education. His lectures drew pupils and physicians from all over the world, with his knowledge reaching as far away as China. His most famous guests were Peter the Great and Voltaire, and he was friends with Linnaeus. For someone so renowned during his lifetime, most physicians remember Boerhaave not for his contributions to medicine but for the condition that bears his name—Boerhaave syndrome—which is the name for the rupture of the esophagus due to violent cough or vomiting.

While Boerhaave may have been the most celebrated physician of the century, his Swiss pupil Albrecht von Haller (1708–1777) was even more influential. This bona fide genius had a hand in many disciplines— mathematics, botany, language, science. He was also a prolific letter writer who frequently communicated with the leading scientific figures of Europe, such as Linnaeus. He dismissed the Linnaean system in favor of his own. He wrote a 71-page poem called *Ode sur les Alpes,* "Ode to the Alps" (1773), an early contribution to the movement known as Romanticism. He attempted to translate the Mesopotamian language of the Chaldeans. In medicine, like Jean Fernel 200 years prior, Haller published a massive multi-volume synthesis, *Elementa physiologiae corporis humani,* "Physiological Elements of the Human Body" (1759–1766), which contained all the known information about human physiology up until his time. His experimental work on the physiology of nerves and muscles is his greatest contribution, but he also showed precisely how the pumping mechanism of the heart worked, and he proved that the heart had autonomous muscular control. He explained the respiratory mechanism of the lungs and published his own research into human anatomy and embryology. In true Enlightenment fashion, he was an encyclopedist, having cataloged much of the available scientific literature in the four-volume *Bibliotheca medicinae practicae*, "Library of the Practice of Medicine" (1776–1788). There was no limit to his ambition, but his inner turmoil caused him to be his own worst enemy.[32] He was cantankerous, obsessive, and consistently inconsistent. A Jekyll and Hyde, he could be at times courteous and delightful and at other times, misanthropic, short-tempered, or raging.[33] Although Haller was one of the great geniuses in the history of medicine and his discoveries would have a lasting influence on the field, his personality traits got in the way of his forming a school of followers.[34]

Giovanni Morgagni (1682–1771) and the Anatomical Basis for Disease

Cullen, Sauvages, Boerhaave, Haller—each made monumental contributions to the history of medicine. But none of these came close to having the impact of Italian anatomist Giovanni Battista Morgagni. Like Mercurialis, Morgagni was born in Forli, Italy and secured a professorship at the University of Padua. He was the pupil of the great Antonio Maria Valsalva (1666–1723). Morgagni revolutionized medicine with his discovery of the anatomical basis of disease, using directly observable evidence from countless autopsies to correlate ante-mortem symptoms with post-mortem findings. The culmination of his life's work can be found in the single most important medical book published in the eighteenth century, *De sedibus et causis morborum per anatomen indagatis libri quinque*, "On the seats and causes of disease investigated by anatomy in five books" (1761). Published when Morgagni was 79 years of age, *De sedibus* contains the descriptions of nearly 700 autopsy dissections from the meticulous notes that he took over the course of his career. The five books were: (1) diseases of the head and neck; (2) diseases of the thorax; (3) diseases of the abdomen; (4) general disease; and (5) supplemental material. The impetus for the work was a desire in Morgagni to deal with discrepancies that were found in a seventeenth-century text entitled *Sepulchretum: sive anatomia practica ex cadaveribus morbo denatis*, "The Cemetery, or, Practical Anatomy of Corpses Dead from Disease" (1679) by Swiss anatomist Theophile Bonet (1620–1689), to whom Morgagni fully acknowledges he owed a debt for his contributions to anatomy.[35]

The end result of Morgagni's long career was the confirmation through 50-plus years of experiment and observation that disease could be traced back to some part of the human anatomy. For example, Morgagni wrote:

> A man of about fifty-four years of age, had begun, five or six months before, to be somewhat emaciated in his whole body ... a troublesome vomiting came on, of a fluid which resembl'd water, tinctur'd with soot ... Death took place ... In the stomach ... was an ulcerated cancerous tumour ... Betwixt the stomach and the spleen were two glandular bodies, of the bigness of a bean, and in their colour, and substance, not much unlike that tumour which I have describ'd in the stomach.[36]

Morgagni believed that clinical symptoms were "the cry of the suffering organs" and the pathology of those organs could be identified at autopsy. This concept seems simple enough, but prior to Morgagni, disease was not thought of in terms of the localization of pathology. Anatomical considerations did not enter the mind of the physician when formulating a diagnosis. For example, if a person was complaining of belly pain, the old way was to think of the symptom in terms of humoral imbalance, not localized inflammation of the appendix or gall bladder. Morgagni was the first to elevate anatomy to the point at which knowledge of it was indispensable to the practicing physician. Galenic and Hippocratic medicine could not survive much longer after *De sedibus*, because anatomy and practice were not separate entities.[37] Morgagni's anatomo-clinical correlation was based on the notion that the human body was a machine consisting of devices with separate functions (organs) that are connected with one another and work together in order to keep the machine going.[38] To Morgagni, disease was caused by a defect in one of these devices which then affected the overall condition of the machine.

After Morgagni, medicine was directed on a path whereby the correct diagnosis was established because a certain level of precision—taken for granted in today's healthcare—was achieved by the physician in localizing the pathology. Morgagni deserves a place along with Vesalius and Harvey as one of the true giants of the history of medicine, as his discoveries paved the way for the nineteenth-century Viennese anatomical pathologists who would finally localize the "seat" of disease to the skin (see Chapter 14).

John Hunter (1728–1793) and the Birth of Modern Surgery

Modern surgery was born in the eighteenth century with the contributions of John Hunter (1728–1793), one of the most fascinating characters in the history of medicine. Hunter was a Scottish surgeon and the younger brother of William Hunter, a notable physician and obstetrician himself. John never attempted to enter medical school, but thanks to arrangements made by his brother, he apprenticed with two famed surgeons—with William Cheselden (1688–1752) in 1748 and with Percival Pott (1714–1788) in 1751. Since breaking away from the barbers in 1745, surgeons were beginning to garner respect equal to that of physicians. Their dress reflected their higher stature: a red satin coat, knee breeches, and buckle shoes, and a gold-headed cane or even a sword.[39]

Hunter soon became proficient at and obsessed with dissection of any sort. He collected thousands of specimens to demonstrate various anatomical features and diseases of both humans and animals; he kept them in his home and later in a museum (housed today in the Royal College of Surgeons in London). He even once paid a large sum of money to acquire the body of the seven-foot, seven-inch Charles Byrne, better known as the Irish Giant, so that he could exhibit his skeleton in his museum. His knowledge about all subjects of natural history, e.g., geology and zoology, was vast. He preferred experimentation over textbooks, and doing over thinking. He stuck with a career in surgery even when an opportunity presented for him to enter medical school and become a physician.

Similar in temperament to Haller, Hunter was *the* inspiration for both Robert Louis Stevenson's *The Strange Case of Dr. Jekyll and Mr. Hyde* and Hugh Lofting's *Doctor Doolittle*. He was a "gruff domineering ogre" with a no-nonsense attitude toward his craft.[40] There is no better example of his matter-of-fact approach than in this famous quote attributed to Hunter:

> Some physiologists will have it that the stomach is a mill; others, that it is a fermenting vat; others, again that it is a stew-pan; but in my view of the matter, it is neither a mill, a fermenting vat nor a stew-pan, but a stomach, gentlemen, a stomach.[41]

Each of Hunter's surviving written works contains viewpoints remarkably contrary to tradition and ahead of their time. For example, he correctly noted that inflammation was not a disease per se but a response of the body to a disease. Hunter's most significant writings include *Natural History of the Human Teeth* (1771), the first text on the teeth; *Treatise on Venereal Disease* (1786; see Interlude 3); and *Treatise on the Blood, Inflammation, and Gunshot Wounds* (1794), in which he challenged the age-old belief that the bullet should be found and extracted from a bullet wound. Much of his unpublished written material was lost in a fire that took place after his death. His brother-in-law Everard Home (1756–1832), a surgeon himself and the person who performed the autopsy of Hunter, had Hunter's papers and plagiarized them, then he deliberately burnt his source material in order to hide the plagiarism.[42] Home is famous for being the first president of the Royal College of Surgeons and the first to discover that something about the sun other than its heat could induce sunburn on the skin.

If Hunter ever wrote about skin diseases in particular, it was lost in the fire. Besides his work with syphilis and gonorrhea, Hunter's contributions to dermatology include the first report of the excision of melanoma (see Conclusion) and his writings on inflammation. In his 1794 treatise, he wrote extensively about wound healing, including the process of generating new skin in a wound, which he called "skinning." He applied his understanding of the natural world to the human body, deducing that diseases such as cancer followed the same rules or principles as seen in nature:

> The specific qualities in diseases also tend more rapidly to the skin than to the deeper-seated parts, except the cancer; although even in this disease the progress towards the superficies is more quick than its progress towards the centre. The venereal has something of the same disposition with the cancer, although not so much. In short, this is a law in nature, and it probably is upon the same principle by which vegetables always approach the surface of the earth.[43]

Hunter's chief legacy was the way he brought science to surgery. He was known for continually improving upon his procedures based on new self-derived experimental evidence and previous learning experiences. After Hunter, the practice of surgery would be based largely on the doctrine of observation, experimentation, and application of scientific evidence, all in an effort to make surgery safe and effective.[44]

James Lind (1716–1794), Franz Mesmer (1734–1815), and the First Clinical Trials

This survey of eighteenth-century medicine concludes with a few additional words about the beginnings of modern evidence-based medicine with reference to the careers of James Lind and Franz Anton Mesmer. James Lind was a Scottish surgeon who served in the Royal Navy and advanced several different practices meant to improve the health and hygiene of sailors. Scurvy was an extraordinarily common problem for sailors in this period. It manifested as poor wound healing, bleeding skin and gums, brittle teeth and bones, fatigue, and ultimately death due to infection or hemorrhage. Mortality numbers of the period were staggering: two million sailors died between the time of Columbus' voyage and the rise of steam engines in the mid-nineteenth century, and any major voyage could expect to lose half of its sailors to scurvy.[45] While not as deadly as plague or smallpox or malaria, by the mid-eighteenth century, the search for a cure for the always-present scurvy became what Bown describes as "a vital factor determining the destiny of nations."[46]

While serving on the *HMS Salisbury*, Lind decided to conduct an experiment to determine if he could identify a positive impact against scurvy with certain diets. His findings were published in his *Treatise on scurvy* in Edinburgh in 1753:

> On the 20th of May 1747, I selected twelve patients in the scurvy, on board the *Salisbury* at sea. Their cases were as similar as I could have them. They all in general had putrid gums, the spots and lassitude, with weakness of the knees. They lay together in one place, being a proper apartment for the sick in the fore-hold; and had one diet common to all, viz. water gruel sweetened with sugar in the morning; fresh mutton-broth often times for dinner; at other times light puddings, boiled biscuit with sugar, etc., and for supper, barley and raisins, rice and currants, sago and wine or the like. Two of these were ordered each a quart of cyder a day. Two others took twenty-five drops of elixir vitriol three times a day.... Two others took two spoonfuls of vinegar three times a day.... Two of the worst patients were put on a course of sea-water.... Two others had each two oranges and one lemon given them every day.... The two remaining patients, took ... an electary recommended by a hospital surgeon.... The consequence was, that the most sudden and visible good effects were perceived from the use of oranges and lemons; one of those who had taken them, being at the end of six days fit for duty.... The other was the best recovered of any in his condition; and ... was appointed to attend the rest of the sick. Next to the oranges, I thought the cyder had the best effects..."[47]

Lind was the first to conduct a clinical trial in the modern era. Progress moved slowly after he published his results, and another 50 years passed before citrus became a staple in the British seafarer's diet.

The other figure affiliated with early clinical trials is the ignominious Franz Mesmer, a Vienna-trained physician and founder of a theory of disease termed animal magnetism. Influenced by Newton and his work on gravity and the tides, he penned *De planetarum influxu in corpus humanum*, "On the Influence of the Planets on the Human Body" (1766) and, after moving to Paris, *Mémoire sur la découverte du magnétisme animal*, "Memoir on the discovery of animal magnetism" (1779). In the latter work, Mesmer posited that in all living things flowed a magnetic fluid that could be obstructed, causing disease. This fluid could be manipulated by practitioners of a method that became known as mesmerism, from which comes the word "mesmerize." He initially used magnets as a part of these sessions but later discarded them in lieu of his person alone, which he claimed could manipulate the fluid and cure the patient. Invisible forces unleashed by Mesmer initiated a "crisis" in predominantly female patients that was characterized by unusual bodily sensations, crying, fainting, uncontrolled gestures, or violent fits, ending in "profound salubrious effects."[48] Mesmer finished his sessions by playing music with a glass armonica— graduated, spinning glass bowls that produce different musical tones with friction.

Mesmer's magnetic methods generated for him much fame and awe all over Europe, but ultimately controversy ensued. Louis XVI ordered that a commission be established to determine whether animal magnetism was real or imagined. The royal commission, led by Benjamin Franklin and Antoine Lavoisier (1743–1794), who is widely considered the father of modern chemistry, used placebo controls to determine the validity of mesmerism. The commission dispensed bogus 'mesmerized treatments' or, in a crossover manner, secretly administered bona fide materials. If the patients reacted to a bogus treatment or did not react to a bona fide one, the claims would be discounted.[49]

With these trials, mesmerism was debunked, and Mesmer left Paris in 1785. Benjamin Franklin, who invented the armonica that Mesmer used in his sessions, was the same man who effectively ended Mesmer's career. The glass armonica did not survive the eighteenth century after growing concerns that the instrument itself caused the player and the listener to go mad. Mesmerism continued to have many practitioners for the next 50 years, but interest in it eventually waned. It is still practiced today in some countries. The legacy of mesmerism is twofold: it was the foundation for hypnotism and the first major medical practice that was questioned and tested with placebo-controlled trials.

BENJAMIN FRANKLIN'S PSORIASIS

Benjamin Franklin (1706–1790), the great American statesman, inventor, and Founding Father, might just be the most famous American to ever have psoriasis. Worldwide, that designation probably goes to Joseph Stalin (1878–1953), whose dermatologist must have been living on borrowed time between every encounter with his unpredictable patient. For Franklin, we have a letter from his innumerable "papers" addressed to his physician friend John Pringle (1707–1782), in which Franklin, writing in the third person about himself, discussed his psoriasis.[50] His psoriasis (which he called scurf) started on his head as a single spot, and then it improved with treatment, only to spread to other parts of his scalp. In the winter of 1776, he developed boils that healed and formed spots of psoriasis at the sites of his healed boils. This phenomenon is termed the isotopic phenomenon of Wolf. The psoriasis then spread to each arm, the small of his back, and parts of his thighs and legs; they would bleed if rubbed or scratched (Auspitz sign). He soon tried a variety of treatments for his ailment, including a mercurial concoction of unknown composition called Belloste's pills and infusion containing Parisian rhubarb. However, Franklin ultimately determined long warm water baths (as in two hours long) to be more effective than any of these medicaments at loosening the scales. By the end of the letter, he proclaimed that his scalp, legs, and thighs were almost clear, but the psoriasis on his back and sides was stubborn. After bringing his physician-friend up to date on his dermatologic history, he asked if the condition was curable and what medications were capable of doing so. Sadly, even 250 years later, there is no "cure" for psoriasis, but we do have highly effective and very safe medications for this ancient affliction.

France's First Dermatologist: Anne-Charles Lorry (1726–1783)

The foundations for the specialty of dermatology were laid in the eighteenth century and can be traced to the careers of five pioneers: Daniel Turner (1667–1740), Jean Astruc (1684–1766), Anne-Charles Lorry (1726–1783), Seguin Henry Jackson (1752–1816), and Joseph Jacob Plenck (1738–1807). These five men individually made their mark on the study of skin disease and collectively set up a situation whereby at the end of their century, the world was ready for the scientific discipline we call dermatology. Turner has already been dealt with in Chapter 9, and Astruc will be covered in Interlude 3. The careers of Lorry, Jackson, and Plenck, to which we now turn, foreshadowed the dominance of their respective cities in the next century in the field of dermatology: Paris, London, and Vienna.

While Daniel Turner can be named the first British dermatologist, Anne-Charles Lorry is considered the first of France. With an additional interest in mental illness, he is considered a pioneer in the field of French psychiatry, and he wrote a major work on melancholy. The son of a law professor at the University of Paris, Lorry was the pupil of the famous Jean Astruc in the 1740s and became a doctor in 1748. He entered aristocratic circles when he saved the gravely ill infant of the Duc de Richelieu. He cared for the smallpox-addled Louis XV and his son and successor, Louis XVI. He rose to the highest possible status for a physician in France, and by 36 years of age, Lorry was one of the three most famous physicians in Paris.[51] He had a very large practice, and a reputation for generosity, kindness, and wisdom.[52]

Lorry published the first book on skin disease in France in 1777, entitled *Tractatus de Morbis Cutaneis*, "Treatise on Cutaneous Diseases." The 700-plus page tome was written in a glorious and highly stylized Latin and was the last of the major texts of dermatologic importance written in that classical language. In the latter half of the eighteenth century, Latin's almost two-millennium-long reign as the universal language of medicine had nearly ended in favor of the vernacular.

Tractatus de Morbis Cutaneis is a significant work for several reasons. It contains the first known reference to the skin as an organ. Lorry wrote in his lengthy introduction:

> Not only must the skin be considered simply as an envelope, but it constitutes an organ, flowing together with a wondrous variety and adorned with the highest wisdom, not only for utility of the body, but also for the beauty of the appearance.[53]

Lorry was also the first to attempt to classify skin diseases depending on whether they were localized to and arising from the skin or a manifestation of internal disease. The method of Mercurialis and Turner—to divide the diseases of the head from the diseases of the rest of the body—finally had an alternative that made somewhat more sense. Moreover, Lorry's expertise in the realm of nervous disorders gave rise to a novel understanding that skin disease could be psychosomatic, a fact of which the modern dermatologist is well aware. Finally, with Lorry and his long treatise, Paris was well on its way to establishing its own dynasty of dermatologists, which would compete with London and Vienna in the next century.

But Lorry's *Tractatus* also had its problems. His choice of Latin restricted those who could benefit from it to an increasingly narrow intellectual elite, in contrast to Turner's work, which had brought the study of skin disease to the masses. Kaposi wrote that the book was "too learned," and Darier complained that Lorry's descriptions of disease were imprecise and incomplete. And except for the new scheme for organizing diseases, there really wasn't anything original in the whole book; it was a last gasp of Galenic medicine and Aristotelian scholasticism.[54] It may have actually caused major setbacks in the advancement of therapeutics because of its emphasis on risky medications and unsubstantial linkages between the skin and certain organs in various diseases.[55] On the other hand, Pierre Rayer (see Chapter 13), who also recognized the imprecision of Lorry's diagnoses, admired Lorry and praised his *Tractatus* for its "general views, and the broad manner in which the author there regards the study of the diseases of the skin," and noted that "Lorry is undoubtedly superior to all the writers who preceded, and to the greater number of those who have followed him."[56]

As one who was entrenched in the traditionalist aristocracy of the *ancien régime*, the *Tractatus* included few Enlightenment principles. Ironically, he was highly regarded by the likes of Voltaire, one of his most famous patients, presumably because Lorry was a proponent of a simple diet and disapproved of rich foods. In spite of his work's major shortcomings, Lorry, the French bridge between Astruc (see Interlude 3) and Alibert (see Chapter 13), deserves to be remembered simply because his writings and career mark the end of an era. His *Tractatus* was the last book written on the skin in the ancient language of Latin, and Lorry's approach, at least for France, was at the end of a very old way of thinking about skin disease.

HISTORY'S GREATEST DERMATOLOGICAL MYSTERY

The greatest medical mystery in the history of skin disease is the question of the chronic, itchy skin disease of the French physician and revolutionary Jean-Paul Marat (1743–1793). It has been suggested that Marat's failure to enter into the Academy of Sciences instigated his left-wing political views, and Marat, full of resentment, sought eventually to exact revenge on his persecutors.[57] Marat played three main roles during the Revolution: he was the main participant in the September Massacres of 1792, he led a popular revolt against the moderate Girondins in the early summer of 1793, and he edited and published the first journal of the Revolution, *L'Ami du Peuple*, "The Friend of the People," from 1789 until his death.[58] Marat was assassinated in his bathtub in 1793 by the Girondist, Charlotte Corday. The French grandmaster, Jacques–Louis David (1748–1825), painted the scene of the crime in a brilliant, Neoclassical style.

Marat suffered severely for the last three to five years of his life with a chronic, pruritic skin disease. To get relief from the incessant itching, Marat sat in his bathtub for hours and hours out of the day, soaking in medicinal bathwater. He spent so much time there that he would even entertain visitors from the tub. It is well documented that the condition started on his scrotum, groin, and perineum, and then spread all over his body, including his face. Cohen and Cohen thoroughly reviewed all of the postulated causes of his condition.[59] Syphilis is an unlikely diagnosis because it does not typically itch, and scabies itches intensely and can spread in this pattern, but it never involves the face. While psoriasis also can spread in this distribution, it is not known for causing intractable itching and less commonly involves the face. Still, we know that Benjamin Franklin spent a lot of time in his tub for his psoriasis (see Chapter 15). Dermatitis herpetiformis, an autoimmune blistering disease associated with gluten insensitivity (celiac disease), has been suggested as a cause, but that condition does not typically affect the scrotum or face. Cohen suggested seborrheic dermatitis as a potential cause because of the distribution of the skin lesions. A bloodstain on a document recovered from Marat's apartment was tested using metagenomic analysis in 2020; the researchers concluded from the study, which proved that *Malassezia* yeast and *Staphylococcal* bacteria were present on Marat's skin, that super-infected seborrheic dermatitis is the correct diagnosis.[60] However, in the author's experience, seborrheic disease does not typically cause incessant itching and severe seborrheic dermatitis is highly unusual in someone who bathes regularly.

Therefore, we are left with only one possible diagnosis from which Marat could have been suffering: neurodermatitis (lichen simplex chronicus). Neurodermatitis is a chronic skin disease that is characterized by severe itching, eczematous skin lesions, skin infections, and misery. Persons with this condition generally suffer from dry, sensitive skin and experience itching that intensifies with scratching. It can notoriously involve the anogenital area and cause itching of the scrotum and anus (*pruritus scroti* and *pruritus ani*). Skin infections with staphylococcus or herpes simplex virus only make matters worse for the patient. The more a person scratches, the worse it gets, and it can spread all over the body. The link between neurodermatitis and stress is well understood, and one can only imagine the stressful life that Marat led during those dangerous years as the French peoples' angry voice. One can only speculate the degree to which anger and stress caused his disease, but an equally interesting topic of speculation is the degree to which the disease fueled his anger.

Curiously, another important figure of this era, Napoleon Bonaparte (1769–1821), is also said to have suffered with an itchy skin condition for many years. The legend surrounding Napoleon's itching holds that he suffered with *the Itch* (scabies), but Friedman argued the following points against Napoleon having scabies: there are no authentic records to prove that he had this disease; the duration of the illness is too long for that diagnosis; the emperor's cleanly habits suggested he was not at risk for scabies; there is no record his physician Corvisart prescribed him sulfur at any point (sulfur was known to be effective for *the Itch* at this time); his first wife Josephine never had *the Itch* (although his second wife may have had it).[61] Friedman instead argued that dermatitis herpetiformis, as in the case of Marat, was the cause of the itching.[62] It is highly doubtful that two significant figures of the French Revolution both suffered with the same uncommon skin condition.

Dermatology Heralded: Seguin Henry Jackson (1752–1816)

Seguin Henry Jackson was an Edinburgh-trained physician who practiced medicine in London in the latter part of the eighteenth century. In 1792, he published "Dermato-pathologia: or practical observations from some new thoughts on the pathology and proximate cause of diseases of the true skin and its emanations, the rete mucosum and cuticle, etc.," which, along with the tomes of Turner, Plenck, and Lorry, was one of four landmark eighteenth-century texts on skin disease. In his work, Jackson included 12 pages of text on microanatomy of the skin, surpassing the work of his predecessors. His entire work is a treasure trove of information, but the preface, in particular, is a valuable summary of the state of understanding of skin disease at the end of the eighteenth century. First, Jackson lamented the chaos that existed in the understanding of skin disease and the pressing need to get "medical men" educated about it:

> There is, even in the present improved state of medical science, no class of diseases so little understood, or so much in want of a rational pathology, to lead us to a more successful, and ready, practice, as that which should include the various chronic affections of the human skin.[63]

He also wrote a section entitled "Cutaneous diseases are most properly in the province of the physician" and explained:

> Since cutaneous inflammations are considered as either symptomatic of a general affection of the system, or, when idiopathic, as liable to be attended with a considerable sympathetic irritation of the whole habit, it is not much to be wondered at, that so many practitioners should be (and I will add justly) of opinion, that they ought more frequently to fall under the province of the physician than of the surgeon.[64]

His comments concerning the way in which he became interested in the skin and the challenges faced in treating skin disease reveal a discipline in chaos. He noted that he had

> become better informed of the many embarrassing opinions, at different times promulgated by the numerous authors, who have written on the subject, some on particular, others on the general, diseases of the skin, all of whom in the opinion of the medical men who have studied them, subscribe to the difficulty of explaining the nature of, as well as successfully treating, this class of disorders.[65]

While the terms *dermatologia* and *dermato-pathologia* first entered the English language with Jackson's publication in 1792, the word *dermatologia* was first coined by the German-born Calvinist and encyclopedist Johann Heinrich Alsted (1588–1638) in his acclaimed *Encyclopædia* (1630).[66] The word *dermalogie* first appeared in a 1764 French medical dictionary by Jean-François Lavoisien.[67] The word *dermatology* originated between 1810 and 1820.[68] Jackson called for *dermatologia* to be added to the curriculums of medical education:

> To further convince my reader of the difficulties of the subject, it ought to be observed to him, that the minute structure and intimate knowledge of the cutis vera, with its exterior and interior appendages, do not seem yet to be either satisfactorily described from the laborious pursuits of anatomical men, or fully determined on by the reasonings and conjectures of physiologists. They would, in my humble opinion, merit great distinction, and would with great propriety form a separate branch of physiology, under the title of dermatologia: for I very much think that it would be considered as a very interesting part of education, in every school of medicine.[69]

While these proposals were not accepted at the time, Jackson deserves recognition for being the first to call for the formal study of skin disease as a distinct scientific discipline.

Jackson offered a "new pathology" as a way of explaining and classifying skin disease, and while his incorrect assessments never took hold, the very fact that he was trying to offer a new approach is noteworthy. In the introduction, he reviewed the great systems for explaining the cause of disease throughout history: Galenic humoral theory, Paracelsian iatrochemistry, and Boerhaavian iatromechanics. He appeared to idolize Cullen throughout the work, but he lamented that Cullen's system, especially as it related to chronic skin diseases, relied too heavily on principles of humoral medicine to explain the causes of these diseases. Jackson was convinced that the cause of chronic skin diseases, which he termed the impetiginous diseases, was:

> An obstruction to the circulation of the cutaneous and epidermitical [*sic*] extreme vessels, in some way or other occasioned, or supported, by an atony, perhaps even a paralysis of them, constitutes the whole, or principal part, of the pathology of almost all impetiginous affections, or the eruptive diseases, sine pyrexia primaria [without primary fever], which may afflict the human skin: and which vascular atonic state I consider as their proximate cause, and that it has its foundation either on a general debility of the muscular system, or in a partially impaired or disturbed action of the extreme vessels of the stomach itself, and on some occasions, perhaps, of those of the intestinal canal, from a sympathetic connection of all these vessels with those of the true skin, and its emanations.... The skin, when viewed in this, its proper and important light, ought no longer to be called a common integument, but should be looked on as an organ of the first consequence to all the functions of human life, and connected with all its diseases.[70]

He was proud of his accomplishment and had even written in his preface to this 1792 text that he hoped history would be kind to him:

> The author, therefore, requests his reader to consider the following sheets, as holding out an humble effort to be of use to mankind, and it will rejoice him much, if he should in time discover that posterity will in the end be benefited by his early reflections on the subject; for it must still require the united labour and observations of many experienced practitioners, to convince a cautious age, that a sure and solid advantage may be derived from any doctrine, which carries with it the appearance of novelty. The author cannot, on that account, presume to expect very soon to see the old method of treating cutaneous diseases, as far as it is connected with the old pathology of them, generally laid aside, to admit a new one, built on a doctrine very contrary to that on which the present prevailing practice is founded.[71]

Jackson's aspirations were never realized by history, as his contributions have been either forgotten, ignored, or overshadowed by the larger characters that immediately followed him. But after a close inspection of *Dermato-pathologia*, one cannot argue with the proposition that in 1792 dermatology as a specialty was heralded in the pages of Jackson's little text.

Classification by Morphology: Joseph Jacob Plenck (1735–1807)

The drive to name, describe, and classify that was so characteristic of the Enlightenment also led to the formalization of nomenclature and the categorization of skin diseases. Previous systems that organized skin diseases by location on the body did not satisfy the Enlightenment physician's desire for order out of the chaotic nosology. The most significant arrangement for the classification of skin diseases was the morphology-based system of Joseph Jacob Plenck, an Austrian polymath and surgeon. Like Mercurialis and Turner before him, Plenck was a prolific writer. He dabbled in many fields of medicine; he published numerous works on obstetrics, ophthalmology, toxicology, dentistry, venereal disease, human physiology, and food science. During his life, he was renowned all over the world because so many physicians and medical students had his books, which appeared in many different languages (Latin, German, English, French, Italian, Dutch, Spanish, Portuguese, Russian, Lithuanian, and Japanese).[72]

An accurate biography of this important figure has been pieced together by Holubar and Frankl, in some of the best scholarship on the history of dermatology.[73] Plenck was born in Vienna in 1735; his father was a bookbinder. He was educated at the Latin School of the Jesuits and apprenticed to a renowned surgeon named Johann Retter. From 1758 to 1763, he served as an imperial regiment surgeon in the Seven Years' War—the first actual world war—when Austria sided with France in its global conflict with Britain and Prussia. When he returned, he received his diploma as *Magister Chirurgiae et Obstetriciae* (Master of Surgery and Obstetrics) in 1763. Like Turner, he was a surgeon, not a physician. In obstetrics, he was the first to advocate the use of gloves in the childbirth of syphilitic mothers to safeguard the physician. In 1763, he sold his family home after his parents died to purchase a license to practice surgery and a surgical theater. He married twice, in 1764 and again in 1779; his first wife died sometime in the 1770s. He had four sons, all of whom died young, and two daughters. In 1770, Empress Maria Theresa summoned him to the University of Tyrnau in Hungary to serve as surgeon and obstetrician. There, Plenck wrote and published his book on skin diseases. In 1783, he moved back to Vienna to serve as director of military pharmacies, and in 1786, he served as professor of chemistry and botany at the Military Academy of Surgery, "The Josephinum," founded by Emperor Joseph II in the 1780s. He eventually gave up the practice of medicine altogether in order to focus on his writings. In 1797, Plenck was knighted (thereafter von Plenck) by Emperor Francis II, who granted him a full retirement in 1805. Having been afflicted by an illness that left him unable to walk, and after a few years of continued reading and writing, he died in his own home in 1807, survived only by his two daughters. Plenck was buried in the St. Marx Cemetery, near the resting place of his famous neighbor, Wolfgang Amadeus Mozart (1756–1791), who lived around the corner from him near St. Stephen's Cathedral.

Plenck left a legacy of 30 diverse medical and scientific treatises. He burst onto the scene in 1766 with the publication of his "A New and Easy Method of giving Mercury to those Afflicted with the Venereal Disease," after which he became renowned. He stirred a minor controversy with the claim, doubted by some, that mixing mercury with acacia gum, which was later called *mercurius gummosus plenckii*, could lead to a cure of syphilis without the salivation induced by the mercury. Despite garnering some criticism, he ultimately deserves credit for attempting to improve the treatment of syphilis in his time, which some considered more or less successful. William Saunders (1743–1817), who translated Plenck's work on mercury into English, remarked that with Plenck's gum, "salivation, though sometimes produced by it, is less violent, and more easily conquered."[74]

Plenck's various publications have received mixed reviews over the years from medical historians. With his text *On Obstetrics* (1768), used in almost all of the universities after its publication, "Plenck has left us a very exact picture of the state of obstetrics at the end of the 18th century."[75] On his surgical writings, Georg Fischer, another medical historian, wrote in 1876,

> Plenck has no significance as a surgeon and his surgical writings are without scientific value. He was, however, an adroit writer who had the gift of getting hold of the kernel of the science in a way which, for the most part was complete and well-arranged, even though with somewhat exaggerated brevity.[76]

His books were, therefore, perfect for elementary instruction, but they lacked the technical details to make them useful to a seasoned surgeon.[77] Plenck's simplified *Doctrina* was perfect for translation and subsequent medical education in foreign countries such as Japan. His later work on venereal disease entitled *Doctrina de Morbis Venereis*, "Instruction on Venereal Disease" (1779), was the most famous work during his lifetime. But his greatest legacy and the work most relevant to our discussion is *Doctrina de Morbis Cutaneis*, "Instruction on Cutaneous Diseases," which was first printed in 1776 in Latin. By flipping through the pages, one can see immediately from the outline format that this *vade mecum* (handbook) was clearly influenced by Linnaeus and Sauvages. In the preface, Plenck discussed the growing need for such a system because of terminological confusion, as well as his influences and sources of information:

> This little work, which I prepared for the use of my pupils, includes 115 kinds of diseases of the skin. I have diligently described chronic diseases, but in addition I specifically concentrated on the differential diagnosis of febrile exanthems, which are distinguished from one another and from similar diseases. Indeed the treatment of febrile exanthems merely consists of healing the fever from which they flow, which pertains to another sphere of pathology. Certainly I am most grateful for the very celebrated men who recently founded generative systems of diseases; I am indebted to Sauvages, Linnaeus, Vogel, Macbride, Cullen,

Sagar, Hartmann, Lorry, and Daniel, whose systems I used often with very productive results. However I do not think—if you attend to it—that I have done a superfluous work, to which I have directed my mind, corrected, and elucidated.[78]

All of the men to whom Plenck owed his gratitude, except Hartmann and Daniel, have been discussed already. It is unclear to which Hartmann Plenck was referring, but the best candidate was Francis Xavier Hartmann (unknown dates), a Viennese contemporary of Plenck and botanist who recorded a botanical classification system. And finally, the Daniel listed is not Daniel Turner but was likely referring to Christian Friedrich Daniel (1714–1771). A lesser known but nonetheless dedicated nosologist, Daniel wrote *Systema aegritudinum* "System of Diseases" (1781). He is most famous for editing the final edition of Sauvages' *Nosologia methodica* (1791). It is evident from the list that Plenck got the inspiration to categorize skin diseases from others who participated in the classification mania of the Enlightenment.

The full title of the work to which we now turn our attention is *Doctrina de morbis cutaneis qua hi morbi in suas classes, genera, et species rediguntur*, "Instruction on cutaneous diseases in which these diseases are reorganized into their own classes, genera, and species." It was published in 1776 in Latin and underwent an author's second edition in 1783, with German and Italian translations of each edition. The 1783 Latin edition was available for the preparation of this section, and an English translation could not be found.

Both editions are dedicated to Giovanni Alessandro Brambilla (1728–1800), the Italian court surgeon who resided at the court of Maria Theresa and Francis I and who served as personal surgeon to Emperor Joseph II. Brambilla was the one most responsible for establishing Joseph's military medical school (see Chapter 14). He wrote an important treatise on surgical instruments entitled *Instrumentarium chirurgicum militare Austricum*, "Surgical Instruments of the Austrian Military" (1780). Brambilla attempted to improve military surgery, and like Daniel Turner, he tried to elevate the status of surgeons relative to physicians. He saw no difference between external diseases and internal diseases as they relate to cause and advocated for surgeons to manage those external conditions that had internal roots, such as measles and smallpox, that were under the dominion of the physician.[79] He stressed the importance of knowledge of the Latin language to his students. In his front matter, Plenck referred to him as a most brilliant, expert, learned, and celebrated man.

Plenck's classification system (Table 10.1) breaks down 119 skin diseases into 14 categories or classes based on morphology of the skin lesions. Recall that both Mercurialis and Turner looked at skin disease from the standpoint of location on the body, and Lorry, from whether the condition was localized to the skin, or a symptom coming from within. Plenck rejected these regional systems in favor of one that could lead the physician to the diagnosis based on direct observation of the disease. Under each class, Plenck has "genera" (subtypes of classes) and "species" (subtypes of genera).

TABLE 10.1

Plenck's "Classes Morborum Cutaneorum"

Class	Category
I	Macules
II	Pustules
III	Vesicles
IV	Bullae
V	Papules
VI	Crusts
VII	Squammes
VIII	Calluses
IX	Excrescences
X	Ulcers
XI	Wounds
XII	Insects of the skin
XIII	Diseases of the nails
XIV	Diseases of the hair

For example, under the first class, "Maculae," Plenck has six different genera of macules, and each of these genera has 3–12 different species.

While Plenck's approach to diagnosis was groundbreaking, his treatment armamentarium fell in line with the standard therapeutic options of his day, with no significant advancements to note. Like Turner before him, Plenck offered a variety of both internal and external medicaments, frequently recommending both options for many diseases. Internal treatments included purging, mercurials, antimonials, diaphoretics, emetics, venesection, antiphlogistics (anti-inflammatories), Peruvian bark (cinchona bark), fumaria (a flowering plant), and sulphur. His favorite external medicaments included *aqua vegetomineralis* (dilute lead acetate water), *butyro cacao* (cocoa butter), *balnea sulphurea* or *salina* (sulphur or saltwater baths), camphor, and various types of *aqua*, oleum (oils), unguents, lotions, and emplastres.

Plenck added prognostic information when he had a sense of it and made it known to his reader which conditions were generally considered incurable. Throughout the text are numerous footnotes, with reference information for his sources. Plenck seemed to give credit where credit was due, referencing contemporaries, such as Lorry, who were doing similar work. His economically sized book was concise and yet comprehensive.

It is plain from the study of the history of medicine that there is a certain irony that affects the legacy of medical polymaths like Mercurialis—and Plenck is no exception: the broader the scope of a writer, i.e., the more diverse topics he wrote about, the weaker that writer's legacy in any individual field. We know that Plenck probably had little experience diagnosing and treating the diseases about which he wrote in *Doctrina de Morbis Cutaneis*. We know that Plenck was able to transmit little of his literary corpus to following generations.[80] Cazenave (see Chapter 13) was critical of Plenck's disregard for the fact that some of the diseases he described went through stages that would put them into multiple classes in his system. For example, some diseases would start vesicular or pustular and evolve into a crusted or ulcerative stage.[81] Pierre Rayer deemed Plenck's system superior to all those that came before his, but he complained that "crusts and ulcers are never primary changes, they always follow pustules, vesicles, bullae, tubercles, and sometimes squammous diseases. The study of crusts cannot be detached from the alterations which produce them."[82] Riehl, an early twentieth-century Austrian dermatologist, was critical of Plenck's morphological approach to classification because it led to a "wholly forced collection of diseases widely differing in their pathology."[83] Kaposi, a countryman of Plenck and one of the true giants of the nineteenth century, echoed this opinion but did see the big picture of the contribution:

> Plenck's *Doctrina de morbis cutaneis*, like a catechism, impresses one by its concise and convenient axioms as an apparently sure guide which could not be better adopted for familiarizing one with diseases of the skin. Yet, as soon as these diseases were observed again at the bedside of the patient, it was easy to be convinced that they did not manifest themselves in forms as fixed as the definitions of Plenck indicated, but showed very variable pathologic phenomena and consequently deserved being placed, some in one class, some in another.... But the exposition of these precise ideas on the primary lesions of diseases of the skin was nevertheless progress of real value for the future of dermatological studies, in that it suppressed in a definite manner and degree the arbitrariness of the terminology, while facilitating discussion.[84]

In 1933, John Lane argued that Plenck is due credit for the idea of using morphology to classify skin lesions, but without a single original idea in the rest of his work, he cannot get any more credit than that.[85]

To the present author, Plenck deserves to be elevated to the highest tier of the dermatologic pantheon. Keizo Dohi, a student of Kaposi (see Chapter 14), saw the big picture: his work "influenced the future great development of dermatology, through its application by Willan, the genius of dermatology."[86] Perhaps the true legacy of *Doctrina de morbis cutaneis* was its utility to Robert Willan, who never credited Plenck, in his development of a classification system of his own (see Chapter 12):

> Willan drew heavily from Plenck's dermatologic alphabet, altering and greatly expanding it. Nonetheless, it was Willan who breathed life into the nascent specialty of dermatology, fleshing out the bare bones provided by Plenck 20 years earlier. If Willan is remembered as the father of modern dermatology, Plenck should be recalled as its grandfather.[87]

Plenck was indeed an industrious, indefatigable writer and educator who published numerous works across many unique disciplines of medicine and science. His individual writings were simultaneously comprehensive and yet brief, and they were for the most part well-arranged. They were up to date, with the inclusion of the recent reports of his contemporaries. Plenck's approach was not encyclopedic, but cursory, nor was his research in-depth. But, even so, it was ambitious for the purposes of educating his audience. Equally important to recall was his audience—barber or surgeon pupils at the military medical school in Vienna, and later, students across Europe and beyond. If Plenck is judged based on his capacity to educate these students of Europe, then he deserves extremely high praise as one of the most influential educators in the history of modern medicine. If he is judged based on his capacity to impress his contemporaries and direct descendants with a system of classification free from flaws and containing all the correct information, pigeonholed perfectly, then he fails in this task. The modern dermatologist understands what a vast body of knowledge is required to practice the specialty. Plenck attempted to distill this almost insurmountable information into a clear, simplistic system for his students. It is this author's opinion that history has not been kind enough to Plenck for his efforts. Does the first person who attempted to climb Mount Everest and came close to the summit, but failed, deserve criticism for their failings or praise for how far they went?

Little has been said here about Plenck as botanist. Know that he was famous enough in that field to have a plant named after him—*Plenkia populnea*. The plant belongs to the *Celastraceae* (bittersweet) family of plants—a fitting family for him. After studying the life and contributions of Joseph Jacob Plenck to the specialty of dermatology, one cannot help but experience the bittersweet feelings that come with knowing the reality that such an ambitious man might have already disappeared into the oblivion of history.

Five Miscellaneous Eighteenth-Century Contributors

There were five minor contributors to the study of skin disease in the 1700s: Bernardino Ramazzini, Percival Pott, Johann Peter Frank, Gaspar Casal, and Thomas Spooner. The very beginning of the eighteenth century saw the emergence of occupational medicine with the career and writings of Bernardino Ramazzini (1633–1714), the preeminent Italian professor of medicine at Padua. In *De Morbis Artificum Diatriba,* "Discourse on Diseases of Workers" (1700), Ramazzini called attention to the pathogenic influence of occupation and shed some light on industrial conditions at the time. In fact, Karl Marx (1818–1883) referenced Ramazzini in his magnum opus, *Das Kapital*, when dealing with the exploitation of the working class. Considered the father of occupational dermatology, Ramazzini described several occupational dermatoses, including grain itch, syphilis in midwives, chemical burns, and percutaneous absorption of chemicals including mercury as well as cutaneous conditions in metal workers, among other occupations.

The other major development in the history of occupational dermatology took place in London when in 1775, English surgeon Percival Pott (1714–1788) determined that chimney soot causes scrotal cancer. Pott wrote in his *Chirurgical Observations*:

> There is a disease as peculiar to a certain set of people, which has not, at least to my knowledge, been publicly noticed; I mean the chimney sweeper's cancer. It is a disease which always makes its first attack on, and its first appearance in, the inferior part of the scrotum; where it produces a superficial, painful, ragged, ill-looking sore, with hard and rising edges: the trade call it the soot-wart.…In no great length of time, it pervades the skin, dartos, and membranes of the scrotum, and seizes the testicle, which it enlarges, hardens, and renders truly and thoroughly distempered; from whence it makes its way up the spermatic process into the abdomen, most frequently indurating and spoiling the inguinal glands: when arrived within the abdomen, it affects some of the viscera, and then very soon becomes painfully destructive. The fate of these people seems singularly hard: in their early infancy, they are most frequently treated with great brutality, and almost starved with cold and hunger; they are thrust up narrow, and sometimes hot chimnies, where they are bruised, burned, and almost suffocated; and when they get to puberty, become peculiarly liable to a most noisome, painful and fatal disease.[88]

Pott was the first to identify a carcinogen, a discovery that led to the Chimney Sweeps Act of 1788 and increased the legal age for apprenticed chimney sweeps to eight and required that the master sweep provide appropriate protective clothing for the young sweeps. In 1840, an act of Parliament increased the beginning age for apprenticeship to 16. The incidence of chimney sweeps' cancer was always very high inside of England because, as Brown and Thornton have pointed out, "the structural peculiarities of English chimneys, the type of coal used, the lack of efficient protective clothing, and disregard of personal hygiene."[89] In spite of public awareness, the incidence of this type of cancer did not decline in England until the mid-twentieth century.

Johann Peter Frank (1745–1821), a German physician who was one of the most widely traveled physicians of the early modern period, served as advisor to both Napoleon and the emperor of Austria, and he attended Alexander I of Russia as his personal physician. He also held professorships at the Universities of Vilnius and Vienna. He was a pioneer of public health, sanitation, and hygiene, and he wrote a landmark nine-volume treatise on these topics. Frank enters our story with an important publication, released in 1792, entitled *De curandis hominum morbis epitome,* "Summary of the Cure of Human Diseases." In that work, Frank coined the term *urticaria,* and he divided exanthems into *nuda* (smooth) or *scabra* (rough). His major contribution was dividing skin eruptions into the acute exanthems and the chronic efflorescences.

Gaspar Casal (1681–1759) was a Spanish physician who first described the rash of pellagra, which is now known to be caused by a deficiency of niacin (vitamin B3). Casal called it *Mal de la rosa,* and the sun-exacerbated, erythematous rash that affects the chest and neck of persons with pellagra—Casal's necklace—is named after him. His writings on the topic were published posthumously in 1762 under the title *Historia natural y medica de la principado de Asturias,* "Natural and medical history of the principality of Asturia." Asturia is a province in northwestern Spain where many of the local peasants suffered from what was called *lepra asturiensis* (Asturian lepra). Convinced that the condition was not a contagious one, Casal instead promoted the idea that the condition was caused by a dietary deficiency. Cornbread was the basis for the diet of these peasants; in the twentieth century, it was proven that a diet based solely on cornbread could lead to pellagra because bread derived from corn is distinctly low in niacin.

Thomas Spooner is only known for writing an extraordinary treatise on *the Itch,* first published in 1714. Biographical data on this man is non-existent. What we do know from the preface of his treatise on *the Itch,* it is clear Spooner was a well-read practitioner (he quoted Sydenham), but he does not describe himself as a physician or a surgeon, nor is he a fellow of the Royal College of Physicians, since he is not listed on Munk's Roll.[90] Surgeons and other non-physician practitioners of medicine such as apothecaries were prevalent at this time; it is possible that Spooner belonged to this group, and he may have been seeing patients out of his home in the center of London. His work was well received: his treatise had five editions, meaning roughly 15,000 copies overall were printed.[91]

Regardless of the lack of details about his life, Spooner left a legacy with the publication of a work targeting the masses. Itching was a rampant problem in eighteenth-century Europe. There was the itch caused by lice, flea bites, eczema, and impetigo plaguing the population. And then there was *the Itch,* which because of overcrowding related to the population explosion that began in the middle of the eighteenth century, became a significant public health challenge in workhouses and jails, and the residences of the poor.[92] Spooner described it in the following manner:

> The Itch is a filthy Distemper, infesting the External Parts of the Body universally, but more particularly the Joints, and between the Fingers, commonly with Pustulous Eruptions raised upon the Scarf-Skin, by almost unavoidable scratching, occasioned thro' violent itching of the Parts; from these Pustulous Eruptions or little Bladders, when broke, there issues a thin Crystalline Humour, which touching any other Part not yet infected, soon causes incessant itching, and upon scratching, more Bladders to arise.[93]

It is clear that Spooner was describing today's scabies, which used to be known as the "seven-year itch" because it was once believed that it attacks a human population in seven-year-long epidemic waves. Perhaps the nickname actually reflects the length of time a person used to suffer with it. Like Turner, he was unaware of the itch mite as the cause of the "distemper" but did correctly acknowledge the contagiousness of this illness, which is among the most contagious illnesses treated by dermatologists:

> And so Contagious is the Itch of either sort, that lying in Bed with a Person troubled with it, or in the Sheets an itchy Person has lain in, or to wipe one's Hands with the same Cloth, or draw on a Glove such a Person has worn, or even to have Linnen washed with the Linnen of one afflicted with the Itch, is sufficient to catch the Distemper and as the Famous and Ingenious Dr. Willis says, 'Certainly the Infection of no one Disease is more easily and certainly propagated (the Plague only excepted) than this of the Itch.'[94]

Spooner divides the treatise into three parts: the first focuses on describing *the Itch*, the second on the cause of *the Itch*, and the last on the treatment of *the Itch*. He believed, as Mercurialis did 150 years prior, that *the Itch*, a localized problem, uncured, could lead to what was called *scabies* (scabbiness), a generalized worsening of the situation and which from the descriptions sounds very much like impetigo, presumably from superinfection of constantly scratched skin. This state would then progress, if untreated, into leprosy:

> Scabies or Scabbiness, is a Disease most commonly succeeding an inveterate Itch either moist or dry, for when either kind has continued long, or been ill Cured, so that the very Fountains of the Blood and Juices are corrupted, an inveterate and filthy Scabbiness, quickly follows, which not only affects the Cuticula or Scarf-Skin, as that does, but penetrates deeper, and fixes upon the Cutis or real Skin, which it gnaws and ulcerates, and causes nasty Scabs to cover the Parts.
>
> If it follows the moist Itch, foul Ichorous Matter issues from them, which is very contagious, and infects any found Part it touches; but if it succeeds the dry Itch, there is seldom any Pus issues from the Scabs, which then appear very crusty, dry and nauseous to the sight.
>
> Sometimes a Scabbiness happens when the Itch has not gone before it, but this is not near so frequent as the Scabbiness following the Itch, which as before said, is generally a Preludium to this hateful Distemper.
>
> A Scabbiness is also accompany'd with itching as well as soreness, especially about the Edges of the small Ulcers that void a foul corrupted Pus in the moist kind, and about the crusty Scabs in the dry sort.
>
> An universal Scabbiness, as it is much worse than the Itch for Filthiness and Putrefaction, so it is much more dangerous and difficult to Cure.
>
> If it continues long without being Cured, the Ulcerations increase in number as well as largeness, and the discharge of Matter from them is so great, the Humours continually flowing that way, that the Body being robb'd or drain'd of its moisture, falls of course into a Consumption, which, together with the fatigue the Patient undergoes in the Day time, and want of Rest and Sleep at Night, occasioned by continual alternate itching and smarting, quickly finishes the fatal Catastrophe, and the unhappy Patient is obliged to submit to a miserable Death.
>
> But this must be understood only of the moist Scabbiness, for the dry one, tho' very Inveterate and Malign, yet seldom or never is attended with Death, but first ushers in a poisonous Leprosy, that, if not timely Cured, soon puts a Period to the Patient's Life.
>
> The Leprosy is the most Malignant Distemper that affects the External Parts of the Body, the Blood and Juices being contaminated with its fatal Poison, whence proceeds the great Difficulty of curing it.[95]

The preceding excerpt does not contain any exaggeration; in the absence of the antibiotics and antiparasitical agents we have today for scabies infestation, the natural order of the progression from simple itching to widespread dermatitis and excoriation to sepsis and death was not uncommon in this era, especially among poor individuals who had limited access to healthcare.

In the section on therapy, Spooner conducted a literature review, quoting several of the major medical writers of his day. Purging and bleeding were the mainstays of treatment of *the Itch*, but quicksilver girdles were dangerous and to be worn with caution. He urged "all persons from tampering with outward medicines, for the cure of cutaneous diseases, without taking proper internal remedies also, by the direction of a skillful physician."[96] *The Itch* was correctly identified as, at least in some cases, a venereal disease (intimate contact is known today as a route for transmission of scabies), with a majority of physicians of the opinion that was a disease of the blood related to syphilis or leprosy. Like leprosy, syphilis, and scurvy—conditions to which *the Itch* was often linked—*the Itch* was deemed by society to reflect low moral character in the afflicted.[97]

Summary

Regarding the history of dermatology in the eighteenth century, Anne-Charles Lorry, Joseph Jacob Plenck, and Seguin Henry Jackson published major treatises on skin disease. In so doing, London, Paris, and Vienna were informally inaugurated as centers of excellence for the budding field of dermatology. Plenck's *Doctrina de Morbis Cutaneis* was particularly valuable because the work, inspired by the great classifiers of medicine, contained the first attempt to classify skin disease based on the morphology of skin lesions, the principal methodology still used today. The eighteenth century saw the skin for the first time being referred to, by Lorry, as an organ, with its primary purposes being excretory and sensory, rather than simply an envelope. Jackson called for the study of the skin and its diseases at the medical schools and promoted the management of skin diseases by physicians instead of by the traditional surgeons. Occupational dermatology had its roots in this period, Percival Pott identified the first known carcinogen, chimney soot, as the causeo of scrotal cancer. A syndrome with major skin involvement (pellagra) was for the first time linked to a dietary deficiency. While the eighteenth century pales in comparison to the nineteenth century in its degree of scientific development, it remains a crucial, fascinating transitional period in the history of dermatology.

Interlude 3

Syphilis

Syphilis is another major historical disease with prominent dermatologic manifestations. Of the four maladies highlighted in this text, syphilis is uniquely important in the development of dermatology as a specialty of medicine, and it remains relevant today. Syphilis is an infection caused by the bacterium *Treponema pallidum*, a corkscrew-shaped spirochete with whip-like structures (flagella) at its poles. Syphilis is not the only treponemal disease; there are three others—pinta, yaws, and bejel—that are referred to as the non-venereal endemic treponematoses; all of these are also caused by *T. pallidum*. Known primarily as a sexually transmitted disease, syphilis can also be transmitted transplacentally. It is known to medical students as the "Great Imitator" because it mimics so many different diseases and can affect virtually every major organ system, including the central nervous and cardiovascular systems. As the renowned William Osler famously claimed, "He who knows syphilis, knows medicine."

Throughout history, the highest risk activity for acquiring syphilis was intercourse with an infected prostitute. Approximately three weeks (range: 10–90 days) after the exposure, a characteristically rubbery and painless chancre (ulcer) develops on the genitals, along with swollen lymph nodes in the adjacent inguinal area. The lack of pain is attributed to damage caused by the spirochetes to the free nerve endings in the skin. Because it is painless, the ulcer often goes unnoticed by the patient, and it resolves without treatment in three to six weeks. This stage of the disease is called *primary syphilis*.

About six weeks later (range: one to three months), myriad manifestations can develop in what is known as *secondary syphilis*. As the spirochete disseminates through the bloodstream all over the body, the person develops a papular, scaly rash affecting the face, trunk, and extremities, including the palms and soles, where the lesions have a characteristic red-brown, penny-like appearance. Uncommonly, the rash can have a pustular appearance. At this stage, fever and generalized swollen lymph nodes may appear. If the hairs fall out in small, diffuse patches, the scalp is referred to as having "moth-eaten alopecia." Examination of the oral cavity can reveal infectious white patches called "mucous patches;" when they occur at the corner of the lips, they are called "split papules." Moist warts that develop in the genital and anal area, said to be teeming with spirochetes, are termed "condyloma lata." Ulcerative lesions can develop in immunocompromised individuals; the term for this condition is "lues maligna." Additional systemic effects of the infection at this stage include fatigue, muscle and joint pain, headache, sore throat, uveitis or retinitis, cranial neuropathies, meningitis, osteitis or periostitis (painful bones), glomerulonephritis, and hepatitis. Interestingly, like primary syphilis, these features all resolve eventually without treatment, and the untreated infected person enters into a latent phase, in which they show no signs of the disease. Fortunately, serologic tests exist today that allow for the diagnosis of patients in this latent phase. Finally, it is worth pointing out that even without treatment, the first two stages of syphilis are rarely fatal.

The last phase of syphilis is called *tertiary syphilis*, which tends to occur many years after the onset of the original infection. Tertiary syphilis is much less common today as the available treatments and early testing prevent the progression of the infection to this stage. The three major features of tertiary syphilis are gummatous lesions, cardiovascular syphilis, and neurosyphilis. Gummatous lesions are chronic infectious infiltrations of an organ, such as the skin or liver, which resemble a tumor-like growth; on the skin, the lesions appear as an ulcerated tumor or nodule, or if the nose is affected, it can lead to destruction of the nose. Cardiovascular syphilis involves inflammation of the aorta, the arteries around the heart, or the valves of the heart; it can be complicated by aortic aneurysm, heart attack, or heart failure. Cardiovascular complications are the most common cause of death in syphilis. In neurosyphilis, the brain, as well as the spinal cord and peripheral nerves, is affected by the infection. Brain involvement can present with stroke-like symptomatology or psychiatric disease, including personality changes,

DOI: 10.1201/9781003273622-16

dementia, psychosis, mania, delirium, and depression. Neurosyphilis, formerly known as "generalized paresis of the insane," is caused by chronic meningoencephalitis and resultant atrophy of the brain. Spinal cord involvement, termed "tabes dorsalis," presents with weakness, diminished reflexes, paresthesias, locomotor ataxia, episodic intense pain, urinary incontinence, deafness, eye pain, and visual impairment. Many of these tertiary neurologic features are irreversible and can be misdiagnosed as Alzheimer's disease, multiple sclerosis, or schizophrenia unless the astute clinician remembers that syphilis is the "Great Imitator" and orders the blood test for syphilis.

Penicillin, often in the form of a single intramuscular injection, is a highly effective treatment for all forms of syphilis. While cardiovascular syphilis and neurosyphilis continue to be deadly forms of the disease, syphilis is much less likely to cause death than it did in the pre-penicillin era, and the estimated mortality rate of syphilis at that time was only 10 percent after 40 years of living with the infection.[1] The bottom line is that syphilis today is not considered a particularly deadly disease, making *T. pallidum* one of the more successful human pathogens: the beginning of the infection is painless and often goes unnoticed; the spirochete does not easily kill its host, and with its so-called stealth pathogenicity, it can disseminate itself early and then evade the immune system for years.[2]

Syphilis can be transmitted from mother to fetus at a rate of 60 percent during the primary and secondary phases; the incidence is highest in the third trimester. Transmission is much lower for mothers with latent syphilis and tertiary syphilis. Babies born with syphilis are said to suffer from congenital syphilis, which is classified as early or late, distinguished as occurring before and after two years of age. Congenital syphilis is a devastating disease; if the fetus survives in utero, the child might show the characteristic features of a saddle nose deformity, frontal bossing, syphilitic rhinitis (termed "snuffles"), linear fissures radiating from mouth and nose (termed "rhagades"), jaundice, skin rash, hepatosplenomegaly, various bony abnormalities, and the triad of deafness, malformed teeth, and keratitis, called "Hutchinson's triad."

From the modern dermatologist's perspective, syphilis presents with mild-to-moderate skin lesions and is usually diagnosed in either the secondary stage—by clinical exam and blood test—or in the latent stage, by blood test as a screening for the disease. It is unusual for patients to present to the office with a chancre; the overwhelming majority of cases observed by the author have been patients with an erythematous scaly rash that involved the trunk and extremities, including the palms and soles. However, only in cases affecting the profoundly immunocompromised will some of these other features—such as pustules and ulcers—be seen. It is important to keep that fact in mind as we examine the historical syphilis, a condition that, based on the descriptions and depictions, was apparently much worse than what is seen today—so much worse that one has to at least question whether it was even the same disease.

The Origins of Syphilis

The history of syphilis in Europe is fascinating and brimming with controversy. The story traditionally begins in October 1494, when King Charles VIII of France amassed an army of 25,000 soldiers and invaded Italy for the purposes of realizing a loose claim to the throne of the Kingdom of Naples, controlled by Spain. He waged a brutal campaign and succeeded in conquering the entire peninsula by May of the following year; Italy had not been sacked this thoroughly since the arrival of the Goths in the fifth century CE. Per Fallopius, the outnumbered Spaniards in Naples released their disease-ridden prostitutes on the unsuspecting, lustful French occupiers.[3] But not wanting his forces to be landlocked in southern Italy, Charles set out to return to France in May 1495. On his return to France, his forces pitched a battle with the League of Venice at the Battle of Fornovo on July 6, 1495. Both sides claimed victory, and Charles escaped Italy; meanwhile, Ferdinand of Aragon recaptured the Kingdom of Naples, leaving Charles empty-handed.

Not long after Charles' Italian Wars came the first reports of syphilis in Europe; it was quickly understood that Charles' soldiers were responsible for spreading the disease to the Italian city-states as they laid waste to the peninsula. This new plague was from that time known in Italy as *morbus gallicus* the "French Disease." The first-ever description of syphilis was written in 1495 by Marcello Cumano, a doctor on the side of the League of Venice at the Battle of Fornovo.[4] He wrote about soldiers with millet-like pustules all over the face and body that started on the foreskin or glans of the penis that started as a single, painful lesion, but because of scratching, it evolved into an ulcer. Days later, the afflicted began to experience bone pain in the arms, legs, and feet, and a general eruption of large pustules all over the body, which would last for a year or longer without treatment.[5] The contagious, sexually transmitted nature of the disease was immediately apparent to everyone, and many of the early descriptions of syphilis characterized it as a repulsive and horribly painful condition, particularly in the bones, and responsible for killing thousands of men.[6]

Soon the epidemic spread to France, brought back from Naples by the French soldiers; subsequently, the French called it the "Neopolitan sickness." It reached Paris in 1496, where the famous Hôtel-Dieu was quickly overwhelmed with patients, who were ultimately turned away out of sheer fright of their contagiousness.[7] It reached the Holy Roman Empire that same year, then England the following year; Northern Europe saw syphilis around the turn of the sixteenth century, and within ten years of the Battle of Fornovo, the disease had spread to every corner of Europe.[8] The various countries of Europe continued the novel pattern of naming it after their nearby enemy; for example, the Russians called it the "Polish sickness," the Dutch called it the "Spanish sickness," and the Turks called it the "Christian sickness."

The significant early texts on syphilis were written by the German Joseph Grunpeck (1473–1532), the Spaniards Gaspar Torella (1452–1520) and Francisco Lopez de Villalobos (1473–1549), and the Italians Niccolò Leoniceno (1428–1524) and Giovanni de Vigo (1450–1525). The scholar Joseph Grunbeck had syphilis himself and, in 1503, wrote a terrifying account of his experience. The first sign of the disease for Grunpeck was marked swelling of the penis and then appeared "suppuration over the entire penis and scrotum," which evolved into extensive ulcerations, followed by a pustular eruption all over the body.[9] In the cases, he observed among the soldiers fighting for Emperor Maximilian I, Grunpeck noted that some had a "rough scabies dotted with black and hideous lumps" from head to knees, including the face.[10] The ulceration of the genitals was the worst feature and often led to extreme pain, suicidal ideations, and mockery from fellow soldiers.

Gaspar Torella was a physician for Rodrigo Borgia (also known as Pope Alexander VI) and his illegitimate son Cesare (1475–1507), two members of the famous Borgia family who hailed from Valencia (Spain). The Borgias rose to prominence during the Italian Renaissance and allegedly committed many crimes. Cesare, said to be the most handsome man of his time and the inspiration behind "The Prince" by Machiavelli (1532), was the most famous person of the first decade of the epidemic to acquire syphilis; he did so in 1497. Cesare Borgia was known to wear a mask on his face in public; some say it was to hide facial scarring brought on by his syphilis, while others claim it was to simply hide himself, a public figure. Torella dedicated his Latin treatise entitled *Tractatus cum consiliis contra pudendagram seu morbum gallicum*, "Treatise with advice against *pudendagra* or the French Disease," to his patient Cesare, whom he treated for the disease. *Pudendagra* means "disease of the *pudenda*"; *pudenda* refers to the parts "to be ashamed of." In his text is the first complete case history of syphilis to be recorded, but it is not reckoned to be the case of Cesare.[11]

In 1498, Spanish doctor Francisco Lopez de Villalobos wrote a medical poem entitled *El sumario de la medicina con un tratado sobre las pestíferas bubas*, "Summary of the medicine with a treatise on the pestiferous bubas"; the best translation for the word *bubas* is scabs or chancres. Originally written in Spanish, the poem consists of 74 stanzas containing 10 lines each, and it was translated and rhymed by George Gaskoin in 1870. Both the original work and the translation are classics and contain detailed information about syphilis. Villalobos stated that the incubation period from exposure to what he described as the hard, painless buba (chancre) was 21–26 days, arriving when the morbid matter from the liver is "ejected onto the genitals."[12] Strangely ignoring the obvious venereal aspects of the disease, Villalobos instead blamed the conjunction of Saturn and Mars on the outbreak of the pestilence, like the eyewitnesses of the Black Death did 150 years prior (see Interlude 2). Villalobos correctly characterized the eruption of secondary syphilis and noted that it occurred most commonly on the face, head, palms, and soles. His dermatologic knowledge was vast; he devoted 16 stanzas to describe the eruption and distinguish it from scabies and from the pustular eruptions described by Avicenna, both of which he argued lacked the bone pain typical of *bubas*. He noted that the joint and bone pain of the illness was more intense at night. As an aside, Villalobos was imprisoned during the Great Inquisition after being accused of being a magician. He was later released and found himself in the good graces of the courts of King Ferdinand and his grandson Charles V, the Holy Roman Emperor, both of whom he served as court physician.[13]

The emergence of syphilis in Italy in the context of the Renaissance and its humanist ideals invoked many questions, and the Italians looked to the ancients for answers. Niccolò Leoniceno, a highly influential Italian humanist and physician (see Chapter 8), wrote *Libellus de epidemia quam vulgo morbum gallicum vocant*, "Small book on the epidemic which is commonly called the French Disease" in 1497. It was dedicated to Pico della Mirandola, who had requested that Leoniceno write the text.[14] While a professor at the University of Ferrara, Leoniceno participated in a famous *disputatio* in April 1497 on the nature and origins of the French Disease; the dispute is brilliantly described by Arrizabalaga et al.[15] The debate participants were Leoniceno and two of his colleagues, Sebastiano dall'Aquila (ca. 1440–1510) and Coradino Gilino (1445–1500); each held a differing viewpoint. Leoniceno, who held the authority of the ancients in the highest regard, took the stance that the French Disease was not a new disease, and he believed that within the pages of Hippocrates and Galen could be found descriptions of the disease his contemporaries called the French Disease. He did not care for this name; instead, he stated that physicians had not yet named the disease.[16] He defined the disease as sores that begin in the genital area and spread all over the body, especially the face, causing extreme pain and disfigurement. He believed the sores resulted from the corruption of several humors brought about by a "warm and humid intemperance of the air."[17] Leoniceno's counterparts at the great *disputatio* held different viewpoints. Dall'Aquila tried to establish that *morbus gallicus* was the same as Galen's *elephantiasis*, using Galen's text along with the writings of other authorities such as Celsus and Pliny the Elder as support for his argument.[18] In contrast, Gilino contended that the French Disease was Celsus' *ignis sacer,* which to him was the same as Avicenna's *ignis persicus,* "Persian fire."

Giovanni de Vigo was an Italian surgeon who authored *Practica in arte chirurgica copiosa*, "Widespread Practices in the Surgical Art." It contains the clearest and most complete description of syphilis, which Vigo called the French Disease, in the early sixteenth century.[19] At this time, Vigo and other medical writers, as well as the public at large, generally understood that this disease was new, contagious, transmitted venereally, had diverse cutaneous manifestations, was associated with intense bone pain, and was fatal. This novel disease was the first to start in the genitals and then spread all over the body.[20] Some considered it a severe type of elephantiasis (leprosy), while others saw it as something much worse and different. In many cases, the descriptions of the disease had hyperbolic language describing it as something horrifying or disgusting, as in the following quote from Grunpeck:

> In recent times I have seen scourges, horrible sicknesses and many infirmities afflict mankind from all corners of the earth. Amongst them has crept in, from the western shores of Gaul, a disease which is so cruel, so distressing, so appalling that until now nothing so horrifying, nothing more terrible or disgusting, has ever been known on this earth.[21]

It is difficult to know whether sixteenth-century syphilis really was that ghastly or whether these writers had a penchant for the dramatic. These descriptions surprise the modern clinician familiar with syphilis; extensive ulceration of the genitals, severe bone pain, and fatality are not common features of the syphilis today. Still, there can be no doubt that the syphilis of 500 years ago was something much worse than we can imagine today.

The Great Pox epidemic flourished for almost 50 years in Europe, with 1510–1520 being the peak decade of its spread. However, by the mid-sixteenth century, less deadly strains evolved, and the disease gained a milder course. By 1546, the deadly condition that had once been capable of causing pustules to cover the body and flesh to slough off the face was no longer able to do so, presumably because the spirochetes had evolved to a less deadly version that could transmit itself to more victims.[22] History does repeat itself: a similar phenomenon occurred in the SARS-CoV-2 pandemic.

The mid-sixteenth-century variety of syphilis was associated with fewer pustules and less pain, and writers of the period generally considered the disease less serious, even on the decline to the point at which it might disappear. What caused the decline in virulence? Awareness and fear led people to avoid sexual contact with anyone covered with skin lesions, and so the more virulent strains died off, and the less virulent strains that caused milder symptoms survived. Today, carriers of syphilis are impossible to distinguish from non-carriers except in the short-lived primary and secondary stages, but even in these stages, those infected present frequently with mild or subtle cutaneous changes.

The Disease with Many Names

Up to this point, the term *syphilis* has been used interchangeably with the French Disease, but *syphilis* was not actually coined until 1530. The person responsible for giving syphilis its lasting name was Girolamo Fracastoro (1476–1553). A giant of sixteenth-century intellectual life and former classmate of Copernicus, Fracastoro is best known for his work entitled *De contagione* (see Interlude 4), in which he presented one of the first theories on contagious disease. In an epic three-volume 1300-verse poem entitled *Syphilis sive morbus gallicus*, "Syphilis or the French Disease," Fracastoro penned in book III a tale about a shepherd named Syphilus [*sic*] who was angry with the gods and instead constructed an altar to his king. One of the disrespected gods sent a plague in return:

> In his anger, he charges his rays with pestilential poisons and virulent miasms [*sic*], which simultaneously infect the air, the earth and the waters. At once upon this criminal earth there arises an unknown plague. Syphilus is the first attacked by it, on account of having been the first to profane the sacred altars. A hideous leprosy covers his body; fearful pains torture his limbs and banish sleep from his eyes. Then, this terrible disease—known since then among us by the name of Syphilis—does not take long to spread in our entire nation, not even sparing our King himself.[23]

The word "syphilis" derives from either the Latinized Greek for "pig-lover," from a character in Ovid's *Metamorphosis* named "Sypilus," or it was transmogrified from the word *erysipelas*.[24] The name did not stick to the diagnosis until two centuries later when Daniel Turner revived the term by entitling his English text, "Syphilis;" curiously, the word is never used in the body of Turner's text.[25] Until then, the disease was instead referred to by its various xenophobic monikers or increasingly as the Great Pox, or simply, The Pox, as opposed to the smaller pox (smallpox). Other names for syphilis in the sixteenth and seventeenth centuries were *grande vérole* (French); among the Scots, it was called *grandgore*; the British soldiers referred to it as "The Black Lion;" the Spanish, *las bubas*. However, *morbus gallicus* was the most commonly used name for syphilis in the sixteenth century. Jacques de Bethencourt (1477–1527), a French physician, was the first to associate the disease with Venus, the patron of sexual activity, when he named syphilis *morbus venerea*.[26] The physicians of the Renaissance instead named the disease *lues venerea*. Since *lues* is Latin and means "plague" or "disease," Fernel and Bethencourt were among the first to call it "VD," venereal disease. The two names *morbus venerea* and *lues venerea* dominated the medical literature of the seventeenth century, only to cede to the less scandalous sounding name, syphilis, in the eighteenth century.

The Columbian Theory versus the Pre-Columbian Theory

Scholars have been questioning where syphilis came from for five centuries. Some of the European thought leaders on the Great Pox—particularly the Italian ones mentioned earlier from Ferrara—argued that syphilis was not a new disease, but the general consensus then is that it was. Physicians such as Ambroise Pare blamed widespread impiety and lasciviousness; others blamed the Moors, who were refugees in Italy after scattering from Spain. Still others blamed things like poisoned wells or astrological events such as the conjunction of Saturn and Mars (see Interlude 2).[27] In 1526, Gonzalo Fernández de Oviedo y Valdés (1478–1557), known simply as Oviedo, was the first to propose that the disease had come from the Americas. Oviedo had spent ten years in the New World starting in 1513 and posited that Columbus and his men brought it back with them to Spain and that Spanish soldiers fighting to defend Naples introduced the disease into Italy.[28] Oviedo's writings on the subject initiated the debate between the Columbian theory—there was no syphilis in Europe until Columbus brought it there—versus the pre-Columbian theory—syphilis was present in Europe prior to 1494 but in a milder form of the disease. It is one of the most hotly contested debates among medical historians, and it is very likely that we will never know for certain the factual answer to the question.

The timing of the first outbreak of syphilis supports the Columbian theory since Columbus had returned from the New World in 1493, with the first cases appearing in Europe the following year. Skeletal remains from Hispaniola demonstrate that approximately 10 percent of the native population had the characteristic skeletal signature of syphilis, proving that Columbus' men would have been exposed to a disease that was endemic to the region.[29] New World human remains as old as 8000 years demonstrate the specific osseous changes of treponemal disease.[30] While it may have been impossible for a few men returning to Europe to spark an epidemic, there were over 300 New World female slaves brought to Europe in 1494 and 1495, and there is no doubt that these women were employed as sex workers in Spain—and possibly Italy—around that time.[31] Finally, supporters of the Columbian theory argue that syphilis was so severe a disease in its early decades in Europe because the population had no immunity whatsoever to the organism.[32] If syphilis had been present in Europe before Columbus, the outbreak would not have been as devastating to the infected or have expanded so rapidly throughout Europe.

Opponents of the Columbian theory scoured ancient and medieval writings looking for evidence of the existence of syphilis before 1494; they argued that descriptions of syphilis could be found in the writings of Hippocrates, Galen, Avicenna, and countless medieval texts. Some even claimed that the malady of Job in the Bible was syphilis.[33] Many texts describe the onset of genital lesions (ulcers or pustules) after intercourse. Medieval surgeons such as Roger of Palermo (ca. 1140–1195) and William of Saliceto (1210–1277) discussed the contagiousness of genital ulcers in their writings.[34] We must remember that translation and interpretation of these texts is, for the most part, a subjective process; in many ways, it is impossible to make definitive assessments of a specific diagnosis retrospectively. Genital herpes and chancroid are examples of pustular and ulcerative diseases, respectively, that are sexually transmitted but are not syphilis.

The skin conditions of the Romans known as *mentagra* and that of the Greeks known as *lichen* have both been proposed as potential names for the syphilis of the ancients. As discussed in Chapter 2, Pliny noted that the two conditions were the Roman and Greek names for the same disease. Hudson argued that while *mentum* to the Romans meant the chin, the pubic area was considered "the lesser chin," and by use of the diminutive, mentum turned into *mentula*, "the little chin." Eventually, *mentula* became a euphemism for the penis, and *mentulagra*, a venereal disease of this organ. Thus, *mentagra* was simply a shortened version of *mentulagra*.[35] In this theory, Pliny's *mentagra* is not referring to a disorder of the chin but a disorder of the genital area—and pre-Columbianists such as Hudson believe Pliny was describing syphilis. This euphemistic analysis is one example of the type of scholarship that the pre-Columbianists have relied upon to support the idea of ancient and medieval syphilis.

The pre-Columbianists contend that descriptions of a "venereal leprosy" by medieval medical scholars in the thirteenth and fourteenth centuries support pre-Columbian syphilis. They argue that warnings by medievalists such as Bernard de Gordon (fl. 1270–1330), that lying in bed with a leper could cause leprosy, was in many cases actually referring to syphilis, as leprosy is not a venereal disease. But as previously discussed in the first Interlude, the stigma of leprosy as a consequence of immoral behavior and sexual promiscuity reached its peak in the Middle Ages and may have resulted from the influence of religious beliefs superimposed on medical theory. The word *lepra* and its more modern cousin, *leprosy*, became associated with impurity and all forms of sin, and since lust is one of the seven deadly sins, the Catholic Church would have particularly cast its focus on these negative attributes in persons with leprosy.[36]

Another argument supporting the confusion of syphilis with leprosy in the Middle Ages was the use of mercury, which has no efficacy against leprosy, but was advocated as a specific treatment for leprosy by such important writers as Theodoric Borgognoni (1205–1296) (see Chapter 7).[37] Hudson pointed out that the "leprosy" of ancient and medieval times was contagious, venereal, and susceptible to mercury, while Hansen's disease is not venereal, mildly contagious, and unresponsive to mercury.[38] Thus, the argument is that ancient and medieval leprosy was syphilis.

In the twentieth century, scientists went to European pre-Columbian skeletal remains for answers in an attempt to settle this debate once and for all. While Rothschild concluded there were no osseous characteristics of syphilis in pre-Columbian specimens from Europe, Africa, and Asia, over 50 conflicting reports were published that concluded that syphilis *was* present in skeletal remains in Europe before Columbus' return.[39] In 2011, however, Harper et al., after a careful analysis of each of the reports, "could not find a single case of Old World treponemal disease that has both a certain diagnosis and a secure pre-Columbian date," noting that the reports "lack specific criteria for the diagnosis of treponemal disease, fail to provide information about the dating methods used, and do not include quality photographs."[40] Thus, solid paleopathological evidence for pre-Columbian syphilis does not exist. As for the supposed diagnostic confusion of syphilis and leprosy among medieval physicians, Crane-Kramer reported that there was no confusion: no skeletal remains showing signs of syphilis exist in leprosarium burial grounds of the Middle Ages.[41] The examination of skeletal remains for evidence of syphilis is apparently open to interpretation among paleopathologists.

A third theory has emerged, which is called the unitarian theory, stating that syphilis, yaws, and bejel, all caused by *T. pallidum*, differ in their clinical expression and the way in which they are transmitted according to the geography and environment where the organism thrives. Yaws occurs in warm, humid tropical regions and is spread by skin-to-skin contact, while bejel is found in hot, dry regions and is spread by contaminated utensils and vessels. The theory argues that at some point in the fifteenth century, *T. pallidum* migrated to Europe, possibly after contact by Europeans with African slaves, and syphilis emerged as the primary expression of infection with the spirochete, one that was particularly infectious, damaging, and lethal. The organism evolved for its new European victims who wore clothing and had better hygiene.[42] This theory exonerates Columbus, his men, and their slaves for causing an extraordinary epidemic, which is, after all, difficult to attribute to a small number of people in such a short period of time. A variation of the theory that implicates Columbus states that his men came into contact with yaws, and when yaws was brought back to Europe, the susceptibility of the population—along with different geography, climate, and living conditions of the region—fostered the dissemination of a new, severe expression of infection with *T. pallidum*.

Reactions to the Great Pox

The earliest explanations attributed the disease to a punishment sent from God for sins and transgressions. In his posthumous publication *De luis venereae curatione perfectissima liber*, "A book concerning on the most effective treatment of venereal disease" (1579), the renowned Jean Fernel (see Chapter 8) was the first to apply a rational perspective to understanding the disease and is thereby the single most important voice of his generation on the subject. Fernel was convinced that the disease was new to Europe and imported from the New World. In both the etiology and the natural history of the disease, he shrewdly compared it to rabies and noted the skin as the only protection against the disease:

> No: it does not come from the stars, nor from the soil, nor from water, nor from wine. Like the mad dog's phlegm, it is a contagion; that is, it spreads by contact; and it has this further resemblance to the dog's virus that it requires a broken surface in order to establish itself in the body. The sound skin is proof against it; but the least sore place—a scratch, an abrasion, the tiniest crack—and through that it can enter. As with arrow-poison, the sound skin has to be pierced to let it pass. And, like the mad dog's virus, having entered it lies dormant for a while; then, in its own due time, to travel to the uttermost ends of the body, working its mischief as it goes.[43]

While fears of syphilis were on the minds of the public at large, even concerns of a ghastly disease like syphilis could not deter men from visiting the brothels. Consequently, demands for preventative measures were naturally spurred during the epidemic. Gabriele Fallopio (1523–1562), also known as Fallopius, was an Italian anatomist who demystified the anatomy of the reproductive organs, who named or discovered—in addition to other body parts—the vagina and clitoris, and argued against the commonly held belief that the penis physically entered the uterus during intercourse. While condoms or sheaths had been in use since ancient times, it was Fallopius' knowledge of genital anatomy that brought the condom into the modern era. In his *De morbo gallico* (1564), he described the success in preventing syphilis with a portable linen sheath soaked in a salty, herbal solution and fixed in place with a pink ribbon. After experimenting with the sheath on 1100 men, he claimed, "I call immortal God to witness that not one of them was infected."[44]

Other sheaths from his period were made of goat or lamb intestines and crafted by butchers. The use of condoms both a preventative for syphilis as well as a means of contraception increased in the seventeenth century in spite of the condemnation of the device by Jesuits such as Leonardus Lessius (1554–1623), who stated that the use of the condom was a sin. Syphilis broke out among Charles I's forces during the English Civil War, and condoms made of fish, cattle, or sheep intestine had to be issued to reduce additional losses.[45] Incidentally, the origin of the word "condom" is unknown, but many speculations about its origin exist, including a legend that attributes the word origin to the name of an English physician—a Colonel Condom or Condon—who was employed at the court of King Charles II (r. 1660–1685).[46] Charles, concerned about the number of illegitimate children he had fathered, asked his physician for the contraceptive. Another possibility is that it derives from the Latin verb *condo*, "to preserve."[47] The word did not appear in medical texts until the eighteenth century when Daniel Turner first used it in his discussion of syphilis. Turner, pointing out the unpopularity of the device, wrote:

> The Condum being the best, if not only Preservative our Libertines have found out at present; and yet by reason of its blunting the Sensation, I have heard some of them acknowledge, that they had often chose to risk a Clap, rather than engage *cum hastis sic clypeatis* [with spears thus sheathed].[48]

Mercury versus Guaiacum

In the sixteenth century, there was renewed interest in mercury, which had been used medicinally since ancient times, especially for skin diseases similar in appearance to syphilis such as leprosy; it became a mainstay of treatment for syphilis for approximately 400 years. One of the earliest supporters of mercury as a therapeutic option (termed "mercurialists") was Paracelsus (1493–1541), the Swiss alchemist and physician whose radical views and distrust of the ancients made him one of the founders of modern medicine. Paracelsus rejected the humoral theory of disease and instead proposed that chemicals—specifically mercury, salt, and sulfur—could cure all diseases. Mercury causes sweating, hypersalivation, and diuresis; the mercurialists viewed these effects as the excretion of the syphilitic contagion. Paracelsus believed that three pints of saliva must be generated to achieve the desired therapeutic effect of mercury.[49] Because mercury is the only metal that is liquid at room temperature, physicians throughout history expected great things from this spectacular and unique element. The problem is that metallic mercury is entirely too toxic, even for the most aggressive of Renaissance physicians; therefore, less harmful mercurial salts were used: mercurous chloride (Hg_2Cl_2) and mercuric chloride ($HgCl_2$), the latter being water-soluble and readily absorbed into the body.[50] The mercurous compound (called calomel), when taken orally, was a purgative (laxative), believed to rid the body specifically of that ever-imagined substance, black bile; it was also used as an anti-syphilitic. In addition, calomel and the mercuric compound, known as corrosive sublimate, could be delivered into the body either by means of friction, in which a mercurial salve was rubbed vigorously into the skin to the point of ulceration, or by fumigation, whereby the mercury salt or even elemental mercury was heated and vapors of the substance inhaled in a sauna-like apparatus. Other methods of treatment included the direct application of mercury plasters to skin lesions, corrosive sublimate baths, and subcutaneous injection. However, by the end of the eighteenth century, internal administration of mercury, either by oral or rectal delivery methods, became more commonplace than these external methods.[51]

Mercury treatment spanned a month or longer and led to various side effects and inconveniences. Ulceration of the mouth and throat, swelling of the gums, tooth loss, and constant and excessive production of saliva were just the oral complaints. Persons undergoing mercury treatment had to hide away for the month to avoid the embarrassing giveaway of the salivation in public. Pink disease, also known as acrodynia, is the condition in which mercury poisoning causes red and painful hands and feet. Mercury toxicity can also manifest as nausea and vomiting, diarrhea, abdominal pain, hypertension, tachycardia, kidney damage, hair loss, motor weakness, and dementia and other neuro-psychiatric effects. One wonders how neurosyphilis was distinguished from mercury-induced brain damage during these times.

COULD MERCURY CURE SYPHILIS?

Since heavy metals such as mercury are toxic to bacteria in the lab, it probably did work in some cases. In other cases, the disease likely entered the latent phase, in which none of the skin manifestations of the disease were showing, giving the treating physician a false sense of victory over the infection.[52] Even today, it is not possible to know for sure without a blood test that a person has been cured of syphilis. The most significant evidence supporting the efficacy of mercury against *T. pallidum* was the discovery of the Jarisch-Herxheimer reaction. The reaction, named after the Austrian dermatologist Adolf Jarisch (1850–1902) and the German dermatologist Karl Herxheimer (1861–1942)—both of whom independently described it—is characterized by the symptoms of fever, chills, and the intensification of skin lesions in persons treated with mercury or penicillin. The Jarisch-Herxheimer is believed to result from toxin release from killed spirochetes; therefore, the presence of the reaction after treatment with mercury indicates the success of the intervention. Herxheimer, incidentally, was one of two famous dermatologists who died in concentration camps during the Holocaust, both of whom perished in Theresienstadt. The other was Abraham Buschke (1868–1943).

The anti-mercurialists, who recognized mercury for the poison that it was, put forth an alternative: guaiacum. The powdered wood of the guaiacum tree was first championed by the German scholar Ulrich von Hutten (1488–1523) in his *De morbo gallico* (1519), which was an account of his own experience with the French Sickness and his treatment with the imported wood. Guaiacum (or guaiac) came from Hispaniola, where the local population found the material effective, according to eyewitnesses such as the aforementioned Oviedo. Like mercury, guaiac had laxative and sweat-inducing properties but did not cause severe salivation. Still, the treatment protocol was even more brutal, involving severe diarrhea, residence in a hot room for a biblical 40 days, and strict fasting for that same time.[53]

Mercury and guaiac divided physicians of the period into two camps; for example, Fracastoro favored mercury, while Fernel favored guaiacum. Jacques de Bethencourt, the author of the first French book on syphilis, interestingly named (in translation) "A New Lenten-Like Penance and Purgatory of Expiation for the Usage of Patients Affected with the French or Venereal Disease" (1527), compared the two treatments and concluded that mercury was the better option, noting that the fasting required of the guaiacum protocol was excessive and that guaiacum was less effective and slower than mercury.[54] Guaiac was no longer used to treat syphilis by the end of the seventeenth century, but it is still used today in medicine in the fecal occult blood test (stool guaiac test). A few sensible physicians, such as Ambroise Pare, recognized the dangers of both mercury and guaiac and suggested less toxic plants or woods that were popular at the time because of their diaphoretic and diuretic properties, namely sarsaparilla, china root, wild pansy, and sassafras.

Eighteenth-Century Venereology

In the eighteenth century, venereal diseases such as gonorrhea, syphilis, and chancroid were rampant problems in London and Paris, and it was generally believed, presumably because they were frequently found present in a person at the same time, that all of these diseases were caused by the same contagion. There was little distinction between these diseases in the sixteenth through eighteenth centuries, and all were collectively referred to in many medical texts of the era as simply venereal disease. Although gonorrhea, a bacterial infection of the urethra, was an ancient disease and syphilis was a new one, most practitioners of the period saw gonorrhea as the early, local stage of the disease, and the signs of *morbus venerea* indicated that the disease had spread all over the body.[55] The ulcer of chancroid, another bacterial infection that causes genital ulceration most commonly in persons who have intercourse with sex workers, was not distinguished clinically as different from the chancre of syphilis until the nineteenth century. Opponents of this "unity theory" were in the minority in the eighteenth century, but their numbers did grow eventually; one in particular, Francis Balfour (1744–1818), authored *Dissertatio medica inauguralis, de gonorrhoea virulenta* in 1767, and a small controversy ensued.

The Scottish surgeon John Hunter (1728–1793) found himself at the front lines treating venereal disease in the eighteenth century, and so it follows that an inquisitive thinker like Hunter would experiment with syphilis to attempt to prove his conviction that gonorrhea and syphilis were the same disease. His experiment, performed in 1767, is one of the most famous investigations in the history of medicine, described by Hunter in his "A Treatise on the Venereal Disease" (1786):

> Two punctures were made on the penis with a lancet dipped in venereal matter from a gonorrhea; one puncture was on the glans; the other on the prepuce.[56]

Within a few days, the test subject developed symptoms of gonorrhea; by day ten, a chancre appeared, leading Hunter to conclude that the experiment proved his hypothesis: gonorrhea and syphilis are the same disease.[57] What he did not consider is the fact that his source of infectious material had both diseases. His erroneous result set back progress on the study of venereal diseases for 50 years. Still, Hunter called attention to the induration of the chancre as a key diagnostic feature, and, for all of his efforts, his name was eventually given to the chancre (Hunterian chancre).

WAS HUNTER HIMSELF THE TEST SUBJECT?

A legend surrounding this experiment is that the test subject used by Hunter was none other than Hunter himself. The legend grew from what Qvist called a "completely irresponsible statement" made by a D'Arcy Power at a Hunterian Oration in 1925. Power claimed that Hunter had syphilitic dementia at the time of his death and died from syphilitic coronary arteritis, implying that his famous experiment ultimately caused his demise.[58] Hunter famously died of what appears to be a heart attack after a heated debate in 1793. Qvist argued that syphilis was not the cause as his autopsy showed no evidence of syphilitic aortic disease. Other arguments by Qvist include the following: Hunter had no qualms about using test subjects for inoculation experiments, which he frequently did, and there is no reason to believe this case was different; there is no textual proof in "A Treatise on the Venereal Disease" that he injected himself; he frequently used the pronoun "I" when referencing himself in the treatise, but not in regard to this case's subject; finally, there is no evidence that Hunter exhibited signs of neurosyphilis in his later years. Qvist contended that Hunter died of non-specific atherosclerosis and never contracted syphilis because he inoculated someone else, not himself.[59] The myth that Hunter "was a 'martyr to science' is sheer romantic sentimentality," but writers of popular medical history have largely ignored Qvist's contentions, and the legend lives on to this day.[60]

The English surgeon and first British practitioner to focus his attention on skin disease, Daniel Turner (1667–1740), was an outspoken authority on venereal disease in the first half of the eighteenth century. It has already been mentioned that Turner introduced and reintroduced, respectively, the terms "condom" and "syphilis" in his writings. In addition to his landmark English text entitled *De Morbis Cutaneis* (1714) discussed in Chapter 9, Turner authored an important treatise entitled "Syphilis. A practical dissertation on the venereal disease" (1717). Exploration of this text, written in English, reveals much about the approach of an early eighteenth-century surgeon to what at his time had become a widespread, yet silent, affliction.

During Turner's time, venereal disease had become known as the "secret disease" as everything about the disease was secret: the parts of the body it affected; the secret encounters that led to it, how the illness was kept secret from one's spouses, masks used to keep one's identity secret, quacks paid extra for secrecy, etc.[61] Charlatans took advantage of the desire for secrecy; in the mid-eighteenth century, a chocolate concoction laced with mercury was developed for at-home self-treatment, and a husband could give the beverage to his unwitting wife to prevent her from catching syphilis from him.[62]

The diagnosis of venereal disease had significant moral implications and vice versa—determining the direction of a person's moral compass could influence the diagnosis. The same type of rash, i.e., one with ulcers, sores, or pustules all over the body, would be diagnosed as scurvy in a person with a perceived upright character, while syphilis was diagnosed in a person deemed wanton or unvirtuous.[63] For dermatologic problems, the accuracy of making the correct diagnosis was so poor that physicians had to resort to grading a person's morality to classify the problem in front of them. Such was the healthcare climate in which Turner found himself practicing in the early eighteenth century.

Since syphilis was primarily considered an external disease, surgeons were the principal caregivers for the malady. Turner argued "that the Surgeon is the most proper Person to be consulted" for the management of venereal disease: to "lay open the venereall Abscesses with cauteries, to rub down the Verrucae, to extirpate Caruncles, to lay bare the rotten Bones, for dilating the sinuous Venereal Ulcers," among other tasks.[64] Like most of his contemporaries, Turner believed that there was only one venereal disease, and he divided his treatise into two parts—the clap and the pox—which were the two stages of venereal disease. Turner apparently did not appreciate the fact that a person can, and frequently does, experience multiple sexually transmitted infections at the same time. For Turner, the failure to promptly and adequately treat clap could lead to a bout of syphilis. His clients, driven by fear, sought treatment at the earliest signs of "being clap'd" to attempt to avoid the living nightmare of the Great Pox.[65] Syphilis crossed all boundaries of social class; no one was immune to the risk to health, marriage, and most importantly, reputation, brought about by this disease. Syphilis could cause significant disfigurement by destroying a person's nose; nasal prostheses were developed and utilized to cover the horrible deformity, but wearing such an apparatus would declare to the world the person's underlying affliction. Nasal reconstruction with plastic surgery techniques such as skin grafting that were pioneered by the Italian surgeon Gaspare Tagliacozzi (1545–1599) was not widely available (see Chapter 8). Fear of disfigurement was a powerful motivator to drive people toward treatment, which at the time was horribly toxic, but the great irony is that, apparently, this fear was not powerful enough to keep people of all socioeconomic statuses out of brothels.

In his characteristic prudish and judgmental fashion, Turner defined syphilis as "a venomous or contagious Distemper, for the most part contracted by impure Coition, as least some contact of the Genitals of both Sexes, or some other lewd and filthy Dalliance between each other that way tending."[66] He presented the arguments for and against syphilis as a new disease and seems to side with those espousing syphilis as an ancient disease and a cousin of *lepra*, *elephantiasis*, *psora*, and even the affliction of Job.[67]

In Turner's treatise on syphilis, 26 of the 30 patient cases described resulted in a cure, which Turner defined in several ways: reduction in the pain of either urination or the urethral discharge; drying up of the scabs and pustules; resolution of the swollen lymph nodes; healing of chancres; preservation of the voice; or relief of pain in head and legs.[68] To achieve these successes, Turner, a mercurialist, required his patients to stay in bed for a month. He administered oral calomel for mild forms of the Pox, and for more severe cases, he advocated external application of topical mercurial "unctions." In both instances, salivation was the goal and signaled to Turner that the treatment was working. If the patient did not "salivate" with topical delivery of the mercury, fumigation with cinnabar (mercury sulfide) was the next step. By the 1730s, since the stigma of salivation prompted a month of inconvenient sequestration, salivation fell out of favor among practitioners in London, who deemed it an antiquated approach and its advocates—including Turner—quacks.[69] Mercury remained a mainstay of treating syphilis after Turner's time; however, prescribing it to the point of salivation—a sign of severe toxicity—was no longer the goal.

FAMOUS PERSONS WITH SYPHILIS

A popular topic concerning the history of syphilis is the speculation about which famous historical persons possibly had the disease. The list of noteworthy persons rumored to have had syphilis includes Idi Amin, Ludwig van Beethoven, Al Capone, Fyodor Dostoevsky, Paul Gauguin, Francisco Goya, Adolf Hitler, Scott Joplin, Vladimir Lenin, Abraham and Mary Todd Lincoln, Édouard Manet, Guy de Maupassant, Friedrich Nietzsche, Franz Schubert, William Shakespeare, Henri de Toulouse-Lautrec, Leo Tolstoy, Henry VIII, Ivan the Terrible, Vincent van Gogh, and Oscar Wilde. From the list, one can postulate that both creative genius and murderous tyrannies can result in part from the effects of neurosyphilis.

The story of William Shakespeare (1564–1616) possibly having syphilis is of greatest interest to our study. According to Ross, Shakespeare's writings reveal an "obsessive interest" in syphilis and his knowledge of the disease: the evidence in his last few sonnets and the gossip of his time all point to the suggestion that the bard had syphilis.[70] Shakespeare referenced the disease numerous times in his works, and he called it in various places the Pox, the malady of France, the infinite malady, the incurable bone-ache, and the hoar-leprosy.[71] While no precise reference to genital chancres exists in any of his works, he referenced "embossed sores" in *As You Like It*, and "canker" in Sonnet 95.[72] *Troilus and Cressida* includes references to the secondary and tertiary features of syphilis: "raw eyes," "bone-ache," and "limekilns in the palm" that refer respectively to the uveitis, periostitis, and palmar rash of syphilis.[73] Knowledge of a disease does not equate to personal infection, but Shakespeare may have implied his syphilis in several of his sonnets; for example, his comment in Sonnet 153 about "the seething bath," which refers to the use of hot baths to treat syphilis, suggests he may have experienced this treatment himself.[74] Finally, in his later years, he developed a tremor, agitation, and social withdrawal, suggesting he was in the throes of mercury poisoning.[75]

Jean Astruc (1684–1766)

Only during the intellectual explosion of the eighteenth century could a figure arise that would become both a giant in the history of syphilis and equally famous for his contributions to the textual analysis of the Holy Bible. That person was France's Jean Astruc. Born in the Languedoc region of France, Astruc trained at the University of Montpellier, where he received his medical degree at 19 years of age in 1703 and began his career as a professor of medicine. In 1711, he moved to Toulouse to teach anatomy before returning to Montpellier five years later as a professor of medicine, where he remained for the next 12 years.[76] After a brief stint as the personal physician of the King of Poland, Astruc returned to Montpellier but eventually settled for good at the University in Paris, where he served as royal physician and where he finished his career. He was a well-rounded scholar, prolific writer, and talented educator— a true academician—who is remembered more for his writings and teaching than his own practice of medicine. In addition to applying his sharp scientific mind to medicine, Astruc, the Catholic son of a Protestant-turned-Catholic father, published anonymously a textual and philological analysis of the Book of Genesis, in which he argued that Genesis was based on four manuscript traditions.

Astruc's most outstanding achievement in the field of medicine was his authorship of *De morbis venereis libri sex*, "Treatise of Venereal Diseases in six books" (1736), in which he summarized all known information about venereal disease at the time. In the two centuries prior to Astruc's publication, countless treatises had been written about the disease with the corpus of information scattered and unsystematic. Astruc brought order and coherence to the knowledge concerning syphilis. The original text was written in Latin in six books; it was expanded into nine books in 1740. Numerous editions and translations followed over the next three decades as it became the gold-standard textbook on venereal diseases for physicians throughout Europe. Daniel Turner once wrote that the work "contains not only the most ample collection, but affords the most useful and instructive history of the venereal disease."[77]

Apparently, the feelings were not mutual: Astruc, in his appendix describing authors of texts on venereal disease, expressed his consternation that surgeons such as Turner could be granted licenses to practice medicine without a medical degree.[78] Astruc was famous for his vociferous defense of the physician's status above surgeons and for defending the jurisdiction of internal diseases with external manifestations, such as smallpox and measles.[79] Astruc also disagreed with Turner on the value of the condom, arguing that they enabled promiscuous sexual activity and did not completely protect one from contracting syphilis.

The first volume of Astruc's "Treatise of Venereal Diseases" is dedicated to the history of venereal disease, with the focus mainly on the refutation of the idea of the antiquity of venereal disease, i.e., that syphilis was present in Europe dating back to ancient times. Astruc, instead, believed in the Columbian theory of the origin of syphilis and noted that the disease first appeared in 1494, brought to Europe by Columbus and his men.[80] His research into this topic is extraordinarily detailed and comprehensive, and he presented all available textual evidence for both sides of the argument, only to dismantle the pre-Columbian viewpoint in a somewhat condescending and arrogant manner that would have made Galen proud. His central thesis is that the writers of the late fifteenth and early sixteenth centuries considered it a new disease at the time.

Astruc, like Turner, called syphilis "the venereal disease." On its cause, Astruc was emphatic that syphilis was spread by "coition" or "generation" (i.e., congenital):

> ... it is now known by certain and indubitable Experience, and the unanimous Consent of all Physicians, that the venereal Disease can neither be contracted by an error in Diet, the Fault of the Air, the Abuse of the Non-naturals, or any spontaneous Corruption of the Humours, but solely by Infection and the Communication of it from one that is diseased.[81]

In congenital cases, he believed that either the father or mother could transmit the infection to the fetus, claiming that a "venereal father" could impregnate a healthy mother, who would then birth a "venereal" newborn.[82] Astruc referred to the contagious material by which the disease was transmitted to the healthy person as the "venereal poison":

> There are therefore conveyed from the Diseased into the Sound, certain Seeds of morbifick Matter, which being introduced into a healthy Body in the smallest Quantity, and by insensible Passages, and gradually increasing in Bulk, Form and Efficacy, sooner or later are able to infect and corrupt the whole Mass of Humours. And these Seeds of the Disease are usually, and not improperly, named the Venereal Ferment, Venom, or Poison.[83]

He posited that other contagious diseases, such as smallpox or plague, were transmitted in a similar fashion, but syphilis was different because its venereal venom was "so much more the noxious," causing a disease "more grievous than others."[84] It is apparent that Astruc was not ready for any precursor theory to the microbial theory of disease, and he erred considerably in his disregard of the concept of *animalcula;* he ridiculed those who proposed that "all diseases were produced by *animalcula* in the blood, and different diseases by different *animalcula*."[85] Clearly, these so-called quacks were closer to the truth than Astruc could even imagine.

In regard to treatment of venereal disease, Astruc, a mercurialist, noted the rise and fall of guaiacum, china root, sarsaparilla, and sassafras—all of which received much praise at first but fell out of favor after proving to be too inconvenient and/or ineffective. He devoted a large portion of his text to assessing whether mercurial fumigation or "salivation by unction" was the better method of delivering the mercury, concluding that mercurial unction was the superior method because it offered the following advantage:

> ... not one shall die: but all of them shall be perfectly cured, without Danger of a Relapse, by a Method which is neither more tedious, or troublesome, nay, on the contrary, is shorter, more easy, and agreeable; in which I am confident all who are acquainted with it will agree with me.[86]

Although Astruc felt that dosing mercury to the point of salivation was not necessary to eradicate the disease, the salivation did indicate to the physician the degree of mercury a patient had in his or her body;

thus, the amount of salivation could guide the physician to how much further to push the dose. Therefore, Astruc encouraged salivation, but with caution; the patient should be limited to one or two pints of saliva production per day.

Astruc also considered gonorrhea the first stage of venereal disease, and he also established the chancre as a feature of the first stage, which included all signs and symptoms affecting the genital area. In addition to gonorrhea and chancres, complications included in Astruc's first stage were the *venereal hernia*, an inflammatory swelling of the testicles; a *venereal abscess* in the perineum; the *gleet*, also called the habitual gonorrhea or *stillicidium,* a chronic discharge of what Astruc states is semen; an *obstinate strangury,* a narrowing of the urinary stream, treated with several different techniques to dilate the urethra; *venereal buboes* and their many forms; phimosis and paraphimosis, disorders of the movement of the foreskin; *gangrene and sphacelus of the pudenda*; and various growths on the genitals, including *phymata, porri, verrucae, and condylomata*; and lesions of the anus, termed *cristae, mora, fici, mariscae, and rhagadia,* which represent different-sized growths or fissures of this part of the body.[87] The information regarding the diagnosis and management of each of these features of the venereal disease is extraordinarily detailed and not for the faint of heart.

Astruc appreciated the known fact that the venereal poison could "lurk some time in the blood" without revealing itself.[88] The eventual onset of the Pox, the main feature of the second stage of the disease, marked its "confirmed State" as follows:

> in which not one or two Parts of the Body, or one or more Functions of the animal Economy are disordered, but with which almost every Part of the Body is infected, and all of their natural Offices disturbed. The Nature of this Disease of so wide an extent, and it comprehends such an infinite Number of different Symptoms, that it rather appears to be a World of Diseases than one.[89]

Astruc's discussion of the accurate diagnosis of the second stage of venereal disease in Book IV is genius. He breaks down the signs and symptoms of syphilis into *demonstrative*, which are those signs the patient presently shows, and *commemorative*, which "call to mind the past state of the patient" and generally represent first-stage problems.[90] Under demonstrative signs, Astruc states that the ten signs (see Table I3.1) are pathognomonic, meaning only venereal disease can be the diagnosis.

Commemorative signs, according to Astruc, are a history of the following nine complaints: excrescences of the pudenda; chancres; phimosis and paraphimosis; buboes of the groin; virulent gonorrhea; excrescences and ulcers of the anus; ulcers, inflammation, and excrescences of the breast; ulcers of the lips, mouth, and fauces; and scabs, herpes, pustules, and ulcers of the skin. Astruc concluded this section with his rules for making the diagnosis of the Pox; the rules, which depend on the presence or absence of the above signs, detail whether to "pronounce it to be the Pox," "there can only be a strong presumption of that it is the Pox," "judgement must be suspended for want of evidence," or "it is no pox."[92]

TABLE I3.1

Ten Pathognomonic Signs of Syphilis According to Jean Astruc[91]

Having had sexual contact with an infected person
Having frequent miscarriages, or a history of bringing "squalid, emaciated, scabby, ulcerated, half-rotten" children into the world
Having sickly children which are "strumous, rickety, humped, hectical, and emaciated" or "puny, broken-backed, large-headed, crooked, bandy-legged, variously distorted, and thick-jointed"
Having local venereal disorders such as ulcers, phimosis, paraphimosis, porri, verrucae, condylomata, or buboes
Having local venereal complaints that resist skillful treatment
Having cutaneous features of the Pox, which are, most importantly, venereal spots, tubercles, and pustules, but also "chaps of the hands, falling off of the hair, diseases of the nails, scabs, tetters, herpes, etc."
Having ulcers of the tonsils, fauces, uvula, palate, gums, or internal part of the nose, with collapse of the nasal bones
Having venereal joint or bone pain, worst at night
Having diseases of the bone, such as exostosis, hyperostosis, abscesses, fractures from the slightest cause
Having glandular and lymphatic tumors and gummata

Astruc's treatise was enormously successful because the differential diagnosis of syphilis at his time was unimaginably tricky to sort out, venereal disease was rampant, and so much was on the line for the patient. It is rare to find a book in which a single disease or related group of diseases was so comprehensively covered; with this authoritative work's equal parts of history, diagnosis, and treatment— especially mercurial therapeutics—one cannot fathom a better source of information on the topic for the eighteenth-century practitioner. In addition, Astruc included a lengthy (over 150 pages) annotated bibliography of every written work on his subject. Astruc's *Treatise of Venereal Diseases* should be remembered as one of the single greatest texts in the history of medicine.

After reviewing Astruc's sections on the skin lesions of venereal disease, it is apparent that Astruc's dermatologic knowledge superseded that of his peers and was ahead of its time. In fact, Pusey went so far as to state that Jean Astruc should be regarded as the founder of modern dermatology.[93] Astruc studied the histopathology of the skin 100 years before anyone else. Take, for example, the following passage in Book IV in which Astruc demonstrates a unique appreciation for the correlation between clinical presentation and his own humoralist understanding of histopathology:

> There are two humours of the skin, which readily allow the venereal poison to mix with them, viz. the mucous, which is contained in the spungy [*sic*] cells of the corpus reticulare malpighii, situated immediately under the skin; and the sebaceous, which gently issues from the glands, or rather from the fine vessels or lacunae of the skin. I take no notice of the other two which are likewise discharged by the pores of the skin, viz. sweat and insensible transpiration, because they are too thin, subtle and aqueous, to imbibe, or retain the venereal poison, which is thick and viscid.

> If the mucous humour is infected with the venereal poison, it will contract a greater acrimony, with which it will vellicate the cutis. Hence will proceed frequent itching and tetters [rash]. Then the small fibres, by which the cuticle is tied down to the cutis, being eroded, the loosened cuticle will be raised up into several small bladders, filled with salt serum, which being opened will form small ulcers. Hence the scabies. Lastly, the disorder encreasing, larger exulcerations will be formed upon the skin, with which the cuticle being eroded, and quite dried up, it will fall off like bran. Hence proceeds the dry, furfuraceous pustule, miliary, corroding herpes.

> Since the cuticle is no where thicker than in the palms of the hands and soles of the feet, the mucous humour that is deposited under it, meets with the more difficulty in passing through its pores. Being collected therefore in greater plenty, and remaining here a longer time, it produces so much the greater heat and itching in these parts. Hence the dried cuticle is divided into callous itching clefts and chaps, which discharge an ichor. Nay, sometimes when it is deeply figured, it separates from the skin, and casts off like exuviae.

> When the same humour is infected with a poison of a less virulent and acrimonius nature, it only slightly corrodes the surface of the skin in certain parts of the body, without injuring the cuticle, the vessels of the skin being in some places divided, spue forth small drops of blood, which being blended with the mucous humor, destroys its native clearness. From hence therefore proceed the plain, even, distinct spots of the skin, when the mucous humour is vitiated in several separate parts of the body; but when it happens to many continued parts, the spots are wider, and of greater extent; and they become livid, purple, red, yellow, in proportion to the greater or smaller quantity of extravasated blood, or according to the difference of the color of the blood so extravasated, whether it be black, red, rosy coloured, or yellow, etc.[94]

Without a doubt, this was the most scientific passage ever written about the skin at the time. Dermatology and dermatopathology are inseparable fields; the modern dermatologist is trained to think about skin disease in relation to its microscopic appearance, and Astruc was among the first, if not the first, to discuss the clinical-pathologic correlation of skin disease in his writings. Astruc authorized a collection of his lectures in 1759 entitled *Traité des tumeurs et des ulcères*, which is closer to a textbook on general dermatology that the title suggests. In addition to being the earliest text in French about skin disease, *Traité* contains some of the first discussions of the anatomic localization of the "seat" of various skin diseases within the histologic layers of the skin.[95] This particular work was a prelude to the inauguration of the science of dermatopathology that took place in the 1840s.[96] For this work and the extraordinary work he did with syphilis, Astruc deserves elevation to the highest level in the pantheon of the specialty.

Nineteenth-Century Venereology

At the end of the eighteenth century, gonorrhea and syphilis were still considered one venereal disease, and mercury was virtually the only treatment offered to the syphilitic. Oral administration of mercury made a comeback and eventually replaced the long-considered less dangerous topical or fumigatory methods. Mercury was delivered orally in several ways: a gum form, as calomel, as corrosive sublimate, and in a popular concoction known as Van Swieten's liquor, which contained sublimate dissolved in water and alcohol.[97] Quacks and charlatans were everywhere, promising a cure with their own mercurial syrups, medicated candies called dragees, and anti-syphilitic waters.

Libertinism, exemplified by the lives of the Marquis de Sade (1740–1814) and Giacomo Casanova (1725–1798)—both of whom may have had the venereal disease—was an approach to life that grew out of the Enlightenment (see Chapter 10); the lack of sexual restraint in its participants sustained the transmission of the treponeme throughout Europe, as did the incessant warfare of this era. In addition, sex workers were ubiquitous, as were their willing and paying customers. The governments of England and France attempted to get the pox-riddled sex workers off the streets to squelch the spread of a disease that could decimate an army or embarrass a politician. Squalid institutions such as the Bicêtre and the Salpêtrière in Paris were closer to prisons than the hospitals they claimed to be; the horrors experienced behind their inescapable walls are incomprehensible.

Given the fact that we are describing a disease most commonly assigned to the French in its history, it is fitting that the French physicians of the nineteenth century would carry the torch passed by their countryman Jean Astruc and lead the way toward a better understanding of the disease and its complications. In 1838, the French physician and savant Philippe Ricord (1800–1889) applied his intellect to venereal disease and became the greatest of the syphilologists of the nineteenth century. Born in Baltimore and the son of a Frenchman who escaped the French Revolution to America, Ricord returned to Paris in 1820 and became a student of the great Guillaume Dupuytren (1777–1835). He took a position at Hôpital du Midi, Paris' venereal disease hospital, in 1831, and worked there for 30 years. His most important publication was *Traité pratique des maladies vénériennes* (1838). In addition to distinguishing syphilis from venereal warts and balanoposthitis (infection or inflammation of the glans and foreskin), Ricord inoculated patients with their own purulent material (from urethral discharge or chancres) and categorically established the distinction between syphilis and gonorrhea. Ricord persuasively argued that the syphilitic "poison" was a "virus" and, very importantly, that the symptoms of syphilis followed a strict and orderly chronology. He is credited with coining the three stages of syphilis: primary, secondary, and tertiary.[98] The major fault in his work is the fact that Ricord argued emphatically and erroneously that the secondary manifestations of syphilis were not contagious, even though they had been proven to be relatively early in Ricord's career in 1837 by the Irish surgeon, William Wallace (1791–1837), who inoculated healthy persons with material from the lesions of secondary syphilis to prove his point.[99] Wallace also introduced potassium iodide as a treatment for syphilis.

Ricord's student was the other giant of nineteenth-century French dermatovenereology, Jean Alfred Fournier (1832–1914). Their collaboration as medical teacher and student was second only to Hebra and Kaposi (see Chapter 14) among the many successful teacher-student collaborations in the history of dermatology. Fournier married Ricord's daughter and inherited not only Ricord's private practice but also absorbed Ricord's teaching ability and clinical skill. Drawing from a case collection numbering in the tens of thousands, Fournier made numerous contributions to the study of syphilis at a time of relative stagnation. He wrote dozens of original works on syphilis over the span of three decades; his greatest legacies were a description of congenital syphilis and his seminal and correct assertions, much to the consternation of neurologists of his era, that syphilis was the cause of tabes dorsalis and generalized paresis of the insane.

In 1879, Fournier was appointed to the first professorship of cutaneous and venereological diseases at the Hôpital Saint-Louis in Paris; he achieved the same at the *Académie Nationale de Médecine* in 1880. The French government forced the creation of a combined chair of dermatology and venereology.[100] Fournier elevated Hôpital Saint-Louis, already an esteemed center of dermatological learning, to become the "international capital of syphilology," and the first international congress on dermatology and syphilology was held there in 1889.[101] His greatest strengths may have been twofold: his compassion for the victims of the disease and its implications for marriages and the paramount importance he placed on educating both fellow physicians and medical students, as well as the public, on the ravages of syphilis.[102] Fournier showed little interest in dermatology in his role chairing that department; instead, he devoted all of his energy to the study of syphilis.[103]

Fournier's legacy in the history of dermatovenereology has been somewhat overshadowed by his contemporary across the English Channel, Jonathan Hutchinson (1828–1913).[104] Unlike Fournier whose specialty was a single disease, Hutchinson was a true multi-specialist, dabbling in many different fields, including surgery, neurology, ophthalmology, and pathology; he was even more prolific than his French counterpart, having written almost 1200 articles. He researched and frequently wrote about leprosy, and he obstinately believed the cause of that affliction was the ingestion of decomposed fish. Undoubtedly the British master of nineteenth-century syphilology, legend has it that he saw over a million syphilitics in his career.[105] There are numerous eponymous signs that bear his name, including the Hutchinson's triad (notched incisors, labyrinthine deafness, and ocular interstitial keratitis), which suggest a diagnosis of congenital syphilis. Hutchinson is also credited with designating syphilis as the "Great Imitator."[106] His contribution to dermatology will be described further in Chapter 12, but note that in his description of Hutchinson, Pusey did not consider him a "finished dermatologist,"[107] while Crissey and Parrish argued that Hutchinson's contributions to dermatology and syphilology were the only lasting legacies out of the medical polymath's diverse career.[108]

The last milestone in the history of venereology in the nineteenth century that is worthy of our attention is the discovery of the etiologic agent of chancroid—the bacterium *Haemophilus ducreyi*—by the Italian dermatologist Augusto Ducrey (1860–1940). Ducrey, who studied medicine in Naples, devoted himself to dermatology and infectious disease and served as professor of dermatology at the universities of Pisa, Genoa, and Rome. His research into the microorganism, which was presented at the first International Congress of Dermatology in 1889, was met with skepticism from those who thought chancroid to have a wide variety of causes, such as poor hygiene, frictional trauma, or irritation, but not a specific pathogen. Ducrey needed a lifeline for his convictions to be confirmed, and he got it from Paul Gerson Unna (see Chapter 14), who independently proved that *H. ducreyi* was the etiologic agent in chancroid in 1892.[109]

RADESYGE AND ST. PAUL'S BAY DISEASE

Syphilis is a disease that presents in many forms and permutations, different for each person who gets it. As mentioned previously, the tertiary phase of the disease, which can present years after the primary and secondary phases of syphilis, causes destructive gummatous skin lesions, especially on the face. From 1760 to 1820 in Norway, there was an epidemic of a disease in which these destructive lesions arose on the face, affecting primarily the peasants in the Norwegian countryside.[110] It was not known to be a form of syphilis at the time, and the Norwegians set up hospitals to deal with the growing public health crisis. They called the condition, *radesyge,* which means "bad disease" or "evil disease." A body of medical literature developed in which physicians of this region tried to explain the cause. The blockage of the sweat pores due to poor hygiene, exposure of the skin to smoke and stench, and humoral imbalance were all offered as causes of the disease, and physicians debated whether *radesyge* was a form of leprosy, which had not disappeared from Norway as it had in Europe.[111] In the first half of the 1800s, *radesyge* became known as a "vague and unspecific" disease localized to the skin.[112] A Norwegian physician named Carl Wilhelm Boeck (1808–1875) ended the debate in 1860 when he published *Traité de la radesyge,* with the subtitle, *syphilis tertiaire,* and argued successfully that *radesyge* was "nothing more than an offspring of syphilis."[113]

Another geohistorical disease that may have been related to syphilis—or confused with it— was St. Paul's Bay disease, an infectious disease with prominent skin manifestations that affected the people of Quebec from 1775 to 1790. Named after a town near British-controlled Quebec rather than a body of water, the disease affected thousands of colonists in the region, particularly French ones, with a chronic and debilitating course, but it was not particularly deadly. St. Paul's Bay disease was characterized by periorificial ulcers, swollen, suppurating glands, painful bones, scabby skin lesions and sores all over the body, and destructive nasopharyngeal changes.[114] Medical practitioners immediately considered this horrific illness to be a form of venereal syphilis, and the public health response involved mercury-based medicine in various forms.[115] Epidemiological studies at the time revealed the intra-household spread of the infection, suggesting that St. Paul's Bay disease may have actually been a non-venereal type of syphilis similar to bejel.

Modern Reactions to Syphilis

Prior to the discovery of penicillin, the modern history of syphilis is peppered with four unprincipled efforts to control the spread of the disease, treat the infection, or gain a better understanding of the nature of the condition. The first of these was *syphilization*—the inoculation of sex workers with syphilitic material in order to induce mild syphilis and reduce the transmission of the disease. Inspired by the vaccination movement and first proposed in the 1840s by the French physician Joseph-Alexandre Auzias-Turenne (1812–1870), syphilization was ultimately debunked as dangerous in 1852 when it was shown that the unethical practice did nothing but give people syphilis. In England, experimentation with syphilization took place at the London Lock Hospital in the 1860s, but the investigators ultimately determined that the procedure was too protracted, painful, and disfiguring to make it worthwhile.[116]

Next was *malariotherapy.* Tertiary syphilis—particularly terminal generalized paresis of the insane (GPI)—was a major cause of psychiatric hospitalization in the eighteenth and nineteenth centuries. In 1917, the Austrian psychiatrist Julius Wagner-Jauregg (1857–1940) pioneered malariotherapy, a procedure by which patients with GPI were inoculated with *Plasmodium vivax* parasites—which causes a milder form of malaria—for the purposes of inducing a fever. It had been observed as far back as the fifteenth century by Díaz de Isla that high fever had therapeutic value in the treatment of syphilis, a temperature-sensitive infection. After a few cycles of induced fever, the malaria was eradicated with quinine, and the patients showed improvement in mental status. Six of nine of Wagner-Jauregg's patients either completely recovered or showed dramatic improvement; an international study referenced by Kragh showed 53 percent had a partial or complete recovery.[117] Approximately 13 percent died of malaria from the protocol.[118] Wagner-Jauregg was awarded the Nobel Prize for Medicine in 1927 for his discovery of malariotherapy, also known as pyrotherapy. However, he became a controversial figure in 2004 when it was discovered that, toward the end of his life, he was a Nazi sympathizer and proponent of eugenics and forced sterilization. He had applied to be a member of the Nazi Party, but was rejected because his first wife was Jewish. An Austrian commission scrutinized his life and writings in 2004; and after finding no racial hygiene terminology in his writings about eugenics, then a mainstream international scientific debate, the commission determined that Wagner-Jauregg "should not be seen as a man with a dubious history."[119]

The next regrettable event in the modern history of syphilis is known as the *American Plan,* or the Chamberlain-Kahn Act of 1918. In an effort to prevent the spread of venereal diseases among US troops fighting in World War I, the act gave the US government the authority to isolate any woman suspected of having a sexually transmitted infection (STI). Diseases such as syphilis were rampant among the US military; as many as one in three soldiers could be out of commission with an STI at any given time. In addition to the closure of many of the red-light districts all across the United States, any woman found without an escort within five miles of a military base could be arrested and forced to submit to a gynecological exam. She could be detained (often for several months) until it could be proven that she did not have an STI or until she was cured of the disease.[120] Directed solely against women, the plan resulted in the detainment of over 15,000 sex workers during the war.[121]

The last and most egregious program was known officially as the *Tuskegee Study of Untreated Syphilis in the Negro Male* (1932–1972). In order to learn more about the natural history of untreated syphilis, 600 black men of Macon County, Alabama—399 with syphilis and a control group of 201 without it—were followed for over 40 years and never given any treatment for the disease; they were prevented from receiving penicillin even after it was proven to be effective as a treatment for syphilis in 1947. In exchange for free medical exams and meals, the men willingly participated in this prospective experiment. They were misled into believing that they were being treated for "bad blood," a general slang term for ailments such as anemia and fatigue, and they were given no informed consent as to the true nature of the study. By the end of the study in 1972, 28 participants had died of syphilis, 40 wives had been infected, and 19 children had acquired the infection congenitally.[122] The arguments of scholars who in trying to avoid presentism have attempted to revise the history of the Tuskegee Study have not found many adherents in the mainstream.[123]

As a side note, the Tuskegee Study had been preceded by a retrospective analysis done in Oslo, Norway, from 1891 to 1910. The nephew of Carl Boeck of Hansen's disease fame, Caesar Boeck (1845–1917) was a Norwegian dermatologist who was convinced that all of the available treatments for syphilis were inadequate. He followed 2000 Norwegian syphilitics over time without attempting treatment and kept detailed notes about the natural history of primary and secondary syphilis. The results of 473 of the cases were published in 1929, providing the basis for much of our understanding of the natural history of the disease.[124] Caesar Boeck is also famous for writing the classic description of sarcoidosis in 1899.

DERMATOLOGY'S CONTROVERSY

Albert Kligman (1916–2010), the famous twentieth-century dermatologist, discoverer of tretinoin, and modern pioneer in acne, allegedly conducted unethical pharmaceutical research on inmates at Holmesburg Prison in the 1950s–1970s. It was not uncommon for inmates in the United States to participate in pharmaceutical research at that time. Primarily involved in cosmetic and pharmaceutical testing, the inmates were also exposed, upon the direction of Kligman, to various potentially harmful substances, including dioxin, herpes simplex virus, vaccinia virus, human papillomavirus, and *Candida*.[125] Whether any of the prisoners, who were paid to participate in Kligman's trials, suffered any long-term harm is unclear. In 2000, a lawsuit against Kligman, the University of Pennsylvania where Kligman worked, and Johnson & Johnson was thrown out because the statute of limitations had expired. Penn Medicine issued an apology for Dr. Kligman's research and instituted measures to alter the legacy of Dr. Kligman in August 2021.[126]

The turn of the twentieth century saw significant developments in syphilology, with the Germans making all of the achievements during this period. In 1905, the German zoologist Fritz Schaudinn (1871–1906) and dermatologist Erich Hoffmann (1868–1959) discovered *T. pallidum* in the tissue of a patient's eroded vulvar papule.[127] Hoffman credited Schaudinn—who died a year later of a gastrointestinal amoebic abscess at just 35 years of age—with the discovery, stating that his own role was only as the collector of the material.[128] A year after the discovery of the organism, the first blood test to detect the presence of infection was developed by August von Wassermann (1866–1925). In 1909, the arsenical compound known as salvarsan was discovered at the laboratory of the German Nobel Laureate Paul Ehrlich (1854–1915). Ehrlich had been searching for what he coined the *Zauberkugel*, a "magic bullet" for syphilis, a compound that could kill the microorganism but not harm the rest of the body; Ehrlich also coined the word "chemotherapy," denoting the same idea. Ehrlich's associate, Sahachiro Hata, was testing the 606th compound against the infection when salvarsan, initially known as "606" and Ehrlich's magic bullet, was discovered. Salvarsan hit the market in 1910 and instantly became one of the first blockbuster drugs. It was, however, fraught with side effects (nausea, vomiting, rashes, liver damage, and death) and required a cumbersome preparation process in that it was delivered by an excruciating intramuscular injection into the buttocks. A more stable and slightly less toxic version of the drug called neosalvarsan became available in 1912. It was more effective than mercury in the treatment of syphilis, but it was ultimately replaced by penicillin in the 1940s.

Within a few years of the introduction of penicillin, the prevalence and incidence of syphilis in the United States sharply declined, dropping from a peak of 443 cases per 100,000 people (1944) to 20–30 cases per 100,000 in the 1970s.[129] The incidence rose again in the 1980s and 1990s (to a peak of 54 cases per 100,000) in association with the epidemic of human immunodeficiency virus (HIV). After a nadir of 11.2 cases per 100,000 in 2000, the incidence of syphilis in the United States is steadily rising again. In 2019, there were 129,813 cases reported in the United States (39.7 cases per 100,000 people).

In 1955, the American Board of Dermatology and Syphilology, as it had been known since its inception in 1932, dropped syphilology from its name. With the introduction of penicillin, the decline in cases of syphilis rendered the title semi-obsolete. But when the AIDS epidemic began in the 1970s, American dermatologists, no longer the experts on sexually transmitted diseases, played an insignificant role in the response to this new epidemic.[130] Today, however, dermatologists receive excellent training in sexually transmitted diseases and are equipped with the knowledge and expertise to recognize the "Great Imitator" that is unsurpassed by any other specialty of medicine.

Summary

Syphilis is a disease of many names: "the Great Pox," *lues venerea*, *morbus gallicus*, and the "Great Imitator," among others. The origin of syphilis is a topic of intense controversy. On the one hand, the Columbian theory supporters contend that syphilis did not exist in Europe before the 1490s and was brought to the Old World by Columbus and his men. On the other hand, the pre-Columbianists present much evidence supporting the idea that syphilis was already in Europe dating back to ancient times. Until the discovery of serologic tests for syphilis in the early twentieth century, dermatology and syphilology were uniquely intertwined and inseparable. Many of the nineteenth-century contributors to the progress in syphilology were dermatologists. The wide variety and complexity of the cutaneous manifestations of the disease necessitated expertise in its clinical diagnosis; the indispensability of this expertise was a catalyst in the development of the specialty of dermatology. It must have been an extraordinary challenge to diagnose syphilis in a patient without a confirmatory blood test and then commit that patient to a toxic mercurial or arsenical treatment. Despite highly effective treatment, this 500+-year-old disease does not appear to be going away any time soon, and dermatologists and other clinicians must remain keenly aware of its presence and its myriad dermatological findings.

11

The Nineteenth Century

An Introduction

The modernization of Western medicine spanned several centuries and cannot be attributed to any one event. The evolving process that began during the Renaissance was accelerated by the Scientific Revolution and the Enlightenment, and after hundreds of years and numerous key developments in the nineteenth century, *physica* reached some semblance of today's medicine. We have seen in the previous chapters that the crucial first steps were the discovery of human anatomy and the advancement of surgical ligatures in the sixteenth century, followed by the comprehension of the circulatory system, the invention of the microscope, and the advocacy of therapeutic restraint in the seventeenth century. The eighteenth century saw the redefining of human physiology, the advent of the anatomical basis for disease, and the evidence-based reboot of the surgical discipline. The nineteenth century is for the history of medicine an extraordinary period when the most tremendous leaps forward took place, particularly in the period from 1850 to 1890. In the following section, we will explore the six major historical advancements in medicine during this period: the discoveries of anesthesia and antisepsis, the identification of microorganisms as a cause of disease, the end of the reign of Galenic humoral theory, the rise of women in medicine, and the arrival of formal medical specialization.

Similarly, the study of skin disease slowly advanced to its modern design over the sixteenth through nineteenth centuries. The most important early steps described in the preceding chapters were: the rise of skin disease to the level of a discipline worthy of focus and the first dermatology texts in Latin (Mercurialis) and in English (Turner); the first suggestion that the skin has its own diseases (Jessen); the appreciation of the skin as a structure with greater purpose than simply being an envelope (Lorry); the first attempt at clinicopathologic correlations for skin disease (Astruc); a call for specialization in skin disease and the coinage of the terms dermatology and dermatopathology (Jackson); and the first attempts at a modern nomenclature and classification system of skin diseases (Plenck). In the nineteenth century, the specialty of dermatology as we know it today was born, and that story is the main focus of the next five chapters.

Anesthesia

While the ancients appreciated the anesthetic properties of opium and alcohol, it was the great physicians of the Islamic Golden Age, e.g., Avicenna, Albucasis, and Avenzoar, who first formally wrote about general anesthesia. Avicenna described a sleep-inducing sponge, soaked in opium, applied to the face. The medieval surgeon Theodoric Borgognoni (1205–1296) was among the first to promote the use of an anesthetizing sponge in medieval surgery—one soaked in opium, mandrake, and hemlock. The field would develop no further until after the scientific revolution and the advances in chemistry, specifically regarding the compounds nitrous oxide, ether, and chloroform. Once these advances took place, pain and suffering could finally be alleviated during surgery, effectively doing away with the most barbaric aspect of ancient and medieval medicine.

The earliest pioneer in modern general anesthesia was Sir Humphry Davy (1778–1829), who wrote in 1800 that nitrous oxide, a gas first discovered by Joseph Priestley (1733–1804), could induce reversible unconsciousness and remove pain during surgical operations.[1] He named it "laughing gas" because of its tendency to cause one to giggle; subsequently, laughing gas parties became a popular pastime in the early

DOI: 10.1201/9781003273622-17

1800s, especially in the United States. In 1844, an American dentist named Horace Wells (1815–1848) successfully used nitrous oxide in a tooth extraction, and the gas found its niche in dentistry, where it is still used to this day.

The story of ether anesthesia began in mid-nineteenth-century America and is indeed a strange one. Ether, discovered in 1540 by the German Valerius Cordus (1515–1544), had properties similar to nitrous oxide but was more powerful.[2] Among its advocates were the American surgeon Crawford Long (1815–1878), who first used ether in 1842 to painlessly excise a cyst of the neck but did not publish his work, and the American dentist William Morton (1819–1868), who first publicly demonstrated ether anesthesia in 1846. Morton received all of the acclaims for the discovery and is considered the father of modern anesthesia by some, even though Long used ether successfully four years prior.

Morton's public accolades triggered a rivalry of other claimants for the honors. Charles Jackson (1805–1880), Morton's mentor, claimed that Morton had stolen the idea from him, but Jackson had a habit of claiming he discovered things. Jackson also contended he had discovered the telegraph before Samuel Morse, digestive physiology before William Beaumont, and guncotton before Christian Schonbein did.[3] While Jackson's proponents claim that "the available evidence overwhelmingly backs up Jackson on all counts," his opponents succeeded in marginalizing Jackson with convincing defenses of their claims and attacks on his character.[4] Jackson lost his mind, supposedly from seeing all the honors given to Morton, and ended up in a mental institution.[5]

Another claimant was Horace Wells, who also contended that his work with nitrous oxide in 1844 gave him the real claim to the discovery of anesthesia. His claims failed, however, and Wells, who became addicted to chloroform, ended up committing suicide in jail, his incarceration a result of being found guilty of throwing sulfuric acid on two prostitutes. Morton fell out of favor with the medical community when he tried to get rich from his discovery, and he died of a stroke at 49 years of age.[6] Perhaps Crawford Long is most worthy of the honorific, "the founder of anesthesia."

Anesthesia was quickly adopted as a standard procedure in American and European surgery. Because of ether's irritating effects on the lungs and its tendency to induce nausea, chloroform, discovered in 1831, replaced it as the principal anesthetizing chemical.[7] The most important early proponent of chloroform was James Simpson (1811–1870), a Scottish obstetrician. Since receiving general anesthesia was, as it is today, not without risk, topical anesthesia for dental and minor ophthalmological procedures was introduced later, with cocaine being the first compound used for this purpose. Sigmund Freud (1856–1939) was among the first to recognize its numbing effects, and Merck & Co. began to market cocaine as a topical anesthetic in the 1880s.[8] Today, dermatologists use local anesthesia regularly and can perform elaborate surgical procedures with their patients wide awake.

Antisepsis

The next key development in medicine in the nineteenth century was the advent of antisepsis. Prior to this discovery, infection and mortality rates from surgical procedures were extremely high. Hospitals were very unclean places. In 1795, the Scottish physician Alexander Gordon (1752–1799) was the first to propose that *materies morbi* (morbid substances) transmitted from the physician to the patient was a cause of disease.[9] The disease in question was puerperal fever (childbed fever), a potentially fatal infection now known to be caused by *Streptococcus pyogenes*, the same bacteria that causes the skin infection erysipelas. Decades later, the Hungarian physician Ignaz Semmelweis (1818–1865) observed at the Vienna General Hospital that medical students who went directly from autopsies to the labor and delivery ward had worse outcomes (maternal mortality rate) than midwives who only focused on obstetrics. He first demonstrated in 1847 that the use of chlorinated disinfectants on the contaminating hands of these medical students reduced the incidence of puerperal fever and saved lives. Prior to the emergence of germ theory, however, neither Gordon nor Semmelweis was able to convince the medical community at large that physicians were unintentionally responsible for the death of their patients; therefore, handwashing was ignored. Frustrated by his critics, Semmelweis became so erratic that he ended up in a mental institution, where he spent his last days lamenting the doctors who refused to wash their hands.[10]

It is possible that general paresis of the insane was the cause of his mental illness (see Interlude 3).[11] Interestingly, it was Ferdinand von Hebra, a hero of Chapter 14, who compassionately lured his friend Semmelweis to the asylum under the pretenses they were to tour a new facility. Semmelweis, upon realizing where he was headed, fought with some guards, suffered an injury, and died of an infection in his wounds in a dark cell two weeks later.[12]

The British surgeon Joseph Lister (1827–1912) ultimately convinced the world of the benefits of antiseptic measures to protect surgical wounds from infection. After studying the research of Louis Pasteur (see below), Lister was convinced that airborne germs in unclean hospitals were responsible for surgical complications such as putrefaction, gangrene, and sepsis; if these germs were killed or prevented from entering the wound, Lister believed these complications would be less common. In 1867, Lister published "On the antiseptic principle in the practice of surgery" in the *Lancet*, proving that cleaning and dressing wounds with the antiseptic chemical carbolic acid (phenol) and spraying the surgical instruments and operating room with carbolic lowered mortality rates in amputations (16/35 died without antisepsis and 6/40 died with antisepsis).[13] But surgeons in Europe and the United States were not quick to accept the conclusions of Lister's research, and Lister and his core of backers had to campaign for the adoption of his ideas. It was not until 1875 in Europe and 1876 in the United States that Lister's persistence finally paid off, and Listerian antisepsis had enough supporting hospitals to reach the orthodox status it still holds today.

Surgeons and obstetricians used their unsanitized bare hands to perform surgery until the 1870s, when Lister's measures finally took hold. Gloves came decades later, invented around 1890 when the American surgeon and a founder of Johns Hopkins Hospital, William Halsted (1852–1922), had the first surgical glove created by Goodyear Rubber Company for his chief nurse and fiancée, Caroline Hampton. The reason behind the invention was not antisepsis-related; it was dermatological. Caroline suffered with dermatitis of her arms and hands from contact with mercuric chloride solution used in the surgical prep.[14]

The Germ Theory of Disease

The history of antisepsis is intertwined with the history of the germ theory of disease, and antisepsis represents the first major practical application of germ theory. This union of science and medicine did more to save lives than possibly any intervention in history until that point. Prior to the mid-nineteenth century and dating back to ancient times, a dominant theory behind the source of many diseases held that the cause was miasma or "bad air." It was literally believed that breathing air that smelled bad could make you sick. Miasma theory was strengthened as Europeans became less tolerant of stench in the late eighteenth century.[15] One can only imagine the smells in the air on the crowded streets of London or Paris during the population expansion of the eighteenth century. A competing theory, contagion, ended up on a collision course with miasma in the 1800s. Contagion had been hinted at by the medieval Islamic physicians, first formerly suggested by Fracastoro in 1546, later given a sturdy foundation in 1675, when Leeuwenhoek discovered bacteria, and contagion was heralded again by the Austrian physician Marcus Antonius von Plenciz (1705–1786) in 1762. The theory of contagion suggested that disease could be transmitted from person to person by "animalcules" that caused disease upon entering the body. The debates between contagion and miasma escalated in the nineteenth century.

The Great Stink of London (1858) and the nineteenth-century British cholera epidemics provide the backdrop that ultimately led to contagion replacing miasma under the modern designation, the "germ theory of disease." The Great Stink occurred in central London and resulted from such a massive accumulation of raw sewage in the River Thames—in combination with hot August temperatures—that famed English scientist Michael Faraday (1791–1867) once wrote, the "feculence rolled up in clouds so dense that they were visible at the surface."[16] Suffering the impossible stench, the citizens feared the miasma rising from the Thames as a cause of deadly cholera.

Cholera is a potentially fatal infection of the intestines caused by *Vibrio cholerae*, which manifests as severe watery diarrhea. There were six major worldwide cholera pandemics from 1817 to 1923, with millions of people dying over the course of 100-plus years. In 1858, cholera was undoubtedly on the minds of Londoners since the deadliest cholera epidemic in the city's history had ended eight years prior, with a more minor outbreak occurring in 1854. During that episode in Soho, the London physician John Snow (1813–1858), by using case mapping to trace the outbreak to a specific drinking water supply, effectively ended the outbreak by removing the handle to the Broad Street pump, concluding that contaminated drinking water caused cholera, not miasma.[17] Although he did not identify a chemical or microscopic source of the problem and the world around him was not yet ready for the idea of fecal-oral contamination, Snow's work with public hygiene foreshadowed the great revolution in medicine—the germ theory of disease.

The two men most responsible for proving the germ theory of disease were Louis Pasteur (1822–1895) and Robert Koch (1843–1910). Pasteur was a French biologist and chemist who is also known for his work with the chemistry of crystals, fermentation, pasteurization, and the vaccination for rabies and anthrax. After heat sterilization of broth placed in swan-neck bottles, Pasteur proved that contamination from the air led to a microbial presence in the broth, thus disproving the theory of spontaneous generation that had endured for two millennia, which stated that decay, putrefaction, and fermentation—along with microbial organisms in the body—were spontaneously generated by the *pneuma* within organic substances.[18] Pasteur's conclusion that contaminating germs—and not miasma—were a cause of disease was built on a foundation laid by four influential pioneers: the aforementioned Semmelweis; the Italian Agostino Bassi (1773–1856) who first identified (1835) a fungus that infects silkworms; the German physician Johann Schoënlein (1793–1864) who showed that tinea favosa (favus) was caused by *Trichophyton schoenleinii* (1839); and Miles J. Berkeley (1803–1889) who hypothesized (1846) that the fungus *Phytophthora infestans* was the cause of the Irish Potato Famine (1845–1849).[19]

Pasteur first got involved with microbiology in 1865 when his country was in the midst of an epidemic disease that was killing silkworms. After determining the cause of the demise of the silkworms to actually be two different diseases, each associated with its own microorganism, Pasteur arrived in 1870 at the correct conclusion that all infectious diseases were caused by microorganisms. In 1880, he wrote about what we today refer to as a staph infection:

> It appears that every furuncle contains an aerobic microscopic parasite, to which is due the local inflammation and the pus formation that follows.[20]

The statement is significant for not only mandating the presence of an organism in the lesion but also because Pasteur correctly noted that the mere presence of the foreign invader caused an inflammatory response from the body. His groundbreaking assertions replaced the fallacious, still-thriving notion that the cause of infectious diseases was humoral imbalance.

While Pasteur laid the foundation for the theory, his younger German contemporary and rival, Robert Koch, formalized germ theory into a set of principles known today as "Koch's postulates." A physician and microbiologist, Koch was the first to grow bacteria on culture media. In addition, he identified the bacteria responsible for three critical diseases of the nineteenth century: anthrax, tuberculosis, and cholera. His postulates, published in 1890, served as guidelines for establishing whether a microbe was the cause of a disease. His four postulates were: (1) the microbe is found in all persons or organisms with the disease, but not in the healthy; (2) the microbe is isolated and cultured from a diseased person or organism; (3) introduction of the cultured microbe into a healthy person causes the disease; and (4) the microbe from the inoculated person or organism is isolated and identified as the same as the original microbe.[21] Koch's postulates have since proven to be inapplicable to certain viral diseases, carrier-state bacterial diseases, and treponemal diseases such as syphilis, but they nevertheless remain a starting point for understanding the nature of infectious disease.

Alone together at a frontier, Pasteur and Koch were giants of nineteenth-century science, and the two men developed a tense relationship, which in the early 1880s, erupted into a full-blown rivalry. The antagonism was naturally fueled by nationalistic friction between France and Germany and complicated by language barriers. Today, both men are equally acknowledged for their contributions to germ theory.

Cell Theory and the End of Galenic Medicine

A series of discoveries and new understandings of anatomy, physiology, and pathology over the course of the nineteenth century dealt blow after blow to humoral medicine. This was the era in which biology—the study of life—rose to prominence as a scientific discipline. Intense investigation and observation of all forms of life replaced philosophical (Aristotelian) explanations for biological processes. These events took place during a period represented by the work of the father of evolution, Charles Darwin (1809–1892), and the father of genetics, Gregor Mendel (1822–1884).

The nature and purpose of the cell, first discovered by Robert Hooke (1635–1703) in 1665, was not explained until 1839 when German botanist Matthias Schleiden (1804–1881) and his physiologist colleague Theodor Schwann (1810–1882) published the following principle: all living organisms consist of either a single cell or are made up of cells, the basic units of life. And thus, the era of cell theory began. Cell theory brought the study of anatomy, physiology, and pathology from a macroscopic, fluid-based (humor-based) or even organ-based level to a microscopic one. It was only a matter of time before the physicians and scientists of the nineteenth theory could no longer rectify Galenic theory with the discoveries of the period.

NINETEENTH-CENTURY ANATOMY AND PHYSIOLOGY

The countless contributions from the anatomists and physiologists of the era are beyond the scope of this book, but the most important figures were France's Marie Francois Xavier Bichat (1771–1802), who founded the field of histology by focusing his research on tissues rather than organs; Claude Bernard (1813–1878), the father of modern physiology who firmly established scientific experimentation as the primary means of investigating physiologic principles; Germany's Johannes Müller (1801–1858), author of the most important text on physiology in the nineteenth century; and Friedrich Gustav Jakob Henle (1809–1885), the microscopist who described the hair follicle, named the outer layer of the inner root sheath, and first discovered the *Demodex* mite—in cerumen—in 1841.

Rudolf Virchow (1821–1902), the founder of modern pathology, was a German physician and biologist who added to cell theory in 1855: *omnia cellula e cellula*, "all cells come from [other] cells." While it was an idea he may have plagiarized from Robert Remak (1815–1860), Virchow was an acute observer of the cell in its healthy and pathologic states.[22] He was the first to recognize cancer cells as having arisen from normal cells, and the first to identify and coin leukemia as a disease of blood cells. Virchow elucidated thromboembolic disease, i.e., clots moving from the leg to the lungs. But his greatest achievement was his founding of the field of cellular pathology, epitomized in his publication *Die Cellularpathologie*, "Cellular Pathology" (1858), the most significant publication in the history of medicine since Morgagni's *De sedibus* in the previous century. His efforts to persuade his medical students to "think microscopically" represented a paradigm shift in how physicians thought about disease. While Morgagni localized illness to a specific location in the body, Virchow narrowed the focus even further to a cellular level within that location. After Virchow, there was no longer any room for discussion of the all-of-a-sudden nonsensical concept of humoral imbalance.

Observations of the cell were possible because of the increasingly mainstream use of much-improved microscopes in the academic institutions of Europe, especially Germany. The different anatomical structures of the skin, first gazed upon with the microscope in the seventeenth century, had all been identified by the end of the nineteenth century (see Table 11.1). Many of the discoverers of the skin's microscopic structures were German and disciples of the great Johannes Müller.

TABLE 11.1

Discovery of the Components of Skin

Layers of the epidermis	1665—Marcello Malpighi (1628–1694)	Discovered the stratum granulosum
	1894—Paul Gerson Unna (1850–1929)	
Sebaceous glands	1698—Marcello Malpighi	
Sweat ducts and glands	1664—Nicholas Steno (1638–1686)	Sweat glands (predicted)
	1665—Marcello Malpighi	Sweat pores/ducts
	1833—Johann Purkinje (1787–1869)	Sweat glands (discovered)
	1834—Gilbert Breschet (1784–1845) and Augustin Roussel de Vauzeme (1754–1837)	Sweat glands (discovered)
Fibroblasts	1858—Rudolf Virchow (1821–1902)	
Melanocytes	1819—Giosué Sangiovanni (1775–1849)	First discovered on squid
Langerhans cell	1868—Paul Langerhans (1847–1888)	
Pacinian corpuscles	1717—Abraham Vater (1684–1751)	Vater's research was lost and the corpuscles were rediscovered by Pacini
	1831—Filippo Pacini (1812–1883)	
Merkel cells	1875—Friedrich Sigmund Merkel (1845–1919)	Called *Tastzellen* ("touch") cells
Ruffini corpuscles	1891—Angelo Ruffini (1864–1929)	
Meissner's corpuscles	1852—Georg Meissner (1829–1905)	Both men contended to have discovered independently
	1852—Rudolf Wagner (1805–1864)	
Outer layer of inner root sheath of hair follicle	1841—Jacob Henle (1809–1885)	
Inner layer of inner root sheath of hair follicle	1845—Thomas Huxley (1825–1895)	At 19 years of age

Clinical Medicine in the Nineteenth Century

While the scientists edged closer and closer to a proper understanding of the nature of disease, the clinicians of the nineteenth century increasingly applied an investigative approach to symptomatology, diagnosis, and therapeutics. The greatest clinician of the first half of the century was French physician René-Théophile-Hyacinthe Laënnec (1781–1826), who invented the stethoscope in 1816, and published the first work on auscultation in 1819, thus elevating the physical examination to its position as a crucial step in the diagnostic process. He also wrote the first descriptions of cirrhosis and bronchiectasis and penned brilliant characterizations of several other pulmonary diseases, including pneumonia and phthisis (tuberculosis).

The most exemplary representative of clinical medicine in the latter half of the century was William Osler (1849–1919). Born in Canada, Osler was the first professor of medicine at Johns Hopkins Medical School in Baltimore. In addition to introducing the American medical education system to bedside teaching, Osler made numerous contributions to medicine, including—but not limited to—descriptions of stomach cancer, abdominal tumors, endocarditis, and cerebral palsy. His most famous publication, "Principles and Practice of Medicine" (1892), was, according to Castiglioni writing in 1958, "the leading one-volume textbook on the subject of our time, if not any time."[23] His next-door neighbor and friend in Baltimore was Harvey Cushing (1869–1939), the man who was to neurosurgery what Osler was to general medicine. In addition to his medical achievements, Cushing won the Pulitzer Prize for a two-volume biography of Osler in 1926.[24]

With any talk of the humors obsolete, it seemed inevitable that the archaic therapeutic intervention of bloodletting would see its last days. The practice persisted into the twentieth century and is still used today for blood diseases such as polycythemia, hemochromatosis (excessive iron in the body), and the dermatological condition called porphyria cutanea tarda (see Interlude 2). Some scholars consider the discussion of bloodletting—particularly as a treatment for pneumonia, heatstroke, and six other indications—found in Osler's masterpiece (as late as the 1947 edition) to be his "blind spot."[25] Bryan pointed out, however, that Osler's inclusion of bloodletting reflected the opinions of his era's leading clinicians and do not indicate what he himself actually did for his own sick patients.[26] But by the twentieth century, the reflexive use of bloodletting for many different conditions—a practice that expedited the deaths of George Washington and Mozart and countless others—was no longer mainstream medicine.

Osler's greatest legacy was the inspiration for generation after generation of physicians to be the most compassionate, learned, and hard-working physicians they could be. The physician of today can find no greater role model than Osler, who taught the value of hard work and careful and accurate observation and who demonstrated charm, cordiality, goodwill, and a "deep interest in everything beautiful and noble" that made him one of medicine's greatest leaders.[27]

The Rise of Women in Medicine

In 2022, more women attend US medical schools than men, but for the better part of human existence, the overwhelming majority of medical practitioners were men. The rise of women in medicine began in the nineteenth century. Prior to this time period, women had always been engaged in the healing arts—think of Hildegard of Bingen or Trota of Trotula or the countless midwives, healers, etc., dating back to ancient times—but they were professionally excluded from enrolling in universities. For all but the last 150 years, women could find no place for themselves in a professional world dominated by men, who deemed them psychologically unfit for the vocation, at risk for sterility and hysteria with such intellectual pursuits, and best suited for life in the home as a wife and mother.[28]

Slowly but surely, these male-supremacist sentiments ebbed to the point when the first woman was admitted to a medical school. It took the dispensation of an enlightened despot, Frederick the Great, to get Dorothea Erxleben (1715–1762) admitted to a university in Germany. She graduated in 1754. A trend of admitting women did not follow, however, and it would take another 100 years before women could get a foot in the door of the medical schools of the world. The American pioneer Elizabeth Blackwell (1821–1910) is most often cited as the world's first woman to receive a medical doctorate from a university. She entered medical school at Geneva Medical College in Geneva, New York, in 1847 and graduated in 1849. The first medical schools in the world for women appeared around this time: New England Female Medical College in Boston in 1848 and the Women's Medical College of Pennsylvania in 1850.

Among the first female dermatologists in the world were Scotland's Agnes Forbes Blackadder (1875–1964), Boston's Loretta Joy Cummins (1883–1958), Philadelphia's Rose Hirschler (1875–1940), and New York's Daisy Maude Orleman Robinson (1869–1942). The question of which of these was the first female dermatologist is a matter of debate and depends on whether appointment, residency completion, or board certification is the criterion by which "first" is determined. Orleman Robinson was appointed to New York's Northwestern Dispensary as attending dermatologist in 1905, and Blackadder was appointed as consultant dermatologist at St. John's Hospital two years later. In 1921, Hirschler was the first woman in the United States to graduate in dermatology and is the most famous of the first female dermatologists. She was the first woman in the world to chair a department of dermatology—at Women's Medical College in Philadelphia (1936). Her academic interests included X-ray therapy and syphilis. In 1916, Cummins was hired as an assistant dermatologist at Mass General Hospital, and in 1928, the first woman to pass the board exam. With these women leaders breaking ground, women have made tremendous strides in the field of dermatology over the last century. In the United States, 49.9 percent of practicing dermatologists were women as of 2021, and 61 percent of dermatology trainees are women as of 2018.[29]

Formal Medical Specialization

The establishment of formal medical specialties is the last of the six major developments in the nineteenth century that gave Western medicine at the time a definitively modern quality. We have seen that the ancient Egyptians had their medical specialists, and according to Galen, the ancient Romans also had them.[30] Indeed, specialist healers and so-called experts for specific conditions, many of whom were quacks, performed procedures and peddled their remedies from time immemorial, but specialists among the learned physician elite were practically non-existent since ancient Roman times. While some degree of specialization emerged in Paris in the 1830s, it was not until the latter half of the nineteenth century that the need for specialists in medicine became apparent throughout Europe and in the United States. Two driving forces behind specialization were: the need to expand medical knowledge, which is best achieved by concentrating cases of the same types of diseases for focused physicians to observe; and the need to manage the health of large populations of patients, with the most efficient means of accomplishing that goal being to gather individuals of the same category of disease.[31]

The first specialties were pediatrics, surgery, obstetrics and gynecology, ophthalmology, and psychiatry; each of these fields requires specialized knowledge and is very different from general medicine. The founding of a specialty is generally associated with one or more physicians who either made significant discoveries in the field or devoted most or all of their energies to the specialty. Many of these founders practiced in the nineteenth century, although the father of modern pediatrics, the Swede Nils von Rosenstein (1707–1773), practiced in the eighteenth century. The aforementioned Hunter, Lister, and Halstead have each been called the father of modern surgery. The American J. Marion Sims (1813–1883) is considered the founder of modern obstetrics and gynecology, but his legacy is tarnished by the fact that he experimented on unanesthetized enslaved Black women. The careers of the French physicians Philippe Pinel (1745–1826) and Jean-Marie Charcot (1825–1893) represent the beginning of modern psychiatry and neurology, respectively. The invention of the ophthalmoscope in 1851 allowed for ophthalmology to become a specialty in its own right. Endocrinology started with France's Charles-Édouard Brown-Séquard (1817–1894) but did not reach legitimacy until the discovery of insulin in the 1920s. The American William Beaumont (1785–1853) solved gastric physiology by 1838, but the German Ismar Boas (1858–1938) is considered the first gastroenterologist, having opened a digestive medicine clinic in 1886; he also founded the first journal devoted to gastroenterology in 1895. The invention of the electrocardiogram by Willem Einthoven (1860–1927) in 1895 signaled the birth of cardiology as a specialty. Hugh Thomas (1834–1891) and his nephew Robert Jones (1857–1933) helped establish orthopedics as specialties. Neurosurgery, urology, rheumatology, and nephrology are specialties that developed in the twentieth century.

Quacks

Before we delve deeper into the history of dermatology in the nineteenth century, let us diverge for a brief discussion of a topic that cannot be overestimated as significant in this story: quackery. It is impossible to separate the history of quackery from the history of dermatology, as the two were intertwined. Before dermatology emerged as a formal discipline in the nineteenth century, the surgeons unwillingly shared the responsibility for the care of dermatologic problems with quacks. The term "quack," which refers to a dishonest, untrained practitioner of medicine, is a shorter version of the word "quacksalver," i.e., one who falsely claims that the salves or ointments or oils, such as snake oil, which he or she peddles could be applied to the skin and deliver curative powers. Their treatments were considered dangerous and outlandish. As opposed to the cautious, deliberate, and prudent physician, quacks were deemed to be rash, inconsiderate, and desperate.[32]

Since ancient times charlatans have promised impossible cures that physicians could not deliver and that even the poor could afford. The advent of formal medical education during the Middle Ages did not reduce their numbers; if anything, it forced the quacks to sharpen their skills with the con. Using knowledge of human nature, which puts hope at a premium, quacks from the sixteenth century onward had their heyday. Confidence is everything in medicine; we tend to trust practitioners and salespeople who communicate confidently, regardless of the substance of the message.

There have been several explanations for this phenomenon, with the traditional basis resting on the quack's manipulative nature, coupled with the innate tendency toward gullibility in the populace.[33] Quacks thrived because, in many instances, their treatments actually worked, although success could result from the placebo effect or simply bestowed relief from a largely psychosomatic illness or rampant hypochondriasis. In contrast, the physician's treatments for various diseases were frequently ineffective, and the hypochondriac was all too often quickly dismissed. These imposters existed because they were not regulated. There were many sick people in Europe during the eighteenth and nineteenth centuries, fostering an abundance of different types of non-physician practitioners. Different personality types of patients, with the power to choose their own desired practitioner, allowed for a wide range of types of healthcare providers. Some patients, especially those with venereal diseases, preferred self-medication and the anonymity of the transaction with the quack. Quacks survived because of various economic developments of the period: economic growth, rising personal expectations, the extension of commercialization, consumer spending, and consumer psychology.[34] The medical profession was in part responsible for the free reign of the quack, especially among the lower classes. The doctors lacked the unity to fight these impostors and get laws passed to prohibit their meddling, and "their grave manner, proud mien, robes, use of Latin terms, aloof conduct, and charges intimidated common patients" who often preferred the warmth and feigned compassion of the quack.[35]

But most of all, quacks existed because their spiels, their handbills, their ads, their showmanship, their charisma—it all just worked. The performances were mini spectacles meant to entice, excite, and impress a willing audience.[36] Dressed in garb designed to catch the eye, the quack performed on a mobile stage that gave him some advantage in height. A stooge lured in the crowd with comic relief in front of a stage decorated with various live animal props, surgical instruments, and banners, while music elevated the excitement. Testimonials and fake certificates were posted all around and handed out to the crowd. In this setting, making a deal with at least a small portion of the public was not all that difficult.

Quacks offered cures for two main categories of diseases: the severe and unpleasant chronic diseases such as dropsy, gout, agues (fevers such as malaria), scurvy, consumption (tuberculosis), rheumatism, and the king's evil, as well as diseases that affected appearance such as growths, sores, scabs, ulcers, wounds, swellings, tumors, cancers, ringworms, and facial redness.[37] Beauty creams targeting women promised relief from redness, pimples, roughness, scurf, freckles, and wrinkles, smallpox pits, unwanted hair, and body odor.[38]

At the turn of the twentieth century, "skin-quacks" continued to thrive because they filled a void left by mainstream medicine. As pointed out by Gowing-Middleton in his 1904 treatise, *The Skin and Skin-Quacks*, physicians did not want to be bothered with mundane cutaneous complaints or problems they did not recognize as problems,

> If a lady tells her doctor that she is annoyed to find that her skin is not so clear as it ordinarily is, or if a man consults his medical man about some spots on his face and body, unless there is some regular and well-known skin disease, with very few exceptions the physician will pooh-pooh the matter, will not investigate it, or seek further for its cause: this is I think, to some extent, the explanation of the existence of the host of "Skin-Quacks" who flourish in every large town in England, the United States, and on the Continent, for people are often heard to say, "Doctors really don't understand these things."

> Many of the slighter skin affections are passed over by the regular practitioner as being out of his way, or beneath his dignity to trouble about. And so the lady who is worried about the abnormal yellowness of her Skin, or the man with his blotches, are thrown into the hands of the many charlatans who are always on the lookout for such customers.[39]

Fortunately, as dermatology grew into a popular field to practice medicine in the twentieth century, the relatively minor concerns of the patient, including the cosmetic complaints, were taken more seriously by the dermatologist, whose focus today is every type of defect in the skin, from the severe to the slight, from the medical to the cosmetic. The day of the Skin-Quack is now over. Or is it?

THE ULTIMATE SACRIFICE

Daniel Alcides Carrión García (1857–1885) was a nineteenth-century Peruvian medical student who made the ultimate sacrifice in the name of medical knowledge. Oroya fever and *verruga peruana*, "Peruvian warts," are the acute and chronic forms, respectively, of infection with the bacterium *Bartonella bacilliformis*. The former is characterized by fever, malaise, enlarged liver and spleen, and swollen glands; while in the latter, the afflicted develops numerous red, wart-like nodules all over the body. The infectious disease is endemic to Peru and other parts of South America. Carrión was the first to prove that the two conditions were related as phases of the same disease. He did so by inoculating himself with material from the wart of a patient with verruga peruana. Not long after, Carrión died of Oroya fever. The government of Peru declared Carrión a national hero, and the two diseases he linked are collectively now known as Carrión's disease.

The Rise of Dermatology as a Specialty of Medicine

Dermatology materialized as a specialty in the late nineteenth century. Because events and discoveries were transpiring simultaneously in different locations throughout the West, this history will be organized geographically rather than chronologically. The settings for the story are seven European cities—Florence, London, Paris, Vienna, Breslau, Berlin, and Hamburg—and three American cities—New York, Boston, and Philadelphia.

While its renown for artistic achievement had waned after its flourishing in the fifteenth and sixteenth centuries, Florence had a lasting tradition for contributions to scientific knowledge, starting with the career of Galileo (1564–1642). In 1657, the *Accademia del Cimento* (Academy of Experiment) was founded as one of the world's first scientific societies. In the seventeenth century, Florence and nearby Pisa saw the careers of such scientific giants as Marcello Malpighi, Giovanni Borelli, and Francesco Redi flourish.

In medicine, however, Florence never equaled the nearby centers of excellence in Salerno, Bologna, and Padua. In fact, for most of the three-century-long reign of the Medici family, medical students were moved out of Florence and trained in Pisa. Founded in 1288, the Santa Maria Nuova Hospital is the oldest in Florence—and one of the oldest continuously running hospitals in the world—but it was known more for its artistic decorations than its medical discoveries. It was not until the late eighteenth century that the enlightened despot, Leopold II (1747–1792), Holy Roman emperor and once Grand Duke of Tuscany, assured Florence a place in the history of medicine when he restored the Ospedale di Bonifazio (Bonfacio) there in the 1780s. Sympathetic to the mentally ill, Leopold appointed the like-minded Vincenzo Chiarugi (1759–1820) as medical director of this hospital designated for the insane and incurables. Chiarugi is an important figure in the history of medicine because of his seminal humanitarian reforms in the treatment of mentally ill persons. His efforts, however, have been overshadowed by the actions of the great Philippe Pinel, who instigated comparable reforms in France and brought about a modern, compassionate approach to dealing with the clinically insane.

Concomitant with his particular interest in the management of the mentally ill, Chiarugi also devoted energy to the diagnosis and treatment of skin diseases. Patients with syphilis and chronic skin diseases were deemed incurable; curiously, they found themselves alongside the insane in the Bonifacio Hospital. Years of making rounds on the schizophrenics and the psoriatics fostered expertise in skin disease, and in 1802, the university appointed Chiarugi an honorary lecturer on skin disease and mental illness. In 1810, he became a full professor with the title of "Professor of Cutaneous Disease and Mental Disturbances."[40]

Northern Italy suffered from a pellagra epidemic starting in the mid-eighteenth century, and Chiarugi took an interest in the burgeoning field of pellagrology. Building on the work of several Italian pellagrologists such as Francesco Fanzago (1764–1836) and Giambattista Marzari (1755–1827), Chiarugi was in a perfect position to have a say in the local public health crisis involving a disease with cutaneous and mental symptomatology. In his lengthy treatise on the subject, Chiarugi focused in vivid detail on the skin rash, which he believed was the most distinct feature of the syndrome.[41] While his colleagues compared pellagra to leprosy or scurvy, Chiarugi, using Cullen's classification system, classified it under the class "cachexia," order "impetigo."[42] He correctly recognized the sun's role in the rash and that pellagra was more common in regions where maize was the dietary staple. It would be another hundred years before the etiology of pellagra was fully worked out, but Chiarugi's professorship on skin disease and mental health lent him the weight needed to become an authority on a local public health issue greatly in need of an explanation.

In 1807, he authored a two-volume treatise on skin disease entitled *Trattato teorico-pratico delle malattie cutanee sordide in genere e in specie*, "Theoretical and practical treatise on sordid cutaneous diseases in genus and species." The word *sordide* is an intriguing choice of adjective for skin diseases. Chiarugi explains in the introduction that he chose that word because skin diseases are more or less "abominable" or "despicable," the latter being the best translation of the word *sordide*.[43] The first volume is a general discussion on skin disease: the structure of the skin, its physiology, the causes of skin disease, and its treatment. The second volume, "on skin disease in particular," contains individual chapters on skin diseases, categorized by Chiarugi's system: papular diseases (impetigo and herpes), pustular diseases (psydrachia, rosacea, scabies, ringworm, lepra), vesicular diseases (hydroa, scabies, achor), macular diseases (ephelides, ecchymoses), and organic diseases (nevi, vitiligo).

Vincenzo Chiarugi was the first professor of dermatology, but unfortunately, there was no one to fill his shoes in Florence, and the professorship was abandoned after his death in 1820. Chiarugi's career is significant as it was one of the first examples of specialization in dermatology and an initial attempt to institutionalize formal training in the field.

Summary

By the early nineteenth century, skin disease had risen to the level of a discipline worthy of focus, and the skin had fallen under the dominion of the physicians, who had willingly taken it away from the surgeons. The elevation of the study of skin diseases coincided with an increasing appreciation of the skin as a structure with greater purpose than simply being an envelope, the understanding that the skin could have its own resident diseases, a call for specialization in skin disease, the coinage of the terms "dermatology" and "dermatopathology," and the first attempts at a nomenclature and classification system of skin diseases. The diseases known at the time—herpes, dartres, tetters, impetigo, etc.—were inconsistently defined and unrecognizable for the most part to us today. A first small step toward bringing order to this chaos—the establishment of a professorship—took place in Florence, but it did not last.

12

The British School

The first of three major schools responsible for shaping the study of skin diseases into a formal specialty is known as the British School. In the eighteenth century, Britain was the home of two important surgeons in this story: Daniel Turner, the first dermatologist, and John Hunter, the first modern surgeon. In the last decade of that century, the British physician Seguin Henry Jackson called for the establishment of the specialty in his groundbreaking text, *Dermato-pathologia*. Two years prior to that landmark publication, the Medical Society of London awarded their prize, the Fothergill Gold Medal, to a 33-year-old physician named Robert Willan, who, after 9 years of medical practice, had created a new system of organizing skin diseases. After 18 years of modification, Willan's arrangement emerged in a landmark publication, and his achievement would go down in history as the most significant publication in the history of dermatology.

Robert Willan (1757–1812)

Robert Willan was born on November 12, 1757, near Sedbergh in the Yorkshire Dales of northwest England. He attended the Sedbergh School, where he became a Latin and Greek scholar, also excelling in mathematics. Because he was a Quaker, Willan could not matriculate at Oxford or Cambridge for medical school; consequently, he attended the more progressive University of Edinburgh, and at 23 years of age, he received his doctorate.[1] Led by William Cullen, Edinburgh was a preeminent center of medical education in Europe, and Willan received an education based on the Enlightenment approach to the natural world with direct observation, classification, and analysis. He was influenced there by several other educators: John Hope (1725–1786), an early supporter of Linnaean taxonomy; Alexander Monro (1733–1817), an anatomy professor; and Andrew Duncan (1744–1828), who worked at the Royal Public Dispensary of Edinburgh and once lamented that there was "no satisfactory distinction of cutaneous diseases."[2]

After two years of practice in Darlington, Willan moved to London, where he began working and teaching at the new Carey Street Public Dispensary in 1783. Employment at a teaching hospital in London was difficult to secure at this time, especially for Edinburgh graduates. Willan's Quaker upbringing and the influence of a Quaker physician named John Lettsom (1744–1815) inevitably led to Willan's choice of a philanthropic career in medicine. He focused his efforts on caring for the poor and underprivileged rather than individual achievement or personal wealth.

During these early years on Carey Street, Willan took an interest in skin disease. By 1784 or 1785, he had reached his conclusions about primary skin lesions, the initial distinctive type of lesion that develops in the first stage of a skin disease. He noted that all skin diseases could be divided into categories based on these elementary forms.[3] His biographer Thomas Bateman speculated it may have been Willan's "own extreme accuracy" that "made him feel early and acutely the vagueness and confusion of language, which universally prevailed in this department of medicine, while his attendance at a public institution brought many of these diseases constantly under inspection."[4] His career at the public dispensary gave him tremendous exposure to a wide range of clinical material from which he would develop his taxonomy. Willan's exposure to Enlightenment principles at Edinburgh and his association with the physician William Cullen gave him the tools he needed to bring some order to the chaos.

Established in 1782 and located on Carey Street near Lincoln's Inn Fields in the center of London, the Carey Street Public Dispensary was one of the most respected dispensaries in the city.[5] It served the vicinity of Clare Market, Drury Lane, Temple Bar, Strand, Holborn, Fleet Street, Ludgate, and Black

DOI: 10.1201/9781003273622-18

and White Friars.[6] The dispensary existed at this location until 1806 when it was moved to Bishop's Court on Chancery Lane, and it prospered there until 1850 when it again returned to Carey Street. A public dispensary was a cross between an outpatient clinic and a pharmacy—it was not a hospital or infirmary, and the ill could not be housed there. As hospitals in London during this time primarily cared for the affluent, the dispensaries' main purpose was to "relieve with advice and medicines, the suffering and industrious part of the community, to whom the Physician's fee, or the Apothecary's bill would be absolute ruin."[7] Public dispensaries depended on the sponsorship of the upper class for financial backing. In the case of the Carey Street Dispensary, the Duke of Sussex financially supported the healthcare establishment and, interestingly, was named its president. The dispensary movement in England grew out of a "philanthropic impulse" of the eighteenth century; it was a cheaper institution to run than a hospital and could handle a larger number of patients. Sixteen public dispensaries were established in London from 1770–1792.[8] For those too ill to go to the dispensary, the dispensary doctor risked his life to enter the home of the afflicted, displaying bravery and heroism that was taken for granted at the time and essentially forgotten by posterity.[9]

An inspection of the by-laws of the public dispensary on Carey Street reveals that the purpose of the dispensary was to relieve the poor with medicine and medical advice, that patients from any quarter could be received there, and that patients in the vicinity of the dispensary could even be visited at their homes if their condition required it.[10] The physician risked his life when calling on feverish patients in their own home, as smallpox was rampant in this era. All of this care was gratis, including the medications provided. Physicians who worked there had to be a fellow, candidate, inceptor candidate, or licentiate of the College of Physicians, and surgeons had to be a member of the Royal College of Surgeons (RCS). One of the physicians would attend the dispensary every Monday, Tuesday, Thursday, and Friday, with the surgeon there on Wednesday and Saturday. The apothecary, required to be licensed with the Company of Apothecaries, compounded and dispensed medications prescribed by the physicians or surgeons; he could serve as a backup to the physician and surgeon and attend any case that occurred in the absence of these doctors. Patients could receive the cowpox vaccine, introduced by Edward Jenner in 1796, on Wednesdays and Saturdays at 12:00 p.m. Records of the Carey Street Public Dispensary reveal that an average of 3000 patients per year used its services.[11] Approximately 50,000 lower class citizens of London were cared for annually by the city's 16 dispensaries.[12]

The dispensary was administered by a hierarchy that included a president, several vice presidents, a treasurer, auditors and trustees, and governors. The governors were the gatekeepers of the clinic. A governor was any benefactor who donated annually one guinea to the treasury of the dispensary; if he donated ten guineas, he could become a governor for life. These governors received the privilege of recommending patients for admission and could subsidize 15 patients each year for each guinea donated.[13] Without a sponsoring governor, patients were not otherwise able to receive care at the clinic. There were some restrictions to note: (1) those with venereal diseases were generally not admitted, unless they had a special recommendation, and they could only be admitted once under any circumstances; (2) persons who received care at the dispensary upon discharge were to deliver a letter of thanks to the recommending governor, and failure to do so would lead to forfeit of future care at the dispensary; (3) once admitted, the patient could be dismissed at any time by the physician or surgeon and would need another letter of recommendation to receive care beyond three months.[14]

Rich in cutaneous morbidity, the Carey Street Public Dispensary was undoubtedly the best possible place for a physician like Willan to thrive for 20 years, gather his data, and develop his classification scheme. The crowded vicinity of the dispensary, with its squalor and its unhygienic citizens, must have been a breeding ground for skin disease.[15] At least for English dermatology, the Carey Street Public Dispensary is where it all began.

Willan developed the idea to classify skin diseases in the same way one would organize plants—by their appearance. It was this early work that Willan submitted to the Medical Society of London and for which he received the Fothergill Medal. His system evolved during the 1790s, and by 1797, Willan had defined seven orders (categories) of skin diseases; he would later add an eighth. Starting in 1798, Willan published installments, each containing one of his orders, over the next ten years (1798, 1801, 1805, and 1808). This work was called *Description and Treatment of Cutaneous Diseases*, and the installments contain some of the earliest color depictions of skin diseases. For the copper engravings to illustrate his diseases, Willan hired such famed artists of the era as Sydenham Teast Edwards (1768–1819), John Boyne (1750–1810), William Thomas Strutt (1777–1850), and Isaac Cruikshank (1756–1811).[16]

In 1808, Willan published *On Cutaneous Diseases, Vol. 1*, the first of two planned volumes, which was composed of the first four previously published installments. The orders of cutaneous diseases contained within that volume were *papulae, squamae, exanthemata*, and *bullae*. It was a gorgeous quarto volume that presented color depictions (33 of them) of skin diseases—a novel idea—and Willan became the author of the first dermatologic atlas.[17] Willan died before he could publish the remaining four orders (*pustulae, vesiculae, tubercula*, and *maculae*). Thomas Bateman (1778–1821), who arrived at the Dispensary in 1802 and quickly became Willan's colleague, assistant, and protege, provided the posthumous completion of Willan's magnum opus a year after his death (see below).

After reviewing the confusing history of the dermatological terminology of the Greeks, Latins, and Arabians, Willan recognized that modern writers did little to clear it up and, if anything, added to the confusion. In reference to these modern writers, Willan wrote:

> They not only give us various interpretations of the accounts left us by the ancients, but have perverted the sense of many passages, especially the Greek authors. They employ the same terms in very different significations. They also make artificial, and often inconsistent arrangements, some reducing all the diseases under two or three genera, while others, too studious of amplification, apply new names to different stages or appearances of the same complaint. Those who attempt to theorize on the subject are seldom clear and satisfactory; but, even should the praise of ingenuity be due some of their speculations, little approbation would, I apprehend, be given to plans of classifying diseases founded on hypothesis, not on symptoms or characteristic appearances.[18]

Prior to Willan, the language of dermatology was in total chaos:

> the words *leprosy, scurvy, herpes, scabies, dartres* and some other appelations have become so indefinite, as to be merely synonyms of cutaneous disease. Even the more scientific inquirers, whose knowledge of diseases was not always equal to their learning, or whose learning fell short of their pathological skill, have interpreted the generic and specific appelations of the ancients in various senses. They have not only differed, for instance, in their acceptation of general terms, such as of the words *pustule, phylctaena, exanthema, erythema, phyma, phlyzacium*, etc., but the particular appelations *lichen, psora, herpes, impetigo, porrigo, scabies*, and many others have been arbitrarily appropriated to very different genera of disease.[19]

Consequently, Willan stated that he endeavored:

1. to fix the sense of the terms employed by proper definitions
2. to constitute general divisions or orders of the diseases from the leading and peculiar circumstances in their appearance, to arrange them into distinct genera, and to describe at large their specific forms or varieties
3. to class and give names to such as have not been hitherto sufficiently distinguished
4. to specify the mode of treatment for each disease[20]

The idea to classify skin lesions by morphology was entirely Plenck's, not Willan's. Willan never credited Plenck in his work, but Bateman corrected this omission in 1814:

> It seems probable, indeed, that Dr. Willan was indebted to this work of Professor Plenck for the groundwork of his classification; since his definitions, as well as his terms, accord accurately with those of the Hungarian nosologist.[21]

By reducing the number of orders to eight, Willan's system was stricter and leaner and followed the laws of classification more precisely. Willan's system executed a botanical principle that grouped plants in the same category, provided they had at least one observable feature in common; in the case of skin diseases, that feature is the elementary lesion.[22] Recognizing that crusts and ulcers typically resulted from the progression of other lesion types, such as *bullae*, Willan did not have separate orders for crusts or ulcers. He gave exanthems, such as measles, their own order and put all growths of the skin under a single heading, *tubercula*. Bateman contended that Willan's system lacked the confusion found in Plenck's system where different stages of the same disease fell into different classes.[23]

The simplifications enacted in Willan's arrangement proved to be a major improvement, and the system worked better than that of Plenck. The system's greatest strength, however, was not how the orders were arranged but the precision of Willan's definitions of the diseases.[24] Willan was the first to emphasize clear and accurate characterizations of diseases, and from his studies, a uniform nomenclature was introduced. Virtually all of the 119 skin diseases he described, both the old and new ones, were given first-rate, updated definitions and descriptions. He revived ancient dermatologic words—e.g., the "eczema" of Aetius and the "impetigo" of Celsus—and assigned them new meanings for the nineteenth century. His nomenclature enabled dermatologists to "write and converse respecting them [cutaneous diseases] with perspicuity, by fixing the meaning of the terms which they employ."[25] At long last, physicians who treated skin diseases finally had a language with which to characterize what they were seeing and to communicate "with precision, the information which we acquire, and therefore [the nomenclature] contributes directly to the advancement of knowledge, or at least removes an otherwise impediment to its progress."[26] Furthermore, specific terminology for specific problems could prevent therapeutic errors, such as:

> the gross misapplication of the remedies of the petechial or sea-scurvy, which have been prescribed for the cure of inflammatory, scaly, and pustular diseases, merely because the epithet, scorbutic [related to scurvy], has been vaguely assigned to them all.[27]

The key to making the correct diagnosis was to identify the primary lesion and classify it according to one of Willan's eight orders.[28] The development and promotion of this fundamental skill—the starting point in any dermatology training program—is another of Willan's great legacies. Bateman attributed Willan's success to his ability "to detect, like an accomplished artist, the minute peculiarities in the appearance of these diseases, which escaped the notice of ordinary observers."[29]

On Willan's magnum opus, the nineteenth-century French giant of dermatology Pierre Rayer (see Chapter 13) wrote:

> The great characteristics of Willan's writings are the impress they bear of the scientific spirit that guided him in his researches; the great precision, and the purity of his descriptions; the particular pains he takes to select well, and to use judiciously, his technical expressions; lastly, the sound judgment he displays in the interpretation of the ancients.[30]

Willan is remembered for several significant contributions. He wrote original and accurate descriptions of numerous skin diseases, including pityriasis versicolor, pemphigus, erythema infectiosum, lupus vulgaris, erythema nodosum, ichthyosis and ichthyosis hystrix, herpes simplex, herpes zoster, tinea capitis, Henoch-Schonlein purpura, rosacea, and senile pruritus.[31] Willan's description of what he called *pompholyx diutinus* is bullous pemphigoid.[32] His greatest feat may have been collecting all of the various types of dermatitis and giving them the general name, eczema.[33]

Willan was the first to accurately describe psoriasis as we know it today, under the term *lepra vulgaris:* "characterized by scaly patches, of different sizes, but having nearly a circular form" and which "sometimes appears first at the elbow, or on the forearm, but more generally about the knee."[34] "Willan's lepra" is the condition we today call chronic plaque psoriasis. In the section that followed, under the heading Psoriasis, Willan listed 11 types of "scaly tetters" that are the variants of today's psoriasis, including guttate, nail, and erythrodermic forms of psoriasis. Thus, "psoriasis," derived from the Greek word *psora*, which meant any itchy skin condition, and unused since the writings of Galen, entered the nomenclature of the budding field of dermatology as the specific term for what we today know to be psoriasis:

> I think it also necessary, in the present series of them, to express the scaly Psora by a distinctive appellation: for this purpose, the term Psoriasis, which the Greek writers themselves employ, seems in all respects, suitable. The disease to be thus entitled is characterized by a roughness and scaliness of the surface, sometimes continuous, sometimes in separate patches, of various sizes,

but of an irregular figure, and for the most part accompanied with rhagades, or fissures in the skin. From the Lepra, it may be distinguished not only by the different form, and distribution of the patches as formerly stated from the Greek writers, but also by its cessation and recurrence at certain seasons of the year, and by the disorder of the constitution with which it is usually attended.[35]

The term *lepra* was eventually absorbed and abandoned under the general term psoriasis when the leprosy bacillus was discovered in the 1870s.[36]

Willan was a public health advocate and as a contemporary of the vaccine pioneer Edward Jenner, he was an ardent supporter of vaccination.[37] He deplored the living conditions of the poor in London and strove to correct the problem through public health initiatives; one such initiative was the establishment of a 15-bed fever hospital in 1802 to isolate and treat Londoners with typhus, particularly rampant at this time, as well as smallpox and scarlet fever. General hospitals refused to admit patients with contagious diseases, so Willan saw the need for special facilities for these patients.[38]

Willan was an early advocate of preventative medicine and favored bathing and cleanliness as proper prophylaxis for skin diseases.[39] He painted a grim picture of skin disease among the poor in London:

And how are the poor, without accommodations for the purpose at home, to clear their bodies from the dirt, dust, and unctuous or adhesive substances, which their various employments fasten on them? There being no provision in any part of the metropolis for washing and bathing, they quietly suffer the penalties annexed to the want of cleanliness, as disagreeable smells, perpetual irritation with chaps and fissures of the skin, boils, and eruptions of inflamed pustules, the Itch and the Prurigo, the Lepra, the dry Tetter, the running Tetter, the Dandruff, and the Scald-head.[40]

While he was a master diagnostician, Willan was weak on therapeutics, even in the opinion of Bateman, who wrote about the paradox:

As a practitioner, he was a close and faithful observer of diseases, and by the peculiar quickness with which he detected their characteristic appearances, however obscured by complication, he had obtained a copious store of sound experience; yet it has been remarked that he did not always prescribe with that vigour and decision, which so much discriminative talent would have authorized.[41]

Willan preferred to recommend baths and fresh air, along with the avoidance of alcoholic beverages, and he had little faith in drugs and other treatments of his time.[42] His supposed weakness may have been rooted in an intelligent skepticism about the treatments at his disposal. Willan's knowledge about "treating the whole patient" served him well and fostered in him some healthy distrust in the traditional treatments of the surgeons and other practitioners who managed skin diseases in the late eighteenth century.

Willan resigned after 20 years at the dispensary in 1803. After his departure from Carey Street in 1803, Willan continued to work in a private practice setting for eight more years. By 1809, Willan had reached the highest level of professional success in Britain, exemplified by his election to the Royal Society. He touched many lives professionally, having educated more than 40 young physicians during his career.[43] Bateman recognized that the indefatigable Willan "never quitted the metropolis for any consideration of health or pleasure, during a period of thirty years."[44] His life, however, would soon be cut short. In 1811, he developed hemoptysis, presumably tuberculosis-related, which prompted him to move to Madeira, Portugal, seeking a healthier place to live. However, he soon died and was buried in Funchal on April 7, 1812, at 55 years of age. He did not survive to see the impact his studies and writings would have on the field of dermatology. In the year of his death, Willan was described in *Gentleman's Magazine* as:

one of the best and noblest of human kind, possessed of every virtue that can ennoble and adorn …. In his profession he was beloved almost beyond example …. He possessed almost every intellectual attainment that can be comprised within the finite compass of the human mind …. In addition to his great merits as a physician, and as an accurate and classical writer, he was one of the most amiable of men, a sincere friend, a good husband and an affectionate father. He was in truth a model of the perfect human character; a benevolent and skilful Physician, a correct and sound philosopher, and a truly virtuous man.[45]

Thomas Bateman noted:

> By the death of Dr. Willan, the profession was deprived of one of its bright ornaments, and of its zealous and able improvers; the sick, of a humane, disinterested, and discerning physician; and the world of an estimable and upright man. By his exterior deportment in public, indeed, he was far from rendering justice to his own character. His early education, his studious mode of life, and retiring disposition, prevented that display of his various and extensive knowledge, in mixed society, which delighted the privacy of a small circle of friends, and which was dispensed with much playfulness and simplicity of manner. In all the relations of domestic life, indeed, he was an object of general esteem and attachment. The gentleness and humanity of his disposition were equally conspicuous in the exercise of his professional duties; in the patient attention with which he listened to the complaints of the sick, whom, in his fullest occupation, he never dismissed from his presence dissatisfied with the brevity of his inquiries; and in the liberality with which he imparted his assistance, yet refused the remuneration to which he was entitled, when the circumstances of the patient appeared to render it oppressive.[46]

The modern physician—of any specialty—could greatly benefit from studying the life and career of Robert Willan.

Thomas Bateman (1778–1821)

The legacy of Robert Willan would not have been fully delivered to posterity had it not been for the posthumous advocacy and support of Willan by his protege, Thomas Bateman. Figures such as Turner or Plenck had no Bateman to carry on their legacy; hence, their accomplishments are largely forgotten. Like Willan, a native of Yorkshire and trained at Edinburgh, Bateman arrived at the Carey Street Dispensary in 1802. He received a licentiate from the Royal College of Physicians in 1805, but he was never offered a Fellowship in the Royal Society. After Willan's departure, Bateman became a physician of the Dispensary and had the same special interest in skin diseases.

After Willan's death, Bateman purchased the copyright of Willan's work as well as his watercolor drawings. In 1813, Bateman finished the task of publishing the second half of Willan's orders of diseases in a complete work entitled *A Practical Synopsis of Cutaneous Diseases According to the Arrangement of Dr. Willan*. This slim volume is possibly the most critical text in the history of dermatology, with 11 editions issued before 1850 and translation into 5 languages. Its fame reached as far as St. Petersburg, where the tsar of Russia ordered several copies and rewarded Bateman with a valuable ring to symbolize imperial approval.[47] Bateman followed up *Practical Synopsis* in 1817 with *Delineations of Cutaneous Diseases*, an atlas containing 70 color prints, which also completed Willan's work from an illustration standpoint. *Delineations* is the first in a long line of impressive dermatologic atlases—to the present author, underappreciated works of art—of the nineteenth century.

Bateman is remembered in his own right for genius as both a physician and a medical writer, but in the preface of *Practical Synopsis*, Bateman made it abundantly clear that credit was due to Willan, and Bateman had no qualms about giving it. He wrote that the work should not "be considered as the completion of that [Willan's] original work" but, instead, "an abstract of the classification proposed by that respected author, together with a concise view of all the genera and species, which he intended that it should comprehend."[48] While the first four orders in *Practical Synopsis* came directly from Willan's work, Bateman stated that the remaining four orders were subsequently derived from "personal experience and research, but principally from a constant intercourse with Dr. Willan, upon the subject of these diseases, during a period of ten years, while his colleague at the Public Dispensary."[49] It seems likely that Bateman made a more substantial contribution to the classification system than his modesty inferred.[50] Willan and Bateman's eight orders can be found in Table 12.1.

Bateman is credited with the original descriptions of solar purpura, alopecia areata, molluscum contagiosum, ecthyma, papular urticaria (which he called *lichen urticatus*), sycosis barbae, and erythema multiforme; in addition, the establishment of eczema as a dermatosis is the direct result of Bateman's presentation of Willan's views.[51] As far as Bateman the man, Bateman was held by his contemporaries in the highest regard

TABLE 12.1

The Eight Orders and Their Genera, According to Willan and Bateman

Papulae (I)	Squamae (II)	Exanthemata (III)	Bullae (IV)	Pustulae (V)	Vesiculae (VI)	Tubercula (VII)	Maculae (VIII)
Strophulus	Lepra	Rubeola	Erysipelas	Impetigo	Varicella	Phyma	Ephelis
Lichen	Psoriasis	Scarlatina	Pemphigus	Porrigo	Vaccinia	Verruca	Naevus
Prurigo	Pityriasis	Urticaria	Pompholyx	Ecthyma	Herpes	Molluscum	
	Ichthyosis	Roseola		Variola	Rupia	Vitiligo	
		Purpura		Scabies	Miliaria	Acne	
		Erythema			Eczema	Sycosis	
					Aphtha	Lupus	
						Elephantiasis	
						Framboesia	

for his professionalism, judgment, integrity, and knowledge.[52] He hosted many physicians at his clinic from all over Europe, readily sharing his knowledge with anyone who came to learn, and leaving a lasting impact. For example, Bateman mentored Ireland's first dermatologist, William Wallace (1791–1837), who then returned to Dublin and established the Dublin Infirmary for the Treatment of Diseases of the Skin in 1818.

BATEMAN'S SPIRITUAL RENEWAL

Bateman's last years are noteworthy in that he was "born again" in the spring of April 1820. In the pamphlet entitled *A Brief Memoir of the Late Thomas Bateman* (1821), possibly written by Rumsey, we can learn about Bateman's renewed spiritual life:

> Dr. Bateman had been expressing to me his conviction that he could not live much longer, and complaining of the dreadful nervous sensations which continually harassed him; and then he added, 'but all these sufferings are a just punishment for my long skepticism, and neglect of God and religion." This led to a conversation, in the course of which he observed, that medical men were very generally skeptical; and that the mischief arose from what he considered a natural tendency of some of their studies to lead to materialism. I replied, that the mischief appeared to me to originate rather in their neglect to examine into the evidence of the truth of the Bible, as an actual revelation from God; because, if a firm conviction of that were once established, the authority of the Scriptures must be paramount; and the tendency of all inferior studies, in opposition to their declarations, could have no weight. He said, he believed I was right, and that he had in fact been intending to examine fully into the subject, when the complaint in his eyes came on, and shut him out from reading. Our conversation ended in his permitting me to read to him the first of [Thomas] Scott's "Essays on the most important Subjects in Religion," which treats of "The Divine Inspiration of the Scriptures." He listened with intense earnestness; and when it was concluded, he exclaimed, "This is demonstration! Complete demonstration!"[53]

Bateman struggled with poor health for the last five years of his life. In 1818, he experienced mercurial erethism (neurotoxicity) after treatment for failing sight in one eye, and he died a few years later from an epidemic fever he presumably caught at the London Fever Hospital.[54] Bateman's life was even shorter than Willan's and ended at 42 years of age in 1821. Bateman's contemporary biographer, Rumsey, wrote:

> He was a sound scholar and an accomplished physician, wanting nothing to adorn and complete the character proper to his rank. He loved learning for its own sake. Science was to him as his daily food; and the exercise of his art, whether in private or in public, was in the strictest sense professional, so as to exhibit altogether, with such qualifications, a character of great value in itself, and much interest to all who have the good of the medical professional at heart.[55]

Thomas Addison (1793–1860)

The Willan-Bateman doctrine of diagnosing and classifying skin diseases based on morphology—henceforth referred to as Willanism—found staying power for two reasons: it was passed down to the physicians who took up the torch at the Carey Street Dispensary, and the doctrine spread to the continent where the so-called French Willanists promoted its adoption in French hospitals. The most important of Willan and Bateman's disciples in London was yet another graduate of Edinburgh, Thomas Addison (1793–1860). Addison was Bateman's pupil starting in 1816 but took over the dispensary in 1819. Addison shared Bateman's enthusiasm for skin disease, and his dermatologic training under Bateman made him an unmatched authority in London in the period after Bateman. At Guy's Hospital, Addison founded a Department of Dermatology in 1824. He supervised Joseph Towne (1806–1879) in the creation of wax models designed to demonstrate skin diseases. Subjecting himself to much ridicule at the time, he proposed that the small yellow bodies on top of the kidneys—the adrenal glands—had life-giving functions; he was later shown to be correct and is credited with the discovery of adrenal insufficiency.[56] He was among the first to link skin diseases with internal diseases when he showed that adrenal insufficiency is associated with diffuse hyperpigmentation of the skin. He was the first to describe xanthomas and morphea.[57] He was seen by his students and peers as a master diagnostician, perhaps because his training in dermatology made him a "master of observation, of the art of inspection."[58]

As a person, Addison was shy and nervous on the inside, haughty and proud on the outside; he was not well liked by his colleagues.[59] He is not known today as a major figure in the dermatology annals, presumably because Addison never wanted to be seen as a specialist in the skin, since there was much prejudice against specialization at the time.[60] For most of his career he battled depression, and between that and his innate shyness, his resultant behavior "deprived him of the affection and understanding of certain colleagues."[61] He retired in 1860, revealing that "a considerable breakdown in my health has scared me from the anxieties, responsibilities and excitement of my profession."[62] A few months later, Addison flung himself from the roof of his house. The obituary stated that he had "laboured under the form of insanity called melancholia, resulting from overwork of the brain."[63]

Anthony Todd Thomson (1778–1849), James Startin (1806–1872), and Jonathan Green (1788–1864)

Anthony Todd Thomson was the last of the line of Edinburgh-trained, dispensary-employed physicians who ensured that the impact of Willan and Bateman would last for decades. Thomson, born in Edinburgh, lived in colonial America for a time while his Loyalist father served as Postmaster-General in Georgia, but they returned to Edinburgh when the American war was lost. After graduating medical school, Thomson moved to London where he worked at a dispensary, gaining much experience with the diagnosis and treatment of skin disease. He secured a professorship at University College London, focusing his career on therapeutics, botany, and skin diseases, and started a first-of-its-kind, albeit unofficial (until 1861) skin disease clinic attached to the university. He is most famous for editing the seventh edition of Bateman's *Practical Synopsis* (1829), which included many of the depictions from Bateman's *Delineations* but on a smaller scale.

London did not have hospitals dedicated to skin disease patients until the 1840s. The dispensary was the principal venue for dermatologic care in Britain in the first half of the nineteenth century. Willan, Bateman, Thomson, and other graduates of Scottish universities found themselves excluded from the "conservative and inbred teaching hospitals," and the founding of hospitals for specific diseases, such as skin diseases, was resisted by the establishment.[64] It was not until 1841 when James Startin, not of the Edinburgh lineage, founded the first skin disease hospital at London Wall; it was later moved to Blackfriars. The Blackfriars skin disease hospital soon became the leading postgraduate center for dermatology training in Britain for the next 80 years.[65] The other claim to fame of Startin, an underappreciated educator in the history of dermatology, was that it was he who wooed the hospital's most famous physician, Jonathan Hutchinson, to its staff (see below). Hutchinson was most responsible for the elevation of Blackfriars to the highest echelon of skin disease hospitals in the world.

A surgeon of minor import in this era was Jonathan Green. After serving as a surgeon in the Royal Navy, Green became interested in skin disease upon visiting Hôpital Saint-Louis in Paris, a renowned institution for the treatment of dermatologic conditions (see Chapter 13). He was an admirer of French dermatology, especially Rayer and Biett, having himself spent time at Hôpital Saint-Louis where he was impressed by the use of vapor baths as a treatment for skin disease.[66] He authored *A Practical Compendium of the Diseases of the Skin, with Cases* (1835), but it did little to advance the specialty or clear up any diagnostic chaos:

> In Green's Diseases of the Skin a table of synonyms gives lepra as synonymous with alphos, vitiligo, morphoea, lepra alphoides, and also leuce and Greek elephantiasis! When psoriasis is noted to be synonymous with lepra, melas, ecthyma, psora leprosa, pityriasis, psora (= scabies) or scabies sicca (= lichen), terminological "confusion now has made its masterpiece."[67]

John Wilson (Unknown Dates)

An even more obscure surgeon who wrote about skin diseases in this era was John Wilson, for whom little biographical data exists. He authored *A familiar treatise on cutaneous diseases; exhibiting, a popular view of their respective symptoms; detailing the limits of secure self-treatment; and illustrating the perilous abuse of indiscriminate remedies* (1813). Similar to the writings of Daniel Turner, this text is an extraordinarily good read, and as it was completely uninfluenced by Willanism, it gives us an idea of the state of knowledge before Willan's system was adopted.[68] Instead of using Willan's nomenclature, Wilson writes of pimples, pustules, scabs, blotches, and tetters. Wilson was one of the first to advocate bathing, noting,

> When perspired matter, or other filthy accumulations, are allowed on the skin, we may easily conjecture that such will become the cause of cutaneous disease; especially where the surface is irritable. How many of us, who claim consideration as personally delicate, scarcely wash the entire surface of the body during a life! And when cutaneous affection seizes us, shall we be surprised at its occasional inveteracy? ... In what relates to clothing and appearance the British are the neatest people on earth; why, then, not extend their care to cleansing the very surface of the body? If we have not an example in our neighbours, let us hold one forth. It is a matter of national concern.[69]

Wilson's text tells us about views toward skin disease of the common man and woman in this era, noting that "purity from cutaneous disease is considered so essential to our kind reception in the world, that many dread the deformity of a blotch more than the occurrence of a moral ill."[70] Wilson promoted himself as a defender of the layperson, who—desperate to avoid the stigma of a visible skin disease— might resort to the "empirical," topical treatments of the quack or worse, concoctions developed through self-experiment, applied at home by the patient in private, without the guidance of a surgeon or physician. He explained his concerns:

> In devoting my attention exclusively to the treatment of cutaneous disorders, I have been witness to so many evils resulting from the private misapplication of remedies, that I presume my labour might be profitably applied, in soliciting attention, to a point intimately involving the public welfare; and, if possible, impressing on the community a sense of the dangers to ensue from empirical practice. Throughout the following pages I shall endeavour to 'rather repress than encourage the private exhibition of Medicine, because I am sensible that such practice generally leads to unsuccessful result. I shall state the limits beyond which prudence will not advance, and earnestly entreat my Readers will do me the justice to believe, that I have led them to the very verge of prudential self-aid. My object is to deter the sufferer from becoming the victim of self-experiment; and I have considered it safer to dictate what may be innocently done, in each

form of cutaneous disorder, than, by an arbitrary interdiction of all authorized means, endanger the consequences of provoked hardihood .... I beg it should be understood throughout, that the main purport of this Work is, to convince those, who are not professionally bred, that they cannot wade deep in physic without increasing the risks of life, and that, if there is any class of diseases peculiarly delicate and dangerous, it is that which occupies the present pages: it is the most liable to busy intermeddling, and therefore the most fruitful source of empirical evils.[71]

Wilson's comments about the complexion of a woman's face versus that of the man tell us much about the dynamics between the sexes in the late eighteenth and early nineteenth centuries:

> Females more especially suffer; their personal appearance being too often their only recommendation to our sex .... Deprived, as females are, by the universal consent of society, from actively selecting objects of union, they must necessarily be much dependant on exterior aids for establishment in life. Divines and Philosophers may descant on the innate beauty of moral worth; and, while the understanding yields implicit conviction, the feelings alone shall disobey the conscientious dictate: so perverse indeed is the human heart, that it will turn, with disgust, from a few pimples on a countenance beaming forth every moral beauty that can adorn the female character.[72]

By comparison, here is Wilson's view on skin disease of the face in men:

> Men, at all periods of life, are necessarily exempted from the operation of the causes last alluded to, and are perhaps less liable to cutaneous disorders, of the constitutional kind, on parts that are visible, than the tender sex; and I fear it may be too justly asserted, that many of those they do suffer by are but the effects of their own indiscretions. Men have many means of enjoyment, if excess can be termed such, or at least are in the habit of gratifying many propensities in which females are not allowed to indulge; these are but the too frequent avenues of disease in varied form. The table, the bottle, and all the concomitants of midnight orgies, are prolific in creating diseases of the skin. The pimpled face of the bacchanalian is a proverbial distinction of excess, yet, with all these provocations to disorder, men suffer less by cutaneous derangement in the earlier stages of life; and, when they do so suffer, they are usually less anxious for its removal; although in the higher ranks any superficial deformity, in either sex, is an evil that delicacy demands should be dispelled, yet still men have not that powerful incitement to study personal aspect, which is so imperative with females. The man of pleasure will often glory in his red nose and pimpled face, as the index of a character, entitled to the appellation of a good jolly fellow.[73]

Samuel Plumbe (1795–1837)

Willanism had its British dissidents; the most famous of these was Samuel Plumbe. Born in Wantage, Oxfordshire, Plumbe took a surgical apprenticeship in London at St. Thomas Hospital and was ultimately admitted to the RCS in 1815. His first forays into dermatology were successful: a well-reviewed essay on *Ringworm of the Scalp, Scalled Head, and Other Forms of Porrigo* (1821) and a paper entitled *On Diseases of the Skin* (1822); the latter publication earned him the Jacksonian prize, issued by the RCS.[74] The 26-year-old surgeon was well on his way to becoming a renowned member of the dermatological pantheon, but the success of the Willan-Bateman system ultimately overshadowed Plumbe's contributions; he is now all but forgotten by posterity. During his life, however, he stood out among his peers for his keen observation, original ideas, and persuasive writings, and he was the most important figure in dermatology in Britain after Bateman's death.[75]

In 1824, Plumbe published *A Practical Treatise on the Diseases of the Skin*, a treatise that is noteworthy for several reasons. In that work, Plumbe tried to offer an alternative to classifying skin diseases by morphology; his system used etiology as the basis of differentiating skin diseases. It contained original lines of thought and did not conform to the orthodox Willanist school. It is evident in his preface that Plumbe respected Willan for his innovations but vocalized his disagreement with Willan's morphology-based system and cumbersome nomenclature. His main complaint with Willan's arrangement was that the morphology of a given skin disease is not static—it changes as the condition progresses—and so it made no sense to him to classify skin diseases this way. He explained:

> A classification of the external and ever-changing forms of the accumulated secretion of disease on the surface—one day a pimple, the next a vesicle, on the third a scab, or crust, the fourth a falling scale, the fifth a red spot! This might have served the purpose at the time for want of a better, but to pronounce it a better classification than one founded, whether with solid foundation or not, by its originators, on etiology, or the *causes* external and internal, of the cutaneous diseases, would be manifestly absurd .... It is impossible to fail to notice in the classification of Willan and Bateman, the adoration of precedent in their adoption of Plenck's arrangement as a starting point. Willan could have known little indeed, practically, of the subject, when he first began to direct his attention to it, even as an author; and it is really surprising that he did not at the commencement see the great and fundamental deficiencies of that system.[76]

To Plumbe, the nomenclature of Willan and Bateman consisted of too many diseases and "those endless distinctions without real differences, which have been made by this author [Willan], as being calculated to discourage the student rather than promote knowledge of the subject."[77] For example, he made an important point when it came to the distinction between eczema and impetigo, two terms that were not clearly defined by Willan and that were confused for over 50 years after Willan's death. Plumbe recognized that the eruptions that Willan and Bateman had described as impetigo were characterized as minute vesicles on an erythematous base and therefore more appropriately designated as eczema than impetigo since they were not pustular.[78]

Plumbe's system had five categories of disease:

1. Due to local peculiarities of the skin (including acne)
2. Due to chronic inflammation of the vessels secreting the cuticle (psoriasis and pityriasis)
3. Due to deranged digestive organs (favus, lichen, prurigo, urticaria)
4. Due to a mixed character (impetigo, scabies)
5. Due to diminished tone of the vessels in the skin (purpura, pemphigus)[79]

The problem with Plumbe's system is that, unlike morphology that is undeniable, Plumbe organized skin diseases according to his theory-based categories, which were inherently speculative. Plumbe's ideas as to the cause of skin disease were his own creation, and some were bizarre and decidedly unmodern.[80] Willan's system lasted because it was concrete; there is no room for abstraction in scientific classification. Morphology could not be questioned or conjectured and was, therefore, the only tried-and-true method for categorizing skin diseases.[81] Plumbe, the champion of etiological classification, failed to convince his morphologist brethren. The French Willanist, Biett (see Chapter 13), delivered a brutal takedown of *Practical Treatise*—in the most tactful way possible—as told in this account recorded in the *Lancet* (1827):

> Biett saw some gentleman smiling at the mention of Monsieur Plumbe, and made a full stop in the middle of the ward, to explain himself. "Gentlemen, you laugh because I speak of Monsieur Plumbe, but on my honour I assure you that I speak disrespectfully of no man, personally; I have a duty to perform here, and a part of that duty is to caution you against the erroneous opinions of men who have appeared as writers on the diseases of the skin; I know nothing of Mr. Plumbe; but I know, and I repeat now what I have before so often repeated, there is no book more replete with error, or containing more incorrect representations of the subject to which it is devoted, than this work of Monsieur Plumbe; in short, Gentlemen, its tendency is to carry back the study of dermoid pathology to the state in which it lay in the dark times of the middle age."[82]

Plumbe described psoriasis and did more than anyone else to merge Willan's designation of *lepra* and *psoriasis* under a single heading, noting that the two conditions were one and the same. His work with psoriasis was so significant that it was suggested in 1949 that psoriasis be given the eponym "Willan–Plumbe syndrome."[83] Plumbe also correctly described acne and proffered his very modern understanding of the pathogenesis of the pimple:

> In its simple and most trifling form, the disease consists merely of obstruction of the sebaceous follicles, in consequence of their contents becoming too hard to pass readily to the surface. Inflammation of the follicle, and the production of what is called a pimple results, and is soon followed by the formation of matter; the follicle is destroyed by this process, the matter is discharged, a little redness remains for a day or two, and the part returns to the healthy state.[84]

In addition to his contributions to the subjects of acne and psoriasis, Plumbe wrote extensively about a growing public concern among children in schools and hospitals: ringworm of the scalp, which he called "porrigo" and we call today tinea. It was a rampant nineteenth-century pediatric ailment, and Plumbe was the acknowledged authority in London on tinea.[85] He promoted forceps-epilation of infected hairs in the scalp. Prior to Plumbe's method, the pitch helmet was utilized for the purposes of removing infected hairs. That method involved the application of an adhesive resin to the entire scalp, which was then left in place for two to three days. The resin would dry and stick to the hairs and, upon its removal, forcibly pull out both infected and uninfected hairs. If removed too aggressively, it could lead to the ghastly complication of avulsion of the scalp away from the skull.[86] On the other hand, Plumbe's method was directed toward only the diseased hairs and was more acceptable to the patient.

Moreover, Plumbe is to be recognized for linking skin disease with overall health since he was keenly aware of the importance of diet and hygiene as it relates to skin health. Plumbe's section on anatomy and physiology of the skin was complete and perceptive, especially when considering Plumbe had no microscope, nor knowledge of the cellular structure of the skin.[87] Finally, Samuel Plumbe has been described as a

> simple, meek, and unassuming man, imbued with an intense interest and zeal for his profession, who undoubtedly preferred labor at his studies in an unimportant dispensary service to publicity and who emerged into the public eye only at intervals with publications of genuine worth and the highest scientific merit. He was not possessed of a burning ambition to obtain high posts at hospitals and universities, and his modest and humble character can be recognized in his works.[88]

Miscellaneous Contributors in the Era of Willan, Bateman, and Plumbe

Some lesser-known physicians wrote about skin diseases in the first half of the nineteenth century, and many of these were inspired by Willan. Bernardino Antonio Gomes (1768–1823), the first Portuguese dermatologist, wrote a 171-page treatise with a title translated as "Dermatological treatise or succinct and systematic description of the diseases of the skin in accordance with the principles and observations of Dr. Willan and Dr. Bateman and including the medicines recommended by the latter and other famous authors" (1820). The German, Ludwig-August Struve (1795–1828), penned *Synopsis morborum cutaneorum secundum classes, genera, species et varietates*, "Overview of skin diseases according to their classes, genera, species and varieties" (1829). In that work, he distinguished between diseases that involve no difference in color or structure of the skin and diseases characterized by changes in color, structure, or both.[89] The German, Friedrich Jacob Behrend (1805–1889), authored "Pictorial representation of non-syphilitic skin diseases accompanied by systematic written commentaries" (1839). Robert Froriep (1804–1861), another German physician, published Bateman's *Delineations* and pictures from other atlases, in installments known as *Atlas der Hautkrankheiten*, "Atlas of Skin Diseases," (1829–1841). Finally, Pierre Prosper Francois Baumes (1791–1871), a French physician, published his own theories of the origin of skin diseases in a work entitled *Nouvelle dermatologie*, "New Dermatology" (1842). His theory that "fluxions" (inflammations or swellings) were responsible for many skin diseases found no adherents, but Baumes is frequently found as a reference in many nineteenth-century French dermatologic texts.[90]

THE CLAIM OF TILESIUS

Robert Willan is recognized as the first to publish depictions of skin diseases. However, a German physician, naturalist, and explorer named Wilhelm Gottlieb Tilesius von Tilenau (1769–1857) once claimed that his friends, teachers, and acquaintances could all testify that he was illustrating skin diseases for ten years before Willan got the idea to do so.[91] After graduating in 1801 from the medical school in Leipzig, where he also took classes to learn how to draw, Tilesius devoted much of his energies early in his career to the study of skin disease. He practiced medicine in Leipzig for the first few years after graduation, where he gained much interest and experience in skin diseases. His talent for the illustration of skin diseases was evident as early as 1793. He was particularly interested in rare diseases, and the naturalist in him strived to capture the disease, like the finding of a rare bird, with a drawing. His most famous depictions were of ichthyosis hystrix, known as "Porcupine Man," and of neurofibromatosis. He took great pride in his work, which he saw as necessarily done by the physician, not the professional artist, because physicians drew with a better sense of the pathological characteristics.[92] Tilesius received many honors from the court of Tsar Alexander I. He accompanied the successful Russian expedition aboard the *Nadezhda* and *Neva* as they circumnavigated the globe in 1803–1806, the first such journey for Russia. On that adventure, Tilesius encountered many exotic creatures and peoples; his experience formed the basis for years of future writings on zoology and comparative anatomy. This very interesting person was significant in the history of dermatology for his early advocacy for the clinical illustration of skin diseases.

Erasmus Wilson (1809–1884)

After the careers of the big three—Willan, Bateman, and Plumbe—of the early nineteenth century, dermatology in Britain waned somewhat while thriving "schools" were becoming established in Paris and Vienna. Unlike those competing locales and their continuous lineages of genius, London had no real heir of Willan and Bateman; original ideas became scarce and had to be imported, e.g., the translation from French into English of Rayer's "Treatise on Skin Disease" by the prolific Scottish physician-writer Robert Willis (1799–1878) in 1841 (see Chapter 13).

The reason for the lack of interest in skin disease was that specialization in the skin in London was regarded with suspicion; treatment of skin diseases was still mainly in the hands of quacks.[93] Furthermore, the microscope was not widely used, and the cellular structure of the skin was still unknown to the British physicians.[94] Also, cutaneous medicine was connected with venereal medicine, and Victorian morality prevented many medical men from entering into a professional subdiscipline where they risked losing the respect of their colleagues for serving a population who were deemed immoral. A final cause for lack of specialization is that in 1840 there were no official facilities in London—like the Hôpital Saint-Louis in Paris or the skin disease clinics of the General Hospital in Vienna—dedicated to caring specifically for skin diseases; those would come later in the 1850s and 1860s. Startin had founded the aforementioned charity clinic dealing with skin disease in 1841, but it struggled for many years before getting moved in 1850 and renamed the Hospital for Diseases of the Skin at Blackfriars.[95] Indeed, Britain had physicians from time to time who wrote treatises on skin diseases, but by the mid-nineteenth century, London was ripe for someone to take up the torch for dermatology and be Britain's answer to Rayer, Bazin, and Hebra.

That man was William James Erasmus Wilson, known to us by his last two names and truly one of the most extraordinary figures of nineteenth-century Britain. The son of Admiral Nelson's Fleet Surgeon, Wilson, was born in London and attended medical school there where he achieved recognition for his meticulous dissection abilities and artistic anatomical drawings.[96] He started his career as an anatomist and surgeon, disciplines which he could teach as well as he practiced. His first publications were texts on anatomy and surgery. He joined the RCS in 1831, was elected a fellow of the RCS in 1843 for his work with the *Demodex* mite, and at just 35 years of age, Wilson achieved that ultimate status symbol of the British gentleman, Fellowship of the Royal Society (1845).

Wilson had managed skin diseases in his general practice in the late 1830s, but it was Thomas Wakley (1795–1862), a friend of his father and the founder of the *Lancet*, who suggested to Wilson around 1840 that he take up skin diseases as a special interest.[97] Wilson, who assisted Wakley as a sub-editor of the journal, exhibited a preference for treating skin disease as well as sympathy toward the poor, in the vein of Robert Willan. Wakley once told Wilson "to acquaint himself with them [skin diseases] so well that when he entered a room the company would start to scratch themselves."[98] With no dispensary or hospital clinic at his disposal, Wilson had to acquaint himself with skin diseases solely in his private practice, which catered to the wealthy but was often visited by the poor.

In 1842, Wilson wrote of his skin specialization: "It is a branch of medicine to which I have given some years of thought, and the mature study of which I henceforth devote my life."[99] Wilson later lamented the "discourtesy and injustice" that he received at the hands of the profession for daring to investigate cutaneous pathology.[100] He staved off criticism of his specialization for the better part of his career. As late as 1875, a *Lancet* reviewer described specialists as not only ignorant but also immoral: "The exclusive practice of some small speciality tends to perpetuate and increase ignorance, if it does not already deprave professional morals."[101]

In the 1840s, Wilson's fame skyrocketed—not because of his surgical skills or his dermatologic pursuits, but because of his involvement in the John White flogging affair of 1846. White was a private in the British Army who was flogged 150 times with cat o' nine tails for assaulting his superior, a sergeant. A month later, White died of pneumonia, and an investigation ensued. While the army doctors did not link the two events, Wakley, as coroner, commissioned Wilson to perform an autopsy and examine the records. Wilson concluded and later convinced a jury that the flogging induced a chain of events that led to White's death, and after this controversy, flogging was abandoned as a means of disciplining soldiers in Britain.[102] This high-profile case brought much notoriety to Wilson.

Wilson soon produced a major dermatological publication together: *A Practical and Theoretical Treatise on the Diagnosis, Pathology, & Treatment of Diseases of the Skin, Arranged According to a Natural System of Classification* (1842). The title was shortened in the second edition to *On Diseases of the Skin* (1847) and underwent six enormously popular editions, the last in 1867. This textbook was his most famous work and consisted of his own observations as well as a compilation of the observations of Willan, Bateman, Plumbe, Green, Biett, and Rayer.[103] He offered yet another classification system that did not gain any traction at the time. He divided skin diseases into the following four headings: diseases of the *derma* (the true skin or dermis), diseases of the sweat glands, diseases of the oil glands, and diseases of the hair follicles. Since it was believed that the epidermis was a product of the dermis, and changes in the epidermis were thus caused by disease in the dermis, Wilson did not think that the epidermis had its own unique diseases. Under each of these four headings, Wilson had several pathology-based subcategories. For example, for diseases of the derma, the categories were inflammation, hypertrophy of the dermal papillae, disorders of the vascular tissue, disordered sensibility (included itching), and disorders of the chromatogenous function of the derma (included pigmentary diseases).

Wilson's atlas, *Portraits of Diseases of the Skin* (1847), containing Wilson's own disease renderings, is one of the most magnificent dermatologic atlases of the nineteenth century. He also founded the first British journal of dermatology—*Journal of Cutaneous Medicine*—in 1865, which "served as an organ for Wilson's papers, his pungent editorial comments, and his dictatorial editorship."[104] The journal ran out of money after only four years but got new life in 1888 as the *British Journal of Dermatology*. Wilson published a student handbook on skin disease that same year. His bibliography is among the most extensive of any physician writer of the nineteenth century.

Wilson's most important publication was written not for the physician but for the general public. In a pocket-sized work entitled *A Practical Treatise on Healthy Skin* (1845), later known as *Healthy Skin*, Wilson delivered a first-of-its-kind, science-based message to the layperson: appreciate your skin, take care of it or else suffer a deplorable skin condition, and know that the study of skin disease has become a science. He included messages to his reader such as "beware the popular remedies for ringworm."[105] The work is even today a delight to read, especially because the language was written with the layperson in mind. The work as a whole represents the best opportunity for us to learn what a nineteenth-century practicing dermatologist told his patients.[106] For appealing to the masses in what was deemed a publicity stunt, Wilson garnered much criticism, and the work may have actually intensified the dislike of the wider medical profession for those who specialized in the skin.[107] But it did draw people to the office for skin problems and put skin health on the minds of the public in a unique way. In this manner, Wilson did more for dermatology than any other figure of the nineteenth century.

In *Healthy Skin*, Wilson preached that skin cleanliness was a sign of health and that removing dirt, sweat, and other waste material excreted on the surface of the skin was a necessary task for maintaining the health of both the skin and the body as a whole. It had been believed for many centuries that the skin's primary function was waste elimination, and in 1835, the first complete synthesis of the anatomy and physiology of the skin was published, and this function of the skin finally had a scientific basis. The publication was *Nouvelle recherches sur la structure de la peau* (1835) by the French comparative anatomists Gilbert Breschet (1784–1845) and Augustin Roussel de Vauzeme (1754–1837). Wilson introduced the layperson to these details of the anatomy of the skin. He also discussed ways of keeping it healthy, e.g., bathing, and the horrors of what could happen to the skin—the gory details of skin disease—when its health was neglected. He likely startled his reader with a discussion of such topics as the *Demodex* mites living in follicles, a discussion that the present author has daily with patients and always finds to be an awkward conversation.

Wilson described the "very minute cylindrical tubes"—the sweat ducts—coursing through the skin to expel noxious compounds.[108] He famously calculated the combined total length of every sweat duct in the body, in what was the most often-quoted passage of the book:

> The number of square inches of surface in a man of ordinary height and bulk, is 2,500; the number of pores, therefore, 7,000,000, and the number of inches of perspiratory tube 1,750,000, that is, 145,833 feet, or 48,600 yards, or nearly twenty eight miles.[109]

Wilson captured the imagination of his readers with this passage because he drew an analogy with the sweat ducts to something presently on their minds: the sewerage pipes of the city.[110] The sanitation movement of the 1840s—the effort to deal with widespread squalor in London in order to prevent disease—was underway; thus, the timing was perfect for Wilson's message.[111] Wilson convincingly argued that blockage of these perspiratory conduits, resulting from both external dirt and the build-up of internally sourced excreted waste, could lead to a wide variety of problems. Wilson's solution was a public health initiative of bathhouses so that persons of every socioeconomic status had access to clean water for bathing. The public heard his message: bathe or risk your health. The goal was not only clean streets and clean homes, but also clean skin and a clean body. Wilson admitted in the preface to *Healthy Skin* that his conviction that skin hygiene could prevent skin disease had plenty of advocates that preceded him, but Wilson's fame gave so much credibility to the argument that he made the bath fashionable in England.[112]

Wilson had once written that a popular mid-nineteenth-century British product called Pears Soap was an excellent cleansing agent. His comment would unknowingly result in one of the most successful advertising campaigns of all time, benefitting Pears greatly, and the company produced advertisements with Wilson's name all over them. The endorsement of Pears Soap drew more ire from his colleagues for Wilson allowing the commercial exploitation of his name and reputation.[113] With the bathhouse campaign and the soap endorsement, he was criticized by his professional colleagues who not only loathed what they saw as shameless self-aggrandizement, but they also disapproved of the popularization of medical knowledge. Wilson defended himself in the *Lancet* in 1864:

> However much I may join in the regret of my friends at the use thus made of my name, I see no means of escaping it. It has happened to others as well as myself, and we see daily the names of eminent men associated with popular remedies of various kinds prepared from their prescriptions. I can only say that I have not encouraged this practice in my own instance.[114]

Wilson appeared to be the powerless victim, unable to stop the use of his name. We cannot know if he was saving face or actually irritated by the exploitation, but the man never gave us any reason to distrust the words out of his mouth or pen.

Published in his journal in 1867, Wilson's classical description of lichen planus was his most significant contribution to the corpus of knowledge on skin disease. Culled from 50 cases, his description was complete with all the varieties, such as the mucosal and annular forms. He also described exfoliative dermatitis, erythema nodosum, trichorrhexis nodosa, roseola, and the spider angiomas of liver disease; he wrote extensively about leprosy. His description of neurotic excoriations laid the groundwork for our understanding of psychosomatic skin disease. His writings on scabies and *Demodex* were among the best in Europe.[115] He was the first to estimate the number of hairs on the human head, which we know today to be about 100,000.[116]

While clearly brilliant, Wilson erred for many years in his nonacceptance of the parasitic nature of certain skin diseases such as favus, ringworm, and pityriasis versicolor, and he blamed ringworm on poor nutrition, ignoring the scientific arguments from his peers both at home and abroad for 20 years or more after the discovery of *Trichophyton* and *Microsporum*.[117] In *Healthy Skin*, he mistakenly chose to share his view with the public that ringworm was noncontagious.[118] Some of Wilson's contemporaries viewed his reluctance to accept fungus as the cause of tinea as an indication that Wilson was too set in his old-fashioned ways to appreciate the new mid-nineteenth-century science of the skin. However, a review of the 1852 third American edition of *On Diseases of the Skin* reveals that this was simply not the case. For example, he quoted Gustav Simon (see Chapter 15) often in the work and frequently discussed the microscopic aspects of the skin and its diseases throughout the text. In the preface, he declared a rather modern approach to the study of skin disease:

> The study of diseases of the skin offers a natural division into two parts—a scientific and practical part. The former embraces all that belongs to structure, physiology, and pathology; the latter, the application of the results of these investigations to the treatment and cure of disease. Conceiving that no real improvement could be made in the practical department of the subject in any other way than through the advancement of the scientific portion, I have continued to bestow much attention and labour on the microscopic examination of the cutaneous tissues.[119]

It would be a challenge to find a more modern way of thinking about dermatology at this time. Furthermore, he demonstrated his acceptance of the itch mite as the cause of scabies, when he wrote:

> I am thoroughly convinced, and so long as I possess that conviction, shall ever continue to maintain that the Acarus is the sole and only cause of scabies, and that every eruption, however acuminated and well-defined its vesicles, if it be deficient in the living cause, is not scabies.[120]

Wilson was not antiquated in his thinking, and in other ways, he challenged the status quo of his time. He was openly critical of Willan's system:

> The artificial classification of Willan is open to the serious objection of assembling together, in the same class, disorders of the most opposite kind, and of separating different phases of the same disease. Thus, the association of purpura with rubeola and scarlatina; erysipelas with pemphigus; ichthyosis with lepra; scabies with variola and porrigo; eczema with varicella and vaccinia; acne with verruca; and naevus with ephelis, is opposed to every principle of affinity of disease.[121]

CLEOPATRA'S NEEDLE

Wilson had many diverse interests outside of medicine. He was a published Egyptologist, and the most famous non-medical story about Wilson involves his enthusiasm for all things Egyptian.[122] In 1878, Wilson organized and paid out of his own pocket to have the obelisk known as Cleopatra's Needle (ca. 1450 BCE) moved from Egypt to London. It had twice been offered as a gift from the Egyptian government to the British people—for the brilliant naval victory over the French in 1798 at the Battle of the Nile—but the donation was declined due to the cost of moving it. Wilson's plan was to float the needle in a case from Alexandria to London. Along the way, a violent storm caused the case to separate from the boat, and six sailors died in the process. The case containing the Needle was found floating off the coast of Portugal three months later, and the journey continued successfully. One can only imagine the pride Wilson felt when he saw the Needle erected along the Thames, where it still stands today.

Travel was another of Wilson's passions, both for leisure and for professional pursuits. He often combined business with pleasure in his journeys. He once went to Eastern Europe to satisfy his desire for knowledge of certain skin diseases, such as leprosy, not seen in his home country. He also visited the clinics of Hebra (see Chapter 14), the details of which are scant.[123] We do know that he held his Viennese counterpart in high regard, as this excerpt from *On Diseases of the Skin* implies, for dealing with the lepra versus leprosy confusion:

> The term Lepra—der Aussatz in German—signifies the eruption, the great eruption. It is synonymous with leprosy, THE leprosy, the ancient leprosy, that which has since been called elephantiasis. Therefore, let us bestow the term lepra where it rightfully belongs, or reject it altogether. The trivial affection which we at present call lepra has no single point of comparison with leprosy. We cannot but admit the truth of this argument, and we cannot, also, but recognize in an instant the monstrous absurdity of calling a comparatively insignificant disease by so portentous a name. Let us suppose a patient addressing his medical adviser: "What is the name of my complaint, Doctor?" And now I will ask any medical man to whom this question has ever been addressed, to reflect on the pang which has gone through his entire frame before he has brought himself to give the only possible answer—"Lepra." "What!" exclaims the startled patient, "Leprosy?" And then the apologetic response—"No, not leprosy; lepra." And the medical man can only hope that the patient will not go at once to his dictionary, and find out that either the dictionary is wrong or the doctor. Now Hebra cuts the Gordian knot. Eczema he calls eczema; lepra, lepra; and that very common affection which we at present term lepra, he calls psoriasis. The change is simple, the reasons for it important. We cannot do better than adopt it. Moreover, it suits the spirit of the British bulldog to call things by their proper names, and we are too noble in our nature not to recognize and value the intellect of our foreign brethren.[124]

Wilson was very wealthy, both from his professional dealings with his affluent patients and from several shrewd investments in gas and railroads, and he was in no way parsimonious.[125] Sir James Paget, the famous British surgeon, commented that he lived modestly.[126] His generosity, both toward the poor and toward society in general, were legendary. He frequently gave away his expertise to the indigent who sought it and even gave these patients his own money to buy their treatment. Wilson was also philanthropic, kind, and compassionate toward the less fortunate, and his specialization never got in the way of his physician-ness—treating the whole patient.[127] While his philanthropic deeds might be seen as publicity-seeking efforts, an obituary argued to the contrary:

> His generosity to poor patients who came to consult him was very great, not only prescribing for them gratis, but supplying the means for carrying out the treatment, and that not only after he became wealthy, but even at a time when he could ill afford to be generous. The amount of good he did privately will probably never be known, as he was one of whom it may truly be said, that he never let his left hand know what his right hand did—so unostentatious was he in regard to his charity.[128]

He endowed the Chair of Dermatology at the RCS and the Chair of Pathology at Aberdeen. He paid to restore a church where he was tutored in his youth. Upon Wilson's own death and later his wife's, the bulk of his fortune was bequeathed to the RCS. He once rescued a suicidal woman from drowning in a local canal and was afterward dubbed a hero by the Humane Society.

Unlike Willan, however, Wilson did show ambition for public recognition. His name eventually became synonymous with skin care and appeared on every bottle of popular hair tonic.[129] Wilson's personality echoed that of Alibert: flamboyant, extroverted, self-seeking.[130] His writing was grandiose and loquacious to the point of exasperation: "he wrote more nonsense than most men."[131] As a lecturer, he was mediocre. He could be scathing about his French contemporaries: after viewing a French moulage (wax model) labeled as pityriasis rubra pilaris but what he argued was actually lichen planus, he noted:

> [the moulages] do not enhance our respect for the present state of dermatological science in France. We think it is a good deal behindhand and especially lacking in regard to pathological considerations and its professors know apparently little of the labors of foreign writers.[132]

Wilson's place in the higher levels of the dermatologic pantheon is secure, but exactly where he fits is open to debate. The statements in Wilson's 1884 *Lancet* obituary—that Wilson "knew more about skin diseases than any man of his time. He cured when others failed to cure."—raise the question of how he compared to his Viennese counterpart Hebra.[133] Other appraisals of his contributions were not so kind, contending that he "added little to pathology or therapeutics, and not a little to confusion by changing terminology"; a review of his widely read textbook in the *Glasgow Medical Journal* (1864) argued that his text was representative of a "low ebb" in dermatology in Britain.[134] However, Wilson was indeed a great figure who did more for dermatology than any other nineteenth-century British dermatologist except Robert Willan. Besnier stated that he "above all had that rare merit, even rarer at the present time, of being a doctor and a dermatologist."[135] Wilson's spectacular life was affirmed in 1881 when Queen Victoria knighted him at age 72, but soon after, he suffered from that worst of fates for a dermatologist: blindness.

While Willan and Bateman were the founders of dermatologic specialization in Britain, Wilson's career represents the advance of dermatology into the mainstream of British medicine. He was dermatology's greatest promoter. His aptitude, zeal, prolificity, and dominant personality allowed him to achieve respectability for the specialty of dermatology. His philanthropy and benevolence inspire the modern physician to give more to humanity than what is provided inside the exam room.

DARWIN'S DERMATITIS

Charles Darwin (1809–1882), the British naturalist and geologist, circumnavigated the globe from 1831–1836 aboard the HMS *Beagle*, and upon returning from his famous voyage, a life of chronic illness began for the 27-year-old Darwin. Just a few of his many physical complaints over the years included chest pain, heart palpitations, headaches, muscle spasms, tremors, malaise and exhaustion, vertigo, visual disturbance, abdominal pain, and nearly constant vomiting. In addition to these internal symptoms, Darwin had a history of dermatological problems. The first time Darwin complained of skin problems was in 1828 when he had to cancel a trip to Edinburgh because of sore lips.[136] Before departing on the HMS *Beagle* in 1831, he wrote to his sister that his hands were "not quite well."[137] After returning from his journey around the world, Darwin developed full-blown eczema and, later in 1847, the dreaded complication that commonly affects persons with severe eczema—boils.[138] His son commented after Darwin's death how "his skin erupted with boils, rashes, and eczema."[139] Darwin noted on several occasions how his eczema was related to his other ailments.[140] His eczema was so bad at one point that his friend Joseph Hooker claimed that during "his violent eczema of the head, he was scarcely recognizable."[141]

Much has been written about Darwin's health, and various speculations from retrospective diagnosticians exist about the causes of Darwin's innumerable ailments. Crohn's disease, lactose intolerance, systemic lupus erythematosus, cyclic vomiting syndrome, and Chagas disease have all been postulated as etiologies. Chagas disease (American trypanosomiasis) is a parasitic illness endemic in South America that Darwin could have contracted while in that part of the world. The exact cause or causes of his various symptoms remain open to debate, but it is likely that Darwin's skin problems were chronic, recurrent dermatitis (eczema) with a strong neurogenic component. It appears that Darwin also suffered from anxiety, panic attacks, and depression for most of his adult life, and chronic forms of eczema (neurodermatitis) in adult patients are very frequently associated with stress and mental illness. His other complaints—the cyclic vomiting, the chest pain, the palpitations—can also be explained by psychosomatic illness.

The Brothers Fox: William Tilbury (1836–1879) and Thomas Colcott (1849–1916)

A new, modern era for dermatology in Victorian Britain that was heralded by the career of Erasmus Wilson was cemented by two men every bit as brilliant as himself: William Tilbury Fox and Jonathan Hutchinson (see below). William Tilbury Fox (1836–1879) was the son of a physician and elder brother of the famous British dermatologist Thomas Colcott Fox. After receiving his MD in 1858, Tilbury Fox embarked on a career in obstetrics, but five years into that field, he switched to dermatology. It was his interest in mycology and the skin that led to the career change.[142]

In contrast to Willan, who worked at the public dispensary, and Wilson, who worked in a private practice, Tilbury Fox found no place in London in which to study skin disease, as dermatologic specialization was still frowned upon by the broader medical community. Consequently, he teamed up with Erasmus Wilson to found the St. John's Hospital for Skin Diseases in London in 1864. But they both resigned from the special hospital after just 12 days, stating in a letter to the *Lancet* that the excuse was a disagreement with a colleague over his career focus on spermatorrhoea, which was the discredited, nineteenth-century male counterpart to hysteria.[143] By 1866, Fox was working in the skin disease department at Charing Cross hospital; two years later, he found a more permanent home in the dermatology department at University College Hospital in London.

Tilbury Fox was a complete dermatologist, equipped with excellent clinical skills as well as a curiosity for new discoveries on the continent, which he imported into England.[144] He revived Willanism and took a hard-line position that defended Willan's eight lesion types as the only eight types possible in nature.[145] He was also an ardent constitutional pathologist, making him somewhat of a cross between Willan and Bazin (see Chapter 14). Unlike Hebra, who shunned the patient's history and focused on only that which he could himself confirm, Fox held on to every word of the patient, as he was of the opinion that the entirety of the patient's story—diet, environment, and habits—was as important in determining both the diagnosis and treatment plan as the physical exam findings. In the end, Hebra's approach endured because constitutional pathology had no scientific basis.

Fox's greatest achievement was the description of the modern concept of impetigo contagiosa, which he separated from eczema as a distinct and very different entity, and established its contagiousness and distinction from each of the meanings that the word *impetigo* had held since the time of Celsus.[146] He is also credited with the first descriptions of dyshidrosis, urticaria pigmentosa, lymphangioma circumscriptum, and dermatitis herpetiformis, and he wrote articles on molluscum, prurigo, and acne. His publication list is among the most impressive of the period. His first publication, *Skin Diseases of Parasitic Origin; Their Nature and Treatment Including the Description and Relations of the Fungi Found in Man* (1863), was a remarkable first entry into the growing corpus of dermatologic literature of nineteenth-century Europe. In that work can be found the first description of kerion, which Fox knew to be a type of fungal infection. He misbelieved that only one kind of pathogenic fungus existed and that the patient's constitutional state determined both the clinical picture and the morphology of the fungus under the microscope.[147]

A year later, Fox issued his textbook, *Skin Diseases: Their Description, Pathology, Diagnosis and Treatment with a Copious Formulary* (1864), which enjoyed major success for many decades. He journeyed to India in 1864 where he became interested in tropical medicine, which resulted in two major publications on endemic skin diseases of India (1872; 1876). Expertise in these diseases was in high demand, given the vast size of the British Empire and frequent contact of the British people with tropical diseases.[148] His work in India taught him that both morphea and leukoderma (*leuce*, white spots) had nothing to do with leprosy; he debunked that age-old belief in his writing on endemic skin disease.[149] His *Lectures on Eczema, Its Nature and Treatment* (1870) was a pioneering treatise on an important, developing concept. He published the *Atlas of Skin Diseases* (1875), which was a revised version of Willan's atlas. He died of heart disease while vacationing in Paris at just 43 years of age, presumably the end result of an illness such as rheumatic fever, acquired on a study abroad in Egypt. As a man, Tilbury Fox was "virtuous, able, industrious, and popular."[150] What greatness in the field of dermatology he accomplished in such a short life, and what equal greatness the world was likely deprived of by such an early death.

Perhaps it was through the career of his younger brother that Tilbury's legacy lived on. After a career as a world-class cricket player, Thomas Colcott Fox joined his older brother in the specialty of dermatology. "Tommy" became a careful observer and master diagnostician whose reputation was as esteemed across the Channel as it was at home; Besnier (see Chapter 14) was once heard to say that "we think the world of Dr. Fox," referring to the younger.[151] Although he never authored a textbook as did his brother, Thomas did collaborate with Tilbury on many projects, including the *Epitome of Skin Diseases with Formulae for Students and Practitioners* (1876). His first appointment was at the Victoria Hospital for Children, and pediatric dermatology became a unique interest of his. He was the first to describe granuloma annulare as the "ringed eruption" in 1895, although the name is credited to his countryman, Radcliff-Crocker (see below); he was the first in Britain to discover tuberculosis as the cause of erythema induratum; and he did some investigative work in mycology, particularly with *Microsporum species*. A gifted, kind, and jovial teacher, the younger Fox was a childless dog lover, inconsolable when his dog died after three long days of Fox himself nursing the dog following a dog fight.[152] He was said by one of his contemporaries to be "the rock upon which modern dermatology was founded."[153] Indeed, the two Foxes were extraordinarily influential in the history of dermatology.

Jonathan Hutchinson (1828–1913)

Jonathan Hutchinson, who has already been introduced in the Interlude on syphilis, helped Wilson legitimize the specialty of dermatology in mid-nineteenth-century Britain. The son of Quakers and an heir to no medical tradition, the young Hutchinson took the surgical route to a career in medicine with plans of medical missionary work. It was the influence of the physician Thomas Laycock (1812–1876) and the surgeon James Paget (1814–1899) who swayed him from that career and toward London academia.[154] Hutchinson was first employed as a surgeon at various hospitals in London, including St. Bartholomew's Hospital, Blackfriars Hospital for Skin Diseases, and the London Hospital. He was a classmate of Joseph Lister.

Hutchinson went on to become one of the most respected physicians of the nineteenth century, and his accomplishments were many: a professorship and later presidency at the RCS (1877), fellowship in the Royal Society (1882), knighthood (1908), and presidencies of various medical societies, including the ophthalmological society and neurological society. Hutchinson was "the last multispecialist," one who dabbled in many different fields of medicine, including surgery, ophthalmology, neurology, syphilology, and leprology.[155] His interests outside of medicine were diverse; he gave weekly educational lectures at his home in Haslemere on varied topics: natural history, maps, charts, historical portraits, and history.[156] A genius with an encyclopedic memory for both the medical literature and his case log, Hutchinson gained experience with skin disease drawn from an enormous private practice that was perhaps only rivaled by that of Wilson.

Among his greatest contributions in dermatology was the Hutchinson sign of melanoma of the nail apparatus, which states that when melanotic pigment is present on the skin fold around the nail, pigmented streaks within the nail itself are concerning for melanoma. He also described arsenical keratoses, juvenile springtime eruption (hydroa aestivale), rodent ulcer, keratoacanthoma, angioma serpiginosum, and countless other dermatologic entities. Hutchinson has more eponyms than possibly anyone in the history of medicine, including a triad, syndrome, facies, two signs, pupil, disease, freckle, mask, etc. He correctly recognized that inheritance is an important factor in determining risk for skin diseases, such as psoriasis, eczema, and acne. Like Tilbury Fox, he tended to side with Bazin on the view that constitution played a major role in the cause of skin disease.

MORTIMER'S MALADY

In 1869, Jonathan Hutchinson may have been the first to describe two cases of sarcoidosis: a 58-year-old coal-wharf worker with a 2-year history of progressively worsening, purple, symmetrical skin plaques on the legs and hands that were neither tender nor painful; and a 64-year-old woman who presented with raised, dusky red skin lesions on the face, forearms, the lobule of the ear, and the bridge of the nose.[157] In keeping with his tendency to name conditions after the person afflicted with it, he referred to the latter as "Mortimer's malady." These types of cases may have inspired Hutchinson's contemporary/fellow physician/neighbor, Sir Arthur Conan Doyle (1859–1930), to make skin disease a basic plot ingredient in his story, *The Adventures of the Blanched*

Soldier (1926). In that story, a dermatologist enters the last scene and diagnoses the patient—who had convinced himself he had leprosy because of his scaly skin lesions of a bleached color—with "pseudo-leprosy," a term that is not in use today. The differential diagnosis of such skin lesions includes vitiligo, eczema, ichthyosis, tinea versicolor, leprosy, mycosis fungoides, and sarcoidosis. As pointed out by Sharma, Doyle and Hutchinson must have known one another and exchanged ideas at meetings of the London Medical Society.[158] Hutchinson attended these meetings regularly, and Dr. Conan Doyle practiced near the office of the Medical Society of London.

Hutchinson was not immune to criticism. While he predicted the existence of the spirochete in syphilis some 25 years before it was discovered, he persisted in his belief that the consumption of rotting fish was the cause of leprosy and not a bacterial infection.[159] He was decidedly obstinate in his views. Others have criticized him as overzealous and that he added to the confusion as a "freelance, giving any dermatosis that was unknown to him a name."[160]

Hutchinson's seminal descriptions were published in the *Archives of Surgery*, a journal he himself founded in 1889 and for which he was the sole contributor. The 11 volumes of *Archives* journals (1889–1900) contain many classics of dermatology. Not all of his contributions to the journal were dermatologic ones; he also contributed innumerable texts on surgery and ophthalmology. According to his biographer, Robert Jackson, his writings contained "catchy, descriptive terms, his use of patients' names for diseases, his belief in the effectiveness of illustrations, superb clinical observation but faulty conclusions, and a lack of humor."[161] William Osler, that Johns Hopkins giant, pointedly characterized the value of Hutchinson's work:

> He is the only great generalized specialist which the profession has produced, and his works are a storehouse upon which the surgeon, the physician, the neurologist, the dermatologist and other specialists freely draw. When anything turns up which is anomalous or peculiar and cyclopaedias are dumb, I tell my students to turn to the volumes of Mr. Hutchinson's Archives of Surgery, as, if it is not mentioned in them, it surely is something very much out of the common.[162]

If the quantity of dermatologic publications is the criterion for assessing influence, with an estimated 600 of his 1200 published articles having a dermatologic subject, Hutchinson was, without a doubt, the most influential physician of nineteenth-century dermatology. But his eye for the new was strictly focused on new diseases, not theory or treatment. With his phenomenal intelligence and diligence compared to his contemporaries, he was a seemingly superhuman, prolific polymath—like Plenck—but not an intensely focused "finished dermatologist," such as Wilson or Hebra or even Fox, and is therefore overshadowed by these men.[163]

But his career did fully span the period of modernization of the specialty of dermatology, and he was both a major player in the developments and a witness to them:

> Dermatology is no longer to be regarded with senseless prejudice, as a mere matter of giving arsenic and prescribing ointments and lotions, nor, as some, only a stage more enlightened, think, an arena for endless debate as to the arbitrary application of pedantic names or older or newer coinage. We have got beyond the old classification, and we are ceasing to be merely empirical therapeutists. We claim for dermatology a foremost place as a branch of scientific medicine, and without hesitation I assert of it that beyond all others it offers attractions to the student of laws of disease in general, and to the seeker after the causes which disturb health and local nutrition.[164]

Speaking to the British Medical Association in 1890, Hutchinson discussed the status and the future of the specialty, and his advocacy demonstrated a passion that cannot be questioned for the specific field of dermatology:

> The dermatologist has before him two principal duties; first, the all-important and paramount one, to cure or relieve those who consult him for skin diseases; and next, to add to the general knowledge of pathology by the study of the phenomena which are brought under his

observation ... [We] have also to some extent found out that the shortest road to successful therapeutics, even in our own department, lies not in toilsome empiricism, but in the attempt to understand rightly the laws under which these diseases are evoked.[165]

Unusual because he specialized in multiple fields, Hutchinson cautioned against focusing solely on the skin in his statement that "the aim of all true-hearted specialists should be to break down the walls of their specialism."[166] Hutchinson spoke a truth: knowledge about internal medicine and other fields can be very useful to the dermatologist.

Finally, on the future of the specialty, Hutchinson stated:

> In the further prosecution of dermatological studies we must, if I mistake not, work mainly on two lines .... We must in the first place avoid narrowness and specialism, and secondly, we must develop to the utmost our knowledge of details. The younger of our recruits need be under no feelings of discouragement that there is but little left for them to do. In truth, only the foundations have as yet been laid. In every direction, more minute examination is needed. Although, according to some of our critics, subdivision has already gone too far, it must, according to my appreciation, be taken much further yet. Not a single skin disease can be mentioned that does not include under its name varieties which need to be separately grouped and separately examined if we would arrive at a truthful estimate of its causes and real nature. So far from these subdivisions making the subject more complex, they are really the only means to its simplification .... We want then, I think, the careful examination and record of clinical facts. No cases should be placed together which are not exactly alike. All possible aids must be invoked. The microscope, the photographic camera, the artist's pencil, and above all the trained eye and pen of the skilled and patient observer must be brought into full use ...
>
> Above all, in order that dermatology should prosper as a part of medicine, it is, I think, essential that we should learn to use our names lightly. Unquestionably we must have names for the groups of phenomena with which we have to deal. We must never for a moment forget, however, that those names do not designate entities which are complete in themselves, and that for the most part we apply them to conditions which in themselves are symptoms or combinations for symptoms. We must be for ever seeking for conceptions which, in dealing with the reality, shall go much deeper than the name which has come into use. Nothing has more impeded the progress of dermatology, nothing makes its study more repellent to the student, or its knowledge more difficult of attainment than the habit of giving an arbitrary name to every little group of phenomena, treating that name as if it represented a substantive and isolated reality, and insisting that the facts of disease shall be made to group themselves in accordance with our conventional nosologies.[167]

Henry Radcliffe Crocker (1845–1909)

The career of the last figure that deserves mention represents an excellent culmination of a century of British developments in dermatology and proof that the efforts of Wilson, Fox, and Hutchinson were not in vain. Henry Radcliffe Crocker was the greatest dermatologist in Britain at the turn of the twentieth century. His career in dermatology began in 1876 when he received an appointment at the skin department of University College Hospital in London. Upon the death of his mentor, Tilbury Fox, he was named head of the department in 1879. The University College Hospital was the premier educational institution for dermatology in London at this time. The clinic had been established by Anthony Todd Thompson in 1828, but the department of dermatology was not founded at University College Hospital until 1859 under the direction of William Jenner (1815–1898), the personal physician of Queen Victoria. While Tilbury Fox had elevated the department to a status on par with the unofficial competition in Paris and Vienna, it was Crocker who enriched and consolidated the department to become a world-renowned center of excellence in dermatology at the end of the century.

Crocker named granuloma annulare and described angiokeratoma, erythema elevatum diutinum, lichen spinulosus, and many others, and he was the first to implicate micrococci as the cause of impetigo.[168] Crocker is significant for being the first of the British dermatologists to incorporate the scientific advancements of histopathology in his practice and teaching, and his recognition of the value of the microscope is seen throughout all of his works. He called attention to the epidemiology of skin disease; the order of prevalence of skin diseases reported by Crocker gives us an idea of the typical caseload of a dermatologist of his era: eczema, acne, scabies, psoriasis, seborrhea, impetigo, urticaria, dermatitis venenata (contact dermatitis), tinea, alopecia, pediculosis, pruritus, verruca, and ecthyma.[169] This list is surprisingly similar to the diagnoses seen in dermatology clinics today.

Like Fox and Hutchinson before him, who were similarly influenced by Bazin, Crocker believed that giving attention to both the general health and diet of the patient was crucial in the management of skin disease patients; in his mind, most skin diseases were secondary to internal diseases. To Crocker, dietary disturbance was the most important risk factor for skin disease; to his way of thinking, disturbances such as intestinal irritation from unhealthy food led to "reflexes" generated in the gastrointestinal tract that affected the skin adversely.[170] His views on diet and skin disease were very influential for the better part of the twentieth century, as were his general beliefs that a dermatologist should treat the whole patient rather than focus solely on the skin. He administered both topical and systemic treatments, and his approach was "a synthesis of the approach of Erasmus Wilson, who relied mainly on systemic therapy, and of the Vienna school, which emphasized topical care."[171]

JOSEPH MERRICK, "THE ELEPHANT MAN"

Crocker is famous in part for being the first to propose a diagnosis in the case of Joseph Merrick (1862–1890); unfortunately, he is better known as the Elephant Man. Merrick was presented by his physician Frederick Treves (1853–1923) as having elephantiasis at a meeting of the Pathological Society of London in 1885. Treves had found Merrick at a sideshow run by Tom Norman and then befriended the severely deformed man and became his doctor.

On Merrick, Crocker wrote:

> An extraordinary case of the kind was brought to the Pathological Society by Treves. I had an opportunity of examining the patient there, and at a show, in which he was exhibited as an "elephant man." The bulk of the disease was on the right side; there was an enormous hypertrophy of the skin of the whole right arm, measuring twelve inches round the wrist and five round one of the fingers, a lax mass of pendulous skin, etc., depending from the right pectoral region. The right side of the face was enormously thickened, and in addition there were huge unsymmetrical exostoses on the forehead and occiput. There were also tumours affecting the right side of the gums, and palate, on both legs, but chiefly the right, and over nearly the whole back and buttocks; the skin was immensely thickened with irregular lobulated masses of confluent tumors of the ordinary molluscous tumour characters. The left arm and hand were small and well formed. The man was twenty-five years old, of stunted growth, and had a right talipes equinus, but was fairly intelligent. The disease was not perceived much at birth, but began to develop when five years old, and has gradually increased since; it was, of course, ascribed to maternal fright during pregnancy.[172]

Crocker proposed that Merrick suffered from dermatolysis (cutis laxa) and bony deformities, brought about by a nervous system disorder. A few decades after Merrick's death, it was proposed incorrectly that Merrick actually had suffered from von Recklinghausen's disease (neurofibromatosis), and this diagnosis stuck with Merrick for most of the twentieth century. At present, it is believed that Merrick's correct diagnosis is a rare disorder called Proteus syndrome.[173]

Incidentally, the origins of the sideshow, also called the freak show, can be traced to the eighteenth century, but it reached its zenith as both a widely popular exhibition and a commercially successful business operation in the 1880s and 1890s in Victorian London and New York City, led by the showmen Norman and PT Barnum, respectively. At these shows, unfortunate persons displayed their various disabilities and deformities, many of which were dermatological. Joseph Merrick was perhaps the most famous, but other skin conditions were represented, including congenital generalized hypertrichosis, hirsutism, albinism, ichthyosis, and acromegaly. Through a present-day lens, the sideshow has been looked back upon as exploitative and cruel, and while that is an anticipated view, we must remember that at the time, the sideshow was a means by which these less-fortunate individuals willingly sought and secured a substantial payment for exposing their vulnerabilities to the world—a world that would otherwise disallow them any income by traditional means.

Crocker's greatest legacy was *Diseases of the Skin* (1888), the most highly regarded dermatology textbook in English for several decades; the third and final edition released in 1903 was a colossal 1466 pages.[174] It is the first textbook in this history that a present-day dermatologist would describe as having a distinctly modern feel. A contemporary of Crocker, Arthur Whitfield (1868–1947), called it "the best work on dermatology that has been produced in any language," and in 1976, the work was described as the "Old Testament of our discipline ... written in lucid classical English."[175] Through this text, it is evident that Crocker represents the first fully modern English-speaking dermatologist, complete with an appreciation for the clinical and histopathological aspects of skin disease. According to his obituary,

> Dr. Radcliff Crocker's very high position as a dermatologist was won alike by his general knowledge of medicine, his particular skill as a clinician, and notably by his admirable contributions to the literature of dermatology. He was one of those teachers who seems destined to exert an influence over the medical education of his country far outside the walls of his own hospital, for he possessed an abundant literary energy, a clear method of exposition, and a profound zeal for the science he spent his life advancing.[176]

Summary

The date March 8, 1790, represents the birthday of British dermatology. That was the day when the Medical Society of London awarded Robert Willan the Fothergill Gold Medal for his novel system for classifying skin diseases. The first four orders of his eight-order system, which was based on the morphology of skin lesions, was published 18 years later in *On Cutaneous Diseases* (1808), the most famous dermatological text of all time. His protege, Thomas Bateman, issued the other four orders in *A Practical Synopsis of Cutaneous Diseases* (1813). Willan's and Bateman's approach to diagnosing skin diseases became known as Willanism; it spread to France largely through the efforts of Laurent-Theodore Biett (see Chapter 13). After Willan and Bateman, dermatology in Britain waned until the 1840s with the career of William James Erasmus Wilson, who brought dermatology into the public consciousness with his *Healthy Skin* (1845), a fascinating text about skin care written for the masses. After Wilson, Tilbury Fox, Jonathan Hutchinson, and Henry Radcliffe-Crocker solidified dermatology's position among the burgeoning specialties of medicine in Britain. Medical specialization occurred later in Britain because the gentleman-physicians of the Victorian era considered the word *specialist* synonymous with *quack*.

13

The French School

Willanism spread from London to the mainland of Europe largely due to the efforts of one man, the aforementioned Laurent-Théodore Biett (1781–1840). Biett was born in Switzerland and completed his medical education in Paris. In 1816, Biett was asked by a wealthy French family to accompany a young man, in a medical capacity, to London. As Biett was himself employed at a dispensary in Paris at the time, he toured the Carey Street Dispensary and there met Thomas Bateman, who taught him the Willanist doctrine.[1] Impressed by some aspects of the system, Biett was the first to bring this doctrine to Paris, thus establishing a lineage of so-called French Willanists. Biett's pupils were "all ears," but his famous mentor was not listening.

Jean-Louis-Marc Alibert (1768–1837)

That mentor was Jean-Louis-Marc Alibert. Born in Villefranche-de-Rouergue in Aveyron in the south of France, Alibert first embarked on a career in the priesthood; however, the French Revolution and its dispersal of all religious orders forced a change of plans for young Alibert. After a period of career uncertainty, Alibert did the natural thing a young man his age would do: head to the big city. Having been influenced by several prominent Parisian physicians, he settled on a career in medicine and entered medical school at an age later than was usual for his time—at twenty-seven. While enrolled at the University of Paris, Alibert experienced an insufficient education due to the turbulence of the last decade of the eighteenth century, but he did cross paths with the great Philippe Pinel, to whom he dedicated his thesis on fevers in 1800. Although the greatest scientist of the period, Antoine Lavoisier (1743–1794), was murdered by the revolutionaries in 1794, scientific pursuit eventually found its advocates within the French government. Medical schools had been abolished in 1792 and were undergoing a period of reconstruction, so Alibert's education was chaotic and inadequate—based on lectures and not clinical patient care.[2] His grades for one of his terms revealed a weakness in "external pathology."[3]

Alibert's inexperience with skin disease would soon be resolved. His first professional appointment after medical school was adjunct physician (1802) at the Hôpital Saint-Louis, where he received the same level of exposure to skin pathology that Willan had received at the Carey Street Dispensary. Founded by Henry IV in 1607 and open since 1611, the 1100-bed, prison-like Hôpital Saint-Louis, which was originally ordered for sequestration of bubonic plague patients on the outskirts of Paris, had become by 1800 a facility for patients with chronic diseases. With dermatologic therapeutics so ineffective at this time, a preponderance of patients with intractable skin diseases—such as syphilis, leprosy, cutaneous tuberculosis, scurvy, ringworm, scrofula, ulcers, and eczemas—occupied the hospital. Rather than request a less daunting assignment, Alibert sunk his teeth into the task and soon realized he had found his professional niche.

Other than what he had learned from reading the *Tractatus* of his countryman Lorry, Alibert could not have had much knowledge about skin disease in 1800–1801. He was entering a deserted, uncharted territory of medicine, but he appeared nonetheless to relish the opportunity that a skin-disease hospital would afford him for fame and glory in a discipline that had yet to be formalized; he "fancied himself as an explorer in the vast unknown land of skin diseases."[4] Alibert approached his mission in dermatology with great zeal—and equal pride. Inpatient dermatology allowed him to evaluate skin diseases as they changed from day to day, and he quickly became a master of not only diagnosis but also the course of the disease, which he considered equal in importance to the morphology. This distinction separates Alibert from Plenck, whose source material was books, and Willan, who worked at an outpatient clinic.[5]

DOI: 10.1201/9781003273622-19

Alibert's career elevated Hôpital Saint-Louis to the preeminent facility for dermatological care in France and the birthplace of the French school of dermatology, founded by Alibert. To correct an over-crowding problem, Alibert quickly limited the admissions at St. Louis to only persons with skin diseases. He wrote to his intern Giron,

> Be inflexible against those parasites who wish to invade our hospital beds. Be firm in the Pavilion, be active, be inexorable, and admit to my service only cases of skin disease.[6]

Skin disease became the only concern of the hospital by order of the council of administration of hospices in Paris on November 27, 1801.[7] That same year, Alibert began to lecture on dermatologic topics in a small amphitheater on the campus of Saint-Louis. As his audience grew, he took his interactive lecture series outdoors to a courtyard under the lime trees. Depictions of skin diseases were suspended from the trees behind Alibert, and live patient presentations were offered when Alibert found interesting patients on the streets of Paris and invited them to the demonstrations.[8] The patients, displayed on platforms, bore the name of their disease in one-inch letters across the chest.[9] He once tried to impress upon his audience the extreme degree of scaling that occurs in exfoliative dermatitis by throwing a bucket of scales on the occupants of the front row seats.[10] Alibert's dynamic teaching style brought him fame that soon spilled over into the general public, and laypersons, finding the lectures curious and then fashionable, attended these lectures with great zeal. Succeeding in making dermatology fascinating to anyone who would listen, Alibert was Mercurialis reborn.

His first of three masterpieces, *Description des maladies de la peau*, "Description of Skin Diseases," was published in 12 sections starting in 1806. The work is historically significant, not only because it was written in French instead of Latin but also because of its stunning artistic impressions of skin disease. The first edition, completed in 1814, was dedicated to Alexander I of Russia, as Alibert was a staunch supporter of monarchy in general, but not of Napoleon.[11] The book sold for 600 francs and was expensive to both produce and purchase and was almost financially ruinous, costing him his wife's entire dowry of 100,000 francs. When she died eight months after their marriage, he was compelled to return the money to her father.[12] The work was very well received by his peers, but it was too costly to be accessible for most. A less-expensive text-only version was completed in 1818.

In 1813, Alibert appointed his best pupil of 12 years, the aforementioned Laurent-Theodore Biett, as an adjunct physician of the hospital; a year later, Biett became the head of the newly founded dermatology outpatient clinic. When the Napoleonic era ended, and the Bourbons were restored to the throne of France in 1815, Alibert, at this point quite famous in France, was appointed royal physician to the king, Louis XVIII. With his time devoted to the king and his own private practice, Alibert turned over the supervision of Hôpital Saint-Louis to Biett. When Louis XVIII died in 1824, Alibert was retained as the personal physician of his successor, Charles X, who made Alibert a baron in 1827 in honor of his service to Louis XVIII. After that monarch fled for England in 1829, Alibert was able to return to his position as Chief Physician at Hôpital Saint-Louis after a 13-year-long break.[13]

The Hôpital Saint-Louis to which Alibert returned was a house divided, having been infiltrated by the cult of Willan. While Alibert was away, Biett had introduced Willan's system to the hospital. In addition, Biett's students and fellow Willanists—Pierre Louis Alphée Cazenave (1795–1877) and Henri Édouard Schedel (1804–1856)—had published a book in 1828 containing Biett's lectures entitled, *Abregé pratique des maladies de la peau*, "Abbreviated Practice of Skin Diseases." This book became the bible of French Willanism and is one of the most important dermatologic texts of the nineteenth century. Alibert's return was marred by the surprise and pain of learning the extent to which ideas that were not his own had been accepted by his former students.[14] Biett tried to convince Alibert of the tenability of the morphological approach to classification, but Alibert defended his own system, and the two eventually became estranged. Alibert respected Willan and his precise descriptions of skin diseases but thought that the elementary lesion was not the complete picture by which to characterize these diseases; i.e., he thought that the Willanist system was too artificial.[15] He was not alone in his convictions, and a rivalry between the *Alibertistes* and the *Willanistes* ensued in France. Unlike Willan, however, whose prize student was loyal to him even after his death, Alibert's once-favorite pupil, Biett, transferred his allegiance to the other side.

Fully prepared to defend his beliefs, Alibert gave a presentation on April 26, 1829, in which he explained his entire understanding of skin disease. It was in this lecture that Alibert's method of organizing skin diseases was revealed to the world as the *Arbre des dermatoses*, "Tree of Dermatoses." The *Tree* represents Alibert's attempt at a "natural" nosology: the smallest branches represent species (68), the next larger branches, genera (25), and the largest branches, orders (3). He brought the botanical basis of Linnaean classification to a whole new level, and he introduced a new nomenclature. His groupings were based not on a single criterion, such as morphology, but instead took into account cause, course, duration, appearance, and response to treatment, and how these diseases related to one another and how they affected the body as a whole.[16] According to Alibert, skin diseases could only be recognized after their complete development had been observed, not by the artificial approach of analyzing the elementary lesion.[17] Upon completion of Alibert's presentation, the audience applauded, which brought Alibert to tears as he addressed them with great appreciation for supporting him and his doctrine.[18] The Protestant introvert Biett delivered his own presentation a few days after the Catholic extrovert Alibert, and he argued in convincing fashion that the Willanist system was more precise, practical, and natural.[19] Alibert, with his gift for rhetoric, did not falter, and the two men bickered contentiously with one another for eight more years.

Alibert's *Tree* was published in both of Alibert's other masterpieces, *Monographie des Dermatoses* (1832) and *Clinique de l'Hôpital Saint-Louis* (1832), the latter containing 62 extraordinary color plates of dermatoses, which are some of the most beautiful images of nineteenth-century dermatology. The spectacular representation of the *Tree* made Alibert internationally famous, but the bottom line is that without a clear understanding of the cause of each skin disease and the relationship between these skin diseases and the whole body, during the period in which he lived, it was impossible to classify skin diseases on any logical Linnean basis other than by their morphology.[20] The result is that to the modern dermatologist, Alibert's *Tree* is entirely useless, bizarre, and full of errors.[21]

Alibert's additional contributions to the nascent field of dermatology were numerous and varied. He described several new diagnoses in various publications throughout his career: dermatosis, dermatolysis, tinea amiantacea, syphilid, mycosis fungoides, seborrhea, keloid, and the Aleppo boil (leishmaniasis).[22] His descriptions were dressed up in a heavily stylized French that is difficult to render properly in English.[23] Like Willan, Alibert promoted Jennerian vaccination and appreciated the risks of certain occupations on skin health.[24]

THE ITCH MITE DISCOVERED, AGAIN

In contrast to Willan and Bateman (and the Willanists) who blamed *the Itch* on some contagion, Alibert was convinced that the rampant skin disease was caused by the sarcoptes mite.[25] Recall that the discovery of the mite by Bonomo and Cestoni in the seventeenth century was forgotten and the writings about it lost at this time. In 1812, the chief pharmacist at Hôpital Saint-Louis, Jean-Chrysanthe Gales (1783–1854), who was studying *the Itch* and the itch mite upon the recommendation of Alibert, claimed to have discovered the itch mite within vesicles of patients with *the Itch*, but no one could reproduce his findings. Twenty-two years later, one of Alibert's medical students at Saint-Louis, a Corsican named Simon Renucci, officially demonstrated in 1834 that the sarcoptes mite was the cause of what is now known as scabies, thus proving Alibert's conviction to be true. Renucci told his colleagues of a peasant woman from his native Corsica who was particularly adept at extracting the itch mite, and according to Alibert, Renucci could repeat the task himself over and over again to demonstrate to physicians and scientists the presence of the mite in persons with scabies, much to Alibert's delight.[26] The fact that it took so many centuries for the medical community to become convinced that the mite exists is a testament to how difficult it is to find the mite in the skin of infested patients. Still, this re-discovery of the scabies mite was the most crucial dermatological discovery in the first half of the nineteenth century, and it occurred in Alibert's domain; 60 percent of all skin disease patients in Europe at the time had the disease.[27] Mite skeptics did exist after Renucci's discovery, and they held out until the efforts of Hebra fully convinced the world several decades later (see Chapter 14).

Alibert's personality afforded him success in life as much as his position and intellect did. His magnificent speaking ability, frequent use of similes and metaphors, and cheerful zeal for his craft made dermatology a fascinating subject for his audience. He was indefatigable, imaginative, brilliant, witty, and wise. He was an all-around kind and agreeable person, a social being, and fond of the finer things in life, e.g., the arts, poetry, and, in particular, beautiful women. He, like Lorry, was a Catholic conservative of the *ancien régime*, most comfortable with the Bourbons in control. Pompous and proud, yet knowing when to be deferential, he respected his charity patients—his "jewels"—with courtesy and benevolence. His demeanor differed strikingly from his cold, somber, and practical counterpart, Biett.[28]

In the end, Alibert and his Tree did not impact the field of dermatology as much as the work of Willan and Bateman, in part because his system had major flaws and in part, because the French Willanists—excluding Biett, who was always respectful of his mentor—were unkind to Alibert, even to the point of ridicule. Perhaps the words of Bateman best summarize Alibert's work: "a splendid and pompous performance ... which however is altogether destitute of method," and "the merit of his publication belongs principally to the artists, who he has had the good fortune to employ."[29] In 1837, Alibertism lost its leading advocate when Alibert himself died of gastric cancer at 69 years of age with a fortune of 600,000 Francs.

It was Alibert's enthusiasm for the topic of skin disease in general that was his greatest legacy, as it engendered much interest in the new scientific discipline. Before Alibert, the medical community of France had been either indifferent to or discouraged by the bizarre multiplicity of skin lesions that they faced as clinicians.[30] Alibert changed this perspective; he brought a certain coolness to the study of the skin, and after him, many emulators and rivals came forth, and interest in the skin and its diseases has not since died down.

The French Willanists in Control

After Alibert's death, the Hôpital Saint-Louis continued as the headquarters of French dermatology, with the Willanists becoming even more influential there. Biett was not as forceful a character as Alibert, but his clear, concise, and practical manner, along with wise, calm, and deep-thinking demeanor, led some of his disciples to believe that Biett was the true founder of the French school.[31] Among his contributions is the description of the collarette (Biett's collarette) of scale around lesions of syphilis as being a distinguishing feature between syphilis and psoriasis. He was among the first to describe lupus erythematosus, under the name *erythème centrifuge*. Rare for his time, Biett was equally interested in dermatologic therapeutics as he was in classification, and he administered a diverse armamentarium of aggressive treatments, including arsenicals, alkalis, baths, vesicants, caustics, purgatives, and phlebotomy.[32] He never had time for writing, but the aforementioned book of his lectures by Cazenave and Schedel was a very important work.

The dermatological torch of Hôpital Saint-Louis was passed after Biett's death in 1840 to his pupil, Cazenave, who carried forth Willan's doctrine as modified by Biett. Cazenave was to Biett what Bateman was to Willan. Cazenave explained the Willanist approach to the diagnosis of skin diseases in the preface to *Abregé pratique des maladies de la peau*: first identify and recognize the elementary lesion; then compare the disease to other diseases with the same elementary lesion; next, observe the location, form, and evolution of the lesions; and finally, arrive at a diagnosis.[33] Translated into many languages, Cazenave's and Schedel's text did more to advance Willanism in Europe and the United States than the work itself of Willan and Bateman. By the mid-nineteenth century, the leaders of dermatology in Europe generally agreed that the search for the elementary (primary) lesion was the first step toward making the diagnosis. However, not all agreed that the Willanist principle of classifying by elementary lesion was the best method for classifying skin diseases. Some of these physicians took a pathologic approach to classification, others an etiological one, and still others, an internal health-based or diathetic (constitution-based) approach.[34]

Cazenave made several of his own contributions to the history of dermatology and syphilology. He founded the first journal devoted to the study of skin disease entitled *Annales des Maladies de la Peau et de la Syphilis,* published from 1843–1852. He authored an important treatise on diseases of the scalp,

Traité des maladies de cuir chevelu (1850); in that work are detailed descriptions of ringworm and alope-cia areata, the latter of which he was the first to associate with vitiligo. His greatest personal contribution, however, was his work with cutaneous lupus. In an 1851 journal can be found the first description of lupus erythematosus, which Cazenave coined in order to rename Biett's *erythème centrifuge,* and which coin-cides with what modern dermatologists refer to as discoid lupus. While he did not distinguish this type of lupus from other forms of lupus (such as lupus vulgaris, a kind of cutaneous tuberculosis), he did divide lupus erythematosus into the superficial, deep, and hypertrophic forms that are still recognized today.

Schedel, on the other hand, made little in the way of contributions besides his coauthorship. What is known about him is that he was trilingual in French, English, and German and thus capable of traveling through the dermatology clinics of Europe; his death was inauspicious; he fell off the side of a mountain while hiking in the Alps.[35]

The legacy of scientific achievement in the field of dermatology at the Hôpital Saint-Louis was car-ried on in the career of Camille-Melchior Gibert (1797–1866). Gibert was another pupil of Biett's and therefore a Willanist, but not to the same degree as his contemporary Cazenave, and Gibert remained on good terms with Alibert.[36] He was appointed head of the dermatology department at the hospital in 1840, and he soon after resumed the outdoor lectures there that made Alibert famous. Dry and unemo-tional, Gibert was known for being a gifted speaker and for his ability to explain complicated issues in a straightforward manner.[37] His most remarkable contributions were his authorship of the first description of pityriasis rosea in 1860, a description that was "photographic in its accuracy and completeness."[38] While the description of the herald patch of that eruption would come later, Gibert's description of pity-riasis rosea was at the time a crucial revelation, because the rash shares many features in common with the eruption of secondary syphilis. Gibert's demonstration of the contagious nature of the skin lesion of secondary syphilis—by inoculation experiments in 1859—was also significant; he succeeded in proving the great Parisian syphilologist Philippe Ricord wrong in his contention that the lesions were not conta-gious. Gibert's notable publications were *Manuel des maladies spéciales de la peau*, "Manual of Skin Diseases" (1834), *Manuel pratique des maladies vénériennes*, "Manual of Venereal Diseases" (1837), and *Mémoire sur les syphilides*, "Memoir on Syphilis" (1847).

The last of the so-called French Willanists at Hôpital Saint-Louis was Marie-Guillaume-Alphonse Devergie (1798–1879). The son of a humble Parisian hospital employee, Devergie entered a career in med-icine and focused most of his early energies on legal medicine and forensics—entrance and exit wounds, sane versus insane, asphyxia from coal gas, the morgue, etc.—fields of which he is considered France's founder.[39] His focus on dermatology coalesced after being appointed head of the Hôpital Saint-Louis upon the death of Biett in 1840, placing him as a contemporary of Cazenave and Gibert—a position he would hold for 24 years. A master morphologist and careful observer, Devergie emphasized in his writings the importance of arriving at the exact diagnosis, and he made greater distinctions between elementary forms based on color and configuration than his predecessors did.[40] His most famous contribution to the history of dermatology was his seminal description of a psoriasis-like condition called pityriasis pilaris in 1857; it got its modern name—pityriasis rubra pilaris—much later. He was also the first to describe the nummular (coin-shaped) type of eczema, and he took Willan's pioneering description of eczema and modified it using four criteria: redness, itching, secretions, and punctate openings of the surface. Devergie gained fame for his expertise with eczema, and his criteria became the diagnostic standard for his time.[41] Devergie's most important dermatological publication was *Traité pratique des maladies de la peau*, "Practical treatise on the diseases of the skin" (1854), but even more important than that work were his publications on medico-legal theory and forensic medicine. As a man, Devergie has been described as inflexibly honest, stiff, and stubborn, but though off-putting to many, he was respected by everyone.[42]

Pierre Rayer (1793–1867)

The next French physician to come to prominence was a true giant of mid-nineteenth-century medicine in France: Pierre François Olive Rayer. Unlike the previous physicians discussed, Rayer never worked at Hôpital Saint-Louis. He was born in Saint-Sylvain and earned his medical degree in Paris in 1818. Overcoming the professional obstacle that was his marriage to a Protestant, his resume reveals a more diverse career than that of his peers, having been affiliated first with Hôpital Saint-Antoine, then Hôpital de la Charité, and subsequently dean of the school of medicine at the University of Paris. He served two French monarchs: Louis Philippe (r. 1830–1848) and Louis Napoleon (aka Napoleon III, r. 1852–1870). He could navigate a laboratory as well as he could a clinic. His varied professional interests included anatomic pathology, comparative medicine, and diseases of the kidney, the latter field of which he is considered a major forerunner. He authored an important three-volume monograph entitled *Traité des maladies des reins*, "Treatise on diseases of the kidneys" (1837–1841), one of the most significant works in the history of nephrology and possibly his most important overall contribution in the history of medicine. In addition, Rayer dabbled in microscopic pathology; along with Casimir-Joseph Davaine (1812–1882), he was the first to observe and describe the microorganism in the blood of diseased sheep that would later be known as *Bacillus anthracis*. It was Robert Koch who later proved that this organism was the cause of anthrax. Rayer also convinced the world that glanders, a fatal disease of horses, was contagious to humans.

Rayer began teaching dermatology at Saint-Antoine in 1825. He wrote an authoritative treatise on skin diseases that was first published in 1827 with the title *Traité théorique et pratique des maladies de la peau fondé sur de nouvelles recherches d'anatomie et de physiologie pathologiques*, "Theoretical and practical treatise on skin diseases based on new research in pathological anatomy and physiology." A second edition accompanied by a 40-plate atlas appeared in 1835. Considered one of the true classics in the history of the specialty, this combination of an encyclopedic text and a glorious atlas enjoyed a long stint as one of the most comprehensive texts on skin disease in the nineteenth century. It was Rayer's greatest dermatologic legacy: his expansion and modification of French Willanism into something uniquely his own, packaged into a masterpiece that became a global export. The work went to Britain, Vienna, Germany, and the United States—places where his work was more popular than in his home country and where he would not have to compete with Biett, Cazenave, Gibert, and Devergie. Rayer's text represents a considerable leap forward from the time of Willan.

In the introduction, Rayer gives his reader a sense of the knowledge required for the study of the skin in the mid-nineteenth century:

> In a word, every day's observation proves more and more satisfactorily, that the study of diseases of the skin cannot be detached from that of general pathology, and of the multifarious morbid conditions with which they have such numerous and varied relations. A knowledge of these diseases, in fact, implies familiarity with general infections, hereditary predispositions, the effects of regimen, mode of life, etc.; it concludes acquaintance with the maladies which have preceded them, knowledge of the internal lesions which accompany them, appreciation of the organic changes which follow certain eruptions, prescience of the affections which are apt to supervene on their disappearance, etc.[43]

Rayer's history of dermatology in the introduction to *Traité théorique et pratique* reveals an author with an expert knowledge of the path taken thus far by the men who came before him; this author holds in the highest regard Rayer as a fair judge of dermatology's forefathers. He noted that the "great merit of the work of Turner is its positive and practical character," containing a doctrine Turner supports with cases from his own practice.[44] Rayer thought highly of Lorry, whom he deemed "undoubtedly superior to all the writers who preceded, and to the greater number of those who have followed him."[45] Rayer sided with the Willanists over the Alibertists, but he did not accept Willan's ideas without argument, and he offered his own original ideas in his work.[46] He wrote about eczema and distinguished the chronic from the acute forms of that disease. He is credited with the first correct descriptions of xanthelasma, ecthyma, adenoma sebaceum, cheilitis exfoliativa, and black hairy tongue. His attempt to classify skin diseases was reasonable and started with four groups: (1) diseases of the skin proper; (2) changes in the accessory organs of the skin; (3) foreign bodies, animate and inanimate; and (4) skin changes secondary to other diseases.

Rayer was one of France's most famous and distinguished citizens.[47] He lived modestly and took care of the poor as well as the elite; he did not particularly desire to care for the latter.[48] Rayer was a well-rounded, popular physician, but being such was not necessary for his self-esteem as his experimental work was more important to him than his clinical.[49]

Ernest Bazin (1807–1878) and *Diathesis*

The zenith of French dermatology in the nineteenth century was reached during the career of Pierre-Antoine-Ernest Bazin.[50] Born outside Paris in a small community called Saint-Brice-sous-Bois, Bazin was a high achiever who entered a career in medicine following the footsteps of his father and grandfather. An intern at Hôpital Saint-Louis in 1834, Bazin attended Alibert's lectures and was an eager acolyte in Biett's clinics. His volatile personality and disregard for the rules of academic promotion cost him the opportunity for a professorship at any of the universities, which gave him a slight chip on his shoulder for the rest of his career.[51] Bazin bounced around the other hospitals in Paris before returning to Hôpital Saint-Louis in 1847, where his soon-to-be opposition—Devergie, Cazenave, and Gibert—was entrenched.

In 1850, Bazin was charged with the care of all patients at the hospital with scabies, which was generally hundreds of people at a time, as the condition was so miserable that the desperate populace turned to the hospitals for relief.[52] Although the Alibertist Renucci had shown that the scabies mite was the cause of the eruption of scabies in 1834, Cazenave and his Willanist colleagues were not yet convinced. Convinced that Renucci was correct, Bazin contended rightly that the mites infested the entire skin surface, save the head, and showed that an ointment called Helmerich ointment (tragacanth gum, potassium carbonate, sulfur sublimate, glycerin, and essence of lavender, lemon, peppermint, clove, and cinnamon) applied to the skin from the neck down to the toes eradicated the mite and expedited the treatment protocol, which he had decreased from 40 inunctions to 2.[53] Bazin's approach to managing scabies, a forgotten protocol imported from Germany and revived by Bazin, was nothing short of revolutionary, and by the mid-1850s, patients with scabies were no longer admitted to the hospital for this problem, thus freeing up much-needed beds for patients with other concerns.[54]

Bazin next applied his intellect to *les teignes* (tinea capitis), another major public health crisis in nineteenth-century Paris. Since its inception, 300 of the 1100 beds at Hôpital Saint-Louis were reserved for children with tinea, who were sequestered in the hospital for a very long time until the condition spontaneously resolved or they submitted to the epilation of infected hairs. The majority of these cases were called *favus*, a condition unfamiliar to the North American dermatologists of modern times but rampant in nineteenth-century Europe. Epilation was first implemented at Hôpital Saint-Louis by the Mahon brothers, two non-physician practitioners who were directed to treat the children of the community who came to the hospital with ringworm of the scalp. Over a twenty-year period, the Mahon brothers treated 40,000 children with their technique, which accomplished the removal of the hair by means of a depilatory pomade concocted by secret formula, possibly containing slaked lime, soda, and lard. The junior Mahon brother penned the first-ever treatise on ringworm of the scalp entitled *Recherches sur le siège et la nature des teignes*, "Investigations on the site and nature of ringworm," (1829).[55]

In the 1830s, German scientists Johann Lukas Schönlein (1793–1864) and Robert Remak (1815–1865) and the Hungarian David Gruby (1810–1898)—the pioneers of medical mycology—had made the revolutionary discovery of a "vegetable parasite" (an early term for fungus) within the lesions of favus and named it *Achorion*. Of these three, Remak was the first to discover the microorganism, but he refused any credit, instead, he gave all of the glory to his mentor, Schönlein. Other genera of fungal organisms that were discovered around this time—by Gruby—were *Trichophyton*, *Microsporum*, and *Candida*. Gruby contended that alopecia areata, an autoimmune disease of the hair follicles that has nothing to do with fungus, was caused by *Microsporum*. This last contention created much confusion and may have resulted from Gruby, a microscopist, confusing the nomenclature and mistaking alopecia areata with "black dot" tinea capitis.[56] The excellent work by these three men with cutaneous fungus was carried on in the 1840s by Carl Ferdinand Eichstedt (1816–1892) who discovered the microorganism (a yeast) responsible for tinea versicolor (pityriasis versicolor). These pioneers worked with microscopic pathogens decades before the germ theory of disease was introduced.

Bazin was the first significant clinician to become convinced of Gruby's research—that ringworm was caused by *Trichophyton*, that favus was caused by *Achorion*, and that alopecia areata was caused by *Microsporum*—at a time when his colleagues, especially Cazenave and Devergie, were slow to warm up to the idea.[57] Only in the case of alopecia areata was Bazin, and many other famous dermatologists of the century, wrong. It was not until the end of the century when Lucien Jacquet (1860–1914), using inoculation experiments, proved that alopecia areata was not caused by a fungus, and when Raymond Sabouraud (1864–1938) definitively sorted out the causes of the various types of tinea capitis. But Bazin deserves credit for being the first to categorically prove that ringworm of the scalp—and of non-hair bearing areas also—was a superficial fungal infection. Bazin treated tineas successfully with epilation of the infected hairs followed by application of corrosive sublimate and cade oil (juniper tar). Bazin's scientific research with tineas paved the way for excellence in mycology by the succeeding generations at Hôpital Saint-Louis.[58] His success with the treatment of scabies, ringworm, and favus effectively made him the top dermatologist in Paris by 1855, but his ideas continued to meet bitter opposition from Cazenave and Devergie.

Bazin's most prolific years were in the period from 1853 to 1862 during which he wrote his five masterpieces: on ringworm (1853), on scrofula (1858), on parasitic skin diseases (1858), on syphilis (1859), and on generic skin diseases (1862). He wrote about the conditions we refer to today as molluscum contagiosum, acne necrotica, acne keloidalis, hydroa vacciniforme, seborrheic dermatitis, mycosis fungoides, leukoplakia, and angiokeratoma. In Bazin's body of writings, he described almost every existing skin disease, many of which were formerly named by other writers after his death.[59] Among his most outstanding contributions were his writings on the cutaneous manifestations of tuberculosis, including scrofula and erythema induratum (of Bazin); he was the first to contend that the former was related to tuberculosis and the first to describe the latter, a condition which to this day bears his name. He did not shy away from the challenging aspects of his specialty; he wrote about factitial diseases, chronic diseases, and such complex topics as eczema. Bazin also laid some of the groundwork for Fournier's efforts with syphilis (see Interlude 3) and described malignant syphilis.[60] He never penned a complete textbook on skin diseases as many of his contemporaries had.

Bazin was a tall, cranky man who was self-made and lived a simple life in a modest home. A frank and outspoken person, if not abrasive and sarcastic, he freely criticized his colleagues, especially when irritated by their not accepting his views.[61] He was kinder to his patients and his students than he was to his colleagues.[62] He was a master diagnostician, but therapeutic relief of the suffering of the patient was his highest priority.[63] He admired the works of Lorry, and he approved of the work of Plenck, Willan, and Bateman, but he disagreed that morphology was the best method of classifying skin diseases. His ideas had great influence abroad; for example, he left an impression on the founder of dermatology in Spain, José Eugenio Olavide (1836–1901).

Bazin's doctrines are, for the most part, incomprehensible even to the modern dermatologist, but the following is an attempt to make some sense of his beliefs. First, he differed from his contemporaries in that he viewed skin diseases as symptoms and believed that the principal task of the clinician was to determine the cause of the symptom (ailment) by looking at the whole body. To Bazin, there was no such thing as diseases confined to the skin, only skin lesions, which he referred to as affections; as summed up by his students, Bazin believed "the lesion is not the disease."[64] Second, although he recognized the importance of evaluating the morphology of skin lesions, Bazin saw Willan's classification as too limited, and he felt that it ignored the transitions between various forms of the same disease.[65] His approach was "to bring together the diagnostic method of the Willanists and the philosophical overview of the Alibertists."[66] Third, he cared nothing about grouping conditions together that looked alike, but instead focused on skin lesions that were specific for a certain causative ailment, such as syphilis, and ones that were common to several different pathologic states. Finally, and most importantly, he organized skin diseases into those due to external causes and those caused by four internal, whole-body constitutional disease states that he called "diatheses:" (1) scrofula; (2) syphilis; (3) arthritism; and (4) herpetism. This so-called Bazinical tetralogy was the centerpiece of his system, and Bazin argued that most of Willan's diseases were manifestations of one of these four diatheses. To Bazin, even an asymptomatic person was still in the grip of a disease, and the future course for that person was predictable by their diathesis.[67]

Bazin did not invent the concept of *diathesis*, but he was its greatest advocate as it related to dermatology. *Diathesis* first appeared in the Hippocratic corpus where it meant "temperament," or what we today would call "constitution," i.e., the state of the body that makes it acquire certain diseases.[68] By the time of Galen, *diathesis* signified a sickly condition or disposition of the body. The word appeared sporadically in the medical writings of the Middle Ages and the Renaissance, but the concept did not become a popular topic until the end of the eighteenth century, especially in Paris. There were 14 diatheses at one point in the early nineteenth century: scrophulous, herpetic, cancerous, gouty, syphilitic, verminous, scorbutic, gangrenous, variolous, measles, mucous, inflammatory, bilious, and serous.[69] The concept competed with the new wave of interest in localizing pathology to a part of the body that started with Morgagni's anatomic basis of disease concept. The history of diathesis represents the struggle between localized disease and general health, between humoral theory and the anatomical basis of disease, and between treating the disease and treating the whole patient.[70]

An advantage of Bazin's system is that each of his four diatheses was linked to unique mineral therapies that were supposedly effective: mercury and iodides for syphilis, cod liver oil and ferric iodide for scrofula, sodium bicarbonate and antimony for arthritism, and arsenicals for the herpitides.[71] Various hydrotherapy spas, which differed in the mineral content of the water, were prescribed based on the requirements of the diathesis. The problem, however, is that while his first two diatheses were reasonable constructs, the other two were products of his imagination, resulting in destructive, polemical criticism leveled against Bazin, especially from Devergie.[72] Diathetic ideas were supported during his time, even in England, but no one accepted arthritism and herpetism diatheses. No slouch, Bazin held his own in the quarrels with the Willanists but ultimately found himself all alone with his tetralogy, and by the end of the nineteenth century, the concept of diathesis in general was debunked and abandoned. Today, the word survives in dermatology only in relation to the concept of atopy, or the atopic diathesis, i.e., the predisposition one has to atopic diseases such as eczema, asthma, and hay fever. Yet, as we learn more and more about the relationship between skin disease (for example, psoriasis) and certain predisposing factors such as obesity, metabolic syndrome, and diabetes, perhaps the concept of diathesis deserves a reinvestigation.

Bazin was the giant of mid-nineteenth-century French dermatology, and his place in the upper echelon of the pantheon is secure. He can be placed there merely on the basis of his work with scabies, mycology, and cutaneous tuberculosis—especially scrofula, allowing us to overlook the abject failure that was his diathetic system. He was a brilliant, aggressive, impatient, imposing, and dismissive man. Above all else, he tried to integrate the budding field of dermatology with the holistic viewpoint of Hippocratic medicine. Perhaps Brocq, to be discussed shortly, best described Bazin's career and legacy when he said,

> For the great mass of physicians, Bazin is merely the discredited author of the diatheses: but for us, the dermatologists of France, he is the most marvelous dermatologic genius who has existed. Those not familiar with his works consider him as a theorist who deforms the facts at will so as to mold them according to his own ideas. The truth is that he was a sagacious and minute observer, guided by a rigorously scientific method. Here is his profession of faith as set forth in the preface to the first edition of his Lessons on the Parasitic Skin Diseases, "The true nosologist does not set forth from physiology, or anatomy, or pathological anatomy in order to study diseases and to classify them by a simple and natural method, he starts out with the patient and observation is his torch."[73]

Alfred Hardy (1811–1893)

Bazin's closest friend and supporter was a colleague, Pierre Louis Philippe Alfred Hardy (1811–1893), a native Parisian and pupil of Alibert who finished medical school in 1836 and arrived at Hôpital Saint-Louis in 1851, where he worked until 1876. Soon after arriving, Hardy became a staunch backer of Bazin and his ideas on parasitic skin disease.[74] Although Hardy and Bazin worked together on many projects and disagreed constantly on virtually every issue, they admired one another.[75] Like Bazin and Alibert before him, Hardy appreciated the Willanist doctrine but attacked that system as inadequate, preferring instead to characterize and organize skin diseases by their true nature and etiology and to incorporate this information into the context of general medicine. To Hardy, the classification of skin diseases "as though they obey specific medical laws" did not matter, nor did the arrival at a precise diagnosis matter; what mattered was knowing to which diathesis the disease belonged.[76] Hardy held these beliefs to the extent that he became the most vocal existential threat to dermatology as a specialty.

Hardy and Bazin were "lumpers" in an epic struggle with the Willanist "splitters." Hardy's approach would have made Alibert proud, but he was astute enough to get rid of Alibert's unconventional nomenclature and divide skin diseases into ten groups: (1) the macules and the deformities; (2) the local inflammations; (3) the parasitic disorders; (4) the eruptive fevers; (5) the symptomatic eruptions; (6) the *dartres* comprising eczema, lichen, psoriasis and pityriasis; (7) the scrofulids; (8) the syphilids; (9) the cancers; and (10) the exotic disorders.[77] With this system, Hardy had resolved the conflict between Willan and Alibert conflict by promoting the best ideas of both sides.[78]

Hardy shared Bazin's enthusiasm for the diathetic theory of disease, and he is famous for writing about what he called the "dartrous diathesis" in *Leçons sur les maladies dartreuses professées à l'hôpital Saint-Louis*, "Lessons on dartrous diseases taught at the Hôpital Saint-Louis" (1862). An English translation by Piffard entitled "The Dartrous Diathesis, or Eczema and Its Allied Affections" (1868) was available for review. The concept of *dartres* is another confusing topic of nineteenth-century dermatology, but it is an important one. *Dartre* is a French word that vaguely means a chronic skin disease and is derived from the ancient Greek words *dero* (to skin or flay) and *derma*.[79] The English equivalent of *dartre* in the eighteenth and nineteenth centuries was "tetters." Willan had done the medical world a favor by expunging "tetters" from the technical vocabulary, but Alibert did not do the same with *dartre*. Hardy promoted *dartres* in his writings and even gave it a clear definition:

> those affections of the skin of different elementary lesions which are often transmitted hereditarily, are reproduced in an almost constant manner, and present as their principal symptoms, itching and a disposition to spread to new areas. They are chronic in course, and although they are accompanied by ulceration they heal with no residual scarring.[80]

In another fine example of lumping, Hardy had effectively placed under one heading all chronic scaly skin conditions that were not associated with syphilis or tuberculosis and that were difficult to distinguish from one another—psoriasis, eczema, lichen, pityriasis, etc. Hardy believed that all these "dartrous" affections belonged together because they all reflected the same underlying disease.[81] In the preface to his translation of Hardy's work on diathesis, Piffard noted that Hardy "believes that many of the affections which have hitherto been considered as distinct and isolated are in reality connected by the closest ties of affinity, and that they are but different manifestations of a common constitutional condition or diathesis."[82]

Hardy's *dartres* was, therefore, the collection of symptoms of a "dartrous diathesis," which he described as the state of a person who is for the most part healthy, but suffers with chronic dry skin and itching even without an eruption. Hardy's dartrous diathesis differed little from Bazin's herpetism diathesis.[83] The dartrous person has a good appetite and eats a larger quantity of food than the average person. Their skin is easily excited by excessive consumption of alcohol, and by insomnia, frictions, and irritating chemicals, among other triggers.[84] While some of these associations may be true for the person suffering from eczema or psoriasis, we know today that eczema and psoriasis share very different immunologic, genetic, and environmental risk factors which preclude being grouped together. Predictably, Hardy's *dartres* diathesis did not survive beyond his lifetime.

Hardy's association with Bazin tarnished his legacy somewhat at home and among the broader, skeptical dermatologic community in Austria, Germany, and the United States.[85] Devergie waged war with words against the two men, who Devergie believed were jeopardizing 60 years of progress in the specialty with what amounted to figments of their imagination.[86] Energized and fully prepared to defend his stance, Hardy attacked Devergie for the invention of countless new skin diseases all based on minor discrepancies in appearance. Hardy also disparaged treatments that were geared toward the morphology (antipapular, antisquamous), not the underlying nature of the problem.[87] History decided the winner of this epic battle; by the 1880s, the diathetic approach to skin disease had been laid to rest in France. As evidenced in an updated textbook on skin disease in 1886, Hardy remained convinced that the approach of Bazin and himself was still the superior method.[88] The British giants Erasmus Wilson, Jonathan Hutchinson, and Tilbury Fox all held moderate diathetic views in their writings and lectures.[89] Note that we know today many skin diseases emerge on the surface, driven by various mechanisms from within the body, while others arise from and are confined to the skin.

Hardy authored several other texts in the 1860s that contained the lessons on skin diseases he taught at Hôpital Saint-Louis (scrofulids, syphilids, etc.). Hardy and his student M.A. de Montméja are credited with the creation of one of the first photographic atlases for dermatology in 1868, *Clinique photographique de l'Hôpital Saint-Louis,* which contained 50 photographs, many of which were hand-colored. Sixteen of the photos were of syphilis, with the mycoses, acne, scabies, impetigo, eczema, and alopecia also represented.[90] A few years earlier, the British surgeon Alexander John Balmanno Squire (1836–1908) published his photographs in *Photographs (Colored from Life) of the Diseases of the Skin* (1864–1866). Squire is also noteworthy for his introduction of chrysarobin as a treatment for psoriasis.

Described as a vivacious, authoritative, and frank educator, Hardy was known in the clinics for the clear, precise, and simple manner he applied to his craft, all qualities that endeared him to his students.[91] He had a long, successful career, capped off with the presidency of the First International Congress of Dermatology in Paris in 1889 and an honorary presidency of the following International Congress held in Vienna in 1892. In the history of French dermatology, Hardy's name is lost in the shadows of Alibert, Biett, and Bazin, but during his lifetime, he was a giant in the field.

Willanism proved to be one of the more tenacious medico-scientific concepts to come out of England in the nineteenth century. When it was put to the test in France, Willanism's morphology-based splitters survived the challenges from the Alibertists and the lumpers, i.e., the defenders of diathesis, Hardy and Bazin. Absence any true understanding of the nature and cause of skin diseases, morphology remained the only fact-based distinction with which to classify them. Until the nature and cause could be even partially ascertained by medical science, the splitters had won; dermatology was, at least for the time being, going to have a lengthy, nitpicking type of nomenclature. One could argue that it still does to this day.

Miscellaneous Late Nineteenth-Century French Contributors

The exceptional progress in advancing dermatology that took place in the early and middle decades of that century at Hôpital Saint-Louis did not decline after the retirement of Ernest Bazin in 1873. Legend after legend in the history of the specialty worked at that hospital, and it will be shown that there were many more illustrious physicians to follow. We have already discussed in the Interlude on syphilis, the legendary Jean-Alfred Fournier (1832–1914), who worked at Hôpital Saint-Louis starting in 1876.

Charles Lailler (1822–1893) succeeded Camille Gibert as head of Hôpital Saint-Louis in 1863 and is credited with two important contributions.[92] He was a founder of the aforementioned *Musée des moulages de l'hôpital Saint-Louis,* which had evolved from a smaller museum and library developed by Devergie in 1867. The museum contained watercolors of skin diseases painted by Devergie and numerous wax moulages of various skin afflictions created by Jules Baretta (1833–1923). Baretta was discovered by Lailler to be extraordinarily talented with artistic representations of fruit and hired him for the museum. The museum helped reestablish the influence that had been lost to the Vienna school.[93] The 3500 moulages contributed by Baretta quickly became famous, and the educational museum became a destination for dermatologists from all over the world. Having been designated a historical monument in 1992, one can still visit *Musée des moulages de l'hôpital Saint-Louis* today. Baretta was not the first to produce dermatologic moulages; that designation goes to German physician Franz Heinrich Martens (1778–1805). The British counterpart to Baretta and Martens was Joseph Towne (1806–1879), who spent his entire career making moulages at Guy's Hospital, London. Before the heyday of the dermatologic photographic atlas, moulages were the primary method for learning the appearance of various skin eruptions for students of dermatology.

The other contribution of Lailler was the establishment of *École des Teignaux* on the campus of Hôpital Saint-Louis in 1886. Both the basic type of tinea of the scalp and the more severe disease, favus, were so rampant in the nineteenth century that Lailler founded a special school where children with tinea, who were routinely excluded from the classroom, could go to receive an education, meals, and treatment for the infection. At this outpatient "Tinea school," the students' scalps were inspected daily, and the infected hairs were plucked with forceps; these efforts attempted with some success to mitigate the spread of the disease. The school was renamed *École Lailler* in 1894 and is especially significant because it was in the school's laboratory where the famous mycologist Raymond Sabouraud (1864–1938) made major advancements in the knowledge about tineas. The school existed until the 1950s when the antifungal medication griseofulvin came out and dramatically turned the tide against the rampant tineas.[94]

Jean Baptiste Émile Vidal (1825–1893) was a "rock star" of Hôpital Saint-Louis in the last decades of the nineteenth century. An extraordinarily successful and able clinician, the contributions of this very stylish and popular man were his description of lichen simplex chronicus and introduction to his colleagues of the histopathological principles of the Vienna school.[95] Vidal collaborated with Henri Leloir (1855–1896) on many of his works, and Louis Brocq (see below) was one of his disciples.

François Henri Hallopeau (1842–1919) was France's answer to the prolific Jonathan Hutchinson. Hallopeau wrote 800 publications, which constitutes a record if compared to Hutchinson's 600.[96] In those works can be found the coinage of the word trichotillomania, a description of pemphigus vegetans that earned him an eponym for that condition, the first report of lichen sclerosis et atrophicus, and innumerable articles on virtually every skin disease.

Pierre Adolphe Adrien Doyon (1827–1907), the lone famous late nineteenth-century French dermatologist who practiced not in Paris but in Lyon and Uriage, founded the *Annales de Dermatologie et de Syphilologie* in 1869, the first journal devoted to skin disease in France since Cazenave's *Annales* in the 1840s. Rather than shape the journal into a repository for his own ideas and discoveries, Doyon created a truly international journal, complete with translations of abstracts and reports from foreign authorities.[97] Fluent in German, Doyon translated Kaposi's *Vorlesungen* (see Chapter 14) and in the process, brought together France and Germany, who were previously divided by nationalistic differences.[98]

Ernest Besnier (1831–1909)

Finally, the story in France concludes with the careers of three French giants of *fin de siècle*. It was during these careers that dermatology in France became definitively modern. The first, Ernest Henri Besnier, was born in Honfleur, France and moved to Paris for medical school, from which he graduated in 1857. For the first 15 years of his career, he was both an internist and an epidemiologist of great repute, and in 1870–1871, he served as a military physician in the Franco-Prussian war.[99] After Bazin retired, Besnier left behind his career in internal medicine and started a career in dermatology at Hôpital Saint-Louis on January 1, 1873. With little formal experience in the field but familiar with the works of Wilson and Bazin, the 41-year-old Besnier was mentored by Charles Lailler and Alfred Hardy, quickly becoming a fine clinician, bench researcher, and budding pathologist.[100] Besnier applied his internal medicine knowledge to his craft and, like his British contemporary Crocker and his French predecessor Bazin, sought constitutional etiologies for skin diseases.

Over the course of the 1860s, dermatology in France had fallen behind the innovative, scientific dermatology department in Vienna led by Kaposi. In 1882, Besnier, in an effort to reform the French school, asked Doyon, who had professional ties to Hebra and Kaposi, to write a report on the modernized Viennese department and publish it in the *Annales*.[101] Besnier soon realized that the dilapidated conditions of the wards called for an upgrade, which he then secured. The outdated conditions of the facilities were symbolic of the retrospectively viewed intellectual stagnation under Bazin and Hardy. What his department needed were some modern laboratories, and he succeeded in bringing them to Hôpital Saint-Louis, having recognized that histopathology, bacteriology, and mycology laboratories were essential components for both dermatology patient care and education. Besnier was the most important early advocate in the French school for the implementation of histopathology as standard practice in dermatologic investigations. He invented the word "biopsy," having written about the skin biopsy as early as 1879.[102] Inspired by his Viennese counterparts, he advocated for the use of topical medications.[103] With these reforms in place during the prime of his career, Besnier's clinics drew students from all over the world. He pushed for dermatology training as a part of the general education of medical students.[104] He proved to have a vast knowledge of the available literature and stayed abreast of the cutting-edge advances of his time.

Besnier was an inspiring, gifted teacher and indefatigable practitioner but a relatively less-prolific writer compared to the other pioneers in this chapter. Beeson described Besnier as a punctual, modest, cautious, and moral man with a well-dressed, stern appearance and piercing glance, and who preferred science over the arts and his home life over travel.[105] When on vacation at Trouville, he never failed to call on his childhood nurse and reveal his soft side:

> on seeing her, we are told, his usual reserve vanished, and he threw himself into her arms in a most touching manner. He was not ashamed to stroll along the beach with this good peasant woman, who was greatly delighted at her boy's striking success.[106]

Besnier's greatest legacy was his seminal description of atopic dermatitis (1892), but his work with sarcoidosis and description of lupus pernio (1889) was also masterful. In addition to his collaboration with Doyon on the skillful translation of Kaposi's text (1881), he contributed articles to Doyon's *Annales* and coauthored a massive, four-volume encyclopedia of dermatology entitled *La pratique dermatologique* (1900–1904), to which he contributed a 300-page chapter on eczema. His characterization of atopic dermatitis holds true today: itching, which comes and goes and leads to scratching, which causes nonspecific skin lesions such as eczema and lichenification.

Along with Vidal and Fournier, Besnier instituted a Thursday session, analogous to our modern-day "Grand Rounds," in which interesting cases were presented and discussed amongst the faculty. These rounds evolved in 1889 into the French Society of Dermatology, of which Besnier served as president for ten years.[107] At this time, Besnier was the undisputed master of dermatology in France, and at the international meetings of the 1890s, he appeared, according to his biographer Thibierge, *primus inter pares*, "first among equals."[108]

Upon his death in 1909, a former student of his, J.J. Pringle, wrote:

> No one who ever attended his clinics can forget the tender thoroughness with which every patient was examined, the grace and accuracy of the language in which all points were demonstrated or elucidated, the unflagging and disinterested zeal of the master's labour, and the delicate—and withal affectionate—irony which he displayed towards his pupils."[109]

Louis Brocq (1856–1928)

The second giant is Louis-Anne-Jean Brocq (1856–1928). Born in the south of France, Brocq was educated in Paris, where he was influenced early in his career by Ernest Besnier and Emile Vidal, the latter someone for whom he showed a particular fondness.[110] Good things were foreshadowed in the young Brocq by his thesis on exfoliative dermatitis (1882), and after an internship at Hôpital Saint-Louis, his career as a dermatologist burgeoned in the early 1890s at the dermatology clinics at La Rochefoucauld Hospital and Broca Hospital in Paris. In spite of suffering from the "perpetual martyrdom" of tuberculosis for the better part of his life, he simultaneously managed a huge private practice, hospital rounds, and scientific research.[111] It was not until 1905 that he achieved "the ambition of his life": he returned, by appointment, to Hôpital Saint-Louis.[112] He served as president of the French Society of Dermatology and Syphilology in 1919. He retired a year later, but he continued to publish works during his retirement. An avid art collector, Brocq and his wife donated over 300 items to the Museum of Agen (southwest France) before and around the time of his death in 1928.[113]

Every present-day dermatologist is familiar with Brocq and his numerous descriptions and eponyms. He was the principal contributor—over 553 pages—to the monumental *La pratique dermatologique* (1900–1904) along with Ernest Besnier and Lucien Jacquet (1860–1914). He wrote seven other major books on dermatology. How he found time to write such voluminous texts is one of the great historical mysteries of time management. In addition, Brocq wrote 300 articles on dermatology on a wide variety of topics: parapsoriasis, bullous diseases, keratosis pilaris, pseudopelade, the first fixed drug eruption—to antipyrine (phenazone), congenital ichthyosiform erythroderma, eczema, the herald patch of pityriasis rosea, angiolupoid sarcoidosis, and the use of coal tar in dermatology.[114] His greatest work may have been with pruritus and lichenification, having continued the progress made by his mentor, Vidal.[115]

Some might argue that Louis Brocq was the greatest dermatologist whoever came out of France, if not the wider world. Brocq was an extremely talented teacher and diagnostician who, like Besnier, drew students from all over the world. He had a powerful personality, a dominant authority, and a somewhat cold appearance. There is no better way to appreciate the greatness of this man than by reading the words about him from the men who knew him. Pusey praised his meticulous ability and uncanny diagnostic and analytical skills.[116] B. Barker Beeson (1883–1961), who once had the good fortune of seeing Brocq in action at his clinic in Paris, wrote in an obituary, that he was "tall and slender, with flashing black eyes" and under a "stern exterior he had a heart of gold and was most loyal to his friends and pupils."[117] Ernest Graham-Little (1867–1950), British dermatologist and Member of Parliament, called the Frenchman Brocq an "example of the French genius at its best" and "one of the acutest observers of his time," and claimed that "no man of his time was more beloved."[118] His most famous and loyal pupil, Lucien-Marie Pautrier (1876–1959), remembered Brocq for his clear and structured mind, exceptional memory, honesty and impartiality, careful consideration of debated issues, and the authority and eminence he radiated, noting that Brocq was at least the equal of Besnier, if not superior to him.[119] It is fitting to conclude this section with something Brocq once said of dermatologists: to be a good one, one must be a "visualist, a patient and discerning analyst, a prudent clinician, a finished physician."[120] How far had the specialty come from the days in which practitioners of the skin were mainly regarded as quacks!

Jean Darier (1856–1938)

The life and career of the third giant, Ferdinand-Jean Darier (1856–1938), takes the story of French dermatology in the nineteenth century to its conclusion. Darier's ancestors were French Protestants who fled France upon the revocation of the Edict of Nantes in 1685 and settled in Budapest, Hungary, where Darier was born. He acquired a perfect knowledge of the German language in these early years and then moved with his family to Geneva, where he learned French. Darier remained there until he reclaimed his French ancestry in 1877 by moving to Paris for a medical education at the College of France, which he completed in 1885.[121] For the first half of his career, Darier was a histopathologist, influenced by Fournier; it was not until 1906 that Darier, influenced by Besnier, settled on skin disease as his main focus. He worked at Hôpital Saint-Louis from 1909 until his retirement in 1921.

Darier was gifted with a keen eye for observation, both clinically and microscopically. As he was a combination of a dermatologist and dermatopathologist, Darier's greatest legacy was his demonstration of the value of the skin biopsy for dermatologists. Although Besnier had understood its important, the skin biopsy at the turn of the century was still not valued by every dermatologist as a useful diagnostic tool. It was Darier, through publications and lectures, who convinced his countrymen of the value of this test. To continue to promote dermatopathology even after his death, Darier founded a Museum of Histology at Hôpital Saint-Louis.[122]

His landmark discovery was the condition named after him and the American James White (see Chapter 15)—Darier–White disease, also known as Darier's disease, or keratosis follicularis—on which he reported in 1889. It is interesting that Darier, who discovered the classic histopathologic features of this disease—called "corps ronds and grains"—erroneously concluded that these bodies were parasitic organisms, specifically a protozoa that he named *Psorosperma*.[123] White contended that the bodies were dyskeratotic epithelial cells, but found Darier's argument convincing. Eventually, a colleague of White was able to prove that White was correct, and Darier withdrew his claim about the bodies being parasites.[124]

Darier's other contributions were descriptions of eruptive syringomas, pseudoxanthoma elasticum, subcutaneous sarcoidosis (Darier-Roussy sarcoid), erythema annulare centrifugum, dermatofibrosarcoma, the "Darier sign" of urticaria pigmentosum, and the concept of tuberculids, a type of which he considered sarcoidosis. In fact, Darier appeared to have described sarcoidosis at the same time as did Caesar Boeck (1845–1917), a Norwegian dermatologist.[125] Darier contributed the first two introductory chapters on the anatomy, physiology, and general pathology of the skin in Besnier's and Brocq's four-volume *La Pratique Dermatologique*. In 1909, he published his own textbook, *Précis de Dermatologie*, a very successful text that was translated into Spanish, English, and German and underwent four editions;

each disease contained a histopathologic description.[126] A *precis* is a concise or abridged statement or a summary, and it was significant because of its clear, detailed descriptions of disease.[127] Darier edited and contributed to the eight-volume *Nouvelle Pratique Dermatologique* (1936), the largest French text on dermatology in the twentieth century. By his retirement in 1921, Darier was one of the most famous dermatologists in the world—because of his textbooks, his numerous publications, and his lectures at international meetings. As a result of the spectacular careers of Darier, Besnier, and Brocq, as well as Fournier and Sabouraud, dermatology in France had returned to its former glory in the era of the French Willanists, and it was standing firmly on a distinctly modern footing.

Summary

Jean-Louis Alibert was to France what Robert Willan was to Britain. It all started in Paris at the Hôpital Saint-Louis because of the efforts of this one man. Alibert's outdoor lectures, wordy books, and breathtaking atlases all promoted the same outcome: dermatology was a legitimate discipline of study in France. To Alibert, skin disease could not be boiled down to its morphology alone; other factors—the overall health of the patient, the duration and course of the eruption, and how the eruption responded to treatment—were equally important, if not more. But Alibert's ambitious system, as depicted in his famous *Tree of Dermatoses*, was bizarre, if not non-sensical, and the French Willanistes defeated the Alibertistes. Willanism became the unofficial approach of the budding French School headquartered at Hôpital Saint-Louis. A series of French Willanists followed Biett and Cazenave—Gibert, Devergie, Rayer. The zenith of the French school occurred in the 1850s with the career of Ernst Bazin and his colleague, Alfred Hardy, both of whom pushed the diathesis theory, which stated that all skin diseases were reflections of overall internal health, which when abnormal, can be categorized into one of four diatheses. Their theory reached Britain and found some support with Wilson, Fox, and Hutchinson, but the late nineteenth-century giants of French dermatology—Ernest Besnier, Louis Brocq, and Jean Darier—who were equipped with microscopes and skin biopsy instruments, took dermatology in a more scientific direction.

Interlude 4

Smallpox

Following leprosy, plague, and syphilis, smallpox is the last of the four major historical diseases with dermatologic implications to be discussed, and it was the deadliest and most dreadful of them all. Unlike the three previously described infections, which were caused by bacteria, smallpox is caused by a virus, that lifeless matter consisting of genetic material surrounded by protein that hijacks living cells to clone and disperse itself. The viruses responsible for smallpox are relatively large and known as *Variola major* and *Variola minor* and belong to the orthopoxvirus genus of DNA viruses that also includes cowpox. *Variola minor* was responsible for a less common and less deadly form of smallpox known as alastrim; our attention is focused on *Variola major*.

Smallpox can be transmitted by inhalation of respiratory secretions from an infected person or by direct contact with infectious material on the skin or on fomites, such as tabletops, bedclothing, and doorknobs. No vector such as a flea or rat is needed. The virus then multiplies in its new victim for an asymptomatic incubation period of 10–14 days, allowing for travel and spread of the disease to other communities before the prodromal period begins. Fever, malaise, frontal headache, and back pain are the first symptoms of smallpox. After two to four days, the virus enters the bloodstream and disseminates all over the body, concentrating in the small vessels just under the surface of the skin; it is during this phase that the rash first appears and when the patient is most contagious. First, the lesions appear as red macules (flat spots) in the oral cavity, and then they spread to the face and other areas with many sebaceous glands. The face at this point has a look and feel of a severe sunburn. Then, the lesions travel to the extremities, relatively sparing the torso; this pattern of distribution is termed centrifugal. The next phase is characterized by the skin lesions becoming raised to form papules having a plateau-like surface; in these first two phases, the rash looks very similar to measles. Then, in the third phase, the lesions accumulate fluid and become vesicular, like small blisters, with a characteristic umbilication (central depression) that confirms the diagnosis to the clinician. Finally, the vesicles turn yellow as they are filled with pus, giving the most striking appearance of the disease while emitting an offensive odor. The vesicles and pustules can occur discretely (separated from one another) or confluently (interconnect with one another to form large networks or lakes of pustules); the confluence of lesions is associated with a much worse prognosis. The face is affected more than any other skin surface. If a person reaches it before expiring, the last phase is marked by scabbing over of the lesions and a high probability of survival but not until the last scab falls off is the patient no longer contagious.

The above description of smallpox is for the ordinary subtype of the disease, which accounts for 90 percent of cases. Other forms include a modified subtype, which is mild and occurs in previously vaccinated persons; the flat or malignant subtype, in which the lesions are not raised above the surface of the skin, but a fulminant course is expected; and the hemorrhagic subtype, an almost uniformly fatal version associated with cutaneous and mucosal hemorrhage.

Smallpox is easily distinguished from chickenpox because the vesicles and pustules are monomorphic (somewhat identical to one another), whereas the vesicles of chickenpox appear at varying stages of development. In addition, chickenpox differs from smallpox in that chickenpox is less apt to scar the skin and erupts in a centripetal distribution (trunk worse than extremities) as opposed to the centrifugal distribution of smallpox. In its early stages, smallpox can be indistinguishable from measles, but measles never forms vesicles or pustules.

The oral smallpox vesicles and pustules erode, exposing the deeper layers of the oral cavity, resulting in extreme discomfort with eating or talking. Starvation-induced weight loss is not uncommon. Cadaveric facies, wasted appearance, and loss of muscle strength and tone are typical. Blindness as a

DOI: 10.1201/9781003273622-20

consequence of blistering of the ocular surface is not uncommon. The patient emits a fetor, which has been described as "oppressive" and "the sweetish, pungent smell of rotting flesh."[1]

Post-mortem examination reveals virtually no part of the body is spared.[2] Delirium, septic shock from staphylococcal superinfection of skin lesions, pneumonia, and other internal organ damage imparted a mortality rate of 20–40 percent. Plasma loss through the skin leads to cardiovascular collapse.[3] The whole ordeal is extraordinarily painful; then, when the scabs come, monumental itching ensues, and scratching worsens the scarring. The afflicted at their peak of pustule formation was a truly horrific sight to behold; it was commonplace to hide any mirrors in the home from the patient.[4] Physicians who treated this condition in the seventeenth and eighteenth centuries considered it the worst disease a person could experience and referred to it as the "Speckled Monster." As far as the history of dermatology goes, no skin disease comes close to being as awful as this one.

Those who survived the month-long illness were constantly reminded of their suffering with horribly disfiguring, deep scars on their face for the rest of their lives; the only comfort was the knowledge that this could never happen again. The scarring was either discrete pockmarks or confluent areas that resembled dark tissue paper.[5] The scars were deeper and wider than acne scars, and a moderate case had 250 pocks.[6] The psychological and emotional devastation must have been enormous. In the eighteenth and nineteenth centuries, the scarring had devastating social implications for the person; a scarred face implied a flawed character. Depression and suicide were common long-term sequelae.

The Origins of Smallpox

The history of smallpox is uncertain, but the current knowledge suggests that it originated around 10,000 BCE in Africa, and from there it spread to India and China.[7] Evidence from the well-preserved mummy of the Pharaoh Ramses V (twelfth century BCE; see Chapter 2) places the disease in pharaonic Egypt. In 1911, paleopathology of the affected skin in another contemporary mummy showed the typical dome-shaped vesicles in the epidermis that one would expect to see in smallpox.[8] The written record on smallpox did not begin until well into the Common Era—Hippocrates did not even mention it—but medical historians, knowing smallpox existed in ancient Egypt, have attributed the disease to several famous epidemics in ancient Greek and Roman history: the Plague of Athens (fifth century BCE), the Antonine Plague (second century CE), and the Plague of Cyprian (third century CE) (see Interlude 2).

Epidemics of smallpox in Europe clearly started sometime between the fifth and seventh centuries CE, and the story of smallpox around that time centers on three bishops.[9] The earliest and most famous person to suffer from smallpox in the first millennium CE in Europe was Bishop Nicaise of Rheims (fifth century CE), who survived the illness but soon after was beheaded by the invading Huns. His martyrdom eventuated in sainthood, and St. Nicaise became the patron saint of smallpox sufferers; a tenth-century prayer to him was "O St. Nicaise! Thou illustrious bishop and martyr, pray for me, a sinner, and defend me by thy intercession from this disease. Amen."[10]

St. Gregory, Bishop of Tours (538–594) wrote the first European description of smallpox circa 573 CE; the following are his words describing the pestilence, as quoted by Robert Willan (see Chapter 12):

> Last year, the state of Tours was desolated by a severe pestilential sickness (Lue Valetudinaria);— such was the nature of the infirmity (languor), that a person, after being seized with a violent fever, was covered all over with vesicles and small pustules (vesicis ac minutis pustulis). The vesicles were white, hard, unyielding, and very painful. If the patient survived to their maturation, they broke, and began to discharge, when the pain was greatly increased by the adhesion of the clothes to the body.—In this malady, the medical art did not avail without the assistance of Saint Martin; for many were restored, who sought a benediction from his holy temple. Among others, the Lady of Count Eborin, while labouring under this pest, was so covered with the vesicles, that neither her hands, nor feet, nor any part of the body, remained exempt, for even her eyes were wholly closed up by them. When nearly at the point of death, she received some of the water, in which the tomb of the blessed saint had been washed at the Lord's Passover.—This having been taken as a drink, and applied to her sores, the fever abated, the discharge from the vesicles was made without pain, and she was soon after healed.[11]

The passage erases any doubt that smallpox was in Europe in the early Middle Ages. It also emphasizes the front and center position of religion in a person's dealings with the disease in this period of history.

The last bishop to highlight here was Bishop Marius of Avenches (532–596), who was the first to coin the term *variola* around 570 CE. Smallpox was initially called *variola*, which is derived from the Latin words *varius,* meaning "various" or "variegated" or "spotted," or from *varus*, which means "pimple." Incidentally, the term smallpox was coined in the sixteenth century in France to distinguish smallpox, which caused small lesions and affected children more than adults, from the Great Pox (syphilis), which was characterized by larger lesions and affected adults primarily.[12] The term *pox*, long-held to be derived from an Anglo-Saxon word *pocca*, meaning sack or bag, may have originated around 1000 CE to refer to any pustule or eruption of the skin.[13]

Smallpox in the Middle Ages

Variola became a topic of discussion for medical writers starting in the early Middle Ages. Aaron of Alexandria (seventh century CE) was the first physician who wrote descriptions of variola and measles. His work, "Pandects," a collection of medical books written in Syriac, survives only within the pages of Rhazes' *Liber continens*.[14] Rhazes (854–925 CE) was the first to differentiate smallpox from measles as two distinct illnesses in his seminal treatise, "On Smallpox and Measles" (910 CE). Rhazes' treatise on smallpox was published in various languages a record 35 times between 1498 and 1848, making it one of the most revered and referenced texts in the history of medicine.[15]

Rhazes characterized the prodrome of both these illnesses:

> a continued fever, pain in the back [a distinguishing feature of smallpox per Rhazes], itching in the nose, and terrors in sleep … then also a pricking which the patient feels all over his body; a fullness of the face, which at times goes and comes; an inflamed colour, and vehement redness in both cheeks; a redness of both the eyes; a heaviness of the whole body; great uneasiness, the symptoms of which are stretching and yawning; a pain in the throat and chest, with a slight difficulty in breathing, and cough; a dryness of the mouth, thick spittle, and hoarseness of the voice; pain and heaviness of the head; inquietude, distress of the mind, nausea, and anxiety [the last four more pronounced in measles] … heat of the whole body, an inflammed colour, and shining redness and especially an intense redness of the gums.[16]

Rhazes believed that measles was more dreadful than smallpox, excluding the capacity of smallpox to blind the eye, which is not a feature of measles. His treatise on smallpox concentrates on treatment: there are chapters on preventing the pustules, managing the throat and eye, drying up the pustules, removing the scabs, dealing with the scars, dietary recommendations, and bowel advice. Rhazes made a point that bloodletting in the early stages, as the above symptoms are surfacing, was the most important treatment for smallpox. The treatise closes with the prognosis based on the appearance of the pustules:

> And as to those [pustules] which are of a greenish, or violet, or black colour, they are all of a bad and fatal kind; and when, besides, a swooning and palpitation of the heart come on, they are worse and still more fatal. And when the fever increases after the appearance of the pustules, it is a bad sign; but if it is lessened on their appearance, that is a good sign. Doubled pustules indicate an abundance of the matter of the disease, and if they are of the curable sort [white, large, few in number], they portend recovery; but if they are of the mortal kind, they portend death.[17]

Rhazes offered a more precise differentiation of the clinical features of these eruptions in *Liber continens:*

> The difference between the two I have found to be, that the Measles are red, and appear only on the surface of skin, without rising above it, while the Small-pox consists of round eminences. When these eminences appear, fix your attention on them, and if you are in doubt as to the disease, do not express any opinion about it for a day or two; but when there are no eminences, you must not give as your opinion that the disease is Small-pox.[18]

Rhazes pointed out that an entity designated as smallpox does not appear in the Galenic corpus, but Rhazes believed that Galen was the first to describe smallpox and that his description was lost in translation, i.e., the Greek term for smallpox was erroneously translated to denote acne.[19] The fact that Rhazes considered smallpox to be a disease of childhood implies that smallpox was endemic in his part of the world at the time of his writings. Endemic diseases are always present in the community, and children are more susceptible to them because the adults are immune since they already experienced the ever-present disease in their own childhood.

Rhazes stated that smallpox arose "when the blood putrifies and ferments" because of excess moisture in the blood.[20] Rhazes used the analogy of fermentation—with its fizzling effect on grape juice in the production of wine—to explain smallpox; the pustules result from the bubbling.[21] Children were believed to be more susceptible to this disease because their blood was thought to be hotter and wetter than that of young adults; the blood cools and dries with age. Moist, pale, and fleshy bodies were considered more susceptible to smallpox than lean, bilious, hot and dry ones, which were considered more susceptible to measles. Smallpox, to Rhazes, was a benign childhood cleansing process. Older persons could get smallpox, but less commonly so, and the cause was exposure to "pestilential, putrid, and malignant constitutions of the air."[22]

Avicenna (980–1037) concurred with Rhazes that smallpox developed from the blood coming to a boil but elaborated on what he saw as three possible causes of the boiling: (1) a natural cleansing process whereby the blood tries to rid itself of residual maternal menstrual blood that was present since the time in the womb; (2) consumption of bad foods that thins and weakens the blood, which in turn is boiled to strengthen itself and rid itself of excess moisture; or (3) an external "cause" enters the body and then the blood, causing it to boil.[23]

Reactions to Smallpox in the Early Modern Period

Girolamo Fracastoro (1478–1553), in his *De contagionibus et contagiosis morbis et earum curatione*, "On contagions and contagious diseases and their treatment" (1546), was the first to formally suggest that smallpox was caused by a contagion. He applied his idea of *seminaria* (small seeds) to smallpox and proposed that a person with smallpox could transmit his disease to another person through these *seminaria* with direct contact, through clothing, or even from a distance. Following Avicenna's lead, Fracastoro believed that the *seminaria* of smallpox had a special affinity for the trace of menstrual blood that supposedly taints the fetal blood *in utero,* triggering its expulsion from the body:

> The pustules presently fill up with a thin sort of pituita and matter, and the malady is relieved by these very means ... for this ebullition is a kind of purification of the blood .... That is why almost all of us suffer from the malady, since we all carry in us that menstrual infection from our mother's womb. Hence this fever is of itself seldom fatal, but is rather a purgation .... Hence when this process has taken place, the malady usually does not recur because the infection has already been secreted in the previous attack.[24]

Fracastoro, like Rhazes, appreciated smallpox as a benign cleansing process that all persons experience after contact with someone or something containing the contagion. Fracastoro's theory of contagion was largely overlooked, and the menstrual blood portion of his theory died with the writings of Mercurialis, who pointed out that if the theory was correct, then smallpox should have existed in the Americas prior to the European encounter; that Cain and Abel should have had smallpox, and that other mammals should also get smallpox.[25] Jan Baptist van Helmont (1578–1614), a disciple of Paracelsus and an iatrochemist from the Spanish Netherlands, promoted smallpox as a contagious disease 50 years after Fracastoro, but it was not until the eighteenth century that the medical world was convinced of this fact. Interestingly, the word *seminaria* persisted in the medical language in the centuries after Fracastoro's writing and was eventually translated as "germs" instead of "seeds."

Thomas Sydenham (1624–1689), the English Hippocrates, observed in one of his many masterpieces, "Smallpox, 1669" that therapeutic intervention against the disease, to which the affluent had greater access, often led to worse outcomes than letting nature take its course—the obligatory approach of the poor.[26] His clinical examination guided his therapeutic approach, which was minimalistic. He specifically recommended withholding treatment for persons with what he called discrete smallpox, in which the lesions are separated from one another. For persons with confluent lesions, Sydenham, like Rhazes before him, noted that the likelihood of death was greater—treatment would be offered, including the cold regimen (see below). Sydenham was the first to differentiate smallpox from measles in the early modern period. He did not acknowledge smallpox as a contagious disease; instead, he promoted a miasma theory and attributed the cause to be "some peculiar constitution of the atmosphere."[27]

Herman Boerhaave, an admirer of Sydenham, thought that Sydenham's description of smallpox could not be improved upon. As the most esteemed physician of eighteenth-century Europe, Boerhaave's legacy in the history of smallpox is that he convinced the world that smallpox arose from a contagion that could be disseminated from persons with the disease.[28] He stated, in his "Aphorisms concerning the knowledge and cure of diseases," that smallpox was

> catch'd from another who had it first by a contagion: which at first seems to be in the air, and transferr'd into the lungs, mouth, nostrils, gullet, stomach, and intestines ...[29]

On the one side was Boerhaave, with his contagion hypothesis, and on the other was Sydenham, with his miasma theory. Miasma versus contagion was a battle that would be fought until the nineteenth century, but by the middle of the eighteenth century, scholars generally accepted that smallpox was a contagious disease.

Boerhaave was a man before his time in his suggestion that the experience of smallpox leaves something in the body that prevents subsequent infection.[30] The mechanism of this acquired immunity was not easily explained, however.[31] James Drake (1667–1707) was an English physician, iatrophysicist, and Fellow of the Royal Society who promoted a novel theory explaining the fact that smallpox never returned for a second time:

> I conceive therefore that the Alteration made in the Skin by the Small-Pox, at whatever Age it comes, is the true Reason why the Distemper never comes again. For the distention, which the Glands and Pores of the Skin suffer at that time, is so great that they scarce ever recover their Tone again, so as to be able any more to arrest the Matter [which Drake refers to elsewhere as thin salt humors] in its Course outward long enough, or in such quantity, as to create those Ulcerous Pustules which are the very Diagnosticks [sic] of the Small-Pox. For tho' the same Feverish Disposition shou'd, and may again arise in the Blood, yet, the Passages thro' the Skin being more free and open, the Matter will never be stopt so there, as to make that appearance, from whence we denominate the Small-Pox.[32]

The same explanation for non-recurrence of disease was also applied to other skin diseases such as leprosy, measles, scarlet fever, and erysipelas. Note that the terms he used—distention, arrest, and tone—are typical iatrophysicist lingo.

Thomas Fuller (1654–1734), a British physician, promoted a different theory in his "Exanthematologia: Or, An Attempt to Give a Rational Account of Eruptive Fevers, Especially of the Measles and Small Pox" (1730), that explained the acquired immunity of smallpox. Fuller posited that all persons contained a substance known as *ovula* (eggs), which are expelled from the body through the skin after they are contacted by the contagion that enters the body. In Fuller's hypothesis, external male elements enter the body and fertilize the internal female elements and deplete them, and "thenceforth new etiological agents will fall upon sterile soil."[33]

Fuller wrote about and supported the popular, imaginationist belief that smallpox could be triggered by the sight of someone with the disease or "simply by having their 'Fancy' overtaken by fearful images of the threat of smallpox."[34] He further described this phenomenon:

> When a Person is taken with a thorough pannic [sic] and Fright, and thinks of nothing but Infection, that extraordinary Perturbation and Terror may form the Spirits into such Species, and create such an Alteration of the Particles of the Body, as will directly and peculiarly act upon the latent ovula as effectively as an actual Contagion might do.[35]

Finally, James Kirkpatrick (1692–1770) was an eighteenth-century British physician in colonial America who espoused the idea that smallpox caused lasting immunity because it depleted something from the body called *pabulum* (Latin for "food" or "fodder"). He believed that smallpox failed to re-infect because "its seeds were sown in an exhausted soil."[36]

Prior to the twelfth century, major smallpox epidemics in the West were relatively uncommon, but the Arab expansion and the Crusades accounted for its spread from Egypt and the Middle East to Western Europe during the Middle Ages.[37] At that time smallpox was capable of causing widespread death in unsuspecting, non-immune populations, but reports of major smallpox epidemics in the Middle Ages are scarce. In 1241, 20,000 of Iceland's 70,000 people were killed by the disease as it was introduced there for the first time from Denmark.[38] Smallpox eventually became an endemic, fact-of-life childhood disease in most of Europe, which served as the world's reservoir of the infection.

Smallpox in the New World

In the New World, colonists and conquistadors brought the disease to the Indigenous populations, causing massive unintentional genocide. Not long after the first occurrence of smallpox in the Americas in 1507, its detrimental effects on the populations could be seen; as many as one-half of the Aztec people were wiped out by the disease, which materially aided the Europeans in their settlement.[39] The Incas experienced similar catastrophe. In North America, Indigenous peoples were so susceptible to the disease that the colonists opted to import Africans for slavery, as they were more resistant to smallpox than local populations.[40] But the unforeseen consequence of importing relatively less susceptible African slaves was the importation of the smallpox virus itself along with them into the United States.

AMHERST'S SMALLPOX BLANKETS

In the Americas, smallpox exposure among the native peoples was not always accidental. Sir Jeffery Amherst (1717–1797), commander-in-chief of the British forces during the French and Indian War (1754–1763), allegedly distributed blankets contaminated with smallpox scabs in the winter of 1763 in the hopes of infecting the native American population surrounding Fort Pitt, which had seen an outbreak of smallpox that year. Records show that Amherst was not the first to order smallpox blankets dispersed as biological warfare in the vicinity of Fort Pitt, but he got the idea from one William Trent, a land speculator who had actually carried out the act in the preceding summer.[41] In the following letter from Amherst to Colonel Henry Bouquet, it is evident that Amherst supported biologic warfare against the native population, but there is no evidence this evil deed was ever carried out:

Amherst: "Could it not be contrived to send the Small Pox among those disaffected tribes of Indians? We must, on this occasion, use every stratagem in our power to reduce them"
...

Bouquet: "I will try to inoculate the _____ by means of blankets that may fall in their hands, taking care however not to get the disease myself" ...

Amherst: "You will do well to try to inoculate the Indians by means of blankets, as well as to try every other method that can serve to extirpate this execrable race." [42]

Since Amherst is now viewed as a contemptible historical figure, efforts have been underway to erase his name on parks, streets, mascots, and other institutions.

Smallpox, which John Adams referred to as the "King of Terrors," was an important factor in the American Revolutionary War (1775–1783). Perhaps Canada would be a part of the United States today if it were not for smallpox, which devastated the Colonial American army as they were besieging an immune British army in Quebec City in 1776. And the siege of the British in Boston (1775–1776) languished a long ten months because of Washington's reluctance to enter the city, fearing smallpox there.[43] In 1779, while the colonists and the British were fighting in the 13 colonies, a joint Spanish-French fleet had an excellent opportunity to invade England, but smallpox crippled the assailing fleet.[44]

A More Virulent Form of the Disease

Modern scientific research has raised doubts that smallpox in Europe prior to the sixteenth or seventeenth century was as virulent or deadly as smallpox that came after that time. Had it been so, it probably would have been given a more daunting name when it was first described in the early Middle Ages. In 2016, researchers who date the divergence of viral subtypes concluded that the strain of severe smallpox contracted by a seventeenth-century Lithuanian child originated in the mid-sixteenth century.[45] They noted that the bills of mortality (mortality records) provide the first clear evidence of severe smallpox in London in 1632. In contrast, bills of mortality from Florence from 1424 to 1458 reveal that only 84 people died from smallpox in that time span.[46] Smallpox that ravaged Europe starting in the seventeenth century was indeed deadlier and more rampant than the earlier endemic and relatively avirulent variety it replaced.[47] Analysis of medical texts before 1600 leads to the conclusion that smallpox before this time was viewed as a merciful childhood disease, given much less attention than plague or syphilis and characterized as benign humoral purification in which the body was expelling morbid matter through the skin.[48] Lastly, it is worth mentioning that the cause of the less virulent form of smallpox in the pre-modern era is not widely believed to be *Variola minor*, which was not described until the twentieth century. *Variola minor* was even less virulent and serious than pre-modern smallpox and may have come about from a post-vaccine mutation.

The deadliest period in the history of smallpox in Europe began in the seventeenth century and peaked in the eighteenth and nineteenth centuries. It overtook the plague, leprosy, and syphilis as the most common cause of premature death during this period.[49] The extraordinary climb in mortality from this disease coincided with Europe's rapid population expansion—from 140 million in 1750 to 250 million by 1845—and increasing mobilization of populations, urbanization, industrialization, and overcrowding.[50] The mortality rate of smallpox during this period was 20–60 percent; survivors had a high probability of being disfigured by scars, and as many as a third were blind.[51] By the end of the eighteenth century, 400,000 Europeans were dying annually from this disease, and about half of the population of Europe was scarred. Smallpox cases were concentrated in the major cities of Europe, with the majority of cases occurring in children. A person might have escaped the disease if reared in the countryside, but migrating to a city as a non-immune adult looking for work was a risky venture.

Anecdotes abound about the way smallpox influence history during this very deadly time.[52] For example, Peter III of Russia (r. 1762) was so disfigured by the disease that his wife, the future Catherine the Great (r. 1762–1796), found him hideous. With no love there, she had him killed not long after he took the throne and then assumed it for herself in one of the great coups of history. Royalty was every bit as susceptible to this disease as the poor. Between 1694 and 1774, smallpox killed Mary II of England, Joseph I of Austria, Luis I of Spain, Peter II of Russia, Ulrika Elnora of Sweden, and Louis XV of France.[53] In Mary II's death and in the death of her son, Prince William, smallpox contributed to the demise of the House of Stuart; her sister, Queen Anne (r. 1702–1714) issued no heir in spite of 17 pregnancies and probably had systemic lupus erythematosus with anti-phospholipid antibody syndrome.[54] Three of her five live births died of smallpox in infancy.[55] In central Europe, the succession of the Habsburg Empire was shifted laterally four times over four generations because of smallpox deaths.[56] Furthermore, the scarring of smallpox had diverse social consequences. For young aristocratic women, especially, a pockmarked face "spelled social death," while prospective nannies had a better chance of getting employment if they were pocked, as they were deemed incapable of transmitting the disease to the children under their care.[57]

The Treatment of Smallpox

The treatment of smallpox in the early modern period entailed the typical therapeutic measures of the time: bloodletting and purgatives. In some cases, leeches were applied to the anus if there was limited normal skin to which the leeches could attach.[58] Sunlight was to be avoided; because it was believed to worsen the scarring, the patient was kept in the dark. Countless unguents, salves, and plasters were used to protect the face from scarring and were written about in the medical texts of the period. To pop or not to pop—the pustules—was the question debated throughout history. The opinion of the most influential medical writer after Galen, Avicenna, was to open the pustules with a golden needle; gold was believed to have greater healing properties compared to other metals. Consequently, the physicians and surgeons of the early modern period who treated smallpox were equipped with golden needles and would painstakingly unroof each pustule at the bedside. In addition, heat therapy was employed in which the febrile patient was wrapped in numerous blankets and kept as warm as possible in stuffy rooms in order to undergo a cleansing sweat; heat therapy was a mainstay until the career of Thomas Sydenham, who convinced the West that a cold regimen was more effective. In cold therapy, the patient was kept in an airy bedroom and given a light blanket and cool beverages. Ice packs to the face and ice-water sponge baths became popular interventions because of Sydenham's influence. These interventions were not administered solely for smallpox, but there was one treatment that was: the Red Treatment.

The Red treatment was an ancient Japanese practice of using red-colored coverings, cloth hangings, garments of caregivers, and objects, including toys for children, to combat smallpox; the practice reached Europe in the twelfth century through the writings of Avicenna and Averroes.[59] The medieval English physician John of Gaddesden (1280–1361), court physician of Edward II and the "Gatesden" of Chaucer's prologue (see Chapter 7), promoted the Red treatment for the King's son and published the success of this remedy in his *Rosa Medicina, or Practical Medicine from Head to Foot* (1314), which happens to be the first medical textbook in English.[60] After Charles V of France (r. 1364–1380) fell ill with smallpox, he was dressed in a red shirt, red stockings, and a red veil, and Queen Elizabeth I of England (r. 1558–1603), a famous sufferer of smallpox, was treated with a red blanket.[61] The dermatologist Niels Finsen (1860–1904), considered the father of phototherapy, argued in 1893 that the Red treatment was more than a medieval superstition. He experimented with red light as a treatment for smallpox and concluded that exposure of the skin to red light "renders the suppuration less severe and less malign" and could protect the skin from pitted scarring.[62] Red treatment fell out of favor in the 1930s and was ultimately debunked as a treatment for smallpox.[63] Interestingly, dermatologists of the twenty-first century use red light to treat acne and several other skin conditions.

Women covered their pockmarks with patches made of black velvet shaped like a flower, a star, the moon, or some other symbol. This trend of masking the scars became commonplace for hiding other blemishes such as acne and evolved into a fashion statement. They applied the patches to the face even in the absence of marks or pimples. One wonders when this fad will return.

Variolation

The story of how the human race ousted smallpox from the world is one of awe, perseverance, and controversy, and it began in Istanbul. Lady Mary Wortley Montague (1689–1762), a true heroine of this tale, was the wife of the British ambassador to the Sublime Porte, the central administration of the Ottoman Empire. At the Ottoman court, Lady Montague witnessed a practice known as inoculation employed by the Turks, which essentially rendered a person immune to smallpox. The Turks had learned about the practice from traders of Circassia in the Northern Caucasus around 1670.[64] It is believed that the practice had originated in India before the Common Era and entered China in the eleventh century.[65] Therefore, the women of Western Asia for centuries had practiced inoculation in which they made an incision in the arms of their children and inserted pustular or scabby material from an infected child into the incision. In this procedure, also known interchangeably as variolation, the virus' unnatural entry through the skin instead of the respiratory tract somehow attenuated the disease. The variolated child, if all went according to plan, experienced most commonly either mild symptoms or no symptoms at all, and they would never get smallpox the more common way.

Desperate to do anything to protect her five-year-old son, Lady Mary Montague, herself a disfigured survivor of smallpox and her brother one of the disease's many casualties, ordered the embassy surgeon, Charles Maitland, to inoculate the boy in March 1718. When she returned to London in 1721, she had her four-year-old daughter inoculated by Maitland in the presence of court physicians.[66] Soon the royal family, intrigued by the prospects of this novel approach, asked for trial runs of inoculation on prisoners and orphans, overseen by the College of Physicians. Impressed by the safety and efficacy of the measure, the first members of the British royal family were inoculated in 1722. Hans Sloane (1660–1753)—physician to Queen Anne and the first two Georges, the successor of Newton as the president of the Royal Society, the founder of the British Museum, and the inventor of chocolate milk—was an important advocate of variolation at the Hanoverian court.

Interest in variolation spread to the 13 colonies, just in time for the Boston smallpox epidemic of 1721. After learning about variolation from his African slave Onesimus, Reverend Cotton Mather (1663–1728) urged widespread variolation in the uninfected, supporting his recommendation with statistical data, which showed that the mortality rate from variolation was much lower than natural smallpox (2 percent versus 14 percent).[67] Many Bostonians resisted the practice, fearing that smallpox would spread from inoculated persons. Violence erupted over the controversy when a crude bomb was thrown into Mather's home. Elsewhere in the colonies, inoculation provoked riots in protest against the local physicians promoting the practice. Ultimately, variolation gained a foothold in the colonies. The data published by Mather made its way back to Europe, and Mather's efforts during the Boston smallpox epidemic in 1721 directly resulted in the rapid adoption of variolation in Europe.[68]

America's founding fathers supported variolation. George Washington's decision to variolate his soldiers, which leveled the playing field with the already variolated Redcoats, was a crucial factor in deciding the outcome of the war. Benjamin Franklin, who lost a son to smallpox in 1736, wrote the following powerful message to parents in his autobiography:

> In 1736 I lost one of my sons, a fine boy of four years old, by the smallpox taken in the common way. I long regretted bitterly and still regret that I had not given it to him by inoculation. This I mention for the sake of the parents who omit that operation, on the supposition that they should never forgive themselves if a child died under it; my example showing that the regret may be the same either way, and that, therefore, the safer should be chosen.[69]

Thomas Jefferson, who once wrote that "the state of medicine is worse than that of total ignorance," was a staunch supporter of variolation.[70]

ABRAHAM LINCOLN'S SMALLPOX

Abraham Lincoln (1809–1865), the 16th president of the United States, contracted smallpox immediately before his famous Gettysburg Address in November 1863 and was coming down with the illness—he had fever, weakness, and headache—while on the train to give his speech. On day four, he developed back pain and a widespread rash that evolved into vesicles. He may have caught it from his son, Tad, and there is no record of Lincoln having been vaccinated against the disease. Long believed to be a mild form of smallpox, more recent research suggests that Lincoln's smallpox almost killed him.[71] His valet, William Johnson, caught the illness a few weeks after Lincoln and died in January 1864. Goldman et al. suggest that Lincoln's doctors had to reassure the public that Lincoln's life was not in jeopardy. The outcome of the Civil War was still unclear in late 1863, and public knowledge that the life of the Union's commander-in-chief hung in the balance might have somehow upset the balance of the war.

Variolation was indeed not without risk; as much as 2 percent died of those variolated died from smallpox caused by the procedure, and the intervention had the potential to trigger an outbreak of smallpox or spread other diseases. Even with isolating the variolated in special smallpox hospitals, the conservative element of the wider European medical community was slow to embrace the practice, arguing it to be too dangerous. Some religious persons deemed it a hubristic intervention against God's plan. However, the fatality rate was significantly lower than that of naturally occurring smallpox.[72] As European royalty continued to die from the disease, variolation found its most powerful supporters in the aristocracy. Marie-Theresa of Austria, Frederick II of Prussia, Louis XVI of France, and Catherine II of Russia are some of the more famous rulers who were variolated and had their children variolated. The latter, an Enlightened despot and one of the most powerful supporters for variolation, had herself, her son, and her court inoculated by an invited British doctor named Thomas Dimsdale in 1768, in an effort to prove to the Russian people that the practice was safe and effective.

One of Catherine's biggest fans, the philosophe Voltaire (1694–1778), found the cutting-edge practice of variolation in line with the forward-thinking principles of the Enlightenment. Voltaire, in his "Letters concerning the English nation" (1733), attempted to persuade his French countrymen that the British practice of variolation saved lives:

> The rest of Europe, that is, the Christian part of it, very gravely assert that the English are fools and madmen; fools, in communicating the contagion of smallpox to their children, in order to hinder them from being subject to that dangerous and loathsome disorder; madmen, in wantonly exposing their children to this pestilence, with the design of preventing a contingent evil. The English, on their side, call the rest of Europe unnatural and cowardly; unnatural, in leaving their children exposed to almost certain death by smallpox; and cowardly, in fearing to give their children a trifling matter of pain for a purpose so noble and so evidently useful …. In a hundred persons that come into the world, at least sixty are found to contract smallpox; of these sixty, twenty are known to die, in the most favorable times, and twenty more wear very disagreeable marks of this cruel disorder as long as they live. Here is then a fifth part of the human species assuredly killed, or, at least, horribly disfigured. Among the vast numbers inoculated in Great Britain, or in Turkey, none are ever known to die, except such as were in a very ill state of health, or given over before. No one is marked with it; no one is ever infected a second time, supposing the inoculation to be perfect, that is, to have taken place as it ought …. The twenty thousand persons who died at Paris in 1723 would have been now alive. What shall we say then? Is it that the French set a lower value upon life? or are the ladies of France less anxious about the preservation of their charms? It is true, and it must be acknowledged, that we are a very odd kind of people![73]

Voltaire's numbers really put the debate in perspective: choose variolation, with its 2 percent risk of dying from variolation-induced smallpox, or accept a 60 percent risk of getting smallpox naturally with a one in three chance of dying if one got it. Opponents argued that variolation killed more lives than it saved, and a spirited debate surrounding inoculation persisted throughout the eighteenth century. Variolation was expensive and not accessible to the poor; consequently, it was never performed on a wide enough scale to reduce the burden of disease in the European population. At the end of the eighteenth century, smallpox was still raging, and with a conservative estimated 20 percent mortality rate, it was the most pressing public health concern in the West.

Vaccination

Enter Edward Jenner (1749–1823). Jenner was an English physician from Gloucestershire who once apprenticed under the great English surgeon John Hunter. He had diverse interests in such fields as zoology (he studied and published research on the cuckoo bird), geology, poetry, and hot air balloons. According to the oft-repeated legend, Jenner's contributions to the history of smallpox began with a conversation between a 13-year-old Jenner and a milkmaid who told him that she could not get smallpox because she had had cowpox. Cowpox was an ulcerative disease of cow udders that caused blisters, pustules, and ulcers of the hand and arm, along with swollen glands and fever, resulting from direct contact with the cow's infected parts. Because milkmaids were known for their beauty and flawless complexion, Jenner subsequently got the idea to variolate a person with cowpox in order to prevent smallpox. The term he used for this process is vaccination, a word that derives from the Latin *vacca*, meaning cow. The practice of vaccination was preferable to variolation because it was much safer and could not trigger an outbreak of smallpox.

The milkmaid legend was completely made up by Jenner's biographer, John Baron, to counter the many assertions that he did not discover the usefulness of cowpox in the prevention of smallpox.[74] Indeed, Jenner was not the first to discover the benefits of cowpox in relation to smallpox; it was actually an English country physician and friend of Jenner named John Fewster (1738–1824) who first announced the following observation at a medical society meeting in 1768: patients who did not react to variolation had a history of cowpox. Jenner learned of the benefits of cowpox from Fewster at that meeting.[75] And someone beat Jenner to the punch with this information: Benjamin Jesty (1737–1816), an English dairy farmer from Yetminster, Dorset, was the first to vaccinate, in 1774, some 22 years before Jenner ever performed the procedure.

It was not until May 1796 that Jenner began to experiment with cowpox. He used fresh cowpox lesions on a young milkmaid named Sarah Nelms, infected by her cow named Blossom, to inoculate the eight-year-old son of James Phipps, his gardener. He took blister material from Sarah's cowpox and scratched it into the skin of the boy. The boy developed a mild fever and axillary discomfort that lasted only 24 hours. In July 1796, Jenner inoculated the boy with smallpox, and when no disease developed, he concluded the boy was protected.[76]

In 1798, Jenner published this case and several other cases in a work entitled "An Inquiry into the Causes and Effects of the *Variolae Vaccinae*, a Disease Discovered in some of the western counties of England, Particularly Gloucestershire And Known by the Name of the Cow Pox." After mixed reviews, Jenner sent out a nationwide survey the next year in the hopes of proving that smallpox resistance was seen in persons with a history of cowpox; with the results of the survey, his theory was confirmed.[77] Jenner's legacy is not that he discovered vaccination, but that he recognized its value; his investigation and publication represent the procedure's greatest advocacy within the scientific community. By 1800, the practice of vaccination had spread across England and subsequently to the rest of Europe and the Americas. By 1801, Jenner had the genius to predict that vaccination would lead to the "annihilation of smallpox—the most dreadful scourge of the human race."[78] Thomas Jefferson, a fervent advocate of vaccination, wrote to Jenner in 1806:

> You have erased from the calendar of human afflictions one of its greatest. Yours is the comfortable reflection that mankind can never forget that you have lived. Future nations will know by history only that the loathsome smallpox has existed.[79]

The obliteration of smallpox that Jenner had predicted took nearly 180 years after the publication of his magnum opus to be achieved.

Although Jenner is considered the "father of vaccines," and by some, the "father of immunology," it has been shown that he was not the first to vaccinate against smallpox. Jesty was not interested in claiming priority over Jenner at the time, and Jenner apparently did not know of Jesty's work until after his experiments with cowpox were published. In 1802, Jenner was granted a financial reward by Parliament for his accomplishments. George Pearson (1751–1828), a physician and rival to Jenner, brought Jesty to London in 1805 to honor him in a ceremony as the true discoverer of vaccination.[80] Jesty's name, however, has largely been forgotten, and all of the honors went to Jenner.

Jenner knew his vaccine worked, but he did not understand how or why; his efforts predated the development of the germ theory of disease. Until viruses were discovered in the twentieth century, it was assumed that smallpox was caused by a bacterium, but unlike in anthrax, diphtheria, cholera, and tuberculosis, microscopists of the late nineteenth century could not isolate an organism in smallpox.[81]

Giuseppe Guarnieri discovered with his microscope the bodies given his name in 1892. These "Guarnieri bodies" were small particles found within epidermal cells of lesional skin, and while he was wrong to identify them as bacteria, he was correct that they were the cause of the disease.[82] Walter Reed (1851–1902) foreshadowed the discovery of viruses by suggesting a "filterable agent" in the blood of yellow fever patients in 1901, but viruses were not actually observed until the invention of the electron microscope in 1931, and the smallpox virus was first distinguished from cowpox and chickenpox with the electron microscope in 1948.

Eradication

The initial method of widespread vaccination was called "arm-to-arm," in which material from the blisters of the arm of a recently vaccinated person was introduced into the arm of the next person. While this method was an efficient approach, it promoted the spread of other diseases. When Britain banned arm-to-arm vaccination in 1898, the source of *vaccinia* was virus promulgated on the flank of a calf. In a later method, threads soaked in cowpox "lymph" were applied to a small incision in the skin. Ultimately, an implantable or injectable form derived from cattle became preferred.

The challenges faced during the eradication campaign included mass production, contamination, and heat-induced degradation of the vaccine during transport. Mass production from inoculated cattle was demonstrated as early as 1842; glycerin was added for germicidal effect in 1891; a heat-stable dried vaccine came out in the 1920s; and the improved freeze-dried vaccine was developed in 1949.[83] The bifurcated needle, which reduced the quantity of vaccine material needed and with which it was much easier to deliver the vaccine intradermally, was invented in 1968. Each of these milestones helped advance the campaign more efficiently toward its goal of total eradication.

Smallpox vaccination was commonplace by the 1830s, but England continued to see outbreaks of the disease. John Simon (1816–1904), a physician and public health official, worked to get the vaccination acts of 1853 and 1867 passed; these acts made vaccination compulsory for all infants of England and Wales in the first three months of life. By the 1870s, more than 90 percent of the infant population had received the vaccine in the first year of life, but by the 1890s, that number had fallen to 66 percent, and by 1907, compulsory vaccination had ended.[84] The decline and eventual abandonment of compulsory vaccination resulted from the anti-vaccination movement that peaked in England in the 1880s. The following arguments against vaccination were the talking points of the movement: vaccination had never been validated scientifically as an effective preventive measure; the vaccine is a form of putrefied animal tissue; obedience to hygienic and sanitary laws was all that was necessary to halt a smallpox outbreak; vaccination can transmit other diseases; compulsory vaccination was a law against liberty; vaccine was a lucrative business for physicians; and vaccination was an attempt to "swindle nature."[85] Anyone paying attention to the anti-vaccination movement of 2021 might notice several of the same arguments being used against the SARS-CoV-2 vaccines. The decline in vaccination in the late nineteenth century had more to do with the success of the vaccination campaign than the activities of the anti-vaccinationists.[86] After 20 years of compulsory vaccination, smallpox was decidedly uncommon in Britain, and people, in general, grew tired of being compelled to get vaccinated.

Smallpox continued to cause staggering mortality well into the twentieth century. In fact, smallpox is estimated to have killed 500 million people in the nineteenth and twentieth centuries, making it the most pressing public health concern of the period.[87] The first country to totally eradicate smallpox was Sweden in 1895, while England and the USSR eradicated smallpox in the 1930s, the United States in 1949, Brazil in 1971, and India in 1975. The last case of naturally occurring *Variola major* was a three-year-old Bangladeshi girl in 1975, and the last person to contract smallpox of any strain was Ali Maalin, a healthcare worker and cook who became ill with *Variola minor* on October 26, 1977, in Somalia. On May 8, 1980, smallpox was declared eradicated from nature everywhere in the world. It is still housed today in special freezers (at −112°F) in two places: The Centers for Disease Control headquarters in Atlanta, Georgia and at a secret laboratory near Novosibirsk, Russia.

Let us conclude with the words of the English physician Robert John Thornton (1768–1837), who wrote in 1805 a description of the devastation wrought by smallpox and the newfound hope of Jennerian vaccination:

> Hence it appears, that had the small-pox seized upon a person more than once during the period of life, the body being susceptible of more than one attack, as is the case with colds, fevers, agues, etc. either the human race would have presented a frightful spectacle of corroded scars and mangled deformity, or, what is more probable, would have become extinct, unless the inventive genius of man, assisted by God's mercy, had found out a mode to lessen the fatality and deformity occasioned by so formidable a disease, either by treatment, or some other means. It is likewise evident from this statement, that all the wars throughout the whole world (an observation worthy the notice of the statesman) have never cut the thread of so many lives as this inexorable devourer of the human race, now happily ... chained down, it is hoped, never more to turn her destructive fury on mankind, and strew the universe with dead bodies, mangled victims, and disconsolate mourners.[88]

Summary

Throughout its long history, smallpox killed approximately one billion people and maimed or blinded an additional billion. Smallpox is second only to tuberculosis as the deadliest infectious disease ever known, and it disfigured more persons than any other disease in history. There is no better example of a pervasive disease with major dermatological manifestations that shaped history, invoked fear and grief, and distressed so many lives with its collateral damage to the beauty of the surface of the human body. Its eradication required the international cooperation of scientists, epidemiologists, surveillance personnel, and public health workers—a true collective global effort over nearly two centuries. Ousting "the Speckled Monster"—Macaulay's "most terrible minister of death"—from the face of the earth is a singular achievement that is perhaps unsurpassed by any other in the history of the human race.

14

The Vienna School and the German Schools

The story moves eastward to central Europe, to the seat of the Habsburg Empire, where the leadership torch in the field of dermatology was passed after 1840—to Vienna. The benevolent despot, Joseph II of the Holy Roman Empire (r. 1780–1790)—son of the Habsburg monarchs Francis I and Maria Theresa, and brother of Marie Antoinette—had established a large hospital in Vienna in an effort to centralize all of Vienna's medical facilities in one place. Known as the *Allgemeines Krankenhaus der Stadt Wien* (*AKH*), or "Vienna General Hospital," it was established in 1784. Attached to the 2000–bed *AKH* were the neoclassical Josephinum and the ominous Narrenturm, or "the fool's tower," one of the first hospitals designated explicitly for the insane in Europe. Destined to become a world-famous medical facility in the nineteenth century, the *AKH* was Joseph's most incredible legacy.

Vienna had a long tradition of having a medical faculty, which had been affiliated with the University of Vienna since its inception in 1365 under the direction of Emperor Rudolf IV. The faculty, however, was never on par with those in Italy and France in the Renaissance and the early modern period. With incessant warfare in the region during the sixteenth and seventeenth centuries, the medical educational system in Vienna reached a deplorable level by the early eighteenth century.[1] It was Maria Theresa (r. 1740–1780) who radically improved the situation. The Habsburgs at the time controlled the Netherlands and its famous medical school in Leiden. Upon the recommendation of Hermann Boerhaave, Maria recruited Gerard van Swieten (1700–1772) of Leiden, celebrated for, among other things, his anti-syphilitic liquor (see Interlude 3). After his appointment, Vienna became increasingly renowned for its excellence in medical training. Van Swieten founded Vienna's first official medical school in 1745 and first modern clinic in 1754. The medical school found its permanent home on the campus of the Vienna General Hospital in 1784 during the reign of Joseph II, and Joseph Jacob Plenck and Johann Peter Frank (see Chapter 10) were important figures of this era.

The approximately 60-year-long period starting in 1745 is known to historians as the First Vienna Medical School. However, Viennese medical education waned in the early nineteenth century, a volatile period in Austrian history that was marked by the Napoleonic wars and the rise of Klemens von Metternich (1773–1859), the Austrian statesman who shaped European politics for 30 years and rejected the liberal spirit embodied in the reign of Joseph II.[2] After several decades of decline due to purging of promising, eminent men from the medical school and their replacement with "servile, politically trustworthy nonentities," the medical school in Vienna unexpectedly rose from the dead—only because of the timely appearance of two Bohemian geniuses: Carl von Rokitansky (1804–1878) and Joseph Škoda (1805–1881).[3]

Rokitansky was one of the founders of the Second Vienna Medical School in the 1840s. After a university education in Prague, he completed his doctorate in medicine in Vienna in 1828. Under the mentorship of Johann Wagner (1800–1832), who had performed the autopsy of Ludwig van Beethoven (1770–1827), Rokitansky became a master prosector and history's first full-time anatomic pathologist. He was the nineteenth-century successor of Morgagni in the realm of pathologic anatomy, having spent the better part of his career correlating findings from tens of thousands of autopsies with the clinical manifestations of disease. His conclusions were published in a magnum opus, the significant, widely read work entitled *Hanbuch der Pathologischen Anatomie* (1842). Unlike his predecessors, who tried to predict pathological findings based on clinical symptoms, Rokitansky worked in reverse, i.e., by explaining the clinical findings from the observed anatomic distortion. In the process, Rokitansky was able to replace the natural-philosophical speculations of German medicine with indisputable facts.[4] In contrast to the widely scattered, decentralized situation of the hospitals of Paris, the centralization of healthcare—and autopsies—in one place in Vienna allowed for the unprecedented potential for scientific investigation.

While Rokitansky was in the autopsy chamber making discoveries such as endometriosis, his counterpart in the clinic, Josef Škoda, was occupied applying this pathologic knowledge to the live patient. Škoda took Laennec's discovery of auscultation and the method of percussion—invented by Leopold Auenbrugger (1722–1809) and advocated by Jean-Nicolas Corvisart (1755–1821)—and succeeded in discovering the clinicopathologic correlation of the heart and lung exam that is still valid today. But Škoda struggled initially to find any supporters of his time-consuming physical exam. In addition, his "therapeutic nihilism," i.e., the non-intervention approach to treating patients, actually had a lower mortality rate than the practices of his bloodletting, purging colleagues. These two factors probably cost the outlier Škoda an opportunity of a professorship early in his career.[5] Rokitansky eventually secured the chair of medicine for Škoda in 1846, and the two men worked together for many years. A combination of individual and cooperative successes could only be achieved at a large-scale institution like the *AKH*, which was by the middle of the century a facility elevated to the highest echelon of medical education and advancements in the Western world.

Ferdinand von Hebra (1816–1880)

Such was the milieu that Ferdinand Karl Franz Schwarzmann Ritter von Hebra encountered upon graduating from medical school in Vienna in 1841. The son of an imperial military officer, Hebra was born in Moravia, a historical region in the eastern part of the present-day Czech Republic, at that time part of the Austrian Empire. Soon after graduating, Hebra, a disciple of Rokitansky, became an assistant to Škoda, whose chest-disease department was, curiously, also in charge of skin disease patients. The three men were sometimes referred to as the "glorious triumvirate."[6]

Paris had led the way toward specialization and scientific accomplishment in medicine in the first half of the nineteenth century, and the German-speaking physicians were witnesses to the success in Paris, as documented by Carl August Wunderlich (1815–1877) in 1841:

> A specialty is a necessary condition for everybody who wants to become rich and famous rapidly.
> Each organ has its priest, and for some, special clinics exist.[7]

After journeying to Paris in 1841 and witnessing its sophisticated dermatologic arena, Škoda, sought a similar center of excellence for Vienna. Thus, he turned over the skin disease wards to Hebra in 1842 and gave him textbooks, counsel, and free rein, with the expectation that Hebra would apply Rokitansky's approach to skin disease, i.e., observe the skin conditions carefully, take samples, and compare and evaluate the data.[8] The *AKH* became a cutting-edge institution where modern, scientific research methods challenged antiquated theories that were ultimately abandoned, and from the investigational labs emerged a new approach to classification, diagnosis, and treatment. In a relatively short time, Hebra founded the Viennese school of dermatology, and by the end of the 1840s, Vienna had become the most effective and renowned teaching institution for dermatology anywhere.[9]

Intolerable to society, the skin disease patients in Vienna had always been sorely neglected, having been regarded with contempt because of their perceived contagiousness, suspicions of having syphilis and leprosy, and assumed incurability due to ineffective treatments, which in some cases could make the situation worse. Consequently, there was never any glory or esteem to be achieved by investigating skin disease; thus, there was no dermatology in Vienna prior to Hebra. But this sympathetic man, like Alibert back in 1800, saw the fertile ground for advances in this field that was the large skin disease ward in front of him. The 25-year-old Hebra proved he had the courage to undertake this heroic task at the *Allgemeines Krankenhaus*, where he spent his entire career. Hebra started lecturing on skin diseases in 1842, but it was not until 1844 that he achieved the assistant professorship needed to legalize his lectures, which were delivered with a witty, straightforward, and practical style, if at times, clumsy, but nearly always warm and humorous.[10]

As in Paris, all skin disease patients were placed in the same ward at *AKH*, separated along with the syphilitics and mentally ill from the general population of sick persons.[11] These patients were housed in an annex called the *Krätzestation*, "scabies station," as all skin disease patients were referred to as having scabies, but the majority of these patients did indeed have actual scabies. Of Hebra's first patients, 2197 out of 2723 had scabies.[12] Like Bazin, Hebra was tasked with treating countless scabies patients in the wards. While the itch mite had been identified a decade prior, the controversy continued as to whether or not the mite was the direct cause of the itch and the eruption. Hebra convinced himself over time—in part, through self-inoculation—that the itch and rash was a local disease caused by the itch-inducing mite.[13] He published his research on the subject of scabies in a text entitled *Über die Krätze*, "On the itch" (1844), and effectively ended the debate about the mite and its relationship to the disease. He concluded that everyone gets scabies if the mites settle on the skin, and the condition is eradicated when the mite and eggs are destroyed. From scabies, Hebra developed and broadened the concept of local diseases of the skin, contending that inflammation in the skin could occur from external irritation and arguing that most diseases of the skin, such as eczema, could in many cases arise from the skin and be limited to the skin. To Hebra, few skin diseases were of a systemic origin, but he did recognize the role of the nervous system in the manifestation of skin disease at a time when no one else did.[14] He advocated skin-directed (topical) treatments such as unguents and did not have the same fear as his colleagues that topical medications could drive the disease into the body.[15]

As the 1840s progressed, Hebra became increasingly dissatisfied with the humoral theory as it related to skin disease, which stated that skin eruptions were caused by an internal imbalance of humor. Though Hebra favored the Willan-Bateman approach, he sought a better system for classifying skin diseases than by their appearance. Hebra applied the principles of the relatively new discipline of anatomic pathology to clinical dermatology and arrived at different conclusions as to how skin diseases originated and how they should be classified. Hebra saw the skin as subject to the same metabolic processes and pathologic principles as the kidney, liver, or any other organ. This novel concept was just emerging in the early 1840s: the skin was not just an organ but an organ with its own specific diseases.

A year later, Hebra published "Attempt to classify skin diseases on the basis of pathologic anatomy" (1845), in which he classified skin diseases neither by region of the body nor by morphology, but by pathological categories, of which there were 12 (see Table 14.1).

Finally, there was a system that resembles the method used in our modern dermatology textbooks. It was a system that was precisely what the burgeoning specialty of dermatology needed at the time—current, simple, comprehensive, logical, and supported and confirmed by the pathologic discoveries of the era—and it incorporated Willan's dermatologic alphabet for its disease descriptions, satisfying the Willanists. In spite of the findings taking place in pathology in Vienna and later in Germany, Hebra's arrangement proved to be impenetrable and irreplaceable for the remainder of the century.

Hebra's career had only just begun, yet he had already settled the scabies controversy, firmly established the concept of local skin disease, and delivered the classification system that would endure for the rest of the nineteenth century. By 1849, he was given an associate professorship, and the outstanding career of this great clinician, teacher, and researcher was underway. As he traveled time and again over

TABLE 14.1

Hebra's 12 Pathological Categories of Skin Diseases

I.	*Hyperemiae cutaneae* (too much blood flow)
II.	*Anaemia cutaneae* (decreased blood flow)
III.	*Anomaliae secretionis glandorum cutanearum* (abnormal glandular secretions)
IV.	*Exudationes* (exudates)
V.	*Hemorrhagiae cutaneae* (hemorrhage)
VI.	*Hypertrophiae* (hypertrophy)
VII.	*Atrophiae* (thinning of the skin)
VIII.	*Neoplasmata* (benign growths)
IX.	*Pseudoplasmata* (malignant growths)
X.	*Ulcerationes* (ulcers)
XI.	*Neuroses* (nerve diseases)
XII.	*Parasitae* (parasitic diseases)

the next 25 years to Hôpital Saint-Louis and the London hospitals, his reputation spread widely through-out Europe and the United States. He took back from Paris an admiration for Alibert, whose penchant for the dramatic Hebra summoned in his own teaching style.[16] He applied his extraordinary mind to virtually every skin disease, precisely defining the known ones and meticulously describing others, such as prurigo, tinea cruris, rhinoscleroma, and lichen scrofulosorum. He once went to Norway, where he coined "Norwegian scabies." His work with erythema multiforme (Hebra's disease) was his greatest legacy as it relates to a single disease. In the realm of dermatologic therapy, he cleaned up the dermato-logic armamentarium by getting rid of hundreds of "useless medications."[17]

JULIUS ROSENBAUM (1807–1874)

Hebra was the most influential advocate of an anatomic-pathological classification and concep-tion of skin disease, but he was not the first. That was Julius Rosenbaum, an obscure German lecturer and physician at the university in Halle. Rosenbaum authored a monograph called *Zur Geschichte und Kritik der Lehre von den Hautkrankheiten,* "A History and Review of the Doctrines of Skin Diseases" (1844). In that work, Rosenbaum criticized Willan for ignoring anatomical considerations in his classification system.[18] Rosenbaum provided the blueprint in his monograph for how dermatology could move forward.[19] Most importantly, he called for an anatomico-pathologic description of Willan's elementary forms, followed by a determination of which parts or structures of the skin are involved in these forms, as well the diseases to which each structure of the skin is prone. Rosenbaum is an underappreciated contributor in the history of dermatology.

Students came from around the world to learn from Hebra and the naked patients he displayed on his rotating platform, choosing Vienna over Paris to fill in any gaps in the knowledge they attained else-where.[20] Hebra taught his students to rely more on the exam than the patient's history when the two were at odds with one another. Facts, not conjecture, were everything to Hebra. His keen eye for recognizing similarities between diseases and distinguishing differences between others must have been awe inspir-ing for his students.[21] He never saw a stubborn skin disease as a hopeless cause, having convinced him-self that getting to the bottom of the cause and an understanding of the pathology could open the avenue to therapeutic success. For a man described as a "short thick-set … with dirty fingers and a dress a good deal the worse for wear," his words overcame his appearance.[22]

During the zenith of his career, Hebra's major publications included *Atlas der Hautkrankheiten,* "Atlas of Skin Diseases" (1856–1876) and *Lehrbuch der Hautkrankheiten,* "Textbook of Skin Diseases" (1860). The former was released in a series of ten installments over 20 years and contained 104 remarkable illustrations by two gifted Viennese painter-physicians, Anton Elfinger (1821–1864) and Carl Heitzmann (1836–1896). The first volume of the latter was initially published as the skin disease volume in Virchow's six-volume "Handbook of Pathology"; and later released in a two-volume work, the first written by Hebra, the second by his successor Moritz Kaposi (see below). That work highlights the separation of primary and secondary lesions for the first time, as well the descriptive dimension we now call distribution—the way in which skin lesions are distributed over the body.[23] Both the atlas and the textbook are classics of nineteenth-century dermatology that influenced physi-cians around the world.

Hebra died on August 5, 1880. During his lifetime, patients and students alike came from all over the world to see him and benefit from his expertise, and with honor upon honor bestowed upon him by both his countrymen and the international community, Hebra had reached a level of fame in the specialty of dermatology that was unmatched in his century. Unlike most of Hebra's British and French predecessors and counterparts, Hebra created something in Vienna that would last well beyond his death: a system of educating students and physicians that was devoted to the perpetuation of his theories and ideals.[24] His lectures, methods, and principles—and his spirit for such—were adopted by his disciples and dispersed throughout the world. Hebra was the perfect amalgamation of the Willanists and Alibertists, and his scientific approach and clinical skill coupled with an extraordinary talent for teaching propelled the budding specialty of dermatology into the modern era. Hebra showed that the size and depth of the subject matter of dermatology was big enough to be pursued as a specialty by physicians.[25]

Bazin and Hardy and their British contemporaries, Wilson and Hutchinson, did not receive Hebra's doctrines with open minds. Their main objection was to Hebra's localization of disease to the skin itself; conversely, skin lesions reflected an internal morbid state, said these contrarians. Hebra's philosophical opponents saw these principles as not only incorrect but also dangerous—this "label of superficiality" was a threat to the intellectual depth of the specialty.[26] How could anyone ever take the specialty seriously if skin diseases were merely surface changes, unrelated to internal morbidity?

The Father of Dermatopathology: Gustav Simon (1810–1857)

Perhaps it was the application of the microscope to skin disease that ultimately proved Hebra was correct in his assertion that the skin had its own pathology (dermatopathology). The founder of the field of dermatopathology was a contemporary of Hebra named Karl Gustav Theodor Simon (1810–1857) of Berlin. Once one of the aforementioned Johannes Müller's many students, Simon took an interest in the microscopy of the skin early in his career, scraping and sampling the skin of his patients and examining it under the microscope. Many of these developments are owed to the major improvements of the nineteenth century in microscopes, including better glass, achromatic lenses (which allowed users to see color), and new methods for illuminating specimens and controlling light. John Riddell, a chemistry professor at Tulane University (then, the University of Louisiana), invented the first practical binocular microscope in the 1850s.

Simon is credited with being the first to publish a report (1842) on *Demodex folliculorum*, the eight-legged microorganism virtually all of us have in our facial follicles, and in the present author's opinion, the cause of most, if not all, cases of papulopustular rosacea. Another of Müller's students, Jacob Henle, discovered the mite a year before him. While chief of skin diseases and syphilis at the Charité Hospital in Berlin, Simon authored the first textbook on dermatopathology, *Die Hautkrankheiten durch anatomische Untersuchungen erläutert*, "Diseases of the skin explained by means of anatomical investigation" (1848). In that work, Simon was the first to correlate the changes in the microscopic structures of the skin with the way each manifested clinically in the patient. In his introduction, he heralded the new field of dermatopathology:

> Skin diseases form a group to be enrolled, too, with those categories of pathology whose challenges have recently and actively engaged attention. Considering the difficulty of the subject and the variety of manifestations to be considered, it was natural that individual investigators sought to reach their goal in varied and diverse ways. Accordingly, many devoted themselves especially to a painstaking study of the external features expressed by these affections, thus more strictly to separate the particular kinds and types from each other; others paid greater attention to causative circumstances. More recently, as our knowledge of the normal structure of the skin was significantly perfected by important discoveries, one soon came to recognize that the method thus far employed could not alone lead to satisfactory results; rather it was unavoidably necessary to find out which components of the cutaneous organ, so organized, showed themselves to be altered in individual skin disease and what was the nature of these changes.[27]

Simon was destined for greatness in nineteenth-century medicine, but his life was cut short due to having contracted syphilis. His behavior alienated his friends, and at just 46 years of age, he died alone of general paresis in a mental hospital. Simon is credited with bringing dermatology to Berlin, founding the so-called Berlin School, equipped with a separate department for skin diseases in 1853.[28] He is an important figure largely forgotten by posterity, but he showed the world the value of the microscope in scientific investigations of the skin. Following in the footsteps of Simon, Carl Wedl (1815–1891) was the first to establish the foundation for excellence in microscopic pathology in Vienna.

Moriz Kaposi (1837–1902)

Of Hebra's many legacies, one cannot ignore his impact on the careers of his students, four of whom particularly stand out for their contributions to the history of dermatology: Moriz (Kohn) Kaposi, Isidor Neumann, Filipp Joseph Pick, and Heinrich Auspitz. Moriz Kaposi (1837–1902) was born with the name Mor Kohn in Hungary to a poor Jewish family. Upon converting to Catholicism in 1871, he changed his name to Kaposi—named after his birthplace Kaposvár—to avoid confusion with many people named Kohn in Vienna.[29] His first name was "Moritz" in the records, but he almost always used "Moriz."[30] After completing medical school in Vienna in 1861, Kaposi started his career in the clinics of Carl Ludwig Sigmund (1810–1883), Hebra's counterpart in the Department of Syphilology at the *AKH*. By the mid-1860s, Kaposi gravitated toward Hebra, who was impressed with the young man's intellect, while Kaposi became increasingly enamored of dermatology. Their professional relationship grew as they started to collaborate on projects such as Hebra's *Lehrbuch*; their ties strengthened further when Kaposi married Hebra's daughter, Martha, in 1869. Legend has it that Hebra turned over his six wealthiest psoriasis patients to Kaposi as a dowry.[31] More interested in literary pursuits than Hebra, Kaposi completed Hebra's *Lehrbuch* in 1876. After Hebra's death in 1880, Kaposi succeeded him as head of the skin disease clinic in Vienna, taking over the care of many of the master's patients, creating much jealousy and discord with his colleagues. William Dubreuilh (1857–1935), Professor of Dermatology in Bordeaux's School of Medicine, once lamented that "he [Kaposi] took Hebra's daughter, house, chair and clientele, leaving the rest to his brother-in-law, Hans von Hebra."[32]

Viennese dermatology reached its zenith under the chairmanship of Moriz Kaposi. Fluent in German, Hungarian, French, and English, Kaposi drew innumerable students from all over the world to his clinics, and Kaposi could speak to these students in their native tongues. Even students from faraway places such as Japan were sent to Kaposi; Keizo Dohi (1866–1931), the founder of Japanese dermatology, studied at Kaposi's clinic during his educational tour in Europe (1892–1898). Kaposi was described as jovial and gentle, yet restless, wise, and gifted with an extraordinary memory, which he applied to the dermatologic literature; on occasion, he was a sharp critic, capable of caustic remarks, which his colleagues feared.[33]

Kaposi was the first in a series of Viennese clinicians who appreciated the microscope and its value to dermatology, as demonstrated by Simon and Wedl and another Austrian pathologist, Salomon Stricker (1834–1898). Kaposi recognized the importance of microscopic examination of skin specimens in the diagnostic workup of the patient. Histopathology figures prominently in Kaposi's writings, especially in his magnum opus, *Pathologie und Therapie der Hautkrankheiten in Vorlesungen für praktische Ärzte und Studierende*, "Pathology and therapy of skin diseases in lectures for practical physicians and students" (1880). Translated into many languages and published in five editions, the *Vorlesungen* is the defining text in dermatology of the second half of the nineteenth century. Its French translation was especially influential. Kaposi's work was edited and translated by Ernest Besnier and Andrien Doyon (see Chapter 13), who created "the first syncretic book of dermatology, away of nationalistic fetishes, errors and eccentricities" and the most influential textbook of dermatology for the next 20 years.[34] *Vorlesungen* was essential reading for any student entering the field of dermatology near the end of the nineteenth century. In addition, Kaposi eventually put together his own atlas, a giant three-volume masterwork entitled *Atlas der Hauthankreiten* (1898–1900). More than 150 publications are attributed to Kaposi, making him one of the most industrious figures in nineteenth-century dermatology.

Kaposi was credited in 1872 with the first description of the sarcoma that bears his name, which he called idiopathic multiple pigmented sarcoma. He also described the varicelliform eruption (eczema herpeticum), xeroderma pigmentosum, acne keloidalis, impetigo herpetiformis, gangrenous herpes zoster, diabetic skin changes, and countless other diagnoses he was the first to describe either clinically or histopathologically.[35] Kaposi was not perfect; he saw no difference between syphilis and chancroid, and he did not recognize lupus vulgaris as a manifestation of tuberculosis.[36]

Kaposi's greatest legacy to the field of dermatology was his early advocacy for histopathology—the advancement of the histopathological examination of skin diseases as a diagnostic and investigational tool. The skin biopsy continues to be one of the most important tasks of the dermatologist in the evaluation of the patient's problem. Like Bateman who followed Willan, or Cazenave behind Biett, Kaposi proved that he could easily fill the big shoes of his mentor, and while Hebra may have founded the Viennese school, Kaposi elevated it to its apex and was its finest representative.

Isidor Neumann (1832–1906) and Filipp Joseph Pick (1834–1910)

Isidor Neumann was another disciple of Hebra and pioneer in dermatopathology who shaped an era. Born in Moravia like his mentor, Neumann graduated from medical school in 1858 and started his career in front of Carl Wedl's microscope. Nearly ten years of work with histopathology culminated with the publication of Neumann's own *Lehrbuch der Hautkrankheiten* (1869), a successful early primer on dermatology and dermatopathology. The work contains excellent depictions of his histopathologic findings. Neumann authored the first text on the lymphatics of the skin (1873) and first described a vegetating form of pemphigus (pemphigus vegetans of Neumann). Among many other dermatologic entities, he delineated the features of photoaging—the aging of the skin brought about by a lifetime of sun exposure—and defined the seborrheic keratosis as a distinct skin lesion. During his lifetime, Neumann was even more famous for his work in syphilology, having replaced Sigmund as head of that department in 1881. His greatest legacy may have been the way in which he effectively ended the separation of the departments of venereology and dermatology; the only distinction remaining was the clinics—Neumann led the venereology clinic, while Kaposi chaired the dermatology clinic.[37] He published his life's work on the treponeme in a monumental text on the subject in 1896. We know less about Neumann's personality and character, but in his obituary, he is described as conscientious and open to factual criticisms, but not a good public speaker.[38] Still, Neumann's broad scope of knowledge of many aspects of dermatology and syphilology set him apart from his colleagues in Vienna.

Filipp Joseph Pick, a pupil of Rokitansky, Skoda, and Hebra, obtained his medical degree in 1860 from the University of Vienna. After working a few years in Hebra's clinic, Pick took what he had learned from the Viennese school and brought it to Prague, where he secured a teaching position and six years later a professorship (1873). He soon proved the contagiousness of molluscum contagiosum, identified the microorganism of tinea cruris, supported the idea that lupus vulgaris was cutaneous tuberculosis, first described trichomycosis axillaris, and first described (at the same time as Herxheimer) acrodermatitis chronica atrophicans, which he called at the time *erythromelia*.[39] His most important achievement was a collaboration with Heinrich Auspitz (see below) to found the *Archiv für Dermatologie und Syphilis*, the first medical journal devoted to dermatology in central Europe, in 1869. Pick put extraordinary effort into the journal, which he edited until his death, and in return, he received the best papers from all across Europe, resulting in his journal becoming the most important dermatologic journal in the world.[40] Pick was not only a master diagnostician but a therapeutics master also; he invented iodoform and the salicylic acid plaster.[41] Pick was considered by some to be Hebra's most brilliant student and a worthy representative to take the teachings of Hebra's *schule* beyond the bounds of Vienna.[42]

Heinrich Auspitz (1835–1886)

Finally, the story of the Vienna school of dermatology concludes with the life and career of Heinrich Auspitz, the last of the physicians trained by the "glorious triumvirate." Also born in Moravia, Auspitz graduated from medical school in Vienna in 1858 and was mentored in Hebra's skin department from 1862 to 1864. Training with Carl Wedl served him well, and Auspitz is remembered for high achievement both at the microscope and at the bedside. Auspitz was gifted, ambitious, and strong-willed, and both Pusey and Goodman proposed that he was the most brilliant of the big four disciples of Hebra.[43]

Auspitz is a somewhat enigmatic and tragic figure, however. With no position for him at *AKH*, in 1872 he established the General Polyclinic with several other physicians, where he directed not only the dermatology clinic but also headed the entire clinic.[44] In 1881, he lost out to Kaposi the inheritance of Hebra's chair, and to Neumann, Sigmund's chair, either of which he was all but certain to receive, but lost due to some last-minute intrigue.[45] While highly intelligent, he was also erratic, impatient, sarcastic, and critical, and consequently, always finishing second professionally. He never immersed himself in Hebra's projects as Kaposi did and often felt passed over by Hebra.[46] He is recognized today for the "Auspitz sign," i.e., the diagnostic phenomenon in psoriasis in which peeling away the scales causes pinpoint bleeding. However, he did not discover it or claim to have discovered it; Hebra and Devergie had written about it, and Turner, Plenck, and Willan also did. He introduced the terms acanthosis and parakeratosis, and he purportedly discovered acantholysis, but that was forgotten and instead attributed to twentieth-century dermatologists.[47] He shunned tradition in lieu of something new, and he constructed his own classification system, published in *System der Hautkrankheiten* (1881), which afforded him fame and in which he attacked his own mentor's system. His system encompassed all aspects of dermatology—the clinical, the physiologic, the pathological, and the experimental—but it failed to grab any supporters.[48] No one used his system. Finally, both his son and his wife died prematurely, as did he; at just 50 years of age, Auspitz passed away from heart disease in 1886.

Auspitz's most influential works were a monograph called *Allgemeine pathologie und Therapie der Haut*, "General pathology and therapy of skin" (1885), and, as discussed above, the *Archiv* he co-founded and coedited with his friend Pick. He invented the curette, the trusty scraping instrument that dermatologists still use to this day. Auspitz was, above all else, remembered for his pioneering in dermatopathology as he was convinced that the microscope was the key to clarifying clinical skin lesions. But perhaps his greatest legacy was his influence on his most famous of pupils, Paul Gerson Unna (see below).

The Breslau School: Heinrich Koebner (1838–1904)

London, Paris, and Vienna were the primary seats of dermatology in the Western world for most of the nineteenth century. But in the 1870s, the fourth epicenter of dermatologic learning sprang up in Europe: Breslau. Located in the historical territory of Silesia, Breslau is known today as Wrocław, Poland. The city has a long, diverse history of having had many different sovereigns: first, the Kingdom of Poland, next, the Kingdoms of Bohemia and Hungary, and then the Habsburg Monarchy of Austria. Maria Theresa ceded the territory of Silesia to Prussia in 1742, and it would remain under Prussian and then German control until 1945.

Dermatology was brought to Breslau by Heinrich Köbner (Koebner). Born in Breslau, Koebner went for a time to Berlin for medical education but completed his doctorate in Breslau in 1859. Koebner was exposed in his medical training to some of the brightest minds in Europe; he was greatly influenced by the pathologists Friedrich Theodor von Frerichs (1819–1885) and the famous Rudolf Virchow, under whom he once studied in Berlin. Not long after his graduation, Koebner spent several months under the tutelage of Ferdinand von Hebra in Vienna, whose personality steered him into a career in dermatology.[49] With his career path set, he sought greater exposure to dermatology in the clinics of Bazin and Hardy in Paris, where Bazin's work with mycology inspired Koebner's lifelong interest in the same. He once showed up at a medical conference with three different types of fungus on his skin, as the result of self-inoculation, to prove that they had three separate causes.[50] In 1861, Koebner returned to Breslau and started a private outpatient clinic for skin disease with an emphasis on medical education, thus establishing the so-called Breslau school. Always conscious of the wider world of knowledge outside Breslau, he sought out information on subjects in which he believed he was deficient, traveling to Norway in 1863 to study leprosy. He was appointed to the University of Breslau in 1869, and a university clinic was established for him there. In the late 1870s, he moved to Berlin for health reasons, i.e., laryngeal tuberculosis. He remained in Berlin until his death in 1904.

Koebner's most noteworthy contribution was the Koebner phenomenon, also known as the isomorphic phenomenon, which refers to the tendency of lesions of psoriasis, lichen planus, and several other skin diseases to erupt—typically 10–20 days later—in skin areas that have experienced trauma. He first reported it in 1872 at a meeting of the Silesian Society of National Culture, although his research was not published until 1876.[51] The case he reported involved a person who developed psoriasis in areas of trauma after horseback riding, particularly overlying a bite of the horsefly.[52]

Koebner was also the first to describe hereditary epidermolysis bullosa, mycotic sycosis barbae (tinea barbae), and quinine-induced drug eruptions. His bibliography consists of journal articles and not treatises; he wrote extensively about mycosis fungoides, pemphigus, leprosy, and syphilis. Koebner's career is significant because his efforts in Breslau represent the first major offshoot from the three main schools; in the case of Breslau, it was a dispersal of ideas from both Vienna and Paris.

After Koebner, Breslau would be the venue for several important figures in the history of dermatology. Oskar Simon (1845–1882) was born in Berlin and earned a doctorate of medicine there in 1868. Like Koebner, Simon went to Vienna to study dermatology under Hebra, and after a stint as a surgeon in the Franco-Prussian War, he returned to Berlin where he practiced the treatment of skin diseases and syphilis, becoming a local authority in those fields. When Koebner left Breslau for Berlin in 1878, Simon succeeded him as professor of dermatology. Simon made a name for himself by describing the histopathology of molluscum contagiosum and the clinical aspects of maculae caeruleae (blue spots).[53] His most important publication was a discussion of the localization of skin diseases (1873). However, his life was cut short by stomach cancer at just 37 years old, causing his contributions to pale in comparison to those of his contemporaries. His legacy is the stability and bright future he provided for the Breslau school after Koebner's death.

Albert Neisser (1855–1916)

Albert Ludwig Sigesmund Neisser, the aforementioned rival of Hansen in the Hansen-Neisser controversy (see Interlude 1), was a Prussian bacteriologist and dermatologist who was born outside of Breslau and spent most of his illustrious career in that city. He received his medical degree in Breslau in 1877 and soon after took a position in Oskar Simon's clinic; two years later, at just 24 years of age, he discovered the gonococcus, a significant milestone in the history of venereology. After a trip to Norway, Neisser published his controversial discovery of the leprosy bacillus in 1880 and moved to Leipzig that same year for a lectureship. He returned to Breslau in 1882 at just 27 years of age to succeed Simon as the director of the dermatology department. He once noted,

> Köbner planted the seed, but if Simon had not been such a skilled gardener who took care of the young plant, the great tree which has been entrusted to me since 1882 would have never developed.[54]

Neisser brought the Breslau school to its zenith, and by the end of the century, Breslau enjoyed its status as one of the premier places in Europe for dermatological education. Neisser had professional relationships abroad, especially with Kaposi and Pick; the trio founded *Deutsche Dermatologische Gesellschaft,* "German Dermatological Society" in Prague in 1889.

Neisser spent most of his career working with leprosy and syphilis. In addition to the controversy with Hansen, Neisser drew much negative attention and censure of himself because of inoculation experiments with syphilis that he performed using four healthy persons. He worked tirelessly to discover the cause of syphilis, even traveling to Java to gather specimens from syphilitic apes. After Schaudinn and Hoffman preempted Neisser with the discovery of *Treponema pallidum* in 1905, Neisser diverted some energies to working with both Wassermann and Ehrlich on their discoveries (see Interlude 3). The University of Breslau named him full professor of dermatology in 1907; his resume at that time almost exclusively demonstrated work in the realm of infectious diseases of the skin.

Neisser's greatest legacy to the specialty of dermatology was the generation of dermatologists he trained at his University Clinic in Breslau. It is said that Neisser taught 35 students who ultimately ran clinics or held professorships in other cities; many of these pupils have names that present-day dermatologists would recognize: Josef Jadassohn (1863–1936), Abraham Buschke (1868–1943), Felix Pinkus (1868–1947), and Max Jessner (1887–1978).[55] Pinkus once praised his mentor as a born leader: he was confident, he had a talent for organizing, an eye for what is essential, and superb speaking ability.[56]

Neisser's industriousness was legendary; he once remarked that "life without work would be unbearingly boring."[57] He was energetic, natural, realistic, and rousing, equipped with a vitality and sense of humor that always got the listener on his side.[58] A student once noted the power Neisser had over people, his personality a spell, a force of attraction.[59] Neisser never had children, but his students, whom he cared for like a father, filled that empty place.[60] He was a dynamic instructor, able to bring refreshing clarity to confusing subjects and to engage otherwise out-of-reach students.[61] In his free time, Neisser enjoyed the arts—paintings, sculpture, architecture, piano, and opera. The art collection on display in his villa, built by a famed architect, was dismantled and destroyed by the Nazis during World War II.[62]

Josef Jadassohn (1863–1936)

Neisser personally requested that upon his death, the best of his students and one-time assistant, Josef Jadassohn, should succeed him as chief of dermatology at the University of Breslau. Jadassohn was born in Leignitz, Silesia and went to medical school in Göttingen, Breslau, Heidelberg, and Leipzig. During his medical school years, Jadassohn became fascinated with the relationship between functional pathology and the pathogenesis of diseases.[63] He started his postgraduate medical career in 1887 in Breslau alongside Neisser, who influenced him to embark on a career in dermatology, a field in which Jadassohn believed he could find the answers to general pathological questions.[64] Jadassohn spent several months at Hôpital Saint-Louis in 1892, where he met and learned from Fournier, Besnier, Brocq, and Darier. He returned to work in Breslau until a position opened up for him in Bern, Switzerland, in 1896. Jadassohn started the Bern school of dermatology that year and thrived at the clinic there for almost 20 years. It was there he greatly influenced the important twentieth-century Swiss dermatologist Bruno Bloch (1878–1933), who later discovered the dopa reaction that allowed for staining of melanin-producing cells. When Neisser died in 1916, Jadassohn had to decide whether to finish what he started in Bern or return to his roots in Breslau; he chose the latter. He spent the remainder of his career in Breslau and superseded any of the former chiefs of dermatology there with his accomplishments. Jadassohn was, without a doubt, the master of the Breslau school, and his return to Breslau marked the elevation of the Breslau school to the top German-speaking dermatology school in Europe, surpassing even Vienna.

Jadassohn's contributions are numerous and encompass virtually every aspect of dermatology. An expert clinician, experimental scientist, deep thinker, and prolific writer, Jadassohn's name is attached to several diseases and seminal descriptions. He is famous for his descriptions of blue nevus, nevus sebaceus, anetoderma, granulosis rubra nasi, pretibial myxedema, and a subtype of pachyonychia congenita, which bears his name. He was among the first to perform experiments in immunology, and he was also a pioneer in immunodermatology. As the "Father of Contact Dermatitis," he invented patch testing, an invaluable test that is still used today. Yet another author of countless publications, Jadassohn edited the 41-volume *Handbuch der Haut—und Geschlechtskrankheiten*, "Handbook of Skin and Venereal Diseases" (1927–1937), the longest work ever published in the history of dermatology.

The Berlin School

The prestigious Breslau school represents the most successful German program for dermatology in the late nineteenth and early twentieth centuries, but it was not the only German school. By around 1850, there were hospital spaces for skin patients in Munich, Würzburg, and Berlin.[65] Of these, Berlin was the most significant, as Berlin was the home of such giants as Rudolf Virchow, Johannes Müller, and Paul Langerhans (1847–1888), the discoverer of the skin cell bearing his name. With such bright minds assembling together, it was only natural that a school of dermatology developed in Berlin. It was first established by Gustav Simon, mentioned previously as the founder of dermatopathology.

Simon's successor at Charité Hospital after his early death was the Berliner and rival of Virchow, Friedrich Wilhelm Felix von Bärensprung (1822–1864). Bärensprung founded a separate skin disease department at the hospital in 1853, where Schönlein had discovered the fungus in favus and still worked. While the German Max Burchardt (1831–1897) was the first to describe erythrasma in 1859, Bärensprung attempted to differentiate erythrasma and tinea cruris. He also distinguished the soft chancre (chancroid) from the hard one (syphilis), and he knew that syphilis, gonorrhea, and chancroid have separate causes. His greatest discovery was the identification of zoster as a disease of the spinal ganglia.[66] He demonstrated time and again that he appreciated the application of the microscope to the field of dermatology, as his mentor had. He wrote three important works: *Beiträge zur Anatomie und Pathologie der menschlichen Haut*, "Contributions to the anatomy and pathology of human skin" (1848); *Die Hautkrankheiten* (1859), his incomplete textbook on skin diseases; and *Die hereditäre Syphilis*, "On congenital syphilis" (1864). The first was an attempt to pick up where Simon left off and represents the last treatise to appear on histopathology of the skin before Unna (see below). His life, too, was cut short; after increasingly erratic behavior and open attacks against his famous rival, he succumbed to general paresis at 42, the same fate of his predecessor, Gustav Simon. While taking a walk on the mental hospital grounds, in a fit of dementia, he jumped into a body of water and drowned.[67] Dermatovenereology was apparently a life-threatening career choice at this time and place. Bärensprung's death overshadowed his life, and he never received the acknowledgment that he deserved. Those that knew him equated him with Hebra.[68]

The zenith of the Berlin school occurred under Edmund Lesser (1852–1918), a student of Hebra and Breslau's Oskar Simon. He took over the chairmanship of the skin and syphilis clinic at Charité in 1896. It was in Lesser's clinic that Schaudinn and Hoffman discovered *Treponema pallidum*. The Berlin school flourished for over 60 years, but it never reached the status of its sister school in Breslau because of the premature deaths of Simon and Bärensprung and because most of Charité's assistant physicians were military physicians ordered to staff the clinic for a brief time.[69]

KARL MARX'S CARBUNCLES

Karl Marx (1818–1883), the German philosopher and author of the *Communist Manifesto* (1848), suffered for many years with "furuncles," "carbuncles," and "boils." The most common cause of these skin lesions is bacterial infection, and in the era predating the advent of antibiotics, it is quite possible that Marx could have been suffering from chronic, recurrent staphylococcal disease. After looking at correspondence published in the 50 volumes of Marx's *Collected Works*, however, the best suggestion of a retrodiagnosis is hidradenitis suppurativa (HS).[70] HS is a chronic, severe, inflammatory skin disease in which the afflicted, who are often smokers, complain of recurrent, sterile abscesses in the creases of the skin, such as the underarms, groin, and perineal areas. The lesions tunnel under the skin or drain outward, causing a significant amount of pain and suffering in the process. Among skin diseases seen in today's dermatology offices, HS is among the most challenging to treat, and for patients with the condition, the poor quality of life associated with the disease often leads to depression and isolation. Marx's "carbuncles" were noted repeatedly to have arisen from the armpits, groins, perianal, genital and suprapubic regions, and inner thighs.[71] Noting the loathing, the disgust, the alienation, and the depression of self-image, mood, and well-being that skin disease, especially HS, can produce, Shuster proposed the very intriguing question: Could Marx's disease have influenced his worldview?[72]

Hamburg: Paul Gerson Unna (1850–1929)

With each of the major schools of European dermatology of the nineteenth century—London, Paris, Vienna, Breslau, Berlin—now described, it may come as a surprise that a final figure from this era, quite possibly the most significant of them all, belonged to none of these schools. He never reached professor status before he retired; only after retirement was he given an honorary professorship. He spoke at various conferences as dermatology's most outstanding "freelance," someone who knew everyone and whom everyone knew.[73] He was the most famous dermatologist in the world for the better part of three decades. That physician was Paul Gerson Unna from Hamburg, Germany.

The son of a physician from Hamburg, Unna carried on his family's strong medical tradition by entering medical school; his education consisted of stints in Heidelberg, then Leipzig, and finally Strasbourg. His training was interrupted by the Franco-Prussian War, in which he fought and suffered a severe battle wound in the thigh; he received a government pension for this injury, monies that he later turned over to his students as prizes.[74] A "born microscopist," Unna's doctoral research, upon the recommendation of his mentor Heinrich Wilhelm Gottfried Waldeyer (1836–1921), was on the histology and development of the epidermis.[75] The thesis explored unconventional ideas, and the criticism that it drew, especially from the German pathologist Friedrich Daniel von Recklinghausen (1833–1910), brought Unna some early recognition. Among other contentions, the controversy stemmed from Unna's proposition that staining reactions of skin specimens could lead to scientific generalizations about the skin and its diseases. Von Recklinghausen and others considered inferences based on staining dead tissue to be false and misleading. Unna was resolute in his convictions, and with time, the doctoral research of 25-year-old Unna was proven to be correct. Today, stains are an indispensable part of the process of examining pathological specimens from any part of the body. Based on his thesis, it was predictive that great things would come from Unna; his idea on stains was nothing short of revolutionary.

After graduating in 1875, Unna went to Vienna and studied under Hebra, Kaposi, and Auspitz, the latter with his brilliant, analytical mind being the most influential of these men on young Unna, especially relating to Unna's interest in microscopy and histopathology. He coauthored with Auspitz in 1876 a study on the syphilitic chancre. In 1878, he returned to Hamburg to work in his father's general practice, but his interest in dermatology spurred him to open a private practice called *Dermatologikum* in Hamburg in 1881. However, due to the rapid growth of his practice, it was moved three years later to Eimsbüttel, a suburb of Hamburg. The facility was equipped with laboratories, inpatient beds, and a home for his family.[76]

With his gifts for teaching, his fluency in English, and his desire for connection with students and physicians, Unna's private compound became an educational destination for students from all over Germany and the world. A spectacular presentation by Unna in English at a Congress in Washington in 1886 on seborrheic dermatitis attracted much attention and probably begged the question in the audience: just who is this man from Hamburg? Not long after, those seeking more from this emerging master could enroll in a formal training program started by Unna in Eimsbüttel in 1888. Participants in his program had to live at the institute for at least six months, pay 1000 deutschmarks for the training, and bring an operating microscope; in return, they received intensive training on every aspect of the skin and its diseases, including four lectures per week from Unna: two clinical, two histological.[77] Unna, in part because of his content, in part because of his fluency in English, was particularly influential on American dermatologists, including the first woman dermatologist, Rose Hirschler (1875–1940) (see Chapter 11). The Americans considered his courses better than similar courses in Berlin and Vienna.[78]

Three publications defined Unna's career: The first, published in 1882, was a dermatological journal Unna founded called *Monatshefte für praktische Dermatologie*, "Monthly Journal for Practical Dermatology." In its pages can be found a demonstration of Unna's industry, enthusiasm, and literary skills within a stream of publications on virtually every topic in dermatology.[79] The *Monatshefte* earned Unna an international reputation, and perhaps no publication did more for the spread of knowledge and for arousing interest in dermatology throughout the world than did this journal.[80] It was renamed *Dermatologische Wochenschrift*, "Dermatology Weekly," in 1885.[81]

The second major publication of Unna's career was his 1200-page magnum opus, which took five years to complete: *Die Histopathologie der Hautkrankheiten*, "The Histopathology of Skin Diseases" (1894). The massive tome contains all available information on dermatopathology that had been accumulated up until the time of its publication, and it was the first text on the subject since Gustav Simon's landmark treatise in 1848. An accompanying atlas arrived in 1897. *Die Histopathologie* is the bible of modern dermatopathology and the achievement of Unna's career that garnered him the most fame.

The preface of *Die Histopathologie* in Norman Walker's 1896 English translation reveals Unna's beliefs about the value of histopathological examination, the state of affairs in dermatology at the end of the 1800s, and Unna's hope for the future of the specialty. On the advantages of the skin as a substrate for investigation and the duty of the investigator, Unna wrote:

> But when, five years ago, the subject was put before me, it seemed to me that there was another and a wider sphere opened, and I soon saw that the work was bound to exceed in extent the other volumes of the system. For, with a few unimportant exceptions, we have, in connection with the skin, two very great advantages. Firstly, we can always get fresh, living material for investigation; and secondly, we are able to observe the part, and to note its relation to the disease as a whole, before excision. This exceptionally favourable position brings with it a two-fold responsibility. The first is clinical. For since it is possible to compare the clinical appearances with the histological details, it is our duty closely to analyse them, to investigate every apparent disharmony and not to rest till we have brought the macro- and micro-appearances into agreement one with the other.[82]

On the present state of the dermatologic literature and the ignorance about dermatopathology as a useful investigative tool, Unna wrote:

> A summary of the literature soon made it evident to me that there was no real histopathology of the skin, that there was but little harmony between clinical and histological detail, and that to the clinician microscopical observation had been more troublesome than useful. It is indeed not to be wondered at, that very eminent dermatologists, even those whose clinical experience is of the utmost value, turn with impatience from present day histopathology, where all the inflammations of the skin seem to be microscopically alike. The fact that, in most dermatological text-books, the microscopical anatomy is merely a sort of ornamental addition, is but too well justified; for when two skin diseases, clinically distinct, give, microscopically, the same appearances, or where the microscope shows differences where clinically none exist, it is clear that something wants elucidation.[83]

On the inadequacy of and contradictory nature of the existing dermatologic literature, he wrote,

> But the majority of publications are too often vague and little characteristic, and many of them, from the insufficient information they give about the seat or stage of the disease, are not only useless, but have actually been applied by other authors to other conditions. This has led to the accumulation of a great number of contradictory statements, which, by their stereotyped reproduction in all literature (especially dissertations), appear under the cloak of science. This is the unfortunate position of the great majority of our most important skin diseases.[84]

Unna did not think it expedient to attempt to rehash or de-confuse the existing literature, but he chose to establish a new foundation on which future generations might build:

> There were thus two methods open to me. I might either content myself with simply repeating the different statements, critically sifting them, and endeavouring to disentangle the great literary confusion, rejecting what was useless, and concluding most chapters with an ignoramus—a somewhat fruitless though not very difficult proceeding. Or, I might attempt, as Gustav Simon did, to work once more through the whole of cutaneous pathology—a labour certainly beyond the power of one individual, and the short period of five years. I have preferred to do this incompletely, and to leave its amplification to the future, rather than to give a mere dreary retrospect...

> With all these adjuvants, it is no longer remarkable that most skin diseases not only do not look alike, but even show such an abundance of histological peculiarities, that their explanation must be for the present postponed. But we may hope, that with continuous improvements in methods,

it will not be long before the histological diagnosis of the different dermatoses is on a level with the clinical. At all events, these new methods, incomplete as they are, have enabled me more thoroughly to understand many old views, and to bring many apparently contradictory statements into accord.[85]

The third career-defining publication for Unna was the "International Atlas of Rare Skin Diseases" (1889–1899), which he coedited with Malcolm Morris of Britain (1849–1924), Louis Duhring of the United States (see Chapter 15), and the aforementioned sidekick of Vidal, Henri-Camille Leloir of France. This multilingual text contained descriptions of its images in German, English, and French and allowed for the dissemination of new observations in clinical dermatology to skin specialists all over the world.

Unna published 500 articles and eight books, many of which were foundational, describing or clarifying virtually every diagnosis. His description of seborrheic dermatitis, widely considered his greatest contribution to clinical dermatology, was recognized as being so exact that the eponym for the disease was given to Unna.[86] He was a historian of the specialty, with his chapter on the history of eczema in his *Pathologie und Therapie des Ekzema* (1903) his greatest historical masterpiece.[87] Unna knew that the Biblical *tsara'at* was not leprosy. By 1900, Unna was the most sought-after instructor of dermatology in the world. That year, he inaugurated a series of three-week-long, intensive lecture courses for dermatologists which encompassed every aspect of dermatology.[88]

Unna's discoveries are myriad. In the realm of histology, he detailed the plasma cell that his mentor Waldeyer had discovered. This work was particularly vital because plasma cells are prevalent in tissue specimens of syphilis, so skin biopsies became an important diagnostic tool in the workup of syphilis at this time.[89] He also described nevus cells, spongiosis, ballooning degeneration, foam cells, the layers of the epidermis, and the degenerative products of collagen and elastin.[90] He was the first to state that the basal cell layer of the epidermis regenerates the other layers, and he defined the statum spinosum and stratum granulosum.[91] He discussed the secretory function of the sweat glands. Unna's knowledge of chemistry, combined with his understanding of the structure of the skin, enabled him to develop several critical stains utilized in the microscopic visualization of structures in both healthy and diseased skin. He was also distinguished in the field of bacteriology as he was among the first to examine *Haemophilus ducreyi* in the tissues of chancroid. He also worked with the leprosy bacillus. He considered bacteria a direct causative factor in eczema, and though rejected by his peers at the time, we know today that bacteria on the skin is an indirect factor in certain types of eczema, mainly atopic eczema. He introduced diascopy in 1893, the use of a glass spatula or slide to visualize how skin lesions changed with pressing the instrument against the skin.[92]

Unna should be considered one of the founders of modern dermatologic therapy. In addition to writing several monographs specifically on treatment, he saw the field of dermatotherapeutics—particularly as it relates to topical therapy—as wide open for innovation. His knowledge of the chemistry and pharmacology of topical interventions and his collaboration with the Hamburg pharmacist Paul Carl Beiersdorf (1836–1896) enabled him to develop many successful topical agents, including Aquaphor, ichthammol, the Unna boot, Basis soap, and several medicated soaps. He worked with sulfur, salicylic acid, resorcinol, anthralin, and chrysarobin to find the best peeling agent for hyperkeratosis and psoriasis. His knowledge of the biology of the skin, coupled with a unique understanding of the pharmacology of topical treatments, allowed for unprecedented developments in the realm of dermatotherapeutics. His masterpiece on therapy was *Allgemeine Therapie der Hautkrankheitin*, "General therapy of skin diseases" (1898).

While Unna was a passive man who let his discoveries speak for themselves, he did not shy away from controversy. Unna was not only admired by many but also had his hostile detractors; Neisser, Kaposi, and other German academics found him irritating and resented the unaffiliated Unna with his unsound ideas and threatening innovations.[93] His friend Darier once stated that Unna had more influence abroad than at home.[94] Yet, Unna stubbornly refused to let go of his beliefs or consider the opinion of others, and he was confident that once enough time had passed, his contributions would ultimately be accepted and appreciated. German academia had no choice but to finally admit Unna into the academic establishment. His career culminated in 1919 with a post-retirement honorary professorship at the University of Hamburg. The secret to Unna's success was a stubborn refusal to depart from his convictions, great self-confidence, and high ethical standards.[95]

UNNA'S DAILY ROUTINE

For a greater understanding of Unna, the man, one can turn to Sigmund Pollitzer's obituary of Unna:

> Unna was somewhat under medium height, and had rather a heavy figure, a noble fore-head, bright eyes and a full beard .... It is obvious that a life so full of work and so extraordinarily productive must have been carefully systematized. During my time in Hamburg, his routine was: breakfast at 7, followed by the morning rounds in the clinic; then the fifteen minute trip to the city, where office patients were seen till noon; then the laboratory visit and discussion with the students; dinner at 1:30, followed by a short rest; then the afternoon rounds and the laboratory; after supper an hour with the 'cello; then study and writing till after midnight. Twice a week, an afternoon was devoted to a visit to the policlinic and discussion of cases. In later years, after Unna had retired from active practice and management of his clinic, he occupied a small cottage in the suburbs where he did his chemical and microscopic work. He acquired the habit of working during the night, retiring at 11 o'clock for a few hours' sleep, then working for two or three hours and then again going to bed. Aside from his studies of philosophic and broad biologic subjects, he lived for dermatology. He rarely visited a theater, he never wasted time over a newspaper. His sole outside interest was music. He played the violin-cello with more than average skill and rarely missed an hour's daily practice, and on Sunday evening there were delightful trios and quartets at his house. He was essentially just and kind. I never saw him lose his poise nor say a harsh or unkind word to any one. In later years, he was in the habit of putting his arm affectionately around the shoulders of a friend or favorite pupil as they walked to and fro in his garden discussing serious problems. In May 1928, he suffered a paralytic stroke, from which he recovered sufficiently to resume his work and to enjoy his beloved 'cello playing. Four days before his death in an attack of influenza, he was adding notes to his manuscripts.[96]

A few remaining facts about Unna are worthy of mention. Unna believed in materialist monism, a philosophy that holds that everything that exists consists of matter, including such concepts as consciousness. He was also an admirer of Darwin, about whose ideas he wrote.[97] He was happily married and the father of four sons and a daughter; three of his sons became dermatologists, and one a pharmacist.[98]

Besides all of Unna's specific accomplishments, the impact of his extraordinary career on the history of his specialty cannot be overstated. In the vein of Erasmus Wilson, Unna's career represents advocacy for the specialty of dermatology as a scientific discipline that few of his contemporaries had equaled. The international speaking, the multilingual, magnificent texts, the basic science foundation of his approach, and the innumerable students whose lives he touched were the means by which Unna continuously engendered interest in dermatology and propelled dermatology into the modern era as a scientific discipline on par with other specialties of medicine. As Hollander expressed, Unna was "the master of an indefatigable dermatologic propaganda," who not only wanted to enlighten the skin specialists in his small circle but also spread dermatologic knowledge throughout the world.[99]

Unna may or may not have been the most brilliant or most hard-working dermatologist of his time, but certainly he was the most well-rounded, a true master of all aspects of dermatology: the anatomical, the biochemical, the clinical, the histopathological, and the pharmacological. His career was one investigation after another in which he applied his knowledge of the basic sciences to the problems of dermatology.[100] It is truly remarkable that he accomplished all that he did without university or institutional support. Only Hebra can claim equal or greater influence on the careers of his pupils. The choice of a "greatest legacy" assigned to Unna is an impossible task, but if forced, it would be to say simply that after Unna, dermatology and dermatopathology were inseparable disciplines—their union is the clinico-pathological correlation—and after Unna, one could no longer exist without the other.

Summary

The most influential of the three European schools of dermatology was the Vienna School, centered at the *Allgemeines Krankenhaus*, the General Hospital. There, Ferdinand von Hebra established a lineage of geniuses that as a group put dermatology on its firmest scientific footing. Incorporating information about the skin and its diseases that was gleaned from the markedly improved microscopes of this era, the appreciation of the skin as having its own resident diseases began in Vienna. Moriz Kaposi, Isidore Neumann, and Joseph Pick carried on the tradition of excellence in dermatology at the internationally famous skin disease clinics started by Hebra, where physicians from as far away as Japan journeyed to learn from the Viennese masters. Heinrich Koebner established an offshoot of the Viennese school in Breslau (modern-day Wroclaw) and Josef Jadassohn elevated the Breslau School to its zenith. A Berlin school was established by Gustav Simon, which was most famous for being the site of discovery of the causative agent of syphilis, *Treponema pallidum*. The freelancer of Hamburg, Paul Gerson Unna, with no university or hospital affiliation for most of his career, was the father of the clinico-pathological correlation, and quite possibly the most important single figure in the history of the specialty.

15

American Dermatology in the Nineteenth Century

For most of the nineteenth century, medicine in the United States lagged behind medicine in Europe. Not until the post-Civil War era beginning in the 1870s, when economic prosperity in the United States allowed for sponsored improvements in universities, did American medicine become increasingly state-of-the-art and begin to rival that of Europe. Dermatology, up until this point a strictly European creation, was born in the United States either in 1869 with the foundation of the New York Dermatological Society; in 1871, with the appointment of the first professor of dermatology at Harvard; or in 1876, with the inauguration of the American Dermatological Society. Prior to these three events, however, two figures had pioneered dermatology in the United States. After some comments on their mid-century contributions, the four principal founders of American dermatology will be addressed.

Noah Worcester (1812–1846)

The first dermatological pioneer in the United States was Noah Worcester, the author of the country's first textbook on dermatology. Worcester, the son of a schoolteacher, was born in New Hampshire. At 15, he went to Harvard and graduated five years later in 1832. Inspired to enter a career in medicine by Reuben Mussey (1780–1866), professor of medicine, Worcester enrolled at Dartmouth Medical School. At this time, medical school in the United States generally consisted of lectures at a college followed by a preceptorship with a local physician. After receiving his doctorate in 1838, Worcester moved to Cincinnati to start a practice. It was not uncommon for those who could afford it to go to Europe to enhance their medical education, so in 1841, Worcester went to Paris to seek additional training from Laennec in percussion and auscultation. During his eight months in Paris, Worcester, who was fluent in French, learned about skin diseases from Gibert and Cazenave at the most outstanding institution for skin disease in the world at the time, Hôpital Saint-Louis.[1] He returned to Ohio "the best trained man in percussion and auscultation in America" and was soon appointed professor of physical diagnosis and pathology at the Medical College of Ohio, only to move to Cleveland a year later for the Chair of Pathology, Physical Diagnosis, and Skin Diseases at Western Reserve University.[2] He contracted tuberculosis, possibly from his wife, who died of the disease a year after their marriage in 1841, and at 34 years of age, he himself was dead.

While in the throes of tuberculosis, Worcester managed to author a treatise on skin disease, the first of its kind in the United States. In 1845, he published *A Synopsis of the Symptoms, Diagnosis and Treatment of the More Common and Important Diseases of the Skin*. Of the texts discussed by the present author from the nineteenth century, Worcester's *Synopsis* is the rarest find. The 300-page tome contains 62 colored illustrations which were reproductions from European atlases. *Synopsis* is on par with any book about skin diseases from that time period.

The preface and introduction of *Synopsis* reveal that Worcester was not a frontier pretender but a science-minded, rational thinker, influenced by the brilliant minds of Europe to whom he acknowledged his indebtedness. He saw his publication as filling a void in knowledge about "this much neglected branch of medicine," lamenting that "in many of our medical institutions, not a single lecture is given upon the nature, classification, and treatment of this interesting class of diseases."[3] The strength of Worcester's text was its rational consideration of skin diseases from a pathologic standpoint and its emphasis on scientific fact and not doctrinal conjectures.[4]

DOI: 10.1201/9781003273622-22

Even in 1845, Worcester believed that poor hygiene was the most common cause of skin disease, but he also understood heredity, contagion, and poor diet as other causes.[5] On food, he wrote:

> Food has a great influence in exciting the eruptions of the skin. The almost universal testimony of physicians shows that the use of the flesh of swine has this effect. Fish is believed to have a similar effect. Crude and indigestible or highly seasoned food, the stimulating drinks, articles of food partially decayed, the use of fat, melted butter, gravies, etc., intemperance in the quantity of even wholesome food, are among the more frequent causes of cutaneous disease.[6]

He knew fungus to be the cause of favus and the acarus as the cause of scabies. Worcester formulated a classification system adapted from the French Willanists in which he established the dichotomy of wet and dry dermatoses: the wet orders were *vesiculae, bullae,* and *pustulae;* the dry were *exanthemata, papulae, squamae, tuberculae,* and *maculae.*[7] In his method, the most proficient path to a diagnosis involved three steps: first, ascertain whether the eruption was initially dry or moist; second, look for the elementary (primary) lesion; and third, if the elementary lesion cannot be determined, "try to learn from the patient or friends the appearance of the disease at first."[8] His emphasis on the elementary lesion demonstrates that he was a devout Willanist. He recognized the value of the systems of Alibert, Wilson, and Plumbe and noted that these were systems that might work for dermatologists with a vast knowledge of the whole specialty, but they were not helpful for beginners trying to make sense of what they saw on the skin.[9]

Worcester's comments on treatment are of particular value as Worcester called for treatments that were based on the pathological nature of the disease, as opposed to treatments with some "fancied specific power," based on humoral theory:

> Let the pathological nature of cutaneous diseases be the carefully studied and remedies applied as experience and reason would dictate in similar diseases of other organs, and much less complaint will be heard of their obstinancy; but frequently no attempt is made to adapt the treatment to the character or stage of the disease, and consequently we ought not to wonder at the result; it is often directed by a physician incapable of giving the pathology of a single eruption; whose whole vocabulary of cutaneous diseases is confined to some four or five vulgar unmeaning names, as "Salt Rheum," "Tetter," and possibly "Herpetic Eruption;" whose whole medical ammunition for their cure consists of some half dozen remedies, administered externally and internally according to some whim or fancied specific power, as Cream of Tartar, Sarsaparilla, internally to "purify the blood;" Arsenic, Sulphur, Corrosive Sublimate prescribed internally as "alterants," and externally as "stimulants;" and some irritating substances made into washes, or still worse, mixed with more irritating rancid lard, under the form of salves and ointments, intended to be applied externally "to dry up the humor."
>
> The great reason that the treatment of cutaneous diseases has generally been attended with so little success, is that we prescribe for them too empirically, and do not pay sufficient attention either to the pathology or to the stage of the eruption.[10]

Worcester's treatments were traditional nineteenth-century treatments for skin disease. He used bloodletting, cathartics, purgatives, laxatives, leeches, sulfur baths, tincture of cantharides, corrosive sublimate, and other tonics, noting that "of all the tonics, no one at the present day, enjoys the reputation that arsenic has acquired in the treatment of chronic cutaneous diseases."[11] Worcester opposed the suppression of eruptions with local remedies, which he viewed as dangerous; an approach with "general" therapies before local ones was the safest protocol. Cleanliness through regular bathing, the importance of a healthy diet, and abstinence from alcohol were also encouraged.

Although *Synopsis* appeared in two editions (1845 and 1850) and was an excellent book, it did not circulate well, failing to get the attention of the East Coast physicians who looked to Europe for knowledge, not to a western outpost like Cleveland.[12] Therefore, because of geography and Worcester's professional disconnection with his eastern brethren, his impact on the foundation of the specialty was minimal to nonexistent.

The Father and Son Bulkley: Henry Daggett (1803–1872) and Lucius (1845–1928)

The second American dermatologist from the first half of the nineteenth century—one whose impact was actually felt—was Henry Daggett Bulkley (1803–1872). Born in Connecticut, Bulkley went to Yale College and Yale School of Medicine, from which he received his doctorate in 1830. Like Worcester, Bulkley then went to Paris to increase his medical knowledge, gravitating toward a career in skin disease after time spent with Biett and Cazenave at Hôpital Saint-Louis. He returned to New York City and started to practice medicine in 1832. In 1836, Bulkley established the Broome Street Infirmary for Diseases of the Skin, the first facility in the United States for the treatment of skin diseases, which, like the Carey Street Dispensary in London, served the indigent and underserved. The infirmary was one of the few such facilities for skin disease in the world at the time. In the first nine days of the infirmary, 246 patients were seen, 231 of whom were suffering from strictly cutaneous complaints, including 11 cases of syphilis.[13] At the clinic, Bulkley began lecturing on skin diseases in 1837, the first formal training for skin disease in the United States, training which focused on the essential teachings of the French school. An eloquent speaker, Bulkley's lectures were published in the *New York State Journal of Medicine* starting in 1840. Because of the single-handed efforts of Bulkley, New York held an exceptionally high place in the development of dermatology. Toward the end of his life, the New York Dermatological Society was organized at Bulkley's home in 1869. It is the oldest dermatological society in the United States.

Although Bulkley wrote many articles and case presentations that were published in medical journals, he never authored a textbook on dermatology. In 1846, however, Bulkley produced an American edition of Cazenave and Schedel's *Abrégé pratique des maladies de la peau* by editing Thomas Burgess' English translation of that French text, known as *Manual of Diseases of the Skin*. Unlike Worcester's textbook, which may not have even reached the hands of New York physicians, Bulkley's *Manual* was a bestseller and the most influential textbook on dermatology in the middle of the nineteenth century. His comments on the very first page about the status of dermatology reveal a specialty with a history of chaos:

> Dermatology seems to many a difficult and uninviting field of study, and the great number of diseases described, together with the somewhat confusing nomenclature and classification often employed, have served to repel rather than attract practical medical man.[14]

Bulkley also edited an American edition (1851) of *Lectures on the Eruptive Fevers* (1843) by the English physician George Gregory (1790–1853), whose textbook on exanthems was, at the time, the finest book on contagious diseases anywhere in the world. As a man, we know more about Bulkley than Worcester from descriptions of him left by his contemporaries.[15] He was not only scholarly and persuasive and charming but also reserved and modest. He demonstrated much sympathy for his patients.

His son Lucius Duncan Bulkley followed in his footsteps with a career in dermatology. Born in Manhattan, Lucius went to Yale for college and Columbia University for medical school; after graduating in 1866, he journeyed to Europe for dermatologic training, where he met Hebra and Neumann in Vienna and Hardy in Paris.[16] His passion for all dermatology knew no bounds. He translated Neumann's *Lehrbuch der Hautkrankheiten* and published it upon his return to New York in 1872. Within a few years of beginning his practice, he started the *Archives of Dermatology*, a quarterly journal. It was not the first journal in the United States on skin disease; that was the *American Journal of Syphilography and Dermatology* started by Morris Henry (1835–1895) in 1870. Lucius was a founding member of the American Dermatological Association in 1876. He founded the New York Skin and Cancer Hospital in 1882 to deal with the multitude of patients with unappealing and malodorous skin diseases who were not welcome at general hospitals.[17] This was the site of the earliest postgraduate training in dermatology in the United States. This facility would become a famous location for advances in dermatology in the next century, and still thrives today (as the Department of Dermatology of NYU). His lectures on skin diseases were very popular with standing room only.

Lucius Bulkley's most important publications were the titles *Eczema and Its Management* (1881), *Acne and Its Management* (1885), *Syphilis in the Innocent* (1894), and *Principles and Application of Local Treatment in Diseases of the Skin* (1907). He was preoccupied with the link between diet and skin disease; his voice was loud in opposition to the acne patient consuming sweets.[18] Bulkley was the first to describe pemphigoid gestationis. He was an outspoken advocate for specialization in medicine, writing that the science and practice of medicine was too vast for any one person to know all of it.[19] He is famous for his controversial views about the dietary origins of cancer and his opposition to the treatment of cancer with surgery. The two Bulkleys were giants of early American dermatology.

James Clarke White (1833–1916)

Dermatology in the United States was officially recognized as a legitimate specialty in 1871 when James Clarke White (1833–1916) of Maine, a graduate of Harvard College and the Harvard-affiliated Tremont Medical School, was appointed as Harvard's—and America's—first professor of dermatology. After graduating from medical school in 1856, White went to the most famous medical school in the world, the one in Vienna, seeking higher learning to increase his competence to practice medicine. There he met the "glorious triumvirate" and later noted about Hebra,

> He was an admirable teacher and no one could forget his clear and convincing method of presenting a subject, and the exhaustive use of abundant clinical material for instruction in diagnosis and therapeutics. It was the perfect system of object teaching given by a master of the keenest observation.[20]

Hebra influenced White to embark on a career in dermatology; in particular, Hebra's teaching style, whereby he demonstrated his analytical and critical thinking skills, impacted White, who would later become America's greatest educator in dermatology.

White returned to Boston in 1857 and opened a general medical practice, but not yet one in which he specialized in dermatology. He also taught chemistry at the medical school during these early years of his career. In 1860, he opened, along with Benjamin Joy Jeffries (1833–1915), the Eliot Street clinic in Boston that offered only dermatological and ophthalmological services. By 1863, White's restriction of his practice to dermatology was complete; he gained more and more experience with treating skin diseases throughout the 1860s, and by 1870, Harvard had opened a skin disease clinic at Massachusetts General Hospital and placed White in charge of it. A year later, he was appointed Professor of Dermatology, a position he would hold for 31 years.

In addition to his promotion of dermatology as a legitimate specialty, White advocated reform in medical education in general, which had been at the time a "proprietary venture, benefitting teachers more than students" who bought tickets to attend lectures.[21] His campaign succeeded with the implementation of a three-year nine-month course with written exams and stricter entrance requirements.[22] White believed that medical education should have two pillars: theoretical knowledge and practical training.[23] By the turn of the century, in large part because of White's efforts, medical education programs—now four years long—improved in the United States and began to resemble the programs in the fine medical schools of Europe. In dermatology, however, the United States still lagged behind Europe with its postgraduate education programs in dermatology and its superior laboratories for basic science research on skin diseases.

White was a prolific writer during his tenure as professor of dermatology. He wrote 125 articles, 50 reviews, 94 editorials, 15 translations, and 8 books or chapters, the most significant of which was his book *Dermatitis Venenata: An Account of the Action of External Irritants upon the Skin* (1887), the first complete work on contact dermatitis.[24] The work is focused on dermatitis which is due to contact with various substances, mainly plant matter, at a time when allergic mechanisms were not yet known. As mentioned in Chapter 13, James Clarke White was the White of Darier-White disease, having described independently the condition known as keratosis follicularis a few months prior to Darier's announcement.

White was a founder and first president of the American Dermatological Association, which met for the first time in Niagara Falls in 1876.

In 1907, White characterized the beginning of his career as a specialist in dermatology as "a long and hard struggle to overcome the opposition, on the part of the general profession, the governing boards of hospitals, and the faculties of our medical schools, to the position of dermatology as an independent department of medicine."[25] The same resistance to specialization felt in Europe was experienced in the United States. But according to White's British contemporary, Malcolm Morris (1849–1924), "judicious and temperate as was his cast of mind, and free as he was from rancorous feeling, White was a good fighter, and one may hope, for his own sake, that he was no stranger to the joy of battle."[26]

Indeed, the battle was won, with all future American dermatologists as victors. While speaking in 1907 at the Sixth International Congress of Dermatology, held for the first time in New York, White noted the advance of American dermatology to the point of equality with its international counterparts:

> We have one hundred and twenty-five professors and teachers of dermatology. We have large and well equipped special laboratories and clinics, perhaps the largest and most magnificent medical school building in the world, and we have produced some admirable and exhaustive treatises and countless papers on dermatology. Most of our teachers have had the advantage of studying our subject with the most distinguished teachers of Europe, living and dead. You see, therefore, that you should find us very much the same as yourselves, and that we meet as equals.[27]

Henry Granger Piffard (1842–1910)

If White was the master of dermatology in Boston, Henry Granger Piffard (1842–1910) was at the same time the master of New York City after Henry Bulkley's death in 1872. Piffard was born in Piffard, a hamlet in western New York named after his ancestors who settled the area. He graduated from the University of the City of New York (now NYU) in 1862 and from the College of Physicians and Surgeons (now Columbia University's Medical School) in 1864. Like Worcester, White, and Bulkley before him, Piffard went to Europe for postgraduate work in dermatology. He spent considerable time in Paris and Vienna, but most of his time was spent at the University College Hospital in London, under the mentorship of Tilbury Fox.[28] It was there that Piffard met another Fox of no relation, George Henry Fox (see below) of New York, who was also there studying dermatology under Tilbury. The two men became close friends for the rest of Piffard's life.

Piffard returned to the United States in 1866 and assumed the role of attending dermatologist at the Bellevue Hospital in New York City, the oldest hospital in America (est. 1736). Piffard's first major publication appeared in 1868: an English translation of Alfred Hardy's "The Dartrous Diathesis." Piffard was a staunch defender of the diathetical ideas of Bazin and Hardy—even to the bitter end of the heyday of the theory. In 1869, he co-founded, along with Henry Daggett Bulkley, the New York Dermatological Society. Two years later, Piffard was appointed visiting dermatologist to the City Hospital's dermatological wards. He received his first professorship in dermatology in 1874 at NYU. By 1875, Piffard had established, along with Lucius Bulkley and George Fox, the first postgraduate course in dermatology in the United States.[29] Graduates of American medical schools no longer had to go to Europe for education in dermatology, and "his lectures, while not gifted with soaring rhetoric, were practical, interesting, and forceful."[30] The course moved to the Skin and Cancer Hospital founded by Bulkley in 1882 and merged with New York University School of Medicine in 1948.[31]

In 1876, Piffard published the second textbook on dermatology in the United States (after Worcester's *Synopsis*): *Elementary Treatise on Diseases of the Skin*. Later, his *A Treatise on the Materia Medica and Therapeutics of the Skin* (1881) was a much-needed formulary of dermatologic medications.[32] He founded another American journal, the *Journal of Cutaneous and Venereal Diseases*, in 1883, an essential journal for cutaneous medicine for almost four decades. This journal still lives on today as *JAMA Dermatology*. His magnum opus was *A Practical Treatise on Diseases of the Skin* (1891), which contained some of the earliest photographic plates in dermatology and set a new standard for illustrating skin diseases in textbooks.[33]

His energy, combined with his brilliant mind, earned Piffard the nickname "Brains" and brought him international recognition.[34] Piffard had diverse interests and countless hobbies, including ballistics, and he was a tinkerer and inventor. His photogenic (light-generating) pistol cartridges, used to facilitate photography of skin diseases, were among his most fascinating inventions. When exploded by a pistol, the cartridges would emit "a magnesium light of great intensity, but momentary duration" allowing for "instantaneous photography at night."[35] One can only imagine the reaction of Piffard's patients as Piffard pulled out his pistol to take a photo of their rashes. The photographs in his *Practical Treatise* were taken using this technique. Piffard also developed variations of surgical instruments, including the dermal curette and battery-powered electrocautery. He was one of the pioneers in the development and application of radiation (both X-ray and ultraviolet) to treat skin diseases, including skin cancer. His invention of an X-ray tube that was safe for the operator earned him his only eponym: the Piffard tube. Piffard's greatest legacies in early American dermatology were his work as a medical educator, his contribution to a growing body of American dermatologic literature, and his advances in medical technology.

George Henry Fox (1846–1937)

Piffard's friend and colleague, George Henry Fox (1846–1937), was another important figure in early American dermatology. The son of a veteran of the War of 1812 and the grandson of a veteran of the Revolutionary War, Fox was born in Saratoga County, NY, and attended college in Rochester, NY. His undergraduate coursework was interrupted by his volunteering for the Civil War, with his service lasting two years.[36] He went to medical school at the University of Pennsylvania and received his MD in 1869. In 1870, Fox then went across the Atlantic for dermatology training where he met Virchow in Berlin; Rokitansky, Hebra, and Neumann in Vienna; Bazin, Hardy and Vidal in Paris; and Tilbury Fox in London. Hebra influenced him more than any other.[37] Fellow students in London included Henry Piffard, Radcliffe Crocker, and the young Canadian William Osler.[38]

Fox returned to the United States in 1873 and started a general medical practice, hoping to make a name for himself as a practitioner of dermatologic complaints in New York. He joined the New York Dermatological Society and was a founding member of the American Dermatological Association in 1876. Fox worked at two different dispensaries in the 1870s where he saw many skin disease patients and applied his interest in photography, collecting photographs of his patient's skin conditions. By the end of the decade, he had a full assortment of pictures to create an atlas of dermatology, which he published as *Photographic Illustrations of Skin Diseases* (1879). His second atlas, *Photographic Illustrations of Cutaneous Syphilis* (1885) completed the whole story of skin diseases.[39]

After his first publication, Fox's professional career skyrocketed, and he was offered professorships in dermatology; he settled into that role at the College of Physicians and Surgeons (now Columbia University) in 1880, where he remained for 26 years. In addition to his groundbreaking photographic atlases, Fox contributed to the corpus of dermatologic knowledge by describing in 1902 the underarm rash of young women known today as Fox-Fordyce disease, along with his colleague John Addison Fordyce (1858–1925). He was also one of several figures to describe matchbox dermatitis, a particularly itchy, obsolete rash caused by contact with the material composing the striking surface of matchboxes.

Fox received all the distinct honors and memberships of the dermatologic societies of his era. He was known to be an able clinician with accurate observational skills and a knack for teaching, all the while looking scholarly and dignified but not arrogant or grandiose.[40] George Henry Fox's long life spanned the entirety of dermatology's beginnings in the United States. His son, Howard Fox (1873–1954), was the founder and first president of the American Academy of Dermatology (1938) and a giant of twentieth-century dermatology.

J.P. MORGAN'S ROSACEA

John Pierpont Morgan (1837–1913), the American financier and magnate who dominated the American banking industry in the latter half of the nineteenth century, suffered by 1888 with rhinophymatous rosacea, better known as rhinophyma. Rhinophyma, a condition that primarily affects men with rosacea, is characterized by an enlarged nose that is engorged with blood vessels, reddish-purple in color, and textured by bulbous protrusions and deep fissures. Morgan's unsightly nose was a source of great insecurity for one of America's most powerful figures. He was never at ease while in public, and he hated to be photographed; he struck with his cane anyone attempting to photograph him. Photographs that were taken of Morgan were touched up to hide from the public his grotesque deformity. One of several biographers of Morgan, Jean Strauss, noted the following about Morgan's personality as it relates to his rhinophyma:

> His social and professional self-confidence were too well established to be undermined by this affliction, but as he became an increasingly public figure, his brusque manner and always searching gaze took on dimensions of defiance, as if he dared people to meet him squarely and not shrink from the sight, asserting the force of his character over the ugliness of his face.[41]

Treatment of his condition—surgical shave of the sebaceous growths—could have been performed at the time, but it is possible that Morgan feared both that a surgical procedure could promote the return of a seizure disorder he had as a child and the public ridicule such a cosmetic surgery might have generated.[42] Other famous persons with rhinophyma include the American actor/comedians W.C. Fields (1880–1946) and Jimmy Durante (1893–1980).

Louis Duhring (1845–1913)

The physicians discussed thus far were instrumental in establishing American dermatology on a firm footing and elevating it to the level of their European counterparts. While each of these men was an excellent clinician and educator, America's version of Unna or Hebra or Brocq or Besnier cannot be found among them. Only one figure from American dermatology came close to that level, and he was not in New York or Boston. The physician to whom the story now turns and the last prominent figure to highlight in this book—the greatest dermatologist of nineteenth-century America—spent his career in Philadelphia. That man was Louis Adolphus Duhring.

Born in Philadelphia, Duhring was the son of a merchant who emigrated from Germany, and by hard work and discerning acuity, he became one of the ten richest men in Philadelphia.[43] The young Duhring attended the University of Pennsylvania (Penn) in 1861 but left in 1863 for a 90-day stint in the 32nd Regiment of Pennsylvania Volunteers when the southern portion of Pennsylvania was threatened by the Confederates.[44] He returned to medical school at Penn in 1863 and received his doctorate in 1867. His first position after medical school was an internship at the Blockley Almshouse, a local hospital for the poor.

Blockley was for Duhring what Hôpital Saint-Louis was for Alibert, and what the *AKH* was for Hebra: a fertile ground for exposure to skin diseases and the development of ideas in a brilliant young physician's mind. While Duhring and ten other interns took care of several thousand sick-poor at Blockley, he quickly showed an interest in skin diseases, and the hospital administration set aside space at the hospital for Duhring to care for skin patients.[45] An accomplished musician, Duhring and his fellow interns who were also musically inclined played in the Blockley Brass Sextette. They played for their friends as well as for the insane asylum patients at Blockley; according to Duhring's colleague, Arthur Van Harlingen (1845–1936), the music had a soothing effect on the insane.[46]

Duhring went to Europe in 1868 where he spent two years—never vacationing, always working to receive additional training in dermatology. His first stop was Vienna where he met the master Hebra, who was so impressed with the young Duhring that he allowed him to accompany him on his dermatologic rounds.[47] Duhring also went to Berlin, Paris, and London, and he studied Eastern diseases in Constantinople and leprosy in Norway.

Duhring returned to Philadelphia in 1870 and opened a dispensary for skin diseases with Van Harlingen. His lectures on skin diseases at the University of Pennsylvania, which began in 1871, were extremely popular and a sign of good things ahead for Duhring's teaching career over the next 40 years. His first paper was an article in July 1870 on "The Pathology of Alopecia Areata."[48] Duhring founded the Department of Dermatology at Penn, the oldest dermatology department in the United States, in 1874. He was appointed clinical professor in 1876 and full professor in 1890. In 1876, a department for skin diseases was opened at Blockley, and Duhring was named visiting dermatologist at that facility, a position he held until 1887. A founding member of the American Dermatological Association in 1876, he served under James C. White as the Association's first vice president and its third and fourth president. During these years, Duhring surrounded himself with excellent assistants; they were, in addition to Van Harlingen, Henry Stelwagon (1853–1919), the author of the first great twentieth-century American dermatology textbook, and Milton Hartzell (1854–1927), for whom the Chair is named today at the Department of Dermatology at Penn.

The year 1876 proved to be an important one for Duhring with his professorship, the side job at Blockley, and the ADA launching; it was also the year the first of eight portions of his *Atlas of Skin Disease* (1876–1880) was released. The atlas, focusing on the more common diseases of the skin, is truly one of the spectacular atlases of the nineteenth century. A year later, Duhring's *Practical Treatise on Skin Diseases* (1877) was published, one year after Piffard's *Elementary Treatise*; it was dedicated to Hebra. The book was extremely successful, having gone through three editions, and with translations into several languages, it was the first American dermatology text to be exported. Through the professorship, the Association, and especially this text, by 32 years of age, Duhring had made a name for himself both nationally and internationally as an excellent clinician, clear and scholarly writer, and gifted educator. He was henceforth the best America had to offer on the international stage of dermatologists.

Duhring's greatest contribution to the history of dermatology was not his textbook; it was the 18 articles he penned from 1884 to 1891 on the topic of dermatitis herpetiformis, a skin condition about which there was much confusion and debate at the time. Also known as "Duhring's disease," dermatitis herpetiformis is an autoimmune blistering disease and one of the itchiest and most miserable skin conditions. Its association with gluten insensitivity and celiac disease was not known at the time. Duhring posited that dermatitis herpetiformis could have papular, vesicular, and bullous presentations but that these presentations were just different forms of the same disease, not distinctly different entities. His opponents, led by Moriz Kaposi, argued that these forms were distinctly different diseases.[49] Duhring's convincing argument, laid out over seven years of erudite scholarship, overcame the opposition, and the varied clinical presentation of dermatitis herpetiformis has been distinctly recognizable ever since.[50]

In the 1890s, Duhring planned a three-volume encyclopedia of dermatology he called *Cutaneous Medicine*. Duhring never liked the word "dermatology"; he preferred instead "cutaneous medicine."[51] The first volume appeared in 1895, and the second in 1898; they represented the product of extraordinary diligence and profuse illustration.[52] A third volume was planned, but it was never published; all of the material for publication, including the manuscript and illustrations, burned in a fire at the Lippincott publishing office in Philadelphia. The project was abandoned after that disaster.

Duhring was a complex man. Around the time young Duhring left Blockley for Europe, he suffered a traumatic life event: his sweetheart and likely future wife died. Duhring underwent a complete change in temperament, from cheerful and sociable to the point that his colleague and friend, Van Harlingen, noted, "I cannot recall any occasion when I have seen him smile or heard him laugh. His absorption in his work was absolute and complete."[53] Duhring remained a bachelor and a loner, and somewhat a miser, for the rest of his life, although he did enjoy on occasion a social life with a few intimate friends. His appearance was meticulous, intelligent, and refined.[54] In 1885, he developed neurasthenia (nervous exhaustion), which culminated in a nervous breakdown, causing five years of absence from his full-time duties at the university for recovery.[55] He suffered further grief in 1892 when his sister and housemate, Julia, with whom he had a very close relationship, died; he asked it be written in his will that he wanted to be buried next to her.[56] His health was never perfect; he frequently fought illness and vague symptoms, including "cardiac irritability and an ill-defined abdominal uneasiness" which persisted until the end of his life.[57] Duhring resigned from all employment in 1910 and died in 1913, with an estate worth 1.25 million, all of which he bequeathed to the University of Pennsylvania. A constricting band around his ileum, a possible cause of his long-term abdominal complaints, was found during his autopsy.[58]

Duhring may have been reclusive and reserved for the better part of his career, but he was not opposed to public speaking. In fact, he thrived in the public arena. The transcripts of many of his addresses as president of the American Dermatological Association are available for review. Of these, his brilliant speech on "The Scope of Dermatology," delivered in 1893 at the 44th Annual Meeting of the American Medical Association, gives us the last word on dermatology in the nineteenth century and a fitting conclusion to the story of the origins of the specialty. In that memorable speech, Duhring defined what dermatology meant to him—its scope, its purpose, and its value. The following series of excerpts from Duhring's speech effectively summarize the state of dermatology at the end of the nineteenth century, show how far it had come from the days of Willan, and reveal the bright future that lay ahead for the specialty. Duhring first defined the purpose of his address:

> What are so-called skin diseases, and what is their nature? Which diseases are entitled to be des-ignated "skin diseases?" Is it possible to separate them from the many general diseases accom-panied by cutaneous symptoms? ... [S]hall the term, "skin disease," continue to be used in its ancient sense? Shall the affections of the skin be looked upon as morbid entities, as diseases whole and complete in themselves and confined to the skin? Or, taking a broader view of the subject, shall they be defined so as to include all manifestations that may occur upon the integu-ment irrespective of the symptoms, cause or nature.[59]

On how skin diseases were viewed throughout history:

> Willan, especially, was an eminent general physician as well as a distinguished dermatologist. His treatment for the commoner affections of the skin was both judicious and successful. But the important questions of etiology and pathology were then for most diseases not at all understood. Very little was known on those subjects. The origin of most disease was regarded as "obscure." ... Affections of the skin were regarded mainly objectively, and were studied much as a model or a picture might be viewed. Beyond the actual expression on the integument they were not closely investigated; the causes were regarded as obscure; and this mode of studying them has held good through decades, up to almost the present date. This method is in no way to be criticized, so far as it goes, but by itself and without the assistance of general pathology, it is far too restricted to meet the requirements of existing knowledge. It fails to recognize the important fact that the integument is a part of the whole organism, and therefore is subject to the great laws of general pathology, and that diseases affecting the integument are not only to be studied as localized areas of disease, but also in their relation to the system at large.[60]

On local diseases of the skin, on widespread diseases with skin involvement, and on diseases of the skin about which it is uncertain whether they are confined to the skin:

> That some diseases are strictly local in all their aspects will be denied by no one, but it is practi-cally often difficult to decide where to draw the line between such affections and those due to influences and causes remote from the skin, as, for example, in the case of the many and often obscure reflex affections.

> On the other hand, it is not difficult with our knowledge of to-day, to give examples of some true skin diseases. Notably among these may be mentioned the local parasitic affections, the inflammations due to numerous external causes, as for example the rhus plant and certain of the hypertrophic, atrophic and neoplastic diseases ... In these affections, and in some others that might be cited, as far as our knowledge extends, the skin is the only organ of the body invaded at any time in the course of the disease.[61]

But while this holds true for a considerable number, there are still many that are in reality widespread diseases, the skin being only one of the organs involved by the process.

As instances of such may be cited the so-called exanthemata, as well as other eruptive fevers, the eruptions due to various poisoned states of the system, as in septicemia, glanders, leprosy and syphilis.[62]

There also exists another group of well-known cutaneous manifestations in which it is difficult to determine whether the process is really confined to the skin, and whether it does not also involve other structures of the body as, for example, the epithelium generally, as in pityriasis rubra and dermatitis exfoliativa. Another group would comprise herpes zoster, pemphigus and the like, where the nervous structures, central or peripheral, are in some way at fault.

Still another class consists of diseases which, while eminently skin diseases, are in some cases at least, dependent upon certain peculiar states of the economy for their existence, as a type of which psoriasis may be given.[63]

On atypical and irregular presentations of skin diseases:

Authors of text-books and systems of dermatology would have us believe that the various diseases may all be arranged and satisfactorily classified, and that they may in all cases be readily differentiated from one another. While this undoubtedly holds true for the majority of cases, ample allowance must be made for atypical, irregular and anomalous forms of disease, of which there occur, I am convinced, more examples than most authors are disposed to admit.[64]

On the scope of dermatology:

I am firmly of the opinion that this branch of medicine should include all morbid manifestations that appear on the skin, whatever may be their cause, their nature and their character. Dermatology has properly to do with the integument and all that pertains to it, and moreover with all the varied causes that may disturb that organ. Thus the exanthematous and the numerous and diverse symptomatic eruptions, whether superficial or deep-seated, fugitive or persistent, are all entitled to a place in the group.[65]

On how knowing the cause of an eruption is every bit as important as identifying the eruption:

The time has arrived when we should endeavor to recognize not only the particular form of eruption, but what is more important, also, the cause which has produced it, upon which success in treatment may depend. Diseases of the skin must be studied from the standpoint of general medicine. It is not possible to comprehend the meaning of certain forms of inflammation of the skin without taking the broadest view of the subject. Thus if we are inclined to regard such diseases as dermatitis exfoliativa, pityriasis rubra, lichen ruber, dermatitis herpetiformis, and the like as mere local cutaneous inflammations we fail to understand the significance of the symptoms. Symptoms and causes must be studied together. The former are elementary, and constitute the alphabet of dermatology, which it need not be stated must be learned. But eruptions in themselves, as mere forms of superficial inflammation, are by no means so important as the relation of the lesions to the causes…. Thus it happens that some diseases are practically uninfluenced by local treatment, and that not until we investigate their possible relations with the general economy do we appreciate their nature…

The objective study of skin diseases is fascinating, and has without question its uses in more ways than one, but it is important that we take steps to advance beyond this elementary stage of knowledge, by attempting to recognize and understand the meaning of the local manifestation. It has been, and still is, too much the custom to study diseases of the skin in the light of pathologic pictures, to name the local manifestation and to so label it as a disease. It is much easier to give the disease a name and to label it than it is to comprehend the process at work. The former is comparatively unimportant for the patient, the latter a point upon which recovery may depend. The nature and meaning of the process in connection with the cutaneous symptoms has not received enough attention, and I believe this to be one reason why the treatment of many of these diseases in the past has been so notoriously unsatisfactory. At all events the relations of the cutaneous disturbance to other structures and to various states of the economy should be much more thoroughly investigated by dermatologists than is the present custom.[66]

On how to be an accomplished dermatologist:

To recognize any one disease, say syphilis, in its varied manifestations on the skin, requires familiarity with all other diseases with which it is liable to be confounded. Therefore, to be an accomplished diagnostician, one must be conversant with every form of eruption to which the skin is liable, including the not rare atypical and aberrant forms. In regarding only the well-known and clearly defined, obvious diseases of the skin as belonging to dermatology, this branch of medicine is not only belittled, but the true meaning of many lesions on the skin is not appreciated. I would insist, therefore, that the manifold and varied changes that take place in the skin due, as we now know, to such a multitude of diverse causes, should be viewed as phases of cutaneous medicine rather than as skin diseases. The idea of this vast array of diseases being morbid entities, for which the integument alone is accountable, must in many cases, at least, be abandoned in favor of the principles of general medicine...

If we would study dermatology with the view of learning all that it can teach us, not only of the skin but of general medicine, we must look in the majority of cases beyond the mere eruption, valuable and important as this is in all cases as a guide to the pathological process at work.... I am of the opinion that the relations of the skin to other parts and functions of the economy are at the present date only partially understood, and that there are many points which will sooner or later be elucidated which will bring cutaneous medicine still closer to general medicine.[67]

On the answer to his original question and the real value of dermatology:

What are so-called skin diseases? ... It is simply this, that our conception of the scope of dermatology must be so widened as to include every pathological manifestation which occurs in the integument, irrespective of the cause or the nature, from a practical standpoint. The great value and importance of dermatology is that it should teach us to know the nature of various processes, as they affect not only the skin but the whole economy. Dermatology should be for the physician as a key with which the skin is made to reveal, in many instances at least, the nature of the process at work in the general system or in special organs, which without this aid might remain obscure. Striking examples supporting this view are noted in syphilis and in leprosy, where the cutaneous manifestations are sometimes the only indication of the presence of these diseases in the body. The recognition of the nature of the cutaneous lesions is often of the greatest value in the general diagnosis.[68]

Along with the aforementioned 1890 lecture by Jonathan Hutchinson (see Chapter 12), Duhring's 1893 address was one of two great speeches from dermatologists in the nineteenth century. While Hutchinson gave specifics on the path to success for dermatology going forward, i.e., embrace the microscope, get scientific, etc., Duhring defined what it is to be a dermatologist, discussed the issue of local diseases and cutaneous manifestations of internal disease, and most importantly, beseeched his colleagues to make it their task to master any and all affections of the skin, including the eruptions associated with internal illness, e.g., measles—eruptions that were historically managed by the general physician. He believed that emphasis on causation over classification would elevate the specialty into a new era in which the dermatologist could shed light on the general health of the patient and could offer treatments that were effective because they addressed the etiology of the problem. Duhring rightly saw the skin as the window into the internal organs, and correctly concluded that diseases in the skin, from the mundane rash such as tinea to the more severe diseases such as psoriasis to the serious paraneoplastic eruptions (internal cancer-associated eruptions), do indeed reveal something about the whole patient. It is up to the dermatologist to make sense of these changes. To the present author, this is the single greatest value of the specialty of dermatology.

Summary

The nineteenth century from a dermatological history perspective can be viewed in two parts: 1800–1840 and 1840–1900. In the former, the two most important developments were the foundation of the London school with the publication of Robert Willan's *On Cutaneous Diseases*, and the inauguration of the Paris school, establishing a century-long dynasty of French greats, starting with Alibert, Biett, and the French Willanists. French Willanism—the modification of Willan's morphology-based classification system and nomenclature by Biett, Cazenave, et al.—withstood many challenges but survived and proved to be the greatest development of this 40-year period. The objective system of organizing skin diseases by their appearance and arriving at a language with which every dermatologist could communicate were necessary initial steps on the path toward modernity.

In the era of 1840–1900, myriad achievements took place which brought dermatology firmly into the modern era. The establishment of the Vienna School in the 1840s by Hebra, who brought science— modern pathologic principles and a pathology-based classification system—to dermatology, was a land- mark event. From Kaposi down to Unna, his disciples were instrumental in fostering the incorporation of the microscope, with its always-improving optical resolution, into dermatologic practice. The advent of dermatopathology and the discovery of tissue stains allowed dermatology to develop both a solid scientific foundation and a diagnostic tool that remains crucial to this day: the skin biopsy. By using the microscope, clinicians were able to prove by mid-century that scabies, ringworm, and favus were all caused by microscopic organisms. After the advent of germ theory a few decades later, bacteriol- ogy allowed for a greater understanding of the pathogenesis of many common skin diseases, such as impetigo. In London, the illustrious careers of Erasmus Wilson, Tilbury Fox, Jonathan Hutchinson, and others helped establish dermatology as a legitimate specialty, denying the anti-specialists any claim to the contrary. In France, the rise of the diathetic beliefs of Bazin and Hardy brought special attention to the fact that skin disease in many cases arises from alterations in constitution. The ascendance of the dermatology journal in the last third of the century allowed for a flurry of articles—out of London, Paris, Breslau, Hamburg, New York—to be published, spreading knowledge all over the world that contained descriptions of new and old skin diseases alike which brought much order to the confusion. The inaugu- ration of local, state, national, and international dermatological societies in the 1870s and 1880s enabled the intelligent minds and the inquisitive students of the specialty to congregate with one another, further disseminating knowledge. Old myths—such as the danger of locally applied treatments and the risk of curing skin lesions because of the fear of driving the disease process inward—were finally abandoned, in large part because of the influence of the Vienna school. Noah Worcester and Henry Daggett Bulkley pioneered dermatology in the United States before it was formalized into a specialty, and these two men cannot be forgotten. The four main founders of American dermatology were James Clarke White, Henry Piffard, George Henry Fox, and Louis Adolphus Duhring, with Duhring the greatest product of American dermatology in the nineteenth century.

16

The Twentieth Century and Beyond

At the turn of the twentieth century, dermatologists could speak the modern language (macules, papules, pustules, etc.) with ease, and they had a lengthy list of diagnoses from which to choose after isolating the primary lesion and applying knowledge of morphology to evaluating the differential diagnosis of that skin lesion. They had a working knowledge of primary and secondary skin lesions, and all of the common skin diseases and many of the not-so-common were known. A skin biopsy could be performed to confirm or deny the clinical diagnosis. Scrapings of skin could also be taken to the microscope for examination of microorganisms. The dermatologist could read textbooks and journals from all over the world and look at photographs of skin diseases in atlases instead of drawings. They could attend conferences and meetings and discuss every aspect of the dermatologic specialty with domestic and international colleagues. The dermatologist at the end of the century could work in a private practice, a public clinic, a hospital ward, or an academic institution. For the dermatologist of the early twentieth century, things did not vary significantly from the way they are today.

The first six International Congresses of Dermatology (see Table 16.1) demonstrate the defining moments when dermatology revealed itself as a fully modernized specialty. The first congress, held in Paris, met at Hôpital Saint-Louis, had 220 attendees and 70 presentations from such speakers as Kaposi, Unna, Radcliffe-Crocker, Besnier, Hallopeau, and Brocq.[1] The speakers shared their experience with treating certain diseases, presented new descriptions, or expounded their opinions on controversial matters regarding the diagnosis of skin disease. Patients with intriguing or rare skin diseases were presented, and time was given for the attendees to examine each case, or they could spend time viewing exhibitions of pharmaceuticals, equipment, and instruments. Syphilis was not ignored at these meetings, as it remained a public health issue at this time. Highlights of these first congresses included presentations on X-ray therapy and its complications, revelatory educational talks about ultraviolet phototherapy by Finsen, delineations of the various types of *Trichophyton* by Sabouraud, and ongoing debates about the nature of seborrheic dermatitis, eczema, and alopecia areata. One can only imagine the enthusiasm, the theatrics, the momentousness, the congeniality on display at these events when the brightest and most famous minds in the history of the specialty were all engaged in listening to each other's presentations and debating with each other at the historical epicenters of dermatology.

Dermatological Therapeutics of the Early Twentieth Century

While the clinical and dermatopathological advances of the nineteenth century were decidedly modern, in the therapeutic arena—because the underlying cause of many skin diseases remained elusive—dermatology was still far away from being able to offer effective, evidence-based, and safe treatments. For example, topical steroids, the go-to treatment for many dermatologic complaints today, were not available until the 1950s. Still, the dermatologist of the early twentieth century did have at their disposal several external and internal treatment options, many of which did work and have been nicely reviewed by Thomsen, the source of the information in the following paragraphs.[2] Indeed, they were more effective than treatments of the era 100 years prior and earlier.

After addressing the general health of the patient by promoting a nutritious, bland diet, regular bathing, and reduced alcohol consumption, the early twentieth-century dermatologist would then correct gastrointestinal dysfunction, which for over two millennia had been considered connected to skin health.

DOI: 10.1201/9781003273622-23

TABLE 16.1

The First Six International Congresses of Dermatology

Date	Location	President
August 5–10, 1889	Paris	Alfred Hardy
September 5–10, 1892	Vienna	Moriz Kaposi
August 4–8, 1896	London	Jonathan Hutchinson
August 2–9, 1900	Paris	Ernest Besnier
September 12–17, 1904	Berlin	Edmund Lesser
September 9–14, 1907	New York	James Clarke White

This dysfunction could be fixed with iron, cod liver oil, quinine, mineral acids, or strychnine. Gentle, regular laxatives (sodium sulfate, magnesium sulfate, etc.) were prescribed for acute inflammatory skin diseases; the days of the violent purgatives were over. After these initial measures were taken, the dermatologist then prescribed medication, and in most cases, both internal and external treatments were offered. The combination of the former, advocated by Wilson, and the latter, advanced by Hebra, provided the best chance of reaching a cure.

Dermatologic internal medications could be divided into four categories: vegetable materials, animal-derived materials, inorganic chemicals, and organic chemicals. Delivered in a tonic (Fowler's solution) or pill form (asiatic pills), there was widespread use of arsenic for skin diseases, specially indicated for psoriasis, lichen planus, pemphigus, and chronic urticaria. Arsenic was capable of causing the following side effects: precancerous keratoses of the palms and soles, general hyperpigmentation, puffy eyelids, conjunctivitis, upset stomach, and liver and kidney disease.

Medications with diuretic properties were used for many chronic inflammations, and quinine was used for pityriasis rubra pilaris, leprosy, chronic urticaria, and furunculosis. Antimony was helpful for acute and subacute eczema, prurigo, and psoriasis. Antipyrine was an antipyretic and analgesic that was used for itching and for the pain of zoster. Oral sulfur was prescribed for hyperhidrosis, furunculosis, and severe acne. Iodine and iodides were useful in tertiary syphilis and tuberculous skin diseases such as lupus vulgaris; mercury, administered most commonly in the corrosive sublimate form, was prescribed for syphilis until the discovery of salvarsan after the turn of the century (see Interlude 3).

The dermatologist had at his disposal a variety of ointments, lotions, oils, liniments, powders, parasiticides, and caustics. There were four categories of local (external) treatments: soothing treatments astringent preparations, antiseptics, and stimulating medications. Benzoated lard was the most commonly used preparation for soothing ointment, but also customary were petroleum fats, white wax, paraffin wax, lanolin, olive or almond oil, cucumber, and cold cream. Astringent ointments contained either lead, zinc, boracic acid, bismuth, or alum. Antiseptic ointments included iodoform, salicylic acid, and carbolic acid (phenol). Stimulating ointments consisted of mercury, tar, oil of cade, thymol, naphthol, chrysarobin, pyrogallic acid, salicylic acid, and sulfur. Soothing lotions contained lead acetate, lead lactate, zinc oxide, calamine, and bismuth. For pruritus, lotions containing liquor carbonis detergens, turpentine derivatives, and salicylic, carbolic, benzoic, and hydrocyanic acids were prescribed. Lotions with both stimulating and antiseptic properties included carbolic acid, tar, thymol, sulfur, calcium sulfide, cantharidin, and/or silver nitrate. Common oils including olive oil, almond oil, linseed oil, cod liver oil, castor oil, and petroleum oils were used to remove scales. Dusting powders, consisting of rice, starch, lycopodium, iris root, and talc, were used to dry the skin. A variety of parasiticides were available to kill mites, lice, and fungus; sulfur was used to kill all three of these. Chrysarobin was thought to be particularly effective against fungus, but the only solution for scalp fungus remained epilation. Lice was treated with stavesacre and various forms of mercury. Caustics were used to deal with indurated or embedded skin diseases, such as lupus vulgaris and various types of skin cancer. Mild caustics included salicylic acid, iodine, mustard, and cantharidin, while the stronger caustics included potash, arsenic, zinc chloride, caustic lime, and silver nitrate. Whether to destroy skin cancers with caustics versus excise them with the knife was a great debate among surgeons throughout history.

Patients took these prescribed medications with little more than the trust in their physician that it was the right thing to do at the time of their illness. However, there was zero regulation of the contents of these medications or the claims of their manufacturers. After the turn of the 20th century, the US government intervened to establish safe and effective treatments for the American consumer. In 1906, President Theodore Roosevelt signed into law the Pure Food and Drug Act, a law aiming to prevent the adulteration of drugs by making it the business of the Bureau of Chemistry (renamed the FDA in 1930) to examine foods and drugs for additives. In 1938, President Franklin D. Roosevelt signed the Federal Food, Drug, and Cosmetic Act into law, banning false therapeutic claims and mandating a pre-market review of the safety of new drugs. These laws were critical final steps in the modernization of healthcare in the 20th century.

Advances in Twentieth- and Twenty-First-Century Dermatology

Since a detailed history of every twentieth-century contribution in dermatology would create a volume as long as this one or longer, the balance of this chapter will focus more on the concepts and developments that have characterized the last 100 years. The history of dermatology in the twentieth and twenty-first centuries is defined in no particular order by (1) the rise of dermatologic surgery; (2) a deeper scientific understanding of the mechanisms of skin disease and a fine-tuning of the diagnostic nomenclature; (3) an endless stream of genuinely great dermatologists and the expansion of dermatology to centers all over the world; (4) the establishment of an ever-increasing number of residency positions for the training of dermatologists; (5) technological discoveries; (6) the addition of cosmetic procedures to the scope of practice for the specialty; (7) a shift toward skin care and preventative measures; and most importantly, (8) the arrival of increasingly more effective treatments.

Skin Cancer and the Rise of Dermatologic Surgery

Dermatology today is a medical-surgical specialty, much like ophthalmology and otolaryngology. Dermatologists perform a variety of surgical procedures and do more surgical excisions of skin cancer than any other specialty. The formal incorporation of surgical procedures into the specialty of dermatology occurred in the twentieth century. The availability and effectiveness of local anesthetics and the increased understanding of the dangers of skin cancer facilitated the addition of surgical procedures to the domain of the dermatologist. Since skin cancer has not been given consideration as a specific topic thus far in this book, let us address its own history with a few brief comments.

The earliest reference to skin cancer comes from the Edwin Smith Papyrus, and it appears that cautery was the preferred treatment of skin cancer for the ancient Egyptians. The Hippocratic corpus, which distinguished ulcerating and non-ulcerating types of skin cancer, contains the coined word *karkinos,* from the Greek word for crab and from which the word carcinoma is derived. The word cancer, in general, referred to ulcerated skin cancers or ulcerated breast cancer in ancient and medieval texts, as the only forms of cancer these peoples knew about were external forms. In Hippocrates' *Aphorisms* can be found advice on treating skin cancer: "Those diseases [cancer] which medicines do not cure, iron [surgery] cures; those which iron cannot cure, fire [cautery] cures; and those which fire cannot cure, are to be reckoned wholly incurable."[3] Writing in the first century CE, Celsus described what today we would recognize as skin cancer and echoed the treatment options of the Hippocratics, noting that early intervention was best, but that a long-standing lesion should be left alone, as the treatment was considered capable of worsening the problem. No advances occurred in the Middle

Ages and the early modern period when it appears that cautery was the preferred method of removing skin cancer, but surgical excision and chemical caustics were also utilized during this period. However, in many cases throughout history, skin cancer was labeled as *noli me tangere,* "touch me not," and left alone because incomplete removal with caustics or some other intervention might aggravate the tumor and make matters worse. Pre-modern skin cancers were more advanced and devastating than they are today, but perhaps they were as not as prevalent, as skin cancer incidence increases with age over 50 years, and life expectancy hovered between only 30 and 40 years for most of human history until the mid-nineteenth century. And who was the first to link skin cancer with sun exposure? That was Unna.

Today, three major types of skin cancer are recognized: melanoma, basal cell carcinoma (BCC), and squamous cell carcinoma (SCC); melanoma is the deadliest of the three. There was no distinction of the different types of skin cancer until the nineteenth century, but the first reports of what we today call melanoma—"fatal black tumors with metastases and black fluid in the body"—occurred in the seventeenth and eighteenth centuries.[4] The Scottish surgeon John Hunter was credited posthumously for the first surgical removal of melanoma in the Western medical literature; in 1787, he excised a soft and black tumor—which he labeled as a "cancerous fungous excrescence"—from the neck of a 35-year-old man.[5] The preserved tumor was determined by histopathology 181 years later to be melanoma.[6] In 1804, Rene Laennec, the inventor of the stethoscope, first coined the term *melanose* in reference to melanoma and has been credited as the first to describe this diagnosis. His publication on melanoma in 1806 drew the ire of his mentor, Dupuytren, who claimed credit for some of the work.[7] Until the word *melanoma* was coined by the Scottish pathologist Robert Carswell (1793–1857) in 1838, the diagnosis was referred to as *melanosis*, implying that the patient typically presented, not surprisingly, with metastatic disease, rather than a single pigmented skin lesion. A diagnosis of melanoma at this time was obviously a death sentence in most cases. The first physicians to provide significant clinical knowledge about melanoma included William Norris (1792–1877), Thomas Fawdington (1795–1843), James Paget (1814–1899), and Oliver Pemberton (1825–1897). Of these, William Norris did more to advance the knowledge about melanoma; its genetic nature, relationship with moles, association with fair skin, metastatic tendency, and amelanotic form were all described by Norris.

For non-melanoma skin cancer in the nineteenth century and into the twentieth century, the two types known today as BCC and SCC were sometimes referred to without distinction as *epithelioma,* as they can look very much like one another. What is now called BCC, the Irish ophthalmologist Arthur Jacob (1790–1874) originally named *ulcus rodens,* "rodent ulcer" in 1827, ending the long run of *noli me tangere* as the name for skin cancer. Because the tumor had the tendency to present as an ulcer with the appearance of having been formed by a rodent's gnawing, Jacob saw the tumor as distinct from other cancerous lesions of the skin and noted its characteristic appearance: "the edges are elevated, smooth and glossy, with a serpentine outline; and are occasionally formed into a range of small tubercles or elevations."[8] The German Carl Thiersch (1822–1895) penned a seminal treatise on *epithelioma* in 1865, noting superficial and deep forms and also the epithelial origins of the tumor.[9] Although Hebra and Kaposi both dealt with this lesion histopathologically as *ulcus rodens*, the name BCC is most often attributed to the German pathologist Ödön Krompecher (1870–1926), in whose publication, *Der Basalzellenkrebs,* "On Basal Cell Cancer," (1903), the best histopathologic definition of BCC was first found.

First described by Percival Pott as arising on the scrotum of the chimney sweepers (see Chapter 10), SCC was confused with BCC and referred to as epithelioma for most of the nineteenth century. In 1912, John Templeton Bowen (1857–1940) brought some clarity to the subject by describing a type of SCC called "squamous cell carcinoma in situ," now called Bowen's disease. While there remains on rare occasion some difficulty to this day in telling them apart, modern dermatopathology can typically sort out these two tumors that originate on the surface of the skin.

The treatment of all types of skin cancer in the nineteenth century was carried out with a variety of options: ligature (tying off the lesion's blood flow with suture), curettage (the use of a scraping instrument), caustics (chemicals to erode the cancerous tissue away), cautery (heat-induced tissue injury), and excision with scalpel or scissors. Of these treatments, caustics were the most common, with the most common caustic used for skin cancer being zinc chloride paste; according to Erasmus Wilson, this procedure was painful but produced the cleanest scar.[10] The first reports of complete excision of what appears to have been BCC came in the preceding century. The French surgeon Jacques Daviel (1696–1762) excised what was very likely BCC in ten patients, followed them over time, and published his results in 1755; all had good results.[11] His dissertation on the excision of carcinomas was lost, and the late-eighteenth and nineteenth-century physicians continued to fear the worst in regard to the prognosis of *noli me tangere*.[12] Excisional surgery was generally avoided unless the lesion was small and contained. With low awareness among the public about the dangers of skin cancer at that time, it is likely that most patients presented with larger lesions than they would today, making surgery the most tenuous option.

As public awareness improved, excisional surgery became increasingly utilized, likely because patients were presenting with smaller tumors, more amenable to a simple excision. Excision has been the mainstay of treating skin cancer since the first half of the twentieth century. Mohs micrographic surgery, a tissue-conserving procedure involving intraoperative, microscopic margin analysis, has been available as a state-of-the-art treatment option for BCC and SCC since Frederic Mohs (1910–2002) revealed his technique in Madison, Wisconsin, in 1936. Curettage with and without cautery, the application of topical medication, cryosurgery, and radiation are other options offered today for the treatment of these tumors. Both radiation and cryosurgery—the use of solid CO_2, liquid oxygen, or liquid nitrogen to destroy skin lesions—were discovered in the last decade of the nineteenth century. Liquid nitrogen (–196°C), the most common cryogen used in dermatology practice today, has been commercially available for dermatology practices since the 1950s. For melanoma, Herbert Snow (1847–1930) and William Handley (1872–1962), recognizing the risk of regional lymph metastasis with that particular type of skin cancer, were important figures in the establishment of the protocols in which wide and deep excision with regional lymph node dissection was the first-line treatment. Wallace Clark (1924–1997) and Alexander Breslow (1928–1980) established the crucial prognostic measurements of melanoma—the Clark level and the Breslow depth—in 1969 and 1970, respectively. While BCC and SCC rarely metastasize, melanoma not uncommonly can. Since the invention of immune therapies, metastatic melanoma is something that a person can survive today.

Etiology, Classification, and the Diagnosis of Skin Diseases

Etiology

The establishment of the germ theory of disease by the end of the nineteenth century had helped explain many of the skin's diseases, but since the majority of skin diseases are not infectious in nature, other scientific explanations were needed. The discoveries in the realms of allergy and immunology, which began at the outset of the twentieth century, paved the way for these explanations, and we can now explain the pathogenesis of many skin diseases (see Table 16.2). Most, if not all, of the advancements took place at the world's academic institutions where medical research is performed. Still, there are numerous skin diseases that continue to mystify us as far as the cause (see Conclusion).

Classification

All modern dermatologists are Willanists in that the first piece of information sought in evaluating any skin disorder is the morphology (appearance) of the primary lesion. But they also pay tribute to Hebra and Unna in their devotion to pathogenesis and dermatopathology. In today's dermatology textbooks, skin diseases are organized by a hybrid system that is based on morphology (Willan), pathogenesis (von Hebra), and dermatopathology. For example, some chapters are organized by diseases that form *bullae* (blisters), while others are arranged by localization of the process to a part of the skin, such as

TABLE 16.2

The Causes of Skin Disease with Examples

Aging	Bateman's purpura, wrinkles, atrophy
Allergic	Poison ivy dermatitis, urticaria, medication reaction
Autoimmune	Lupus erythematosus, bullous pemphigoid, alopecia areata, vitiligo
Deposition	Amyloidosis, calcinosis cutis, porphyria cutanea tarda
External factors	Sunburn, abrasion, burn, frostbite, bites, irritant contact dermatitis
Genetic	Neurofibromatosis, ichthyosis, Darier disease, Hailey-Hailey disease
Follicular occlusion	Acne, hidradenitis suppurativa
Infectious	Impetigo, herpes simplex virus, scabies, cellulitis
Inflammatory/Immune	Psoriasis, eczema, lichen planus, Sweet syndrome, vasculitis
Metabolic	Acanthosis nigricans, Bullosis diabeticorum, Necrobiosis lipoidica
Neoplastic	Seborrheic keratosis, melanoma, angioma, dermatofibrosarcoma
Neurological	Hyperhidrosis, pruritus, scalp dysesthesia, notalgia paresthetica
Nutritional deficiency	Scurvy, acrodermatitis enteropathica, glossitis
Psychological	Delusions of parasitosis, trichotillomania
Systemic disease	Petechiae and purpura, telogen effluvium, Covid toes
Vascular	Venous leg ulcer, edema blisters, rosacea

acne—a disease of the follicles. Still others are arranged by the pathogenesis, as in the case of autoimmune disorders. In addition, other conditions which are manifestations of internal diseases that play out on the skin are given their own sections. As a result, dermatologists are asked to arrange information in their minds according to how the disease looks to the naked eye and how it presents under the microscope, as well as according to the mechanism behind the disease, whether it is a local pathology in the skin, or a reflection of internal health. A further complicating factor is a fact that skin diseases can have regional predilections on the body; for example, some present on the palms and soles, while others prefer the genital region, face, or scalp.

All these varied ways of arranging skin diseases lead one to the following two conclusions: dermatology is a highly challenging field, and there was no clear winner among Willan, Alibert, Bazin, Hebra, and the others as to how to properly arrange skin diseases. Perhaps they are all winners, as our current system is a hodgepodge of all of these arrangements. Our current system evolved during the twentieth century and cannot be attributed to any one person or persons. In many ways, it resulted from a simple impetus: the need to arrange information in textbooks. Finally, it should be pointed out that a specific classification of skin diseases is not overly useful for dermatologists, practically speaking. More important than classification is the formation of a different diagnosis that is morphology-driven, and even more helpful, diagnosis-driven, as the present author's work with this topic has shown.[13]

Diagnosis

Over the course of the last hundred years, article after article has come forth, increasing the body of published dermatologic literature to an enormous size. As it stands today, there are an estimated 2000 different skin diseases, a name for every possible diseased state of the skin. It would require several hundred pages more to tell the story of each of the dermatologic contributors of the twentieth century, but knowing that the task has already been completed with such extraordinary perfection by others, the present author refers the reader to that source.[14] Even so, this history of dermatology cannot stand alone without highlighting some of the most important contributions of the last 120 years (see Table 16.3).

Nearly all of these contributors are giants in the history of dermatology, and many of them have been honored with eponyms for the diagnoses they first described. Dermatologists are fond of eponyms, but it is always a little difficult to decide whether to tell a patient he has "Grover's disease" or "transient acantholytic dermatosis."

TABLE 16.3

Selected Diagnoses with Their Twentieth-Century Describers

Atrophoderma	1923	Agostino Pasini and Luis Pierini
Incontinentia pigmentii	1926	Bruno Broch
Pemphigus erythematosus	1926	Francis Senear and Barney Usher
Confluent and reticulated papillomatosis	1927	Henri Gougerot and A. Carteaud
Pyoderma gangrenosum	1930	Louis Brunsting
Necrobiosis lipoidica	1932	M. Oppenheim / E. Urbach (independently)
Sezary syndrome	1938	Albert Sezary
Benign familial chronic pemphigus	1939	Howard Hailey and Hugh Hailey
Nevus of Ota	1939	Masao Ota
Spitz nevus	1948	Sophie Spitz
Becker's nevus	1949	S. William Becker
Bullous pemphigoid	1953	Walter Lever
Lymphocytic infiltrate of the skin	1953	Max Jessner
Papular acrodermatitis of childhood	1955	Fernando Gianotti and Agostino Crosti
Subcorneal pustular dermatosis	1956	Ian Sneddon and Darrell Wilkinson
Toxic epidermal necrolysis	1956	Alan Lyell
Netherton's syndrome	1958	Earl Netherton
Acute febrile neutrophilic dermatosis	1964	Robert Sweet
Acrokeratosis paraneoplastica	1965	Andre Bazex
Lymphomatoid papulosis	1965	A. Dupont (coined by W.L. Macaulay, 1968)
Transient acantholytic dermatosis	1970	Ralph Grover
Eosinophilic cellulitis	1971	George Wells
Merkel cell carcinoma	1972	Cyril Toker
Dysplastic nevus syndrome	1978	Wallace Clark, R.R. Reimer, and Mark Greene
Paraneoplastic pemphigus	1990	Grant Anhalt

The Most Influential Dermatologists of the Twentieth Century

There are other figures that did more than write the first description of a disease, and these persons deserve special recognition for elevating the status of the field of dermatology to what it is today. The present author begs forgiveness for overlooking any figure deemed more impressive by those still living to attest to it.

United States

William Pusey (1865–1940), the last author to write a complete history of dermatology, was the first great dermatologist of twentieth-century America. As the only dermatologist ever to hold the position of president of the American Medical Association, Pusey was as good a leader as he was a clinician. His areas of interest included X-ray therapy (including the use of X-rays for acne), syphilis, and the history of dermatology. He penned a significant textbook, *The Principles and Practice of Dermatology for Students and Practitioners* (1907).

Marion Sulzberger (1895–1983) trained under Bruno Bloch in Zurich and Joseph Jadassohn in Germany; he held professorships over his 46-year-long career at Columbia, New York University, and University of California, San Francisco. Known as "Mr. Dermatology," Sulzberger's opinion was sought by patients from all over the world, and he held honorary memberships in virtually every dermatologic society in the world. He was as capable a bench researcher as he was a clinician, and his scientific pursuits included sweating, skin physiology, and allergy. His most outstanding contribution was the introduction of topical corticosteroids, along with Victor Witten, in 1951. He also studied the use of oral corticosteroids in dermatology, and his name is attached to incontinentia pigmenti (Bloch-Sulzberger disease).

An author of 16 books, Sulzberger was quite possibly the greatest dermatologist of the twentieth century in any country.

Thomas B. Fitzpatrick (1919–2003) was the Professor and Chairman of the Department of Dermatology at Harvard Medical School and Chief of the Massachusetts General Hospital Dermatology Service for almost 40 years (1959–1987). As the mentor to many of the top dermatologists in America, as well as the editor of one of the specialty's best textbooks, *Dermatology in General Medicine*, Fitzpatrick was *the* world leader in dermatologic education for the second half of the twentieth century. He also deciphered the chemistry of melanogenesis, invented the skin type system that bears his name, developed with his colleagues and introduced to the world PUVA treatment (to be addressed shortly), and generated the criteria, along with Martin Mihm and Wallace Clark, for the early diagnosis of melanoma.

Walter B. Shelley (1917–2009) was a long-time professor of dermatology at the University of Pennsylvania and, later in his career, at the Medical College of Ohio. Like a reincarnation of Unna, Shelley had for his whole career devoted equal parts of his energies to both the clinical and the scientific. He researched virtually every aspect of cutaneous biology (sweat glands, nerves, itch, hair, nails, etc.) and wrote hundreds of papers on his research. He was the first to describe a dozen or more dermatologic entities, including aquagenic urticaria, larva currens, autoimmune progesterone dermatitis, piezogenic pedal papules, and mid-dermal elastolysis. In his books, his greatest attribute—intellectual curiosity—is on full display, and the anecdotal evidence recorded by Shelley in such works as *Advanced Dermatologic Therapy II* (1987) for a time carried as much weight as the peer-reviewed, evidence-based medical articles written by his contemporaries. Such was the mastery this man had over his craft.

Walter Lever (1909–1992) was the first great dermatopathologist in America. Born in Germany and trained at Harvard, Lever's main legacy was the work he did with bullous diseases, having described bullous pemphigoid and cicatricial pemphigoid. He was among the first to contend that the blistering diseases we now know to result from autoantibodies were a consequence of that very cause. Inspired by his German counterpart Oscar Gans (see below), Lever published the first textbook in America on the topic of dermatopathology: *Histopathology of the Skin* (1949).

A. Bernard Ackerman (1936–2008) was the other great dermatopathologist of the twentieth century. Trained in dermatology first, Ackerman worked as a skin pathologist at New York University and Thomas Jefferson University in Philadelphia before affiliating with Cornell and starting the Ackerman Academy of Dermatopathology. He was a prolific writer, having written three dozen books and countless articles on his pathologic discoveries. He literally wrote the book on inflammatory skin diseases; his magnum opus was *Histologic Diagnosis of Inflammatory Skin Diseases* (1978). Famous for his strong opinions and for mentoring innumerable disciples who followed his dogma, Ackerman's fame knew no bounds, and his career did much to set apart dermatopathology as a distinct discipline separate from general pathology.

Britain

Archibald Gray (1880–1967), another of Jadassohn's trainees, succeeded Radcliffe-Crocker at the University College London starting in 1909. With abysmal facilities and with dermatology nowhere near the cutting edge when he took the helm, Gray's skills in leadership and organization ensured that British dermatology would regain a firm footing and maintain it into the second half of the twentieth century. His greatest legacy was the foundation of the British Association of Dermatology in 1920.

Frederick Parkes Weber (1863–1962), although a general physician and a polymath, was one of the most accomplished figures in British dermatology in the first half of the twentieth century. Employed at the German Hospital in London, he wrote over 1200 articles, and his name is associated with several dermatologic entities: Klippel-Trénaunay-Weber syndrome, Weber-Christian disease, Osler-Weber-Rendu disease, Sturge-Weber syndrome, and Weber-Cockayne syndrome.

Geoffrey Dowling (1891–1976) was the greatest British dermatologist of the twentieth century and even more important than Gray in elevating British dermatology out of its nadir. Born in South Africa, Dowling went to boarding school and medical school in Britain. He received appointments at Guy's Hospital and St. John's Hospital before settling at St. Thomas' Hospital for a long stint as senior dermatologist. He trained a generation of superb clinicians, including George Wells, Arthur Rook, Douglas Sweet, and Darrell Wilkinson.[15] His contributions include his work with *Pityrosporum ovale* in seborrheic dermatitis, the co-discovery of reticulated pigmented anomaly of the flexures (Dowling-Degos disease), the advancement of our understanding of dermatomyositis and scleroderma, and the introduction of calciferol as a treatment for lupus vulgaris.

James Arthur Rook (1918–1996) was the most influential British dermatologist of the second half of the twentieth century. Having trained under Dowling, Rook worked for the majority of his career at Addenbrooke's Hospital in Cambridge. His most famous contribution is the "Rook Book," or Rook's *Textbook of Dermatology* (1968), now in its eighth edition. He also wrote very pioneering articles on keratoacanthoma and bullous diseases.

France

After Darier, whose career straddled two centuries, Achille Civatte (1877–1956) took over the reins at Hôpital Saint-Louis in the second quarter of the twentieth century. While well-rounded in all aspects of dermatology, Civatte's passion was dermatopathology, presumably because of Darier's influence early in his career. In addition to identifying the histopathologic bodies that now bear his name, Civatte described the V-shaped, reticular pattern of pigmentation that occurs with photoaging of the neck (poikiloderma of Civatte). He was a pioneer in distinguishing pemphigus from pemphigoid, noting the presence of acantholysis in the former but not the latter.

Henri Gougerot (1881–1955) was another leading dermatologist in France from the 1920s through the 1950s. Gougerot's name is easily recognized by dermatologists; he described confluent and reticulated papillomatosis and Gougerot-Blum disease, as well as tumid lupus erythematosus. Sjogren syndrome was originally called Gougerot-Sjogren syndrome as Gougerot did some of the initial reporting on that disease. He wrote over 2500 articles and contributed to Darier's eight-volume *Nouvelle Pratique Dermatologique*. He and Civatte and the next figure, Degos, along with Albert Sezary (1880–1956) and Albert Touraine (1883–1961), all thrived together at Hôpital Saint-Louis in yet another heyday of dermatology at the famous institution.

Robert Degos (1904–1987) was an equally important figure in French dermatology in the twentieth century. As the French half of Dowling-Degos disease, Degos by mid-century was to France what Dowling was to Britain. This master clinician trained under Gougerot at Hôpital Saint-Louis, where he first discovered a scarce condition called malignant atrophic papulosis (Degos disease). He was a prolific writer, authoring over 1000 articles, and his famous textbook *Dermatologie* (1953) was the leading textbook in French for several decades.

The German-speaking World

Gustav Riehl (1855–1943) was the last of a long, brilliant line of physicians who trained under Hebra and Kaposi, and his work ensured that Viennese dermatology would remain strong heading into the twentieth century. Leo Ritter von Zumbusch (1874–1940) made Munich a center of excellence for dermatology starting in 1915, and he was the first to describe severe, generalized pustular psoriasis. Heinrich Gottron (1890–1974) put Tübingen on the map as yet another center, and in addition to describing the papules that bear his name, he characterized scleromyxedema, verrucous carcinoma, and acrogeria. Frankfurt's Oscar Gans (1888–1983), a student of Unna, was the most accomplished German dermatopathologist of the twentieth century and the author of *Histologie der Hautkrankheiten* (1925), the most widely read book on his craft in the era. Otto Braun-Falco (1922–2018) was the greatest German dermatologist of the latter half of the twentieth century.

Miscellaneous Contributors

The twentieth century saw interest in dermatology increase all over the world, and by mid-century, it was a truly international specialty. Lajos Nékám (1868–1957)—once a research assistant to Kaposi, Lesser, Besnier, Brocq, Hutchinson, and Unna—was the founder of dermatology in Hungary. While proudly boasting an academic tradition for dermatology dating back to the days of Chiarugi in the early nineteenth century, Italy's most distinguished dermatologic figures were Domenico Majocchi (1849–1929),

Celso Pellizzari (1851–1925), Vittorio Mibelli (1860–1910), Aldo Castellani (1874–1971), Agostino Crosti (1896–1988), and Fernando Gianotti (1920–1984). In Croatia, Franjo Kogoj (1894–1983) discovered the pustule that bears his name. In Denmark, Besnier's student Carl Rasch (1861–1938) and Edvard Ehlers of Ehlers-Danlos syndrome (1862–1937) brought the specialty to preeminence there, and Holger Haxthausen (1892–1959) and Svend Lomholt (1888–1949) helped sustain the prestige. Niels Danbolt (1900–1984), the first to describe acrodermatitis enteropathica, was the greatest Norwegian dermatologist in the twentieth century. In Japan, Keizo Dohi (1866–1931), Masao Ota (1885–1945), and Minor Ito (1894–1982) inaugurated a forthcoming century of excellence in dermatology. HaeKwan Kung Sun Oh (1878–1963) established the first dermatology department and clinic in Korea in 1917. In Argentina, dermatology's founding fathers were Baldamero Sommer (1857–1918) and Pedro Balina (1880–1949). As a British colony, India had received British dermatology as early as the end of the nineteenth century, but by the 1920s, India was on its way to becoming a world leader in leprology, venereology, and dermatology. Eventually, Western dermatology reached China and Australia—virtually everywhere—and this list of greatness goes on and on. Who among the myriad world-renowned dermatologists of the early twenty-first century will stand out in the next history of dermatology to be written?

Residency Training in Dermatology

The first American residency programs—where medical school graduates go to get training and certification in their chosen field—were established by Osler, Halsted et al. at Johns Hopkins Hospital in the late 1800s. The American Board of Dermatology, the certifying body for graduates of America's dermatology residencies, was established in 1932. The first board exam took place in 1933, and 20 of the 27 first test-takers passed the exam (26.7 percent failure rate).[16] Residency programs emerged all over the US in the twentieth century, with many of them established in the 1950s; new ones continue to form even to this day. The term *resident* is a throwback to an era when the trainees were expected to *reside* in the hospital, always present and ready for that next educational opportunity to arrive at the hospital. Dermatology residencies in many instances developed as divisions under the Departments of Internal Medicine or Surgery within the large institutions, but today, many dermatology residencies are funded by their own stand-alone departments.

To achieve board certification in dermatology, a medical student must complete a four-year program that consists of a one-year internship in internal medicine or surgery plus a three-year residency in dermatology. Dermatology is now among the most coveted fields in medicine in which to secure a residency position. A career in dermatology is in high demand due to its eight-to-five office hours, competitive income, and job security. In addition, there is a short supply of residency positions in the United States related to a lack of funding for these positions. While the number of residency positions is increasing each year, there were 692 applicants in 2020 for only 538 residency spots, meaning that only 77 percent of medical students who desire to be a dermatologist can accomplish that goal.[17] America's top five dermatology residency programs based on academic achievement are Harvard University, University of California-San Francisco, Stanford University, University of Pennsylvania, and Emory University.[18] Specialty training in dermatology is available in universities all over the world.

Technological Advancements of the Twentieth and Twenty-First Centuries

The twentieth century saw critical technological advancements that significantly elevated the status of dermatology beyond what it was at the beginning of the century. Advancements discussed in this section are phototherapy, lasers, botulinum toxin, and dermoscopy.

Phototherapy

The history of phototherapy begins in 1893 with a publication by Niels Finsen (1860–1904) entitled *Om Lysets Indvirkninger paa Huden*, "On the effects of light on the skin." In 1896, he published

Om Anvendelse i Medicinen af koncentrerede kemiske Lysstraaler, "The use of concentrated chemical light rays in medicine." Finsen believed that light had therapeutic effects on the skin based on his personal experience with sunbathing as a treatment for his own poor health due to Niemann-Pick disease. His electric carbon arc torch emitted a broad spectrum of light; the lens placed in front of the patient's skin determined the wavelength of light that hit the skin. He applied his theory to the treatment of one of the more stubborn skin diseases at the time, *lupus vulgaris.* Finsen won the Nobel Prize in 1903 "in recognition of his contribution to the treatment of diseases, especially lupus vulgaris, with concentrated light radiation, whereby he has opened a new avenue for medical science."[19] He remains to this day the only dermatologist to ever win the Nobel Prize, and sadly, he was too ill at the time to travel to Stockholm to receive his award.[20]

It was only a matter of time before ultraviolet light therapy was applied to other skin diseases, especially psoriasis. In 1923, an American dermatologist, William H. Goeckerman (1884–1954), introduced broadband UVB phototherapy using a high-pressure mercury lamp for the treatment of psoriasis. In his inpatient protocol, crude coal tar was applied to the skin lesions, and UVB was directed on the skin. To this day, Goeckerman therapy is one of the most effective treatments we have for psoriasis, even more effective than our modern biologic treatments in many cases.[21] In 1947, the Egyptian Professor Abdel Monem El Mofty at Cairo University Medical School recognized that an Egyptian weed named *Ammi majus,* used since ancient times, could have therapeutic value when its medicinal contents were applied to the skin of vitiligo and psoriasis patients. The substance—methoxsalen (8-MOP, xanthotoxin)—was eventually studied by Thomas Fitzpatrick (1919–2003) and John Parrish (1939–present) at Harvard Medical School, and in 1974, an oral form (psoralen) was introduced as PUVA (psoralen + UVA). It was FDA-approved for the treatment of psoriasis in 1982. Patients took the oral medication prior to entering a UVA lightbox; the psoralen caused the patient to become more light-sensitive, thereby increasing the therapeutic value of the light. PUVA was a highly effective treatment for psoriasis, but overtime it became apparent that the treatment caused many detrimental effects on the skin, including carcinoma and melanoma. PUVA has been, for the most part, abandoned in modern dermatology practices and was replaced with narrowband UVB therapy beginning in the 1990s. This is the most common type of phototherapy offered in dermatology offices today, and it does not require medication prior to the treatment. Narrowband UVB phototherapy is a safe treatment option for patients with psoriasis, eczema, itching, cutaneous T-cell lymphoma, and vitiligo. It is called narrowband because the bulbs emit a very narrow spectrum of ultraviolet light (311–313 nm), the spectrum of light that is most therapeutic against skin diseases and least likely to burn the skin. Its efficacy for these conditions rivals the efficacy of systemic medications. Ultraviolet therapy works in skin disease by suppressing the immune cells in the skin that are responsible for these diseases. Phototherapy remains an essential component of the dermatologist's toolkit.

Lasers

The next major advancement in twentieth-century dermatologic technology is the laser. "Laser" is an acronym that stands for *Light Amplification by Stimulated Emission of Radiation.* The scientific history of lasers begins with the work of Max Planck (1858–1947) and Albert Einstein (1879–1955). In 1900, Planck discovered the relationship between energy and frequency in radiation, concluding that energy is emitted or absorbed in discrete chunks called *quanta.* Einstein applied Planck's idea to light, discovering the *photon* and formulating the *Quantum Theory of Light* in 1905. Einstein introduced the concept of stimulated emission about ten years later: a photon of a specific frequency can interact with an excited electron, and new photons are generated that have the same properties (frequency, polarization, direction) as the original photon. Einstein's concept was first applied to microwave radiation, and "masers" were developed in the 1950s. Late in that decade, the same idea was applied to visible light and infrared radiation. Experiments by Charles Townes (1915–2015), Arthur Schawlow (1921–1999), and Gordon Gould (1920–2005) led up to the invention of the laser in 1960.

A laser has a solid, liquid, gas, or semiconductor medium that emits photons of a single wavelength light in one direction upon having its electrons "excited" by an electrical current. The first laser, constructed by Theodore Maiman (1927–2007), had a synthetic ruby crystal medium. Once the laser was revealed to the world, widescale research began with the goal of applying laser technology to different aspects of life—CD-ROMs, laser printers, industrial cutting, etc. In the mid-1960s, lasers were first applied to the skin for the purpose of removing tattoos and hair. The first person responsible for the promotion of lasers in dermatology was the American dermatologist, Leon Goldman (1906–1977). Lasers of different media or delivery mechanisms were invented around this time: neodymium (1961), q-switching (1961), argon (1964), alexandrite (1964), neodymium:YAG (1964), carbon dioxide (1964), dye (1967), etc. The exact process whereby lasers perform to selectively remove undesired structures from the skin—the theory of selective photothermolysis—was explained by Rox Anderson (1950–present) and John Parrish in 1980. Anderson and Dieter Manstein in 2004 introduced non-ablative fractional photothermolysis, the technology is used to resurface wrinkled skin by delivering laser energy to the dermis without causing any damage to the epidermis. Now not only hair and tattoos can be removed from the skin, but also pigmented lesions, broken blood vessels, vascular tumors, scars, and wrinkles.

Botulinum Toxin

How the human race harnessed one of nature's deadliest substances for therapeutic purposes is one of modern medicine's most fascinating tales. The substance, botulinum toxin, is a neurotoxin that was first isolated in 1944 from the gram-positive, rod-shaped anaerobic bacterium known as *Clostridium botulinum*. The word *botulinum* is derived from the Latin word *botulus*, meaning sausage, and that word was chosen for the toxin because the first reports of botulism in the eighteenth century involved several persons who died from the affliction after ingesting undercooked blood sausage. Thus, botulinum toxin was first known as "sausage poison." By the twentieth century, it was evident that canned foods contaminated with the bacteria could be a source of botulism. In that disorder, a person ingests the toxin and develops difficulty swallowing, dry mouth, blurry vision, respiratory distress, nausea, vomiting, diarrhea, and paralysis. The toxin interferes with neurotransmitter release at the neuromuscular junction, meaning that nerves cannot innervate muscles. Fortunately, the toxin is easily heat-inactivated, and proper processing of foods prior to canning prevents this deadly form of food poisoning.

After failing to weaponize the toxin as a biological agent during World War II, researchers continued to study it for other purposes; eventually, in the 1960s, it occurred to the American ophthalmologist Alan Scott (1932–2021) to research substances as a treatment for strabismus (malalignment of the eyes). In 1978, Scott conducted a study in which botulinum toxin was injected into the periocular muscles of strabismus patients. After his successes and the successes of several other investigators in the 1980s, botulinum toxin, marketed by Allergan, received FDA approval as a treatment for strabismus, hemifacial spasms, and blepharospasm in 1989. In 1987, two Canadian physicians—an ophthalmologist named Jean Carruthers and her husband Alastair, a dermatologist—noted that periocular injection of botulinum toxin for blepharospasm seemed to rid a person temporarily of forehead wrinkles. After many years of research, the duo published their data in 1996, and botulinum received FDA approval for glabellar wrinkles in 2002. Since that time, botulinum toxin injections for upper face wrinkles have been a trendy and safe procedure that is offered in dermatology offices. Seven million Americans per year receive these injections, and the procedure has one of the highest patient satisfaction rates of any cosmetic procedure. In addition, botulinum toxin injections have received FDA approval for many other indications, including migraine headaches, dystonia, spasticity, laryngeal disorders, urinary incontinence, and hyperhidrosis.

Dermatoscopy

The last major technological advancement in dermatology to highlight in this section is dermatoscopy (or dermoscopy), a development that began in the twentieth century but has accelerated in the twenty-first century. Dermatoscopy is defined as the application of a handheld magnifying device to the surface of the skin for the purposes of evaluating skin lesions or skin diseases. The year 1971 is commonly noted as the year dermatoscopy was introduced in dermatology, although microscopes and similar devices have been used to inspect the skin since the seventeenth century. The first physician to do so was a Frenchman named Pierre Borel (1620–1689), who used a microscope to evaluate the capillaries of the nail apparatus in 1655. Johan Kolhaus (unknown dates) performed the same studies in 1663. In 1878, the German physician Ernst Karl Abbe added immersion oil (cedar oil) to the skin to increase the resolution of skin surface microscopes. Unna's work with diascopy and immersion oil in 1893 pushed that diagnostic technique into the modern era. Collectively, these advances were necessary to bring about the science of dermatoscopy, which burgeoned in the second half of the twentieth century. This brings us to 1971, when the Scottish-born dermatologist, Rona MacKie, introduced the idea that the skin surface microscope was capable of distinguishing melanoma from other pigmented lesions.

Since that time, dermatoscopy has become its own subdiscipline within dermatology, and article after article has been amassing in the dermatologic literature. Today, the modern dermatologist is equipped with this device in hand because it is extremely helpful with the physical examination. It can assist with the distinction of benign and malignant pigmented skin lesions (including melanoma), and it can also be used to diagnose countless benign lesions, BCC, SCC, rashes including psoriasis, types of hair loss, and skin infections and infestations such as scabies—all without a biopsy. Dermatoscopy has tremendous value for the modern dermatology patient: it screens out benign lesions, preventing unnecessary biopsies and reducing the cost of healthcare, and it helps identify problematic skin lesions at an early stage in which a lesion might otherwise appear unproblematic to the naked eye. Practicing dermatology without a dermatoscope may already be analogous to a cardiologist practicing cardiology without a stethoscope.

Cosmetics in Dermatology

Caring about one's appearance is a concern that has existed in humans since the beginning of history. We have seen that cosmetic matters were of major importance to the ancient Egyptians, Greeks, and Romans. The ancient Egyptians left behind bottles of cosmetic lotions and oils as evidence of their obsession with esthetics. The demand for cosmetic services has always been there—recall Crito's list of cosmetic topics (see Chapter 4). Whether the maintenance, promotion, and establishment of beauty in a patient is the professional responsibility of a physician is a subject that has been debated since the Hippocratic era. The ancient physician was inclined to equate beauty with health; medieval physicians (e.g., Avicenna) and Renaissance physicians (e.g., Mercurialis) agreed with this archaic stance. But by the early modern period of the seventeenth and eighteenth centuries, physicians did not wish to be bothered with such insignificant concerns, and the patients desperate for cosmetic enhancement had to resort to quacks to get their cosmetic needs met. Trustworthy cosmetic providers have been in short supply until approximately the last 100 years. The twentieth century saw the rise of plastic surgery and dermatology as the two specialties of medicine in which patients can reliably find these providers. While one impetus for physicians to provide cosmetic services was to offer a safe setting for the public who would otherwise suffer at the hands of an unskilled quack, a competing motivation is that cosmetic procedures are lucrative and leave out the third party—the insurance company.

The main objective of the modern cosmetic patient in the dermatology clinic is to improve the appearance of the aging face. The most popular procedures for that purpose include botulinum toxin injections to relax forehead and periorbital facial muscles that wrinkle the face: injections of hyaluronic acid fillers to fill lower face lines and folds and aged lips; chemical peels to lessen pigmentary changes and fine lines related to sun damage; lasers to remove unwanted brown spots and broken blood vessels; and lasers and other devices to tighten or resurface the face. These procedures are done in an outpatient clinical setting with or without local anesthesia. Unlike some of the procedures performed by plastic surgeons, all procedures done by dermatologists are outside the operating room. Cosmetic procedures such as botulinum toxin injections, dermal filler injections, and laser treatments are now a mainstay of dermatology offices all over the world, and their addition to the dermatologist's repertoire has been followed with an ever-expanding list of services and a multibillion-dollar industry. Some dermatologists make cosmetic procedures their primary focus, while others (such as the present author) focus solely on medical and/or surgical dermatology, and many offer both medical and cosmetic services. These procedures, developed over the last 150 years, are outlined in Table 16.4.

TABLE 16.4

The Introduction of Cosmetic Procedures by Year

Rhinoplasty for cosmetic enhancement	1829
Phenol chemical peel for skin lightening	1871
Autologous fat transfer	1893
Paraffin filler injections	1899
Facelifts introduced	1906–1912
Hair transplantation	1959
Silicone for soft tissue augmentation	1965
Injectable bovine collagen for wrinkles	1981
Tumescent anesthesia for liposuction	1987
Botulinum toxin for glabellar wrinkles	2002
First hyaluronic acid filler for wrinkles	2003
Fractional laser resurfacing for wrinkles	2004
Cryolipolysis for unwanted fat	2007

Skin Care and Preventative Measures

Prior to the middle of the twentieth century, physicians rarely concerned themselves with speaking to patients about skin care and measures to prevent skin problems. Even after 1845, when Erasmus Wilson published *Healthy Skin,* in which he discussed skin care for the masses (see Chapter 12), physicians were not apt to speak about the skin in this way; they were increasingly interested in skin diseases, not skin disease prevention. This began to change in the mid-twentieth century when the era of modern dermatology was underway, and discussing the prevention of skin disease, especially skin cancer, became as important to the dermatologist as the treatment of those same diseases.

The advocacy of protecting the skin from the sun has been the most crucial development in the preventative healthcare of the skin in the last 100 years. The application of various products, e.g., zinc oxide, to the skin to protect against tanning for cosmetic purposes—but not for health reasons—has been done for thousands of years, as the Egyptians used rice bran and jasmine for this purpose.[22] The ancient Chinese, Indian, Egyptian, and Greek peoples all used umbrellas for sun protection. Prior to the twentieth century, clothing covered the skin in Western cultures, largely for reasons of religious piety and morality. As people began to reveal more and more skin starting in the post-WWI era, there arose a need for something that could allow the skin to be exposed to the sun without consequential sunburn.

The first sunscreens were invented in the 1920s and 1930s, and the answer to the question "who invented the sunscreen" varies depending on whether we are discussing effective sunscreen or any substance purported to protect the skin from the sun.[23] In 1932, H.A. Milton Blake of Australia developed a product containing phenyl salicylate (salol). Eugene Schueler, the French founder of L'Oreal, produced a "filtering oil" called *Ambre Solaire* in 1936. Benjamin Green invented a sun-protective substance in 1944 to protect WWII soldiers from the glaring Pacific sun. Not one of these products was highly protective. The first effective sunscreen was invented by the Austrian Franz Greiter in 1946. It was called Glacier Crème, and Greiter famously thought of inventing it after suffering a sunburn while hiking in the Alps. In 1962, Greiter introduced the concept of sun protective factor (SPF), which is defined as the ratio of UVB solar energy required to cause a sunburn on protected skin versus unprotected skin. Para-aminobenzoic acid (PABA) was invented in 1943 and was increasingly used in sunscreens developed in the 1950s and 1960s until it was shown in the 1980s that it might actually increase UV damage. The first UVA sunscreen (avobenzone) was invented in the 1980s. More and more chemical sunscreens have been invented over the last 50 years, but recently many of these substances, such as oxybenzone, have come under scrutiny for safety concerns as it relates to their absorption into the body through the skin. Sunscreens containing zinc oxide and titanium are the most effective and are generally considered the safest. In general, sunscreens protect against the development of melanoma and SCC, but not BCC; they are also the first line of defense against the harmful rays that age the skin of the face.

Today, dermatologists spend a considerable amount of time in each office visit counseling patients on the proper way to care for their largest organ. There are countless skin care products available; some have more evidence behind their promises than others. A simple and evidence-based skin care regimen for the face involves cleansing the face with a gentle cleanser twice daily, the morning application of a moisturizer with a sun-protective factor (SPF 15 or higher) along with an antioxidant lotion that contains Vitamin C, and the nighttime application of a moisturizer along with a retinoid cream. Vitamin C binds the sun-generated free radicals and prevents aging of our skin, while retinoids repair the actual damage from the sun. The earlier in a person's life this routine is started, the more likely a person will appreciate the benefits of it later in life. Other evidence-based products are fluorouracil cream, hydroquinone, and alpha and beta hydroxy acids. The secret to finding the right skin care products, and not modern-day snake oil, is to research the product's ingredients.

Modern Dermatologic Therapy

This brings us to the conclusion of this entire history—modern dermatologic therapy. Dermatologists were for a long time ridiculed for not being able to fix many of the problems faced by dermatology patients, and as with any good joke, there is some truth behind it. That is the case no longer. The most important developments in the modern history of dermatology are the highly effective, targeted treatments we now have available for moderate to severe skin diseases (see Table 16.5). We have come a long

TABLE 16.5

Key Therapeutic Developments in the Twentieth and Twenty-First Centuries

Dapsone for leprosy	1947
Topical cortisone	1952
Benzoyl peroxide introduced	1953
Prednisone	1955
Triamcinolone	1958
Griseofulvin for tinea capitis	1959
Methotrexate	1959
5FU Cream for actinic keratosis	1960s
Doxycycline	1967
Topical tretinoin available	1971
Isotretinoin for recalcitrant nodular acne	1982
Cyclosporine for transplant rejection	1983
First biologics (alefacept and efalizumab) for psoriasis	2003
Etanercept for psoriasis	2004
Infliximab for psoriasis	2006
Adalimumab for psoriasis	2008
Ustekinumab for psoriasis	2009
First immune checkpoint inhibitor for stage IV melanoma	2010
Omalizumab for chronic hives	2014
Ivermectin cream for rosacea	2014
Ixekizumab for psoriasis	2016
Dupilumab for atopic dermatitis	2017
Guselkumab for psoriasis	2017
Rituximab for pemphigus (and other blistering diseases)	2018

way since the days of enemas, laxatives, and bloodletting for skin disease. As of 2022, dermatologists can offer highly effective and safe treatments for almost all of the ordinary and most problematic skin diseases. The introduction of a few medications on the list—especially dupilumab for atopic dermatitis, the IL-17 and IL-23 monoclonal antibodies for psoriasis, and the immune checkpoint inhibitors for metastatic melanoma—are truly historic developments in their capacity to end human suffering with skin disease. Not listed is the momentous repurposing of two older medications, spironolactone and propranolol, which enabled dermatologists to offer effective treatments for two significant dermatologic conditions, hormonal acne, and infantile hemangiomas, respectively. Isotretinoin was the single greatest therapeutic development of the twentieth century.

Conclusion

Skin disease has conceivably provoked more suffering than any other type of disease in history—not only from the pain, itching, and disfigurement but also from the reactions of others who did not understand it. Without any reliable treatments, the average skin disease patient throughout history likely endured rashes, itching, and tumors of an unimaginable severity—and for a very long time. Unlike other types of disease, people know you have skin disease when you have it. Some react with disgust, others with fear of catching the disease, and still others with guilt from being more fortunate and healthier than those affected. We've all heard the phrase "don't judge a book by its cover"; unfortunately, for most of human history, people have been indeed judged by their covers. In addition to the physical aspects of the illness, it is precisely that judgment that makes skin disease so troubling. Because of the social aspects of skin, skin disease can affect one's identity and one's psyche more so than any other category of disease.

In ancient Mesopotamia, if you developed a skin disease, such as psoriasis, eczema, impetigo, herpes, or vitiligo, you would have very likely been considered cursed by the gods for some sin, and if you had the ultimate disease of implied impurity, *saḫaršubbû*, you might have been forcibly driven from the city. In the Jewish tradition, skin disease, collectively known as *tsara'at,* would have brought you a similar fate as outlined in the book of Leviticus. If you were lucky enough to find yourself in ancient Egypt or ancient Greece with your skin disease, you might have been told you had too much *whdw* in your body by the Egyptian *swnw* or an imbalance of humor by the Greek *iatros*. In those places, you might be subjected to all manner of treatments such as enemas, bloodletting, or laxatives, but you were less likely to face ostracism. These ineffective measures must have been demoralizing for the afflicted, in which case, you could make the journey to the asclepeion in Epidaurus and get treated by the priest after a night in the temple, or simply make a votive offering.

In ancient Rome, where cosmetic appearance peaked in value among all ancient peoples, skin disease, especially the dreaded facial disease *mentagra*, was a fate worse than death because of the social stigma and repulsion—the sheer horror—on the face of its witnesses. You cannot hide a skin disease that occurs on the face. The vain (synonymous with Roman) man would spend a small fortune to have his face scarred with cautery to rid himself of such a condition. By late antiquity, persons with severe skin disease were given the label *lepra* and ostracized from the rest of society. An ancient and medieval word, *lepra*, should not be confused with leprosy. In the High Middle Ages, *lepra* became closer in meaning to leprosy (Hansen's disease), and it was deemed necessary to set up courts so that persons with skin diseases could be examined for judicial purposes, with the goal of segregating only the ones having our modern understanding of leprosy. The practice of ostracizing persons with skin disease, carried forth in the Western Christian tradition until the mid-to-late twentieth century, has very ancient origins.

Skin disease might have also closed particular doors for you in society and destined you for other fates—some desired, some not. Consider the young woman who was lucky enough to survive smallpox. Having smallpox scars may have ruined her prospects for marriage, but it increased her marketability as a nanny since the presence of the scars gave away her immune status to prospective families. The politician found to have the Great Pox—syphilis—could lose his job and even his family. So for the better part of human history, skin disease could trigger the possibility of pain, itching, imperfection, depression, embarrassment, ridicule, judgment, unemployment, avoidance, hatred, repulsion, and the ultimate type of suffering, exile.

Four of history's most fear-inspiring diseases—leprosy, plague, syphilis, and smallpox—had skin manifestations as major features, and each of these diseases was explored in this text. Two of them were acute diseases (smallpox and plague), and the other two were chronic. In the acute diseases, skin lesions signaled the distinct possibility that the infected would die, and soon. The skin lesions of plague were the most ominous, while the widespread pustules of smallpox predicted at least a lifetime of deformity in those who were fortunate enough to survive. In leprosy and syphilis, the skin lesions did not forecast imminent death, but with them, the afflicted could anticipate a fate that in many ways was worse than death: moral judgment and ostracization.

DOI: 10.1201/9781003273622-24

One of the primary purposes of this book has been to describe the history of *what* and *when* physicians knew about the skin and its diseases throughout history. Dermatology as a topic of discussion for medical writers has existed for as long as medicine itself. We saw that the Mesopotamians had no word for the skin, but they did write more about skin disease than any other types of diseases in their medical texts. They also had an extensive dermatologic nomenclature that surpassed their contemporaries and even the Greco-Romans that followed them. The Egyptians did have a word for the skin and also wrote expansively about skin diseases; their legacy in the history of dermatology may have been their therapeutic practices, which the Greeks borrowed to some extent. We saw that the Greeks, starting with Hippocrates, laid the earliest foundation for modern dermatology by giving us many of our extant words for skin disease and by establishing the basis for the theory of skin disease—humoral theory—that would become the dominant theory for the explanation of all disease for over 2000 years. The skin at this time was viewed as a fishnet-like envelope equipped with pores that allowed for breathing and passage of impurities from the body. The Romans fine-tuned the terminology of the Greeks and expanded it so that by the end of the Roman Empire, the language of dermatology was in place and would remain the same until the modern era. However, the diagnostic terminology bequeathed by the Romans was chaotic, and skin diseases—much in need of proper nomenclature and classification—were confused with one another until only 200 years ago. The collective Roman medical community, led by Galen, did become aware of one of the skin's many additional functions: tactile sensation. Indeed, the advancement of knowledge about the skin and its diseases stalled at this point and did not proceed much further until the invention of the microscope and its application to the skin by Marcello Malpighi in the seventeenth century.

Thus, in the period between Galen (second century CE) and Malpighi (seventeenth century CE), little advancement in knowledge about the skin occurred. The Middle Ages were, instead, a period of compilation and preservation of ancient ideas for the most part, with a few noteworthy bright spots interspersed. The compilation center of the ancient ideas was in the Byzantine Empire, and the preservation center was in the medieval Islamic world. In the former, Oribasius, Aetius, Alexander, and Paul wrote important medical treatises that contained comprehensive information about skin disease. Later, the Arabic medical writers preserved this ancient knowledge by translating the Greek medical texts of the ancient world and late antiquity into Arabic. These texts were, in turn, translated in the late Middle Ages into the language of medicine at the time: Latin. The efforts to translate these Greek texts into Arabic by the medical men of the Islamic Golden Age almost certainly saved this knowledge since much of the information in these ancient texts would have been otherwise lost for all time had it not been done.

There were some bright spots for dermatology in the Middle Ages. First was Isidore's *Etymologies*, in which the origin of words was cataloged, including nearly all words for skin diseases at the time of its writing in the seventh century. Next was the dermatology of Anglo-Saxon England, which had both northern and Greco-Roman influences. Then, we saw that Rhazes and Avicenna focused much of their attention on skin disease. The former worked out the differences between smallpox and measles, while the latter wrote more pages on skin disease than any other medieval writer. Avicenna's *Canon of Medicine* was the perfect culmination of Galenic and Arabic medicine and the most influential medical text for 500 years after his death. Finally, at some point during the Middle Ages, skin disease fell under the dominion of the medieval surgeon, and it would be the surgeon who was the principal caretaker of the skin until the nineteenth century. We saw several important medieval surgeons write about the skin, none more important than Henri de Mondeville and Guy de Chauliac, as well as the first female authors on skin disease, Hildegard of Bingen and Trota of Salerno.

By the Renaissance, the learned medical men, based in the established universities all over Europe, had discovered the ancient medical texts of Galen, Celsus, and others. While at first these texts did much to satisfy the curiosity of physicians in regard to the body and disease, the concomitant emergence of human dissection as a scientific endeavor led to a questioning of ancient medical knowledge and ultimately to an anatomical revolution that was one of the most important events in the history of medicine. The skin, however, was not included in this revolution, and nothing new as far as knowledge of the skin developed in the fourteenth and fifteenth centuries. And we also saw the first book devoted entirely to skin disease—Mercurialis' *De Morbis Cutaneis*—published in this time period. We noticed that Jan Jessen was arguing a very modern concept at this time: the skin has its own diseases. Still, the skin did not have its revolution until the seventeenth century, when its microanatomy was discovered by

Marcello Malpighi and William Cowper, among others, who applied the newly invented microscope to the skin for the first time and proved that there was more to the skin than meets the naked eye. Not long after, the first "dermatologist," Daniel Turner, arrived on the scene and published practical information about skin disease in the first English treatise entirely on the subject.

The eighteenth century was defined by the Enlightenment, and for medicine, one of the main aspects of this era was an impulse in the learned medical men to classify disease using Linnaeus' approach as a guide. It was during this period that we saw the first efforts to classify skin diseases, and the most success-ful system out of numerous attempts was accomplished by the Viennese surgeon and medical polymath Plenck, who had the brilliant idea to categorize skin diseases by their appearance. The eighteenth century also saw the masterwork on venereal disease by Jean Astruc, the first French book on cutaneous medicine by Anne-Charles Lorry, and the heralding of the specialty of dermatology by Seguin Henry Jackson.

Twenty years after Plenck, Willan and his protégé Bateman attempted their own classification of skin diseases based on morphology—and they were even more successful than Plenck, having constructed a widely influential system. Willan also achieved something that no physician in history had been able to accomplish: he brought order to the chaos that was the dermatologic nomenclature that had been in use since it was bequeathed by the Romans. This ordering of the terminology of skin disease, needed since ancient times, enabled physicians with interest in the skin to communicate with one another using a coher-ent and unambiguous language. Willan was the founder of the British school of dermatology, and his ideas spread to France, where the French Willanists competed with the founder of French dermatology, Jean-Louis Alibert, and ultimately prevailed. Meanwhile, in Vienna, the third epicenter of dermatologic knowl-edge arose in the 1840s, led by the ultimate of influential nineteenth-century physicians who studied the skin, Ferdinand von Hebra. His main contribution was the establishment of dermatology on a firm scien-tific footing. From Vienna, intellectual curiosity in skin disease spread to Breslau, Berlin, and Hamburg, the last of these cities the home of the great Paul Gerson Unna. Although late to the story, we saw that it did not take long for the United States to match Britain, France, and the German-speaking countries, thanks to the efforts of men such as Henry Daggett Bulkley, James Clarke White, and Louis Duhring.

Specialization in medicine is a very modern phenomenon; while the Egyptians and Romans may have had their own versions of specialist physicians, the Western medical tradition dating from Roman times to the nineteenth century did not. Medical specialization first arose in the big cities, with Paris leading the way in the 1830s, then German-speaking cities of Vienna and Berlin in the 1840s and 1850s, and finally London and the American cities in the 1860s and 1870s. After the unification of medicine and surgery in the nineteenth century, dermatology was one of the first fields to develop as a specialty, along with obstetrics and ophthalmology. A major motivation for specialization was academic: to advance medical knowledge by gathering as much possible information and experience about a specific topic and to promote research and teaching of that information.[1] As medical knowledge reached new heights in the nineteenth century, it simply became too difficult, given the limits of human intelligence, for one person to master every aspect of the medical art.[2]

Paris pioneered medical specialization because it had the largest medical school in the world at the time and because it also had a coordinated network of institutions of unprecedented size, the halls of which were filled with physicians interested in research.[3] Although much smaller in population compared to Paris, Vienna followed the same path toward specialization, one paved by state-sponsored scientific research at the *AKH*. The goal was to amass as much medical knowledge as possible. Competition drove specialization to develop in places like Boston and Philadelphia, where private universities introduced specialties to keep up with the economic pressures of the free market that was the educational system in the United States at the time.[4] If Penn had a dermatology department, then Harvard needed one as well. Specialization in dermatology in these three places was "top-down," that is, specialists emerged out of the big institutions.

In contrast, London saw specialties emerge later because it lacked this academic network, and because the gentleman-physicians of London, more interested in private practice than academic specialization, were generalists who felt threatened professionally by specialists.[5] There was also an innate, traditional-ist sentiment within the culture of the academic institutions that a physician should not specialize in one field until he mastered the diagnosis and treatment of disease in all its various forms in all parts of the body.[6] Much to the chagrin of the establishment, specialization in dermatology in Britain did eventually happen, with the main driving force the development of specialty practices, as individual practitioners on the streets of London chose to limit themselves to the care of skin diseases. This "bottom-up" development of dermatologic specialization was a much slower process than on the continent or across the Atlantic, and it was not until the early twentieth century that dermatology as a distinct discipline was embraced by the medical community as a whole in Britain.

A final factor that paved the way for specialization was governmental sponsorship, as in the case of venereology. Venereology emerged as a formal specialty, for the most part, because of public health concerns about the diseases dealt with by its specialists.[7] Syphilis among the military was a matter of national security. Dermatology and venereology were separated in their beginnings, even in Vienna and Paris, where separate hospitals existed for skin disease patients and venereal disease patients. As the need to distinguish venereal skin lesions from nonvenereal ones became increasingly important, dermatology and venereology merged under one umbrella in many of the European institutions by the mid-to-late nineteenth century. In the United States, venereology was hidden within dermatology, its practitioners delivering care for patients with venereal diseases but not identifying themselves with venereology, as the morality of their patients was questioned by society.[8] In Britain, the two fields always remained distinct, and venereologists, like their patients, suffered low status among their peers and did not develop a strong specialist identity.[9]

Let us conclude with Malcolm Morris' speech at the British Medical Association meeting in 1897 in which he explained how dermatology came about in a famous lecture entitled "The Rise and Progress of Dermatology":

> Each of the three great schools which helped to lay the foundations of modern dermatology had certain marked characteristics. The English [school] was essentially clinical, using classification only as a practical help in diagnosis. As observed, the French systematized, striding somewhat impatiently over facts to get at general formulas, which, though plausible on paper, too often broken down in application. The German was pathological, giving attention mainly to the mechanism and occasionally taking too little heed of the causes setting it in motion. Each school had thus the defects of its qualities; but each played an important part in the development of dermatology, and much of what was good in each still survives in the cutaneous medicine of the present day.
>
> Now dermatology is truly international, the different schools which were formerly as separate states having become fused into one scientific commonwealth. This has been accomplished by the translation of representative works of each school into the language of the others; by the multiplication of journals, devoted to this special branch of medical science in which everything of value that is published in any part of the world is gathered up and summarized; by the facilities of communication which make it easy for the scientific pilgrim to visit every dermatological shrine where his devotion is likely to be rewarded with the knowledge of some new thing; and by congresses, those marts for the exchange of scientific wares which have so powerfully aided in the diffusion of knowledge, in the extinction of national jealousies, and in the correction of provincial ways of thought.[10]

THE FOUNDER OF DERMATOLOGY

This brings us to a final question: just who was the "Founder of Dermatology?" If we exclude ancient contributors such as Galen and Hippocrates, there are seven candidates: Mercurialis, Turner, Astruc, Plenck, Willan, von Hebra, and Unna. Of these, Robert Willan is the most common answer to the question. The criteria for such an appellation is open to debate, but to the present author, one criterion should be recognition of that physician or surgeon who devoted all or most of his energies to the skin and its diseases. That criterion eliminates the following candidates from the list: Mercurialis, who produced the first-ever text on dermatology; Astruc, whose contributions were largely in the realm of venereology; and Plenck, who created the first meaningful classification of skin diseases. All of these men were medical polymaths who focused attention on many other fields in medicine.

Another criterion rates the degree of influence on contemporaries and the generations of physicians that followed. While Turner wrote the first treatise on skin disease in English and, in many ways, was the first bonafide dermatologist in history, his career and publications had far less influence on his peers and his descendants than the remaining three men: Willan, von Hebra, and Unna.

If the last criterion involves the physician whose career did more for establishing dermatology on its firmest foundation going forward, with no turning backward, then von Hebra is the best possible answer to the question, with Willan and Unna in a very close second and third place, respectively. Willan's classification system and his ordering of the chaotic nomenclature were much needed at the time, but Ferdinand von Hebra is *the* founder of dermatology because after him, dermatology was a science and one with enough depth that physicians could specialize in it.

The question of "Who was the founder of dermatology?" will continue to be debated. If the question is "Who was the greatest dermatologist in history?" that answer is easier to reach. Unna was the greatest because he was the most complete—clinically, scientifically, therapeutically; von Hebra is a close second, and perhaps, Brocq, Bazin, or Besnier follow.

Future Directions

Imagine if Unna, Hebra, or Willan could see what dermatology is like today, then consider what another hundred years of advancement has in store for the specialty. Perhaps artificial intelligence, the next frontier in science, will allow for the replacement of dermatologists with computers, equipped with mole-analyzing cameras, or robots and their skin-stripping tapes for sampling rashes and moles. A question sure to arise in the not-too-distant future is can the human dermatologist compete with the diagnostic accuracy of the computer? Will humans 100 years from now marvel at the old days when dermatological care was provided by humans and not machines?

Another direction that seems likely is the expansion of telemedicine, which, to some extent, is already here. Patients want virtual visits with their doctors, and while dermatology is more challenging to practice in front of a computer screen instead of a live patient, there is no reason why chronic skin disease follow-ups cannot be performed virtually, and with improvements in video quality, other skin problems can be evaluated as well.

The overwhelming majority of very ill skin disease patients in US hospitals are never seen by a dermatologist because very few US dermatologists actually go to the hospital for consultations. The reasons behind this situation are numerous, but it must be stated that dermatologists bring tremendous value to not only the sick patients in the hospital but also to the payers of these hospital stays. Analysis of the cost savings of hospital stays when dermatology is consulted would likely reveal a substantial reduction in cost and a source for potential incentives to lure dermatologists back to the hospital.

Many of the best treatments for moderate-to-severe skin disease cost tens of thousands of dollars per year. Access to these medications is frequently cost-prohibitive or otherwise obstructed. Very often, patients, especially ones over the age of 65, must choose between living with their disease versus a trial of risky immunosuppressants, while the safer biologic (immunomodulating) drugs cannot be accessed. While the solutions to fixing these high-cost issues will likely remain elusive, it must be declared that dermatology is now in the post-immunosuppressive era of therapeutics.

These concerns pale in comparison to the global problem of poor access to cutting-edge Western medications in countries that lack the healthcare infrastructure of Western nations. We must remember that not everyone with severe acne, psoriasis, and eczema in the world has access to medications like isotretinoin, guselkumab, or dupilumab, and there remains in 2022 much suffering in the world when it comes to skin disease. Improving access to these medications for patients all over the world is an essential goal for dermatology in the next decades.

The most un-talked-about crisis in the United States is the one concerning mental health. Mental illness is increasing at an alarming rate. Any practicing dermatologist can tell you that the relationship between mental health and skin health is a profound connection which we only partly understand.

Dermatologists often find themselves at the front lines of managing mentally ill patients, ranging from patients with delusions of parasitosis to neurotic excoriations to body dysmorphic disorder to trichotillomania to stress-exacerbated skin diseases. It is time for dermatologists to get the training they need to help these patients directly, as the medical system cannot presently handle the burden of caring for all of these patients. We must return to the days of Vincenzo Chiarugi, professor of cutaneous diseases and mental disturbances.

Therapeutically, not uncommon conditions that presently lack highly effective and safe treatment options include mycosis fungoides, severe forms of alopecia areata, hidradenitis suppurativa, granuloma annulare, and vitiligo, but research is ongoing to tackle these diseases. A rapidly effective treatment that turns off the inflammatory cascade that devastates the skin in toxic epidermal necrolysis is much needed. Many of the genetic disorders that affect the skin—the most troubling being epidermolysis bullosa—desperately need remedies.

In regard to etiology, let us hope one of the main points of Louis Duhring's 1893 speech (see Chapter 15)—the specialty must focus on the cause of skin disease—can inspire future generations of skin specialists. Too many of the conditions dermatologists treat are idiopathic, e.g., granuloma annulare, pityriasis rubra pilaris, pityriasis lichenoides, and lichen planus. Will the next century see the mystery behind these bizarre skin affections finally solved?

Many questions remain without answers as dermatology looks to keep up with the evolving discipline of holistic and integrative medicine. As trust in the healthcare system plummets in the midst of the Covid-19 pandemic, we can expect the number of patients looking for alternatives to mainstream healthcare approaches to continue to increase. A frontier of dermatological research has to be the relationship among diet, internal health, mental health, and skin disease. For example, what exactly is the relationship between diet and acne? What are some of the modifiable contributing factors that might help the countless cases of hormonal acne that are seen in dermatology clinics every day? Is hormonal blockade really the only way? For psoriasis, what dietary and lifestyle modifications might decrease the severity of disease? For children who stay indoors now more than ever, and for adults who work from home, how much sun exposure is actually good for them in relation to vitamin D levels, immune health, mental health, and skin health? Are dermatologists doing a disservice by preaching sun avoidance to their patients? These are just some of the many questions that we can hope to have answered in the near future. Perhaps a first step is to bring back the diathesis concept of Bazin and Hardy and establish new diatheses for the modern patient: the metabolic diathesis, the autoimmune diathesis, the psoriasis diathesis, the hormonal diathesis, the neurotic diathesis, etc. Maybe medicine has swung too far away from the days of the Galenists, who knew at least that whole health and dietary moderation were of paramount importance in skin disease. In sum, the future of dermatology involves an intense focus on the etiology and risk factors of skin diseases, and after "breaking down the walls of our specialism," as Hutchinson had put it, it entails an unflinching view not only of the surface of the patient but also of the whole person underneath that surface.

While there is much remaining for us to learn about the skin and its diseases, the physicians of history are owed a tremendous debt of gratitude for bringing order to the chaos that was the (mis)understanding of skin diseases. This book has recounted that long story, and it is hopefully evident by now that the skin was for several millennia one of the most poorly understood parts of the human body and the source of many different types of anguish. Dermatologists now have the knowledge that is needed to make sense of what we are seeing on the skin and communicate that information to the modern patient. We are very fortunate to live in a world where specialists in the skin exist who can spot a potentially deadly melanoma before it becomes a serious problem; who quickly spot that elusive scabies mite in order to precisely identify the cause of one's incessant itching; who can uncover the single mystery chemical in a person's skin care products that might be causing allergic contact dermatitis; who are able to eradicate that severe cystic acne in a self-conscious teenager; who might determine that a patient has liver disease or leukemia or some other internal disease from a skin exam; and who remind everyone to protect their outer covering from the sun and to care for it and cherish it with gentle soaps and emollients. Humanity has suffered long enough with skin diseases, and after four millennia of speculation and discourse and two centuries of intense specialization in the science of the skin, a trip to the dermatologist can now result in a swift and prudent end to these primordial afflictions.

Endnotes

Preface

1 Mark A. Everett, "Erasmus Wilson and the Birth of the Specialty of Dermatology," *International Journal of Dermatology* 17, no. 4 (1978): 352.
2 Dike Drummond, *Stop Physician Burnout* (New York, NY: Heritage Press, 2014), 20.

Introduction

1 Nina G. Jablonski and George Chaplin, "The Colours of Humanity: The Evolution of Pigmentation in the Human Lineage," *Philosophical Transactions of the Royal Society of London* B 372 (2017): 1–8.
2 Jablonski and Chaplin, *Colours of Humanity*, 1–8.

Chapter 1: Ancient Mesopotamia

1 Philo Judaeus. *The Works*, trans. by C.D. Yonge (United Kingdom: n.p., 1855), Philo (20 BCE to 50 CE) was discussing the "rewards" of impiety and lawless iniquity.
2 Thomas Macaulay, *The Complete Works of Thomas Babington Macaulay*, Volume 4 (New York NY: Houghton Mifflin, 1910), 634.
3 Joseph Jacob Plenck, *Doctrina de Morbis Cutaneis: Qua Hi Morbi in Suas Classes, Genera et Species Rediguntur* (Vienna: Apud Rudolphum Græffer, 1783). Preface. Translated by the Author and Dr. Althea Ashe.
4 Louise Cilliers and Francois P. Retief, "Mesopotamian Medicine," *South African Medical Journal* 97, no. 1 (2007): 27.
5 Plinio Prioreschi, *Primitive and Ancient Medicine* (New York, NY: Edwin Mellen Press, 1991), 446.
6 Guido Majno, *The Healing Hand: Man and Wound in the Ancient World* (Delran, NJ: Classics of Medicine Library, 1991), 36–37.
7 Cilliers and Retief, "Mesopotamian Medicine," 27–30.
8 Cilliers and Retief, "Mesopotamian Medicine," 28.
9 Majno, "Healing Hand," 40.
10 Emily K. Teall, "Medicine and Doctoring in Ancient Mesopotamia," *Grand Valley Journal of History* 3, no. 1 (2014): 1.
11 JoAnn Scurlock and Burton R. Andersen, *Diagnoses in Assyrian and Babylonian Medicine: Ancient Sources, Translations, and Modern Medical Analyses* (Urbana-Champaign, IL: University of Illinois Press, 2005), 208.
12 Scurlock and Andersen, "Diagnoses in Assyrian and Babylonian Medicine," 209–245.
13 JoAnn Scurlock, *Sourcebook for Ancient Mesopotamian Medicine* (United States: SBL Press, 2014), 236.
14 Francesca Minen, "Medico-Dermatologic Notions in Mesopotamian Cuneiform Sources," *Antesteria* 7, 21–33 (2018): 25.
15 Francesca Minen, "Ancient Mesopotamian Views on Human Skin and Body: A Cultural-Historical Analysis of Dermatological Data from Cuneiform Sources," *Notes and Records* 74, no. 1 (2020): 125.
16 Scurlock and Andersen, "Diagnoses in Assyrian and Babylonian Medicine," 230.
17 Minen, "Ancient Mesopotamian Views on Human Skin and Body," 26.
18 Francesca Minen, "Medico-Dermatologic Notions in Mesopotamian Cuneiform Sources," *Antesteria* 7, 21–33 (2018): 28. Adapted by the author.
19 Minen, "Ancient Mesopotamian Views on Human Skin and Body," 124.
20 Scurlock, "Sourcebook," 237.

21 Minen, "Medico-Dermatologic Notions," 29.

22 Minen, "Medico-Dermatologic Notions," 30.

23 Minen, "Medico-Dermatologic Notions in Mesopotamian Cuneiform Sources," 27.

24 Leo Oppenheim et al. "La'bu." *The Assyriological Dictionary of the Oriental Institute of the University of Chicago*, Volume 9 (Chicago, IL: University of Chicago Press, 1973), 35.

25 Scurlock and Andersen, "Diagnoses in Assyrian and Babylonian Medicine," 209–245.

26 Minen, "Ancient Mesopotamian Views," 126.

27 Minen, "Ancient Mesopotamian Views," 127.

28 R. Campbell Thompson, "Assyrian Prescriptions for Treating Bruises or Swellings," *American Journal of Semitic Languages and Literatures* 47, no. 1 (1930): 1–25.

29 Majno, "Healing Hand," 46.

30 Majno, "Healing Hand," 46.

31 Personal communication with Dr. Holly Caldwell.

32 Munir A. Bankole et al., "Synergistic Antimicrobial Activities of Phytoestrogens in Crude Extracts of Two Sesame Species against Some Common Pathogenic Microorganisms," *African Journal of Traditional, Complementary, and Alternative Medicines* 4, no. 4 (2007): 427.

Chapter 2: Ancient Egypt

1 Keith Houston, *The Book: A Cover-to-Cover Exploration of the Most Powerful Object of Our Time* (New York, NY: W.W. Norton & Company, 1998), 28.

2 John Nunn, *Ancient Egyptian Medicine* (London: British Museum Press, 2003), 25.

3 Roy Porter, *The Greatest Benefit to Mankind: A Medical History of Humanity* (New York, NY: W. W. Norton, 1998), 48–49.

4 Plinio Prioreschi, *Primitive and Ancient Medicine* (Lewiston, NY: Edwin Mellen Press, 1991), 351.

5 James Henry Breasted, *The Edwin Smith Papyrus: An Egyptian Medical Treatise of the Seventeenth Century before Christ* (New York, NY: New York Historical Society, 1922), 5.

6 Herodotus, *Herodotus*, trans. Alfred. D. Godley (Cambridge, MA: Harvard University Press, 1920), II.77.2; quote: Prioreschi, *Primitive and Ancient Medicine*, 346–347.

7 Prioreschi, *Primitive and Ancient Medicine*, 347.

8 Prioreschi, *Primitive and Ancient Medicine*, 365.

9 William Osler, *The Evolution of Modern Medicine* (New Haven, CT: Yale University Press, 1921), 12.

10 Joan F. Hickson, "Medicine in Ancient Egypt and Its Relevance Today," *Journal of the Royal College of General Practitioners* 21, no. 110 (1971): 512.

11 Prioreschi, *Primitive and Ancient Medicine,* 344.

12 Breasted, *Edwin Smith Papyrus*, xiii.

13 Prioreschi, *Primitive and Ancient Medicine*, 367.

14 Patric Blomstedt, "Imhotep and the Discovery of Cerebrospinal Fluid," *Anatomy Research International* 2014, no. 3 (2014): 2.

15 Porter, *Greatest Benefit*, 49.

16 Hickson, *Medicine in Ancient Egypt,* 511–516.

17 Prioreschi, *Primitive and Ancient Medicine,* 362.

18 *Ancient Egyptian Medicine: The Papyrus Ebers*, trans. Cyril P. Bryan (Chicago Ridge, IL: Ares, 1991), 6.

19 *Ancient Egyptian Medicine*, 7.

20 The two translations used for preparation of this section are the English translation by Cyril Bryan (1930) of Dr. H. Joachim's German translation of the papyrus, and Paul Ghalioungui's new English translation (Paul Ghalioungui, *The Ebers Papyrus: A New English Translation, Commentaries, and Glossaries* [Cairo: Academy of Scientific Research and Technology, 1987]). Ghalioungui extensively referenced a third English translation by Bendix Ebbell (1937) (Ebbell, B. *The Papyrus Ebers: The Greatest Egyptian Medical Document* [Copenhagen: Levin & Munksgaard, 1937]).

21 *Ancient Egyptian Medicine*, 15.

22 Anke Hartmann, "Back to the Roots—Dermatology in Ancient Egyptian Medicine," *Journal der Deutschen Dermatologischen Gesellschaft* 14, no. 4 (2016): 392.

23 Nunn, *Ancient Egyptian Medicine*, 95.

24 Hartmann, *Back to the Roots,* 390.

25 William Allen Pusey, *The History of Dermatology* (London: Baillière, Tindall & Cox, 1933), 12–13.

26 Hartmann, *Back to the Roots,* 393; Ghalioungui, *The Ebers Papyrus,* 31.

27 *Ancient Egyptian Medicine,* 88.

28 *Ancient Egyptian Medicine,* 88.

29 *Ancient Egyptian Medicine,* 90.

30 *Ancient Egyptian Medicine,* 92.

31 Eric Maranda, Brian J. Simmons, and Paolo Romanelli, "Cryotherapy—As Ancient as the Pharaohs," *JAMA Dermatology* 152, no. 6 (June 2016): 730.

32 Ghalioungui, *Ebers Papyrus,* no. 139–164.

33 Ghalioungui, *Ebers Papyrus,* no. 869.

34 *Ancient Egyptian Medicine,* 93.

35 Ghalioungui, *Ebers Papyrus,* no. 714–721.

36 Hartmann, *Back to the Roots,* 394.

37 Susruthi Rajanala and Neelam A. Vashi, "Cleopatra and Sour Milk—The Ancient Practice of Chemical Peeling," *JAMA Dermatology* 153, no. 10 (2017): 1006.

38 Ghalioungui, *Ebers Papyrus,* no. 451–462, no. 464–473.

39 Ghalioungui, *Ebers Papyrus,* no. 771.

40 Pusey, *History of Dermatology,* 14.

41 Nunn, *Ancient Egyptian Medicine,* 95.

42 University of Bonn, "Deadly Ancient Egyptian Medication? German Scientists Shed Light on Dark Secret of Queen Hatshepsut's Flacon," *ScienceDaily,* August 22, 2011.

43 Helieh S. Oz, "Dirt, Saliva and Leprosy: Anti-Inflammatory and Anti-infectious Effects," *Diseases* 7, no. 1 (2019): 1.

44 Hartmann, *Back to the Roots,* 394.

45 Keith Liddell, "Skin Disease in Antiquity," *Clinical Medicine* 6, no. 1 (January–February 2006): 84.

46 Hartmann, *Back to the Roots,* 393.

47 Breasted, *Edwin Smith Papyrus,* xiii.

48 Breasted, *Edwin Smith Papyrus,* xvii.

49 Breasted, *Edwin Smith Papyrus,* 7.

50 Breasted, *Edwin Smith Papyrus,* 505.

51 Breasted, *Edwin Smith Papyrus,* 506–507. Quote is in the public domain.

52 Stanley Jacobs, *Nefertiti's Secret* (lulu.com, 2019), 117.

53 Stanley W. Jacobs and Eric J. Culbertson, "Effects of Topical Mandelic Acid Treatment on Facial Skin Viscoelasticity," Facial Plastic Surgery 34, no. 6 (December 2018): 651.

54 Eve Lowenstein, "Paleodermatoses: Lessons Learned from Mummies," *Journal of the American Academy of Dermatology* 50, no. 6 (2004), 919.

55 Kieron S. Leslie and Nick J. Levell, "Skin Disease in Mummies," *International Journal of Dermatology* 45, no. 2 (February 2006):161.

56 Lowenstein, *Paleodermatoses,* 921.

57 Lowenstein, *Paleodermatoses,* 921.

58 Chris Elliot, "Bandages, Bitumen, Bodies and Business—Egyptian Mummies as Raw Material," *Aegyptiaca* 1 (2017), 26.

59 Karl Dannenfeldt, "Egyptian Mumia: The Sixteenth Century Experience and Debate," *The Sixteenth Century Journal* 16, no. 2 (1985): 163.

60 Elliot, *Bandages, Bitumen, Bodies and Business,* 27–28.

61 Lowenstein, *Paleodermatoses,* 922–923.

62 Eve Lowenstein, "Paleodermatoses: Lessons Learned from Mummies," *Journal of the American Academy of Dermatology* 50, no. 6 (2004): 919–931.

63 Jana Jones et al., "Identification of Proteins from 4200-Year-Old Skin and Muscle Tissue Biopsies from Ancient Egyptian Mummies of the First Intermediate Period Shows Evidence of Acute Inflammation and Severe Immune Response," *Philosophical Transactions: Mathematical, Physical and Engineering Sciences* 374, no. 2079 (2016): 2.

64 Lowenstein, *Paleodermatoses,* 930.

65 Lowenstein, *Paleodermatoses,* 928.

66 Lowenstein, *Paleodermatoses,* 929.

67 Donald Hopkins, *The Greatest Killer: Smallpox in History; with a New Introduction* (Chicago, IL: University of Chicago Press, 2002), 15.

68 Lowenstein, *Paleodermatoses,* 926.

69 Rosalie David, *Egyptian Mummies and Modern Science* (Cambridge: Cambridge University Press, 2008), 211–215.

Chapter 3: Classical Greece

1 Porter, *Greatest Benefit,* 64.

2 Hassan N. Sallam, "Aristotle, Godfather of Evidence-Based Medicine," *Facts, Views, and Vision in Obstetrics and Gynaecology* 2, no. 1 (2010): 11.

3 Porter, *Greatest Benefit,* 65.

4 Lydia Kang and Nate Pedersen, *Quackery: A Brief History of the Worst Ways to Cure Everything* (United States: Workman Publishing Company, 2017), 14.

5 Liddell, *Skin Disease in Antiquity,* 82.

6 William F. Bynum, *History of Medicine: A Very Short Introduction* (Oxford: Oxford University Press, 2008), 5.

7 Vivian Nutton, "Medicine in the Greek World, 800–50 BC," in *The Western Medical Tradition: 800 BC to AD 1800* (United Kingdom: Cambridge University Press, 1995), 21.

8 Nutton, *Medicine in the Greek World,*" 22.

9 Bynum, *History of Medicine,* 6.

10 Paul Strathern, *A Brief History of Medicine: From Hippocrates to Gene Therapy* (New York, NY: Carroll & Graf, 2005), 6–7.

11 Nutton, *Medicine in the Greek World,* 23.

12 Sherwin B. Nuland, *Doctors: The Biography of Medicine* (New York, NY: Vintage, 1995), 7.

13 Bynum, *History of Medicine,* 10.

14 Bynum, *History of Medicine,* 8.

15 Nuland, *Doctors,* 8.

16 Nutton, *Medicine in the Greek World,* 11.

17 Porter, *Greatest Benefit,* 62.

18 Nuland, *Doctors,* 9.

19 Philip van der Eijk, *Diocles of Carystus: A Collection of the Fragments* (Leiden: Brill, 2001).

20 Vivian Nutton, *Medicine in the Greek World,* 36.

21 Vivian Nutton, "Roman Medicine, 250 BC to 200 AD," in *The Western Medical Tradition: 800 BC to AD 1800* (United Kingdom: Cambridge University Press, 1995), 42.

22 Porter, *Greatest Benefit,* 67.

23 Porter, *Greatest Benefit,* 68.

24 Porter, *Greatest Benefit,* 68.

25 Nutton, *Medicine in the Greek World,* 35.

26 Robert Fortuine, *The Words of Medicine: Sources, Meanings, and Delights* (Springfield, IL: Charles C. Thomas, 2001), 30.

27 Rosa Santoro, "Skin over the Centuries. A Short History of Dermatology: Physiology, Pathology, and Cosmetics," *Medicina Historica* 1, no. 2 (2017): 95.

28 Fortuine, *Words of Medicine,* 33.

29 Santoro, *Skin over the Centuries,* 97.

30 Leo Schep, "Was the Death of Alexander the Great Due to Poisoning? Was It *Veratrum album*?" *Clinical Toxicology* 52, no. 1 (2014): 72.

31 John Burnet, "Fragments of Empedocles," in *Early Greek Philosophy* (London: A. and C. Black, 1908), 219.

32 Mieneke te Hennepe, "Of the Fisherman's Net and Skin Pores: Reframing Conceptions of the Skin in Medicine, 1572–1714," in *Blood, Sweat and Tears: The Changing Concepts of Physiology from Antiquity into Early Modern Europe,* ed. Manfred Horstmanshoff, Helen King, and Claus Zittel (Leiden: Brill, 2012), 526–8.

33 van der Eijk, *Diocles,* 299.

34 Jean-William Fitting, "From Breathing to Respiration," *Respiration* 89, no. 1 (2015): 83.

35 Michael Stolberg, "Sweat. Learned Concepts and Popular Perceptions, 1500–1800," in *Blood, Sweat and Tears: The Changing Concepts of Physiology from Antiquity into Early Modern Europe*, ed. Manfred Horstmanshoff, Helen King, and Claus Zittel (Leiden: Brill, 2012), 503.

36 Stolberg, *Sweat*, 503.

37 Hippocrates, *The Genuine Works of Hippocrates*, ed. and trans. and Francis Adams (United Kingdom: Sydenham Society, 1849), 239.

38 T.K. Johansen, *Aristotle on the Sense-Organs* (Cambridge, UK: Cambridge University Press, 1998), 212.

39 Rudolph E. Siegel, *Galen on Sense Perception* (Basel: Karger, 1970), 175.

40 Plato, *"Timaeus" and "Critias,"* trans. A.E. Taylor (London: Routledge Library Editions, 2013), 80–1.

41 Aristotle, *On the Generation of Animals*, trans. Arthur Platt (Oxford: Clarendon Press, 1910), II.6.41.

42 Aristotle, *Problems*, trans. Robert Mayhew (Cambridge, MA: Harvard University Press, 2011).

43 Aristotle, *Generation of Animals*, V.3.3.

44 Plato, *"Timaeus" and "Critias,"* trans. Robin Waterfield (New York, NY: Oxford, 2008), 89.

45 Liddell, *Skin Disease in Antiquity*, 82–3.

46 Ivan McCaw, "A Synopsis of the History of Dermatology," *Ulster Medical Journal* 13, no. 2 (Nov. 1944): 111.

47 William F. Hansen, *Ariadne's Thread: a Guide to International Tales Found in Classical Literature* (Ithaca, NY: Cornell University Press, 2009), 149–50.

48 Katlein Franca et al. "Psychodermatology: A Trip through History," *Anais Brasileiros de Dermatologia* 88, no. 5 (2013): 842.

49 Herman Goodman, *Notable Contributors to the Knowledge of Dermatology* (New York: Medical Lay Press, 1953), 20–1; Alsaidan, Mohammed et al. "Hippocrates' Contributions to Dermatology Revisited," *JAMA Dermatology* 151, no. 6 (2015): 658.

50 Pusey, *History of Dermatology*, 23

51 Liddell, *Skin Disease in Antiquity*, 84.

52 Liddell, *Skin Disease in Antiquity*, 85.

53 Pusey, *History of Dermatology*, 24.

54 Hippocrates and Galen, *The Writings of Hippocrates and Galen*, trans. John R. Coxe (United States: Lindsay and Blakiston, 1846), 401.

55 Gérard Tilles, Daniel Wallach, and Alain Taieb, "Topical Therapy of Atopic Dermatitis: Controversies from Hippocrates to Topical Immunomodulators," *Journal of the American Academy of Dermatology* 56, no. 2 (2007): 295.

56 Scott Norton, "What Caused the Athenian Itch in Hippocrates' *On Epidemics*?" *Journal of the American Academy of Dermatology* 57, no. 6 (2007): 1093–4.

57 Anton Sebastian, *Dictionary of the History of Medicine* (New York, NY: Parthenon, 1999), 302.

58 Pusey, *History of Dermatology*, 24.

Chapter 4: The Roman Empire

1 Bynum, *History of Medicine*, 17–18.

2 Porter, *Greatest Benefit*, 69.

3 Porter, *Greatest Benefit*, 70.

4 Goodman, *Notable Contributors*, 31.

5 Strathern, *A Brief History of Medicine*, 74, Sebastian, *Dictionary of the History of Medicine*, 185.

6 Theodore Rosenthal, "Aulus Cornelius Celsus: His Contributions to Dermatology," *Archives of Dermatology* 84, no. 4 (1961): 614.

7 Porter, *Greatest Benefit*, 71.

8 Vivian Nutton, *Ancient Medicine* (Routledge, 2014), 170.

9 Rosenthal, *Aulus Cornelius Celsus*, 615.

10 Rosenthal, *Aulus Cornelius Celsus*, 615.

11 John T. Crissey and Lawrence C. Parish, *The Dermatology and Syphilology of the Nineteenth Century* (New York, NY: Praeger, 1981), 3.

12 Aulus Cornelius Celsus, *A Translation of the Eight Books of Aul. Corn. Celsus on Medicine*, 3rd ed., rev. and ed. George Collier (London: Simpkin and Marshall, 1840), V.XXVI.20.

13 Celsus, *On Medicine*, V.XXVI.33.

14 Celsus, *On Medicine*, V.XXVI.34.

15 Celsus, *On Medicine*, V.XXVII.1.

16 Celsus, *On Medicine*, V.XXVII.2.

17 Celsus, *On Medicine*, V.XXVIII.1.

18 Celsus, *On Medicine*, V.XXVIII.1–2.

19 Celsus, *On Medicine*, V.XXVIII.7.

20 Celsus, *On Medicine*, V.XVIII.7.

21 Celsus, *On Medicine*, V.XXVIII.14

22 Celsus, *On Medicine*, V.XXVIII.19. Nineteenth-century translators such as Collier translated the word vitiligo as leprosy. The Greek words in Collier's text have been deleted for succinctness.

23 Celsus, *On Medicine*, VI.IV.

24 Celsus, *On Medicine*, VI.II.

25 Celsus, *On Medicine*, VI.V.

26 Rosenthal, *Aulus Cornelius Celsus*, 617.

27 Celsus, *On Medicine*, VI.XVIII.1.

28 John H. Dirckx, "Isidore of Seville on the Origins and Meanings of Medical Terms," *American Journal of Dermatopathology* 29, no. 6 (Dec. 2007): 363.

29 Howard Fox, "Dermatology of the Ancients," in *Transactions of the Section on Dermatology of the American Medical Association* (Chicago, IL: American Medical Association Press, 1915), 30.

30 John H. Dirckx, "Dermatologic Terms in the *De Medicina* of Celsus," *American Journal of Dermatopathology* 5, no. 4 (Aug. 1983): 363.

31 Jeffrey S. Hamilton, "Scribonius Largus on the Medical Profession," *Bulletin of the History of Medicine* 60, no. 2 (1986): 209.

32 Barry Baldwin, "The Career and Work of Scribonius Largus," *Rheinisches Museum für Philologie* 135, no. 1 (1992): 77.

33 Baldwin, *Scribonius Largus*, 79.

34 John M. Riddle, *Contraception and Abortion from the Ancient World to the Renaissance* (Cambridge, MA: Harvard University Press, 1992), 6–7.

35 Gregory Tsoucalas et al., "The 'Torpedo' Effect in Medicine," *International Maritime Health* 65, no. 2 (2014): 66

36 Goeffrey D. Schott, "Whence 'Zoster'? The Convoluted Classical Origins of a Sometimes Illogical Term," *Medical Humanities* 43, no. 1 (Mar. 2017): 15.

37 Fortuine, *Words of Medicine*, 148.

38 Conway Zirkle, "The Death of Gaius Plinius Secundus (23–79 A.D.)," *Isis* 58, no. 4 (1967): 553.

39 Also, botany, medicine, pharmacology, magic, aquatic life, mining and mineralogy, and art history.

40 Pliny The Elder, *The Natural History*. trans. John Bostock and Henry T. Riley (London: Taylor & Francis Group, 1855), Book 1, dedication.

41 Pliny the Elder, *The Natural History*, XXVI.I.

42 Pliny the Elder, *The Natural History,* XXVI.II.

43 Pliny the Elder, *The Natural History* XXVI.III.

44 Ronald Syme, "Governors Dying in Syria," *Zeitschrift für Papyrologie und Epigraphik* 41 (1981), 126.

45 Martial, *Epigrams* (Bohn's Classical Library, 1897), XII.59.

46 Martial, *Epigrams*, X.22.

47 Martial, *Epigrams*, XI.98.

48 Pliny the Elder, *The Natural History,* XXVI.III.

49 Pliny the Elder, *The Natural History,* XXVI.III.

50 Pliny the Elder, *The Natural History,* XXVI.III.

51 Pliny the Elder, *The Natural History,* XXVI.74.

52 Nutton, *Ancient Medicine*, 178.

53 John M. Riddle, *Dioscorides on Pharmacy and Medicine* (Austin, TX: University of Texas Press, 1985), 13.

54 Riddle, *Dioscorides*, 11.

55 Riddle, *Dioscorides*, 42.

56 Nutton, *Ancient Medicine*, 178.

57 Riddle, *Dioscorides*, 25–26.

58 Riddle, *Dioscorides*, 42.

59 Pedanius Dioscorides, *De Materia Medica: A New Indexed Version in Modern English*, trans. Tess Anne Obaldeston (Johannesberg: Ibidis, 2000).

60 Dioscorides, *De Materia Medica*, I.36.

61 Riddle, *Dioscorides*, 52.

62 Riddle, *Dioscorides*, 57.

63 Dioscorides, *De Materia Medica*, I.101.

64 Riddle, *Dioscorides*, 134.

65 Dioscorides, *De Materia Medica*, V.84.

66 Riddle, *Dioscorides*, 33–34.

67 Riddle, *Dioscorides on Pharmacy and Medicine*, 34.

68 Gaspare Baggieri and Melissa Baggieri, "Dermatology: The Stock-in-Trade in Ancient Rome," *Journal of Applied Cosmetology* 29 (2011): 147–152.

69 Arturo Castiglioni, *A History of Medicine* (New York, NY: Knopf, 1958), 220.

70 Bynum, *History of Medicine*, 15.

71 *On the Ideal Physician, On the Ideal Philosophy, On the Elements according to Hippocrates, On Anatomical Preparations, On Dissections of the Veins and Arteries, On the Movements of Muscles, On the Teachings of Hippocrates and Plato, On the Affected Parts, On the Usefulness of the Parts of the Human Body, On the Medical Art, On the Method of Treatment.*

72 Castiglioni, *History of Medicine*, 218.

73 Porter, *Greatest Benefit*, 74.

74 Porter, *Greatest Benefit*, 73.

75 Castiglioni, *History of Medicine*, 219.

76 Nutton, *Ancient Medicine*, 238.

77 Porter, *Greatest Benefit*, 79.

78 Pusey, *History of Dermatology*, 29.

79 Porter, *Greatest Benefit*, 76.

80 Castiglioni, *History of Medicine*, 224.

81 Demetrios Karaberopoulos, Marianna Karamanou, and George Androutsos, "The Theriac in Antiquity," *Lancet* 379, no. 9830 (2012): 1942–1943.

82 Nutton, *Ancient Medicine*, 253.

83 Nutton, *Ancient Medicine*, 243–244.

84 Nutton, *Ancient Medicine*, 248.

85 Jack Edward McCallum, *Military Medicine: From Ancient Times to the 21st Century* (Santa Barbara, CA: ABC-CLIO, 2008), 26.

86 Castiglioni, *History of Medicine*, 221.

87 Castiglioni, *History of Medicine*, 225.

88 Nuland, *Doctors*, 32.

89 Steven Connor, *The Book of Skin* (Ithaca, NY: Cornell University Press, 2004), 13.

90 Santoro, *Skin over the Centuries*, 95.

91 Marjorie O. Boyle, *Senses of Touch: Human Dignity and Deformity from Michelangelo to Calvin* (Belgium: Brill, 1998), 143.

92 Santoro, *Skin over the Centuries*, 99.

93 Pusey, *History of Dermatology*, 30.

94 Galen, *De Tumoribus Praeter Naturam: A Critical Edition with Translation and Indices*, trans. Jeremiah Reedy (Ann Arbor: University of Michigan, 1968), 29–50; Other small "swellings" that develop on the skin include *myrmeciae, acrochordons, psydraces,* and *epinyctidies,* which according to Galen, "are known to everyone." Boils and tubercles are swellings confined to the skin that differ only in degree of hardness. Other similar swellings include the *bubo* and the *phygethlon;* the latter occurs only in the groin or armpit. Hardening of the glands there is called *struma.* Dilatation of the veins is called *cirsos,* which occurs due to weakness of the veins.

95 Charles D. O'Malley, "Dermatological Origins," *Archives of Dermatology* 83 (Feb. 1961): 69.

96 Pusey, *History of Dermatology*, 30.

97 Alissa Cowden and Abby S. Van Voorhees, "Introduction: History of Psoriasis and Psoriasis Therapy," in *Treatment of Psoriasis*, ed. Jeffrey. M. Weinberg (Basel, Switzerland: Birkhäuser, 2008), 2.

98 Nutton, *Ancient Medicine*, 262.

99 Prioreschi, *Primitive and Ancient Medicine*, 303.

100 Prioreschi, *Primitive and Ancient Medicine,* 303.

101 It was published by Valentin Rose in Latin for the first time in 1879; no English translation can be found.

102 Cassius Felix, *Cassii Felicis de Medicina: Ex Graecis Logicae Sectae Auctoribus Liber, Translatus sub Artabure et Calepio Consulibus (anno 447)*, ed. Valentin Rose (Lipsiae: B. G. Teubneri, 1879), II–XXVI.

103 Cassius, *Cassii Felicis de Medicina*, II–XXVI.

104 Porter, *Greatest Benefit*, 70.

105 Porter, *Greatest Benefit*, 70.

106 Castiglioni, *History of Medicine*, 204.

107 Frank Ursin, Claudia Borelli, and Florian Steger, "Dermatology in Ancient Rome: Medical Ingredients in Ovid's 'Remedies for Female Faces,'" *Journal of Cosmetic Dermatology* 19, no. 6 (2020): 1389.

108 Ursin, Borelli, and Steger, *Dermatology in Ancient Rome*, 1393.

109 Richard L. Sutton Jr., *Sixteenth Century Physician and His Methods: Mercurialis on Diseases of the Skin, the First Book on the Subject* (Kansas City, MO: Lowell Press, 1986), 211.

110 Alex E. Wright, Joseph McFarland, and Mohammadali M. Shoja, "Archigenes and the Syndrome of Vertigo, Tinnitus, Hearing Loss, and Headache," *Child's Nervous System* 37, no. 8 (Aug. 2021): 2417.

111 Niki Papavramidou et al., "Ancient Greek and Greco-Roman Methods in Modern Surgical Treatment of Cancer," *Annals of Surgical Oncology* 17, no. 3 (2010): 665.

112 Jack Edward McCallum, *Military Medicine: From Ancient Times to the 21st Century* (Santa Barbara, CA: ABC-CLIO, 2008), 26.

113 Wright, McFarland, and Shoja, *Archigenes and the Syndrome of Vertigo, Tinnitus, Hearing Loss, and Headache*, 2417.

114 Timothy S. Miller and John W. Nesbitt, *Walking Corpses: Leprosy in Byzantium and the Medieval West* (Ithaca; London: Cornell University Press, 2014), 58.

115 Goodman, *Notable Contributors*, 25.

116 Frank N. Magill, *Dictionary of World Biography* (London: Routledge, 2014), 110.

117 Halil Tekiner, "Aretaeus of Cappadocia and His Treatises on Diseases," *Turkish Neurosurgery* 25, no. 3 (2015): 508.

118 Sebastian, *Dictionary of the History of Medicine*, 87.

119 Marianna Karamanou, Kyriakos P. Kyriakis, and George Androutsos, "Aretaeus of Cappadocia on Leprosy's Transmission," *JAMA Dermatology* 149, no. 3 (2013): 292.

120 Goodman, *Notable Contributors*, 28.

121 Castiglioni, *History of Medicine*, 202.

122 Caelius Aurelianus, *On Acute Diseases and on Chronic Diseases*, ed. and trans. Israel E. Drabkin (Chicago, IL: University of Chicago Press, 1951), 823.

123 Aurelianus, *On Acute Diseases and on Chronic Diseases*, 823.

124 John Dirckx, "Dermatologic Terms in the Onomasticon of Julius Pollux," *American Journal of Dermatopathology* 26, no. 6 (2004): 511–513.

125 Horace, *Satires*, trans. Christopher Smart and Theodore Buckley (New York, NY: Harper & Bros., 1863), I.5.62–64.

126 Ortwin Knorr, "Morbus Campanus in Horace, Satires 1.5.62" *Classical Quarterly* 62, no. 2 (2012): 870.

127 Knorr, *Morbus Campanus*, 872.

128 David R. Langslow, *Medical Latin in the Roman Empire* (Oxford: Oxford University Press, 2000), 29.

129 Santoro, *Skin over the Centuries*, 95.

130 Fortuine, *Words of Medicine*, 61.

131 John Scarborough, *Medical and Biological Terminologies: Classical Origins* (Norman, OK: University of Oklahoma Press, 1998), 261.

132 Langslow, *Medical Latin in the Roman Empire*, 315–336.

133 Job 2: 7, Authorized King James Version.

134 Leonard Hoenig, "The Plague Called 'Shechin' in the Bible," *American Journal of Dermatopathology* 7, no. 6 (Dec. 1985): 547.

135 Hoenig, *Plague Called 'Shechin,'* 547–548.

136 1 Samuel 5: 1–6, The King James Version.

137 Thierry Appelboom, Elie Cogan, and Jean Klastersky, "Job of the Bible: Leprosy or Scabies?" *Mount Sinai Journal of Medicine* 74, no. 1 (Apr. 2007): 36–39.

138 Karl Holubar, "Dermatology in Biblical Perspective: An Illustration from the Book of Job," *American Journal of Dermatopathology* 7, no. 5 (Oct. 1985): 438.

139 Deut. 28: 27–28, Authorized (King James) Version.

140 Oumeish Y. Oumeish, "The Cultural and Philosophical Concepts of Cosmetics in Beauty and Art through the Medical History of Mankind," *Clinics in Dermatology* 19, no. 4 (2001): 383.

141 Flavius Josephus, *The Antiquities of the Jews*, trans. William Whiston (London: W. Bowyer, 1737), XXVII.6.5.

142 Flavius Josephus, *The Wars of the Jews,* trans. William Whiston (London: W. Bowyer, 1737), I.33.5.

143 W. Ried Litchfield, "The Bittersweet Demise of Herod the Great," *Journal of the Royal Society of Medicine* 91, no. 5 (1998): 284.

144 Louise Cilliers and Francois P. Retief, "The Illnesses of Herod the Great: The Biblical World," *Acta Theologica* 2005, no. sup. 7 (2005): 289–290.

Interlude 1: Leprosy (Hansen's Disease)

1 Mirko Dražen Grmek, *Diseases in the Ancient Greek World* (Baltimore, MD: Johns Hopkins University Press, 1995), 202.

2 Gwen Robbins et al., "Ancient Skeletal Evidence for Leprosy in India (2000 B.C.)," *PLoS One* 4, no. 5 (May 2009): e5669.

3 Katrina McLeod and Robin Yates, "Forms of Ch'in Law: An Annotated Translation of the Feng-Chen Shih," *Harvard Journal of Asiatic Studies* 41, no. 1 (1981): 153.

4 Miller and Nesbit, *Walking Corpses*, 17.

5 Grmek, *Diseases in the Ancient Greek World*, 166.

6 Grmek, *Diseases in the Ancient Greek World*, 167.

7 Gillian Crane-Kramer, "Was There a Medieval Diagnostic Confusion between Leprosy and Syphilis? An Examination of the Skeletal Evidence," in *The Past and Present of Leprosy: Archeological, Historical, Palaeopathological and Clinical Approaches*, ed. Charlotte A. Roberts. Proceedings of the International Congress on the Evolution and Palaeoepidemiology of the Infectious Diseases 3 (ICEPID), University of Bradford, July 26–31, 1999 (Oxford: Archaeopress, 2002), 112.

8 Andrzej Grzybowski and Małgorzata Nita, "Leprosy in the Bible," *Clinical Dermatology* 34, no. 1 (2016): 6.

9 Grzybowski and Nita, *Leprosy in the Bible*, 3.

10 Lev. 13:1–3 (King James Version).

11 Num. 12:9–10 (King James Version).

12 II Kings. 5:1–27 (The King James Version).

13 Grzybowski and Nita, *Leprosy in the Bible*, 3.

14 Grzybowski and Nita, *Leprosy in the Bible*, 6.

15 Grzybowski and Nita, *Leprosy in the Bible*, 4.

16 Miller and Nesbit, *Walking Corpses*, 10.

17 Miller and Nesbit, *Walking Corpses*, 11.

18 Grmek, *Diseases in the Ancient Greek World*, 167.

19 Pliny, *The Natural History,* XXVI.5.

20 Miller and Nesbit, *Walking Corpses*, 13.

21 Miller and Nesbit, *Walking Corpses*, 13.

22 Aretaeus, *The Extant Works of Aretaeus, the Cappadocian*, ed. and trans. Francis Adams (London: Printed for the Sydenham Society, 1856), Chronic II.13, 368.

23 Aretaeus, *Extant Works*, 368.

24 Aretaeus, *Extant Works*, 369–72.

25 Miller and Nesbit, *Walking Corpses*, 57.

26 Miller and Nesbit, *Walking Corpses*, 25–26.

27 Miller and Nesbit, *Walking Corpses*, 27.
28 Miller and Nesbit, *Walking Corpses*, 21.
29 Justin Donovan, "Leprosy," in *The Catholic Encyclopedia* (New York, NY: Robert Appleton, 1910), 184.
30 Miller and Nesbit, *Walking Corpses*, 73.
31 Richard J. Lucariello and Martin Reichel, "The Leper King," *JAMA Dermatology* 152, no. 7 (2016): 815.
32 Luke E. Demaitre, *Leprosy in Premodern Medicine: A Malady of the Whole Body* (Baltimore, MD: Johns Hopkins University Press, 2007), 34–74.
33 Demaitre, *Leprosy in Premodern Medicine*, 19.
34 Demaitre, *Leprosy in Premodern Medicine*, 22.
35 Crane-Kramer, *Confusion between Leprosy and Syphilis?* 113.
36 Demaitre, *Leprosy in Premodern Medicine*, 103–31.
37 Demaitre, *Leprosy in Premodern Medicine*, 172.
38 Demaitre, *Leprosy in Premodern Medicine*, 163.
39 Demaitre, *Leprosy in Premodern Medicine*, 165.
40 Demaitre, *Leprosy in Premodern Medicine*, 174–5.
41 Demaitre, *Leprosy in Premodern Medicine*, 194.
42 Samuel Johnson, "Leprosy," in *A Dictionary of the English Language* (London: JP Knapton, 1755).
43 Demaitre, *Leprosy in Premodern Medicine*, 220.
44 Miller and Nesbit, *Walking Corpses*, 114.
45 Demaitre, *Leprosy in Premodern Medicine*, 259–77.
46 Verena J. Schuenemann et al., "Genome-Wide Comparison of Medieval and Modern *Mycobacterium leprae*," *Science* 341, no. 6142 (July 2013): 179.
47 Grmek, *Diseases in the Ancient Greek World*, 203.
48 Helen D. Donoghue et al., "Co-Infection of *Mycobacterium tuberculosis* and *Mycobacterium leprae* in Human Archaeological Samples: A Possible Explanation for the Historical Decline of Leprosy," *Proceedings of the Royal Society of London* 272, no. 1561 (February 22, 2005): 389.
49 René Dubos and Jean Dubos, *The White Plague: Tuberculosis, Man, and Society* (New Brunswick, NJ: Rutgers University Press, 1996), 195.
50 Porter, *Greatest Benefit*, 241.
51 Demaitre, *Leprosy in Premodern Medicine*, 30–1.
52 Sangita Ghosh and Soumik Chaudhuri, "Chronicles of Gerhard-Henrik Armauer Hansen's Life and Work," *Indian Journal of Dermatology* 60, no. 3 (2015): 219.
53 Ghosh and Chaudhuri, *Hansen's Life and Work*, 220.
54 Ghosh and Chaudhuri, *Hansen's Life and Work*, 221.
55 Ghosh and Chaudhuri, *Hansen's Life and Work*, 221.
56 Ghosh and Chaudhuri, *Hansen's Life and Work*, 221.
57 John Parascandola, "Chaulmoogra Oil and the Treatment of Leprosy," *Pharmacy in History* 45, no. 2 (2003): 47.
58 Parascandola, *Chaulmoogra Oil and the Treatment of Leprosy*, 47–56.
59 Marc Monot et al., "On the Origin of Leprosy," *Science* 308, no. 5724 (2005): 1042.
60 Marcia G. Gaudet, *Carville: Remembering Leprosy in America* (Jackson, MS: University Press of Mississippi, 2004), 264.
61 Louisiana Department of Health (LDH), Office of Public Health, Department of Infectious Disease, Leprosy Annual Report, 2014.
62 LDH, Leprosy Annual Report.
63 Zachary Gussow, *Leprosy, Racism, and Public Health: Social Policy in Chronic Disease Control* (Boulder, CO: Westview Press, 1989), 155.
64 Hajime Sato and Janet E. Frantz, "Termination of the Leprosy Isolation Policy in the US and Japan: Science, Policy Changes, and the Garbage Can Model," *BMC International Health and Human Rights* 5, no. 1 (2005): 5.
65 LDH, Leprosy Annual Report.
66 Brian H. Bennett, David L. Parker, and Mark Robson, "Leprosy: Steps along the Journey of Eradication," *Public Health Reports* 123, no. 2 (2008): 198.
67 https://www.who.int/en/news-room/fact-sheets/detail/leprosy. Accessed December 17, 2021.

68   P. Narasimha Rao and Sujai Suneetha, "Current Situation of Leprosy in India and Its Future Implications," *Indian Dermatology Online Journal* 9, no. 2 (2018): 83–9.

69   Vidyadhar R. Sardesai, "Leprosy Elimination: A Myth or Reality," *Journal of Neurosciences in Rural Practice* 6, no. 2 (2015): 137.

Chapter 5: The Early Middle Ages

1   Isidore of Seville, *Etymologies: The Complete English Translation of Isidori Hispalensis Episcopi Etymologiarum Sive Originum*, vol. 20, trans. Priscilla Throop (Charlotte, VT: MedievalMS, 2013), xi.

2   Dirckx, *Isidore of Seville*, 581.

3   Isidore of Seville, *Etymologies*, IV.1.1.

4   Isidore of Seville, *Etymologies*, IV.3.1–2.

5   Isidore of Seville, *Etymologies*, IV.4.1.

6   Isidore of Seville, *Etymologies*, IV.6.17.

7   Isidore of Seville, *Etymologies*, XI.1.28 and XI.1.78–80. Throop questioned Isidore's accuracy with these particular etymologies.

8   Connor, *Book of Skin*, 11.

9   Isidore of Seville, *Etymologies*, I.VIII.1–23.

10   Faith Wallis, *Medieval Medicine: A Reader* (Toronto: University of Toronto Press, 2010), 3.

11   Alain Touwaide, "Ravenna," in *Medieval Science, Technology, and Medicine: An Encyclopedia*, eds. Thomas F. Glick, Steven J. Livesey, and Faith Wallis (London: Routledge, 2005), 433.

12   Violet Moller, *Map of Knowledge: A Thousand-Year History of How Classical Ideas Were Lost and Found* (New York, NY: Anchor, 2020), 176.

13   Vivian Nutton, "From Galen to Alexander: Aspects of Medicine and Medical Practice in Late Antiquity," *Dumbarton Oaks Papers* 38 (1984): 2.

14   Wallis, *Medieval Medicine*, 1.

15   Porter, *Greatest Benefit*, 89.

16   Gregory Tsoucalas, Markos Sgantzos, "Oribasius—Pediatric Skin Eruptions and the Origins of the Allergic Reaction to Breast Milk," *JAMA Dermatology* 153, no. 4 (2017): 303.

17   Oribasius, "Books to Eunapius, 4.53.t," as quoted in Laurence Totelin, *Concocting History* (blog), https://ancientrecipes.wordpress.com/2013/11/06/let-the-sun-shine.

18   John Lascaratos, Christos Liapis, and Maria Kouvaraki, "Surgery on Varices in Byzantine Times (1324–1453 CE)," *Journal of Vascular Surgery* 33, no. 1 (January 2001): 197–201.

19   Niki Papavramidou, Anthony Karpouzis, and Thespis Demetriou, "Aetius's Reports on Genital Warts," *JAMA Dermatology* 149, no. 9 (2013): 1118.

20   Robert N.R. Grant, "The History of Acne," *Proceedings of the Royal Society of Medicine* 44, no. 8 (1951): 647–649.

21   John Scarborough, "The Life and Times of Alexander of Tralles," *Expedition Magazine* 39, no. 2 (1997): 53–54.

22   Scarborough, "Alexander of Tralles," 55–60.

23   Prioreschi, *Primitive and Ancient Medicine*, 58.

24   Goodman, *Notable Contributors*, 30.

25   Porter, *Greatest Benefit*, 89–90.

26   Porter, *Greatest Benefit*, 90.

27   Paulus Aegineta, *The Seven Books of Paulus Ægineta*, trans. Francis Adams (London: Sydenham Society, 1844).

28   Paulus Aegineta, *Seven Books*, Book 4, 1.

29   Paulus Aegineta, *Seven Books*, Book 4, 15.

30   Paulus Aegineta, *Seven Books*, Book 4, 30.

31   Paulus Aegineta, *Seven Books*, Book 4, 46.

32   Paulus Aegineta, *Seven Books*, Book 4, 51.

33   Paulus Aegineta, *Seven Books*, Book 4, 65.

34   Paulus Aegineta, *Seven Books*, Book 4, 59.

35   Paulus Aegineta, *Seven Books*, Book 4, 75.

36 Paulus Aegineta, *Seven Books*, Book 4, 79.

37 Paulus Aegineta, *Seven Books*, Book 4, 114.

38 Paulus Aegineta, *Seven Books*, Book 4, 139.

39 Paulus Aegineta, *Seven Books*, Book 4, 150.

40 Nikolaos G. Stavrianeas, Eugenia Toumbis Ioannou, and Faidon-Marios Laskaratos, "Constantine the Great and Leprosy: Fact or Fiction?" *Clinical Dermatology* 27, no. 1 (January–February 2009): 139–141.

41 Rosa M. Díaz Díaz, Tatiana Sánz Sánchez, Maria Martín de Santa Olalla Y Llanes, "Dermatologic Conditions of Eminent Historical Figures," *Actas Dermosifiliogr* (English ed.) 112, no. 4 (April 2021): 354.

42 Eileen Huckbody, "Dermatology throughout the Dark Ages," *International Journal of Dermatology* 19, no. 6 (1980): 345.

43 Robert Mory, David Mindell, and David Bloom, "The Leech and the Physician: Biology, Etymology, and Medical Practice with *Hirudinea medicinalis*," *World Journal of Surgery* 24, no. 7 (2000): 878. It is possible that the word *lǣċe* was originally derived from the Latin, *legere* (to collect or gather, or later, to speak or teach, as in lecture). Interestingly, there is no etymological evidence that the word for leech was the word for doctor because doctors used leeches therapeutically.

44 Thomas O. Cockayne, *Leechdoms, Wortcunning, and Starcraft of Early England: Being a Collection of Documents, for the Most Part Never Before Printed; Illustrating the History of Science in This Country before the Norman Quest (1864–1866)* (London: Longman, Green, Volume 1, 1864; Volume 2, 1865; Vol. 3, 1866), Volume II, 298.

45 Malcolm L. Cameron, *Anglo-Saxon Medicine* (Cambridge: Cambridge University Press, 1993), 35, 47.

46 Godfrid Storms, *Anglo-Saxon Magic* (Dordrecht: Springer, 1948), 15.

47 Vivian Nutton, "Medicine in Late Antiquity and the Early Middle Ages," in *The Western Medical Tradition: 800 BC to AD 1800* (Cambridge: Cambridge University Press, 1995), 86.

48 Cameron, *Anglo-Saxon Medicine*, 129.

49 Cockayne, *Leechdoms* vol. 1, 39.

50 Cockayne, *Leechdoms* vol. 1, 71.

51 Storms, *Anglo-Saxon Magic* 1, 164.

52 Cockayne, *Leechdoms* vol. 1, 77.

53 Cockayne, *Leechdoms* vol. 1, 107.

54 Cockayne, *Leechdoms* vol. 1, 323 and 337.

55 Felix Grendon, "Charm B-5," *The Anglo-Saxon Charms* (New York, NY: Columbia University Press, 1909), Charm B-5, 195 (Leechbook III.63).

56 Karen Louise Jolly, *Popular Religion in Late Saxon England: Elf Charms in Context* (Chapel Hill, NC: University of North Carolina Press, 2015), 134.

57 Cockayne, *Leechdoms* vol. 3, 343.

58 Cockayne, *Leechdoms* vol. 3, 13.

59 Grendon, "Charm A-9," *Anglo-Saxon Charms*, 171.

60 Cockayne, *Leechdoms*, vol. 1, 35.

61 Freya Harrison et al., "A 1,000-Year-Old Antimicrobial Remedy with Antistaphylococcal Activity," *mBio* 6, no. 4 (2015): e1129.

62 Amanda L. Fuchs et al., "Characterization of the Antibacterial Activity of Bald's Eyesalve against Drug-Resistant *Staphylococcus aureus* and *Pseudomonas aeruginosa*," *PLoS One* 13, no. 11 (2018): 1.

63 Jessica Furner-Pardoe et al., "Anti-Biofilm Efficacy of a Medieval Treatment for Bacterial Infection Requires the Combination of Multiple Ingredients," *Scientific Reports* 10, no. 1 (2020): 1.

64 Liang Jian-Hui et al. *A Handbook of Traditional Chinese Dermatology*, trans. Bob Flaws and Ting-Liang Zhang (Boulder, CO: Blue Poppy Press, 1993), 1.

65 Jian-Hui, *Chinese Dermatology*, 1.

66 Jian-Hui, *Chinese Dermatology*, 1–2.

67 Hu Chuan-Kui, Fang Da-Ding, and Ye Gan-Yun, "Some Sketches on the History of Chinese Dermatology," *Archives of Dermatological Research* 272, nos. 1–2 (1982): 186.

68 Hopkins, *The Greatest Killer*, 18.

69 Arthur Boylston, "The Origins of Inoculation," *Journal of the Royal Society of Medicine* 105, no. 7 (2012): 311.

70 Boylston, *Origins of Inoculation*, 312.
71 Jully Mudang, Anuja E. George, Smitha Varghese, "Major Contributions to Dermatology from India," *Journal of Skin and Sexually Transmitted Diseases* 2, no. 2 (2020): 79.
72 Mudang, George, Varghese, *Major Contributions to Dermatology from India*, 79.
73 Mudang, George, Varghese, *Major Contributions to Dermatology from India*, 79–80.
74 Hopkins, *The Greatest Killer*, 17.

Chapter 6: The Islamic Golden Age

1 Porter, *Greatest Benefit*, 95.
2 Porter, *Greatest Benefit*, 102.
3 Thérèse-Anne Druart, "Al-Razi," in *Medieval Science, Technology, and Medicine: An Encyclopedia*, eds. Thomas F. Glick, Steven J. Livesey, and Faith Wallis (London: Routledge, 2005), 434.
4 Porter, *Greatest Benefit*, 97.
5 Leslie Marquis, "Arabian Contributors to Dermatology," *International Journal of Dermatology* 24, no. 1 (January–February 1985), 62.
6 Marquis, *Arabian Contributors*, 62.
7 Marquis, *Arabian Contributors*, 62.
8 Jacob Primley, "Ibn Sina," in *Medieval Science, Technology, and Medicine: An Encyclopedia*, eds. Thomas F. Glick, Steven J. Livesey, and Faith Wallis (London: Routledge, 2006), 257.
9 Avicenna, *A Treatise on the Canon of Medicine*, trans. Oscar C. Gruner (Birmingham, AL: Classics of Medicine Library, 1984), 239.
10 Avicenna, *Canon of Medicine*, 265.
11 Avicenna, *Canon of Medicine*, 423.
12 Avicenna, *Canon of Medicine*, 427.
13 Avicenna, *Canon of Medicine*, 431.
14 Avicenna, *Canon of Medicine*, 438.
15 Avicenna, *Canon of Medicine*, 439.
16 Avicenna, *Canon of Medicine*, 487.
17 Avicenna, *Canon of Medicine*, 490–491.
18 Primley, *Ibn Sina*, 62.
19 Avicenna, *Canon of Medicine*, 803.
20 Avicenna, *Treatise on the Canon of Medicine*, 806.
21 Avicenna, *Canon of Medicine*, 843.
22 Huckbody, *Dermatology throughout the Dark Ages*, 346.
23 Primley, *Ibn Sina*, 62.
24 Goodman, *Notable Contributors*, 41.
25 David I. Grove, *Tapeworms, Lice, and Prions: A Compendium of Unpleasant Infections* (Oxford: Oxford University Press, 2014), 72.
26 Jorge Romaní, Xavier Sierra, and Andrew Casson, "Dermatologic Diseases in 8 of the Cantigas of Holy Mary of Alfonso X the Learned, Part 2: Genital Mutilation, Scrofuloderma, Scabies, Erysipelas, and the Ailments of the King," *Actas Dermo-Sifiliograficas* 107, no. 8 (October 2016), 664.
27 Alfonso X, *Songs of Holy Mary of Alfonso X, the Wise: A Translation of the Cantigas de Santa María*, trans. Kathleen Kulp-Hill (Tempe, AZ: Arizona Center for Medieval and Renaissance Studies, 2000), 269–270.
28 Moses Maimonides, *The Medical Aphorisms of Moses Maimonides: Translated and Edited by Fred Rosner and Suessman Muntner* (New York, NY: Yeshiva University Press, 1971), vol. I, 66.
29 Maimonides, *Medical Aphorisms*, vol. 1, 67.
30 Maimonides, *Medical Aphorisms*, vol. 1, 81.
31 Maimonides, *Medical Aphorisms*, vol. 1, 77.
32 Maimonides, *Medical Aphorisms*, vol. 1, 192.
33 Maimonides, *Medical Aphorisms*, vol. 2, 17.
34 Maimonides, *Medical Aphorisms*, vol. 2, 20.
35 Maimonides, Medical Aphorisms, vol. 2, 29.

Chapter 7: The Medieval West

1 William Manchester, *A World Lit Only by Fire* (New York, NY: Sterling, 2014), 2.
2 Wallis, *Medieval Medicine*, 73.
3 Jürgen Leonhardt and Kenneth Kronenberg. *Latin: Story of a World Language* (Cambridge, MA: The Belknap Press of Harvard University Press, 2016), 94.
4 Harris, William. *Ancient Literacy* (Cambridge, MA: Harvard University Press, 1989), 267.
5 Eltjo Buringh, *Medieval Manuscript Production in the Latin West: Explorations with a Global Database* (Leiden: Brill, 2011), 291.
6 Leonhardt and Kronenberg, *Latin*, 122.
7 Meg Leja, "The Sacred Art: Medicine in the Carolingian Renaissance," *Viator* 47 (2016): 1.
8 Leja, *Sacred Art*, 2–3.
9 Wallis, *Medieval Medicine*, 73–74.
10 Wallis, *Medieval Medicine*, 73–74.
11 Wallis, *Medieval Medicine*, 94.
12 Meg Leja, "The Sacred Art: Medicine in the Carolingian Renaissance," *Viator* 47 (2016): 1–34.
13 Leja, *Sacred Art*, 6–16 ; (quote) Alcuin, Carmen XXVI, ed. E. Dümmler, MGH Poetae Latini Aevi Carolini 1 (Berlin 1881). Eng. trans. Peter Godman, Poetry of the Carolingian Renaissance (London 1985). 118–119.
14 Francois Retief & Louise Cilliers, "The Evolution of Hospitals from Antiquity to the Renaissance," *Acta Theologica* 26, no. 2 (2010): 224.
15 Leja, *Sacred Art*, 28–33.
16 Wallis, *Medieval Medicine*, 47.
17 Michael H. Shank, "That the Medieval Christian Church Suppressed the Growth of Science," in *Galileo Goes to Jail and Other Myths about Science and Religion*, ed. Ronald L. Numbers (Cambridge, MA: Harvard University Press, 2010), 20.
18 David C Lindberg, *Science in the Middle Ages* (Chicago: University of Chicago Press, 1978), 16.
19 Shank, *Medieval Christian Church*, 21–22.
20 Shank, *Medieval Christian Church*, 25–26.
21 Katharine Park, "That the Medieval Church Prohibited Dissection in Numbers," in *Galileo Goes to Jail and Other Myths about Science and Religion*, ed. Ronald L. Numbers (Cambridge, MA: Harvard University Press, 2010), 43.
22 Park, *Medieval Church*, 45–46.
23 Park, *Medieval Church*, 45–46.
24 Ghosh, *Human Cadaveric Dissection*, 154.
25 Moller, *Map of Knowledge*, 216.
26 Moller, *Map of Knowledge*, 137.
27 Moller, *Map of Knowledge*, 137–138.
28 Nicholas Ostler, *Ad Infinitum: A Biography of Latin* (New York, NY: Walker Books, 2009), 211.
29 Jack Hartnell, *Medieval Bodies: Life, Death and Art in the Middle Ages* (London: Profile Books Ltd, 2019), 19.
30 Michael Shank, "Universities," in *Medieval Science, Technology, and Medicine: An Encyclopedia*, ed. Thomas F. Glick, Steven J. Livesey, and Faith Wallis (London: Routledge, 2005), 495.
31 Moller, *Map of Knowledge*, 170.
32 Armstrong, Dorsey, *The Medieval World* (transcript) (Chantilly, VA: Teaching Company, 2009), 48.
33 Moller, *Map of Knowledge*, 169–170.
34 Moller, *Map of Knowledge*, 180.
35 Moller, *Map of Knowledge*, 194.
36 Georges Androutsos, "Theophilus Protospatharius: Byzantine Forerunner of Urology," *Histoire des sciences medicales* 41, no. 1 (Jan.–Mar. 2007): 41.
37 Wallis, *Medieval Medicine*, 129, 131.
38 Ghosh, *Human Cadaveric Dissection*, 154.
39 Park, *Medieval Church*, 46.
40 Brenda Gardenour, "Hospitals," in *Medieval Science, Technology, and Medicine: An Encyclopedia*, ed. Thomas F. Glick, Steven J. Livesey, and Faith Wallis (London: Routledge, 2005), 226.

41 Gardenour, *Hospitals*, 226.

42 Toni Mount, *Medieval Medicine: Its Mysteries and Science* (Stroud, Gloucestershire: Amberley, 2016), 89.

43 Mount, *Medieval Medicine*, 90.

44 Mount, *Medieval Medicine*, 91.

45 Mount, *Medieval Medicine*, 86.

46 Mount, *Medieval Medicine*, 12.

47 Porter, *Greatest Benefit*, 119.

48 Porter, *Greatest Benefit*, 119.

49 William Manchester, *A World Lit Only by Fire: The Medieval Mind and the Renaissance – Portrait of an Age* (United States: Little, Brown, 2009), 55.

50 Katherine Ashenburg, *The Dirt on Clean: An Unsanitized History* (New York, NY: North Point, 2008), 54.

51 Jerome, *The Principal Works of St. Jerome*. ed. Philip Schaff, trans. W.H. Freemantle (New York, NY: Christian Literature Publishing, 1892). Letter XIV to Heliodorus, 10.

52 Connor, *Book of Skin*, 23.

53 Connor, *Book of Skin*, 22.

54 Paul B Newman, *Daily Life in the Middle Ages* (United States: McFarland, 2018), 152.

55 Connor, *Book of Skin*, 21.

56 Hartnell, *Medieval Bodies*, 90.

57 Marcia Ramos-e-Silva, "Saint Hildegard von Bingen (1098–1179): 'The Light of Her People and of Her Time,'" *International Journal of Dermatology* 38, no. 4 (1999): 315.

58 Katherine Foxhall, "Making Modern Migraine Medieval: Men of Science, Hildegard of Bingen and the Life of a Retrospective Diagnosis," *Medical History* 58, no. 3 (2014): 354.

59 Hildegard, *Causes and Cures: The Complete English Translation of Hildegard's "Causae et Curae Libri VI*," trans. Priscilla Throop (Charlotte, VT: MedievalMS, 2008); Hildegard, *Hildegard Von Bingen's "Physica": The Complete Translation of Her Classic Work on Health and Healing*, trans. Priscilla Throop (Rochester, VT: Healing Arts, 1998), 1998.

60 J. Romaní and M. Romaní, "Causes and Cures of Skin Diseases in the Work of Hildegard of Bingen," *Actas Dermo-Sifiliograficas* 108, no. 6 (July–Aug. 2017): 540.

61 Romaní and Romaní, *Skin Diseases in the Work of Hildegard of Bingen*, 3.

62 Hildegard, *Causes and Cures*, 126.

63 Hildegard, *Causes and Cures*, 128.

64 Hildegard, *Causes and Cures*, 130–131.

65 Hildegard, *Physica*, 62.

66 Hildegard, *Physica*, 162.

67 Hildegard, *Physica*, 42.

68 Porter, *Greatest Benefit*, 129.

69 Maurizio Bifulco, Domenico De Falco, Rita P. Aquino, and Simona Pisanti, "Trotula De Ruggiero: The Magister Mulier Sapiens and Her Medical Dermatology Treatises," *Journal of Cosmetic Dermatology* 18, no. 6 (Dec. 2019): 1613.

70 Bifulco, De Falco, Aquino, and Pisanti, *Trotula De Ruggiero*, 1614.

71 Monica Helen Green, *The Trotula: A Medieval Compendium of Women's Medicine* (Philadelphia, PA: University of Pennsylvania Press, 2001), 50–51.

72 Bifulco, De Falco, Aquino, and Pisanti, *Trotula De Ruggiero*, 1614.

73 Green, *Trotula*, 99.

74 Green, *Trotula*, 101.

75 Green, *Trotula*, 102.

76 Green, *Trotula*, 107.

77 Pusey, *History of Dermatology*, 37.

78 Henry E. Michelson, "The History of Lupus Vulgaris," *Journal of Investigative Dermatology* 7, no. 5 (1946): 261.

79 Teodorico Borgognoni, *The Surgery of Theodoric*, vol. 1 (New York, NY: Appleton-Century-Crofts, 1955), XL.

80 Jeffrey A. Freiberg, "The Mythos of Laudable Pus along with an Explanation for its Origin," *Journal of Community Hospital Internal Medicine Perspective* 7, no. 3 (2017): 196–198.

81 Geoffrey Chaucer, "The General Prologue," *The Canterbury* Tales in *The Broadview Anthology of British Literature Volume 1: The Medieval Period,* Third Edition (United Kingdom: Broadview Press, 2014), 438 (lines 429–434).

82 Huckbody, *Dermatology throughout the Dark Ages*, 346.

83 Henry Handerson, *Gilbertus Anglicus: Medicine of the 13th Century* (Cleveland, OH, Cleveland Medical Library Association, 1918), 30.

84 Handerson, *Gilbertus Anglicus*, 30.

85 Handerson, *Gilbertus Anglicus*, 31.

86 Handerson, *Gilbertus Anglicus*, 31.

87 Handerson, *Gilbertus Anglicus*, 31.

88 Handerson, *Gilbertus Anglicus*, 31–32.

89 Antonio Perciaccante et al., "Scabies Outbreak in the 14th Century: Clues from Correspondence between Poets," *American Journal of Medicine* 129, no. 10 (Oct. 2016): 1136.

90 Perciaccante, *Scabies Outbreak*, 1136.

91 Perciaccante, *Scabies Outbreak*, 1136.

92 Perciaccante, *Scabies Outbreak*, 1136.

93 Hartnell, *Medieval Bodies*, 83.

94 Sanjib K. Ghosh, "Henri de Mondeville (1260–1320): Medieval French Anatomist and Surgeon," *European Journal of Anatomy* 19, no. 3 (2015), 313.

95 Henri De Mondeville, *The Surgery of Master Henri De Mondeville,* trans. by Leonard Rosenman, MD (Bloomington, ID: Xlibris, 2003), 728–729.

96 Mondeville, *Surgery*, 749.

97 Mondeville, *Surgery*, 749.

98 Mondeville, *Surgery*, 755.

99 Mondeville, *Surgery*, 766.

100 Mondeville, *Surgery*, 766.

101 Mondeville, *Surgery*, 767.

102 Pusey, *History of Dermatology*, 39.

103 Mondeville, *Surgery*, 770.

104 Mondeville, *Surgery*, 869.

105 Guy de Chauliac, *The Major Surgery of Guy De Chauliac Surgeon and Master in Medicine of the University of Montpellier,* trans. by Leonard Rosenman, MD (Bloomington, ID: Xlibris, 2007), 90.

106 Chauliac, *Major Surgery*, 44.

107 Chauliac, *Major Surgery*, 139.

108 Chauliac, *Major Surgery*, 188–189.

109 Chauliac, *Major Surgery*, 451.

110 Chauliac, *Major Surgery*, 452.

111 Chauliac, *Major Surgery*, 458–465.

112 Chauliac, *Major Surgery*, 465.

113 Chauliac, *Major Surgery*, 484.

114 Chauliac, *Major Surgery*, 493.

115 Chauliac, *Major Surgery*, 493.

Chapter 8: The Renaissance

1 Porter, *Greatest Benefit*, 170.

2 Jon Arrizabalaga et al., *The Great Pox: The French Disease in Renaissance Europe* (New Haven, CT: Yale University Press, 1997), 62–66.

3 Porter, *Greatest Benefit*, 171.

4 Anthony C. Grayling, *The Age of Genius: The Seventeenth Century and the Birth of the Modern Mind* (New York: Bloomsbury, 2016), 161.

5 Crissey and Parish, *Dermatology and Syphilology*, 7.

6 Grayling, *Age of Genius*, 159–162.

7 Porter, *Greatest Benefit*, 176.

8   Leonardo Da Vinci, *Leonardo Da Vinci's Note-Books*, comp. and trans. Edward McCurdy (New York, NY: Empire State, 1923), 78.

9   Jonathan Jones, "The Real Da Vinci Code," *Guardian*, August 30, 2006.

10 Porter, *Greatest Benefit*, 171.

11 Strathern, *A Brief History of Medicine*, 92.

12 Charles D. O'Malley, *Andreas Vesalius of Brussels, 1514-1564* (Berkeley: University of California Press, 1964), 250.

13 Charles Ambrose, "Andreas Vesalius (1514–1564)—An Unfinished Life," *Acta Medico-Historica Adriatica* 12 (December 2014): 228.

14 Bynum, *History of Medicine*, 31.

15 Ahmadreza Afshar, David P. Steensma, and Robert A. Kyle, "Andreas Vesalius and *De Fabrica*," *Mayo Clinic Proceedings* 94, no. 5 (May 2019): e67; Andreas Vesalius, *The Fabric of the Human Body* (Basel: Karger, 2014).

16 Vesalius, *Fabric of the Human Body*, 471–473.

17 Vesalius, *Fabric of the Human Body*, 473.

18 Joan Lane, *A Social History of Medicine: Health, Healing and Disease in England, 1750–1950* (Taylor & Francis, 2012), 169.

19 Richard Hollingham, *Blood and Guts: A History of Surgery* (New York, NY: Thomas Dunne, 2008), 58.

20 Hollingham, *Blood and Guts*, 101.

21 Ambroise Pare, *The Collected Works of Ambroise Pare*, trans. Thomas Johnson (1634; Pound Ridge, NY: Milford House, 1968), 88–89.

22 Pare, *Collected Works*.

23 Alexander Chalmers, *General Biographical Dictionary*, vol. 14 (London: Nichols, 1814), 216.

24 R. Shane Tubbs, "Anatomy Is to Physiology as Geography Is to History; It Describes the Theatre of Events," *Clinical Anatomy* 28 (2015): 151.

25 G. Rickey Welch, "In Retrospect: Fernel's Physiologia," *Nature* 456, no. 7221 (2008): 446.

26 John M. Forrester and John Henry, "The Physiologia of Jean Fernel (1567)," *Transactions of the American Philosophical Society* 93, no. 1 (2003): 1–2.

27 Forrester and Henry, *Physiologia*, 5.

28 Forrester and Henry, *Physiologia*, 174.

29 Forrester and Henry, *Physiologia*, 149–151.

30 Hannah Murphy, "Skin and Disease in Early Modern Medicine: Jan Jessen's *De Cute, et Cutaneis Affectibus* (1601)," *Bulletin of the History of Medicine* 94, no. 2 (2020), 190.

31 Francesco Cappello, Aldo Gerbino, and Giovanni Zummo, "Giovanni Filippo Ingrassia: A Five-Hundred Year-Long Lesson," *Clinical Anatomy* 23, no. 7 (October 2010): 743.

32 Pusey, *History of Dermatology*, 35, Goodman, *Notable Contributors*, 65, 67.

33 I. Velenciuc et al., "A Renaissance Promoter of Modern Surgery," *Revista Medico-Chirurgicala a Societatii de Medici si Naturalisti din Iasi* 120, no. 1 (2016): 201.

34 Goodman, *Notable Contributors*, 65.

35 Juliana Hill Cotton, "Manardo, Giovanni," in *Dictionary of Scientific Biography*, vol. 9 (New York, NY: Scribners, 1974), 74–75.

36 Goodman, *Notable Contributors*, 68.

37 Michel Angelo Biondo, *M. Angelus Blondus, De Cognitione Hominis Per Aspectum, Etc.* (Rome: Senatus venetiarum privilegio, 1544), 27–29.

38 Pusey, *History of Dermatology*, 43.

39 Filippo Pesapane, Antonella Coggi, and Raffaele Gianotti, "Two Important Italian Scientists of the Renaissance and the First Book Ever Devoted to Nevi," *JAMA Dermatology* 150, no. 7 (2014), 737.

40 Pieter van Foreest, *Observationum et Curationum Medicinalium, Sive Medicinae Theoricae et Practicae Libri XXX, XXXI, et XXXII: De Venenis, Fucis & Lue Venera* (Nuremberg: Wolfgang and Johann Endter, 1676), 52–64.

41 Sutton, *Sixteenth Century Physician and His Methods*, xxviii.

42 Nancy G. Siraisi, "History, Antiquarianism, and Medicine: The Case of Girolamo Mercuriale," *Journal of the History of Ideas* 64, no. 2 (2003): 250.

43 Siraisi, *History, Antiquarianism, and Medicine*, 250.

44 Sutton, *Sixteenth Century Physician and His Methods*, xxviii.

45 Alberto Sanchez-Garcia and Elena Garcia-Vilarino, "Historic Research about the First Dermatology Book and Its Author, Hieronymus Mercurialis," *Indian Dermatology Online Journal* 10, no. 2 (March–April 2019): 212–213.

46 Joseph B. Byrne, *Encyclopedia of the Black Death* (Santa Barbara, CA: ABC-CLIO, 2012), 233–234.

47 Sanchez-Garcia and Garcia-Vilarino, *First Dermatology Book*, 213.

48 Sutton, *Sixteenth Century Physician and His Methods*, 6.

49 Richard L. Sutton Jr., *Sixteenth Century Physician and His Methods: Mercurialis on Diseases of the Skin, the First Book on the Subject* (Kansas City, MO: Lowell Press, 1986).

50 Sutton, *Sixteenth Century Physician*, xxxi.

51 Sutton, *Sixteenth Century Physician*, 5.

52 Sutton, *Sixteenth Century Physician*, 11.

53 Sutton, *Sixteenth Century Physician*, 12.

54 Sutton, *Sixteenth Century Physician*, 13.

55 Sutton, *Sixteenth Century Physician*, 15.

56 Sutton, *Sixteenth Century Physician*, 21.

57 Sutton, *Sixteenth Century Physician*, 28.

58 Sutton, *Sixteenth Century Physician*, 33.

59 Sutton, *Sixteenth Century Physician*, 36.

60 Sutton, *Sixteenth Century Physician*, 36.

61 Sutton, *Sixteenth Century Physician*, 38.

62 Sutton, *Sixteenth Century Physician*, 43.

63 Sutton, *Sixteenth Century Physician*, 44–47.

64 Sutton, *Sixteenth Century Physician*, 51–53.

65 Sutton, *Sixteenth Century Physician*, 53–54.

66 Sutton, *Sixteenth Century Physician*, 54.

67 Sutton, *Sixteenth Century Physician*, 54.

68 Sutton, *Sixteenth Century Physician*, 59.

69 Sutton, *Sixteenth Century Physician*, 62.

70 Sutton, *Sixteenth Century Physician*, 63.

71 Sutton, *Sixteenth Century Physician*, 66.

72 Sutton, *Sixteenth Century Physician*, 68–69.

73 Sutton, *Sixteenth Century Physician*, 78.

74 Sutton, *Sixteenth Century Physician*, 77.

75 Sutton, *Sixteenth Century Physician*, 78.

76 Sutton, *Sixteenth Century Physician*, 80.

77 Sutton, *Sixteenth Century Physician*, 95.

78 Sutton, *Sixteenth Century Physician*, 91, 94.

79 Sutton, *Sixteenth Century Physician*, 93.

80 Sutton, *Sixteenth Century Physician*, 98.

81 Sutton, *Sixteenth Century Physician*, 101.

82 Sutton, *Sixteenth Century Physician*, 104.

83 Sutton, *Sixteenth Century Physician*, 105.

84 Sutton, *Sixteenth Century Physician*, 107.

85 Sutton, *Sixteenth Century Physician*, 109.

86 Sutton, *Sixteenth Century Physician*, 110.

87 Sutton, *Sixteenth Century Physician*, 114–115.

88 Sutton, *Sixteenth Century Physician*, 115.

89 Sutton, *Sixteenth Century Physician*, 121.

90 Dante, "Inferno," *The Divine Comedy of Dante Alighieri*, trans. Henry Wadsworth Longfellow (Cambridge, UK: Riverside Press, 1886), XXIX.70–90, p. 151–152.

91 Sutton, *Sixteenth Century Physician*, 122.

92 Sutton, *Sixteenth Century Physician*, 122, 123.

93 Sutton, *Sixteenth Century Physician*, 125.

94 Sutton, *Sixteenth Century Physician*, 128.

95 Sutton, *Sixteenth Century Physician*, 128.

96 Sutton, *Sixteenth Century Physician*, 128.

97 The subtitle, "Non solum Medicis et Philosophis; verum etiam omnium disciplinarum studiosis apprime utilis," translates as "Not only for doctors and philosophers; especially useful for students of truly all disciplines."

98 Mercuriale, Girolamo, Mancinus, Julius, *De Decoratione Liber* (Venice: Iuntas, 1601), 32. Translated by the author and Dr. Althea Ashe.

99 Nils Krueger et al., "The History of Aesthetic Medicine and Surgery," *Journal of Drugs Dermatology* 12, no. 7 (July 2013): 737.

100 Murphy, *Skin and Disease*, 208.

101 Murphy, *Skin and Disease*, 208.

102 Murphy, *Skin and Disease*, 209.

103 Murphy, *Skin and Disease*, 212.

104 Murphy, *Skin and Disease*, 209.

105 Murphy, *Skin and Disease*, 212.

106 Murphy, *Skin and Disease*, 182–183.

Interlude 2: The Black Death and Other Pandemics

1   Robert J. Littman, "The Plague of Athens: Epidemiology and Paleopathology," *Mount Sinai Medical Journal* 76, no. 5 (Oct. 2009): 456.

2   Charles Collier, *The History of the Plague of Athens: Translated from Thucydides: With Remarks Explanatory of Its Pathology* (London: David Nutt, 1857): 23–26.

3   Burke A. Cunha, "The Cause of the Plague of Athens: Plague, Typhoid, Typhus, Smallpox, or Measles?" *Infectious Disease Clinics of North America* 18, no. 1 (Mar. 2004): 29–43.

4   Manolis J. Papagrigorakis et al., "DNA Examination of Ancient Dental Pulp Incriminates Typhoid Fever as a Probable Cause of the Plague of Athens," *International Journal of Infectious Diseases* 10, no. 3 (2006): 204; Beth Shapiro et al., "No Proof That Typhoid Caused the Plague of Athens (a Reply to Papagrigorakis et al.)," *International Journal of Infectious Diseases* 10, no. 4 (2006): 334.

5   Patrick E. Olson et al., "The Thucydides Syndrome: Ebola déjà Vu? (or Ebola Reemergent?)," *Emerging Infectious Diseases* 2, no. 2 (1996): 155–156.

6   George C. Kohn, *Encyclopedia of Plague & Pestilence* (New York, NY: Facts on File, 2007): 57.

7   Kyle Harper, *The Fate of Rome: Climate, Disease, and the End of an Empire* (Princeton, NJ: Princeton University Press, 2019): 104.

8   Harper, *The Fate of Rome*, 115.

9   Harper, *The Fate of Rome*, 115–116.

10 Harper, *The Fate of Rome*, 136.

11 Harper, *The Fate of Rome*, 137.

12 Harper, *The Fate of Rome*, 141.

13 Kohn, *Encyclopedia*, 74.

14 William Hardy McNeill, *Plagues and Peoples* (New York, NY: Anchor Books, 1998): 132.

15 Ariane Düx et al., "Measles Virus and Rinderpest Virus Divergence Dated to the Sixth Century BCE," *Science* 368, no. 6497 (Jun. 2020): 1367.

16 Harper, *The Fate of Rome*, 141–144.

17 World Health Organization news release, "Measles Cases Spike Globally Due to Gaps in Vaccination Coverage [Internet]," *World Health Organization News Room* (2018). https://www.who.int/news-room/detail/29-11-2018-measles-cases-spike-globally-due-to-gaps-in-vaccination-coverage.

18 Lee Mordechai et al., "The Justinianic Plague: An Inconsequential Pandemic?" *Proceedings of the National Academy Science* 116, no. 51 (2019): 25546.

19 Kohn, *Encyclopedia*, 188.

20 David M. Wagner et al., "*Yersinia pestis* and the Plague of Justinian, 541–543 AD: A Genomic Analysis," *Lancet Infectious Diseases* 14, no. 4 (2014): 319.

21 Giovanna Morelli et al., "*Yersinia pestis* Genome Sequencing Identifies Patterns of Global Phylogenetic Diversity," *Nature Genetics* 42, no. 12 (2010): 1142; Simon Rasmussen, et al., "Early Divergent Strains of *Yersinia pestis* in Eurasia 5,000 Years Ago," *Cell* 163, no. 3 (2015): 571.

22 Nicolás Rascovan et al., "Emergence and Spread of Basal Lineages of *Yersinia pestis* during the Neolithic Decline," *Cell* 176, no. 1–2 (2019): 295.

23 John Mulhall, "Plague before the Pandemics: The Greek Medical Evidence for Bubonic Plague before the Sixth Century," *Bulletin of the History of Medicine* 93, no. 2 (2019): 161.

24 Mulhall, *Plague before the Pandemics*, 166.

25 Mulhall, *Plague before the Pandemics*, 174.

26 Mulhall, *Plague before the Pandemics*, 175.

27 Procopius, *History of the Wars*, 7 vols., trans. H.B. Dewing (Cambridge, MA: Harvard University Press, 1914): Vol. I, 451–473.

28 Procopius, *History of the Wars*, II, XXII.17.

29 Procopius, *History of the Wars*, II, XXII.28.

30 Procopius, *History of the Wars*, II, XXII.30–40.

31 George D. Sussman, "Was the Black Death in India and China?" *Bulletin of the History Medicine* 85, no. 3 (Fall 2011): 319.

32 Boris Velimirovic and Helga Velimirovic, "Plague in Vienna," *Reviews of Infectious Diseases* 11, no. 5 (Sep.–Oct. 1989): 812; Philip Ziegler, *The Black Death* (New York, NY: Harper Perennial Modern Classics, 2009): 17–18.

33 Ziegler, *Black Death*, 17–18.

34 Christopher J. Duncan and Susan Scott, "What Caused the Black Death?" *Postgraduate Medical Journal* 81, no. 955 (2005): 711–717.

35 Duncan and Scott, *What Caused the Black Death?* 317.

36 Duncan and Scott, *What Caused the Black Death?* 317.

37 Duncan and Scott, *What Caused the Black Death?* 317.

38 John Payne, *The Decameron of Giovanni Boccaccio* (London: The Villon Society, 1886): 5.

39 Chauliac, *Major Surgery*, 249.

40 Rosemary Horrox, *The Black Death* (Manchester, UK: Manchester University Press, 2007): 24.

41 Justus F.C. Hecker, *The Epidemics of the Middle Ages*, trans. Benjamin Babington (United Kingdom: n.p., 1844): 10.

42 Timothy S. Miller, "The Plague in John VI Cantacuzenus and Thucydides," *Greek, Roman and Byzantine Studies* 17 (1976): 391.

43 Thomas K. Welty et al., "Nineteen Cases of Plague in Arizona: A Spectrum including Ecthyma Gangrenosum Due to Plague and Plague in Pregnancy," *West Journal of Medicine* 142, no. 5 (1985): 641–646; Mahery Ratsitorahina et al., "Epidemiological and Diagnostic Aspects of the Outbreak of Pneumonic Plague in Madagascar," *Lancet* 355, no. 9198 (2000): 111–113.

44 Thomas Butler, "Plague Gives Surprises in the First Decade of the 21st Century in the United States and Worldwide," *American Journal of Tropical Medicine and Hygiene* 89, no. 4 (2013): 789.

45 Samuel K. Cohn, "The Black Death: End of a Paradigm," *American Historical Review* 107, no. 3 (2002): 715.

46 Cohn, *The Black Death*, 716.

47 Welty, *Nineteen Cases*, 645; Thomas Butler, "Yersinia Infections: Centennial of the Discovery of the Plague Bacillus," *Clinical Infectious Disease* 19, no. 4 (1994): 658.

48 Thomas Butler, "Plague Gives Surprises in the First Decade of the 21st Century in the United States and Worldwide," *American Journal of Tropical Medicine and Hygiene* 89, no. 4 (2013): 658.

49 Stephanie Haensch et al., "Distinct Clones of *Yersinia pestis* Caused the Black Death," *PLoS Pathogens* 6, no. 10 (2010): e1000134.

50 Katharine R. Dean et al., "Human Ectoparasites and Spread of Plague in Europe," *Proceedings of the National Academy of Sciences* 115, no. 6 (Feb. 2018): 1304.

51 Guy, *Major Surgery*, 250.

52 Horrox, *The Black Death*, 116.

53 Guy, *Major Surgery*, 250.

54 Horrox, *The Black Death*.

55 George Hudler, *Magical Mushrooms, Mischievous Molds* (Princeton, NJ: Princeton University Press, 1998): 73.

56 George Barger, *Ergot and Ergotism: A Monograph Based on the Dohme Lectures Delivered in Johns Hopkins University, Baltimore* (London: Gurney and Jackson, 1931): 44.

57 Henry S. Wellcome, *From Ergot to "Ernutin": An Historical Sketch* (London: Burroughs Wellcome, 1908): 22.

58 Wellcome, *From Ergot to "Ernutin,"* 24.

59 Wellcome, *From Ergot to "Ernutin,"* 24.

60 Wellcome, *From Ergot to "Ernutin,"* 33.

61 Wellcome, *From Ergot to "Ernutin,"* 25.

62 Wellcome, *From Ergot to "Ernutin,"* 29.

63 Albrecht Classen, *Bodily and Spiritual Hygiene in Medieval and Early Modern Literature: Explorations of Textual Presentations of Filth and Water* (Berlin: De Gruyter, 2017): 22.

64 Alessandra Foscati, *St. Anthony's Fire from Antiquity until the Eighteenth Century* (Amsterdam: Amsterdam University Press, 2020): 180–182.

65 Wellcome, *From Ergot to "Ernutin,"* 36.

66 Torbjørn Alm and Brita Elvevåg, "Ergotism in Norway. Part 1: The Symptoms and Their Interpretation from the Late Iron Age to the Seventeenth Century," *History of Psychiatry* 24, no. 1 (2013): 16–17.

67 Barger, *Ergot and Ergotism*, 57.

68 Alm and Elvevåg, *Ergotism in Norway*, 16.

69 Barger, *Ergot and Ergotism*, 43.

70 Mary Matossian, *Poisons of the Past: Morals, Epidemics, and History* (New Haven: Yale University Press, 1991): 59–66.

71 Kohn, *Encyclopedia*, 332.

72 Matossian, *Poisons*, 81–87.

73 Jonathan W. Silvertown and Amy Whitesides, *An Orchard Invisible: A Natural History of Seeds* (Chicago, IL: University of Chicago Press, 2010): 64.

74 Wellcome, *From Ergot to "Ernutin,"* 12; Paul L. Schiff, "Ergot and Its Alkaloids," *American Journal of Pharmaceutical Education* 70, no. 5 (2006): 1.

75 Wellcome, *From Ergot to "Ernutin,"* 12–13.

76 Schiff, *Ergot and Its Alkaloids*, 1.

77 Henry P. Albarelli Jr., *Terrible Mistake: The Murder of Frank Olson and the CIA's Secret Cold War Experiments* (Walterville, OR: Trine Day, 2009).

78 Robert E. Bartholomew et al., "Mass Psychogenic Illness and the Social Network: Is It Changing the Pattern of Outbreaks?" *Journal of the Royal Society of Medicine* 105, no. 12 (2012): 509.

79 Alessandra Foscati, *St. Anthony's Fire from Antiquity until the Eighteenth Century* (Amsterdam: Amsterdam University Press, 2020).

80 Í. Corral and C. Corral, "Neurological Considerations in the History of Tarantism in Spain," *Neurosciences and History* 4, no. 3 (2016): 100.

81 Stephen Storace, "A Genuine Letter from an Italian Gentleman Concerning the Bite of the Tarantula," *Gentleman's Magazine* 23 (Sep. 1753): 433–434.

82 Jean Fogo Russell, "Tarantism," *Medical History* 23, no. 4 (Oct. 1979): 409.

83 Russell, *Tarantism*, 409.

84 Russell, *Tarantism*, 409.

85 Russell, *Tarantism*, 422.

86 John Waller, "A Forgotten Plague: Making Sense of Dancing Mania," *Lancet* 373, no. 9664 (Feb. 2009): 624.

87 Kohn, *Encyclopedia*, 76.

88 Waller, *A Forgotten Plague*, 625.

89 Thiago C. Vale and Francisco Cardoso, "Chorea: A Journey through History," *Tremor and Other Hyperkinetic Movements* 5 (2015): 1–2.

90 Paul Heyman, Leopold Simons, and Christel Cochez, "Were the English Sweating Sickness and the Picardy Sweat Caused by Hantaviruses?" *Viruses* 6, no. 1 (2014): 152.

91 Kohn, *Encyclopedia*, 92.

92 Heyman, Simons, and Cochez, Were the English Sweating Sickness and the Picardy Sweat Caused by Hantaviruses? 158.

93 Eric Bridson, "The English 'Sweate' (*Sudor Anglicus*) and Hantavirus Pulmonary Syndrome," *British Journal of Biomedical Science* 58, no. 1 (2001): 1–6.

94 Warren R. Heymann, "The History of Syphilis," *Journal of the American Academy of Dermatology* 54, no. 2 (2006): 110. Outbreaks occurred in 1485, 1508, 1517, 1528, and 1551.

95 Kohn, *Encyclopedia*, 309.

96 Prosper Menière, "Epidemic Miliary Sweating Fever," *Boston Medical and Surgical Journal* 7, no. 23 (1833): 364.

97 Kohn, *Encyclopedia*, 267; Heyman, Simons, and Cochez, Were the English Sweating Sickness and the Picardy Sweat Caused by Hantaviruses? 151.

98 Jacob Kantor, "Plica Polonica: Confusion, Confabulation, and the Death of a Disease," *Archives of Dermatology* 148, no. 5 (2012): 633.

99 Eglė Sakalauskaitė-Juodeikienė, Dalius Jatužis, Saulius Kaubrys, "*Plica polonica*: From National Plague to Death of the Disease in the Nineteenth-Century Vilnius," *Indian Journal of Dermatology, Venereology, and Leprology* 84, no. 4 (Jul.–Aug. 2018): 4.

100 Avi Ohry and Nissim Ohana, "On Plica Polonica and the Forgotten Joseph Romain Louis Kerckhoffs (1789–1867)," *Progress in Health Sciences* 8, no 1 (2018): 211.

101 Kantor, *Plica Polonica*, 633.

102 P.N. Suresh Kumar and Velayudhan Rajmohan, "Plica Neuropathica (Polonica) in Schizophrenia," *Indian Journal of Psychiatry* 54, no. 3 (2012): 289.

103 Elias E. Mazokopakis and Christos G. Karagiannis, "Environmental and Medical Aspects Related to the Sixth Plague of Egypt," *Maedica* 14, no. 3 (2019): 310.

104 John Dirckx, "Virgil on Anthrax," *American Journal of Dermatopathology* 3, no. 2 (1981): 191–196.

105 Boris A. Revich and Marina A. Podolnaya, "Thawing of Permafrost May Disturb Historic Cattle Burial Grounds in East Siberia," *Global Health Action* 4 (2011): 1.

106 Esper G. Kallas et al., "Predictors of Mortality in Patients with Yellow Fever: An Observational Cohort Study," *Lancet Infectious Diseases* 19, no. 7 (2019); published correction appears in *Lancet Infectious Diseases* 19, no. 11 (Nov. 2019): 750.

107 Tini Garske et al., "Yellow Fever in Africa: Estimating the Burden of Disease and Impact of Mass Vaccination from Outbreak and Serological Data," *PLoS Medicine* 11, no. 5 (2014): e1001638.

108 Personal communication with Dr. Holly Caldwell.

109 Kohn, *Encyclopedia*, 384.

110 Didier Raoult, Theodore Woodward, and J. Stephen Dumler, "The History of Epidemic Typhus," *Infectious Disease Clinics of North America* 18, no. 1 (2004): 135.

111 Raoult, Woodward, and Dumler, *History of Epidemic Typhus*, 135.

112 Raoult, Woodward, and Dumler, *History of Epidemic Typhus*, 136.

113 Hans Zinsser, *Rats, Lice and History* (Boston, MA: Little Brown, 1963): 9.

114 WHO data. https://www.who.int/data/gho/data/themes/hiv-aids.

115 See Wei Tan et al., "Skin Manifestations of COVID-19: A Worldwide Review," *Journal of the American Academy of Dermatology International* 2 (2021): 119–133.

Chapter 9: The Scientific Revolution

1 David Brewster, *Memoirs of the Life, Writings, and Discoveries of Sir Isaac Newton* (Edinburgh: Thomas Constable, 1855), 407–408.

2 Jean le Rond D'Alembert, *Essai sur les éléments de philosophie* (1759) (Belgium: Olms, 1965).

3 Robert Liveing, "Clinical Remarks on the Study and Diagnosis of Skin-Diseases," *British Medical Journal* 1, no. 896 (1878): 283.

4 Malcolm Morris, "An Address Delivered at the Opening of the Section of Dermatology. The Rise and Progress of Dermatology." *British Medical Journal* 2, no. 1916 (1897): 697.

5 Claimed by both the Poles and Germans, Copernicus actually resided most of his adult life in the semi-independent, archbishopric of Warmia, which was then a Prussian territory but is now in Poland.

6 Nicolaus Copernicus, *De Revolutionibus Orbium Cælestium*, Book 1, trans. Edward Rosen (1543; Warsaw: Polish Scientific Publications, 1978), 22.

7 Robert Carruthers, *Cyclopædia of English Literature: A History, Critical and Biographical, of British Authors, from the Earliest to the Present Times* (Philadelphia, PA: J. B. Lippincott, 1867), 256.

8 Alan Charles Kors, *The Birth of the Modern Mind: An Intellectual History of the Seventeenth and Eighteenth Century* (Springfield, VA: Teaching Co., 1998), 37.

9 John Locke, *An Essay Concerning Human Understanding* (London: W. Tegg, 1849), 61.

10 Kors, *Birth of the Modern Mind*, 88.

11 Kors, *Birth of the Modern Mind*, 31.

12 Kors, *Birth of the Modern Mind*, 96, 101.

13 William Harvey, *On the Motion of the Heart and Blood in Animals,* trans. Robert Willis (United Kingdom: Bell, 1889), 3.

14 Porter, *Greatest Benefit*, 212.

15 William Harvey and George Morgan, *An Anatomical Dissertation upon the Movement of the Heart and Blood in Animals: Being a Statement of the Discovery of the Circulation of the Blood* (United Kingdom: G. Moreton, 1894), vii

16 Carl Zimmer, *Soul Made Flesh: The Discovery of the Brain—and How It Changed the World* (New York, NY: Free Press, 2004), 240.

17 R.M. Yost, "Sydenham's Philosophy of Science," *Osiris* 9 (1950): 84.

18 Locke to Molyneux, June 15, 1697, in *Familiar Letters between Mr. John Locke and Several of His Friends* (London: Orway's Head in St. Martin's Court, 1742), 176–177.

19 Porter, *Greatest Benefit*, 229.

20 William Wadd, *Mems., Maxims, and Memoirs* (London: Callow & Wilson, 1827), 231.

21 Edward Berdoe, *The Origin and Growth of the Healing Art: A Popular History of Medicine in All Ages and Countries* (London: Swan Sonnenschein, 1893), 382.

22 Kate Kelly, *The Scientific Revolution and Medicine* (New York, NY: Facts on File, 2010), 116.

23 Kenneth Dewhurst, *Dr. Thomas Sydenham, 1624–1689: His Life and Original Writings* (Berkeley, CA: University of California Press, 1966), 60.

24 Thomas Sydenham, *The Works of Thomas Sydenham, M.D.*, 2 vols., ed. Robert G. Latham and trans. William A. Greenhill (London: Sydenham Society, 1848), 15.

25 Sydenham, *Works*, 25.

26 Samuel Hafenreffer, *Pandocheion Aiolodermon in Quo Cutis eique Adhaerentium Partium, Affectus Omnes, Singulari Methodo, et Cognoscendi et Curandi Fidelissime Traduntur: Quod etiam Variis Medicamentis Galenicis, Chymicis, Cosmeticis, aliisque Nobilibus Selectioribus est Illustratum ....* (Tübingen: Germany, 1630), title. Translated by Dr. Althea Ashe.

27 Hafenreffer, *Pandocheion Aiolodermon*, subtitle. Translated by the author and Dr. Althea Ashe.

28 Hafenreffer, *Pandocheion Aiolodermon*, front matter. Translated by the author and Dr. Althea Ashe.

29 Pusey, *History of Dermatology*, 43.

30 Korting, *German Dermatology*, 117.

31 Demaitre, *Leprosy in Premodern Medicine*, 30.

32 Demaitre, *Leprosy in Premodern Medicine*, 202.

33 John R. Kirkup, "Vicary Lecture, 1976. The Tercentenary of Richard Wiseman's 'Severall Chirurgicall Treatises'," *Annals of the Royal College of Surgeons of England* 59, no. 4 (1977): 275.

34 Porter, *Greatest Benefit*, 187.

35 John Frank Payne, *Thomas Sydenham* (London: Unwin, 1900), 48.

36 Dewhurst, *Dr. Thomas Sydenham*, 12.

37 D'Arcy Power, "Richard Wiseman," in *Dictionary of National Biography* (United Kingdom: Oxford University Press, 1900), 247.

38 Richard Wiseman, *Several Chirurgical Treatises* (London: Flesher, 1676), epistle to reader.

39 Wiseman, *Several Chirurgical Treatises*, epistle to reader.

40 Huckbody, *Dermatology throughout the Dark Ages*, 345.

41 Wiseman, *Several Chirurgical Treatises*, 245–247.

42 Larry Dossey, "The Royal Touch: A Look at Healing in Times Past," *Explore—The Journal of Science and Healing* 9 (2013): 124.

43 William Shakespeare and George Clark, "Macbeth," *The Works* (United Kingdom: Macmillan, 1867) Act 4.3, lines 147–158.

44 David J. Sturdy, "The Royal Touch in England," in *European Monarchy: Its Evolution and Practice from Roman Antiquity to Modern Times*, eds. Heinz Duchhardt, Richard A. Jackson, and David Sturdy (Stuttgart: Franz Steiner, 1992), 171–171.

45 Sturdy, *Royal Touch in England*, 171.

46 Thomas Longmore, *Richard Wiseman: Surgeon and Sergeant-Surgeon to Charles II* (London: Longmans, Green, and Co., 1891), 148.

47 William Cowper et al., *The Anatomy of Humane Bodies* (Leiden: Johan Arnold Langerak, 1737). 4th table.

48 Robert F. Buckman Jr and J. William Futrell, "William Cowper," *Surgery* 99, no. 5 (May 1986): 589.

49 Marcia Ramos-e-Silva, "Giovan Cosimo Bonomo (1663–1696): Discoverer of the Etiology of Scabies," *International Journal of Dermatology* 37, no. 8 (1998): 625–630.

50 Richard Mead, *The Medical Works of Richard Mead, M.D., Physician to His Late Majesty K. George II, Fellow of the Royal Colleges of Physicians at London and Edinburgh, and of the Royal Society* (London: C. Hitch, et al., 1762), 656.

51 Ramos-e-Silva, *Giovan Cosimo Bonomo (1663–1696): Discoverer of the Etiology of Scabies*, 628–629.

52 Ramos-e-Silva, *Giovan Cosimo Bonomo*, 629.

53 Ramos-e-Silva, *Giovan Cosimo Bonomo*, 629.

54 Kevin P. Siena, "The Moral Biology of 'the Itch' in Eighteenth Century Britain," in *A Medical History of Skin: Scratching the Surface*, ed. Kevin P. Siena (London: Routledge, 2016), 72–73.

55 Connor, *Book of Skin*, 228–229.

56 Ramos-e-Silva, *Giovan Cosimo Bonomo*, 629.

57 Jeremiah S. Finch, *A Facsimile of the 1711 Sales Auction Catalogue of Sir Thomas Browne and His Son Edward's Libraries* (Leiden: E.J. Brill, 1986).

58 Reid Barbour and Claire Preston, *Sir Thomas Browne: The World Proposed* (Oxford: Oxford University Press, 2008), 279–280.

59 Barbour and Preston, *Sir Thomas Browne*, 279.

60 Thomas Browne, *The Works of Sir Thomas Browne* (London: Pickering, 1835), 42–43.

61 Charles E. Kellett, "Sir Thomas Browne and the Disease Called the Morgellons," *Annals of Medical History* 7 (1935): 468.

62 Ambroise Paré and George Baker, *The Workes of that Famous Chirurgion Ambrose Parey* (United Kingdom: Richard Cotes, and Willi: Du-gard, 1649), 250.

63 Jacques Guillemeau, *Child-Birth; Or, The Happy Delivery of Women: Wherein Is Set Downe the Government of Women, with a Treatise for the Nursing of Children* (United Kingdom: Anne Griffin, 1635), 116–117 (in the Treatise for the Nursing of Children).

64 Kellett, *Disease Called the Morgellons*, 469.

65 Kellett, *Disease Called the Morgellons*, 475.

66 Daniel Le Clerc, *A Natural and Medicinal History of Worms* (United Kingdom, J. Wilcox, at the Green-Dragon, in Little-Britain, 1721), 281.

67 Andrew S. Curran, *The Anatomy of Blackness: Science and Slavery in an Age of Enlightenment* (Baltimore, MD: Johns Hopkins University Press, 2011), 1.

68 Jean Riolan et al., *A Sure Guide; or, The Best and Nearest Way to Physick and Chyrurgery*, trans. Nicholas Culpeper and William Rand (London, 1671), 195.

69 Riolan et al., *Sure Guide*, 36.

70 Erasmus Wilson, *On Diseases of the Skin*, 4th American ed. (Philadelphia, PA: Blanchard and Lea, 1857), xix.

71 Michael J.G. Farthing, "Nicholas Culpeper (1616–1654): London's First General Practitioner?" *Journal of Medical Biography* 23, no. 3 (2015): 152.

72 Nicholas Culpeper, *Culpeper's English Physician: And Complete Herbal* (London: British Directory Office, 1794), xiii–xiv.

73 Culpeper, *Culpeper's English Physician*, Book II, 19.

74 Albert M. Kligman, "Poison Ivy (Rhus) Dermatitis: An Experimental Study," *AMA Archives of Dermatology* 77, no. 2 (1958): 149.

75 Daniel Sennert, *The Art of Chirurgery, Explained in Six Parts.... Being the Whol Fifth Book of Practical Physick*, trans. Nicolas Culpeper and Abdiah Cole (United Kingdom: Peter Cole & Edward Cole, 1661).

76 L.J.A. Loewenthal, "Daniel Turner and 'De Morbis Cutaneis,'" *Archives of Dermatology* 85, no. 4 (1962): 521.

77 Loewenthal, *Daniel Turner*, 523.

78 Philip K. Wilson, *Surgery, Skin and Syphilis: Daniel Turner's London (1667–1741)* (Atlanta, GA: Rodopi, 1999), 34–37.

79 Wilson, *Surgery, Skin and Syphilis*, 51–52.

80 Daniel Turner, *De Morbis Cutaneis: A Treatise of Diseases Incident to the Skin* (London: R. Wilkin, 1736), 4.

81 John E. Lane, "Daniel Turner and the First Degree of Doctor of Medicine," *Annals of Medical History* 2, no. 4 (1919): 367–376.

82 Crissey and Parish, *Dermatology and Syphilology*, 8.

83 Wilson, *Surgery, Skin and Syphilis*, 194–195.

84 Daniel Turner, *Apologia Chyrurgica* (United Kingdom: J. Whitlock, 1695). From the complete title.

85 Turner, *De Morbis Cutaneis*, ii.

86 Turner, *De Morbis Cutaneis,* 310.

87 Turner, *De Morbis Cutaneis,* 312.

88 Turner, *De Morbis Cutaneis,* 80–81.

89 Turner, *De Morbis Cutaneis,* 360.

90 Turner, *De Morbis Cutaneis,* 361.

91 Turner, *De Morbis Cutaneis,* 365.

92 Turner, *De Morbis Cutaneis,* 166, 169.

93 Turner, *De Morbis Cutaneis,* 169.

94 Turner, *De Morbis Cutaneis,* 171.

95 Turner, *De Morbis Cutaneis,* 171.

96 Turner, *De Morbis Cutaneis,* 171.

97 Turner, *De Morbis Cutaneis,* 172.

98 Turner, *De Morbis Cutaneis,* 172.

99 Turner, *De Morbis Cutaneis,* 173.

100 Turner, *De Morbis Cutaneis,* 173–174.

101 Turner, *De Morbis Cutaneis,* 174–175.

102 Turner, *De Morbis Cutaneis,* 178.

103 Turner, *De Morbis Cutaneis,* 175.

104 James Augustus Blondel, *The Power of the Mother's Imagination over the Foetus Examin'd: In Answer to Dr. Daniel Turner's Book, Intitled "A Defence of the XIIth Chapter of the First Part of a Treatise,* De Morbis Cutaneis" (London: John Brotherton, 1729), i–xi.

105 Philip K. Wilson, "'Out of Sight, Out of Mind?': The Daniel Turner-James Blondel Dispute over the Power of the Maternal Imagination," *Annals of Science* 49, no. 1 (1992): 63.

106 Lane, *Daniel Turner*, 370.

107 Wilson, *Surgery, Skin and Syphilis*, 192.

108 Wilson, *Surgery, Skin and Syphilis*, 208.

109 Bateman, *Practical Synopsis*, 148.

110 William Wadd, *Nugæ canoræ; or, Epitaphian mementos, in stone-cutter's verse, of the medici family of modern times* (United Kingdom: Nichols, 1827), 20.

111 Norman Moore, "Daniel Turner," in *Dictionary of National Biography 1885-1900*, Vol 57 (Oxford: Oxford University Press, 1899).

112 Emily Cock, "'He Would by No Means Risque His Reputation': Patient and Doctor Shame in Daniel Turner's *De Morbis Cutaneis* (1714) and *Syphilis* (1717)," *Medical Humanities* 43 (2017): 231–236.

113 Cock, *Patient and Doctor Shame in Daniel Turner*, 236.

114 John Thorne Crissey, Karl Holubar, and Lawrence C. Parish, *Historical Atlas of Dermatology and Dermatologists* (United States: CRC Press, 2013), 10.

115 Patrick. J. Hare, "Daniel Turner (1667–1741)," *British Journal of Dermatology* 79, no. 12 (1967), 661.

116 Alan Lyell, "Daniel Turner (1667–1740) LRCP London (1711) M.D. Honorary, Yale (1723), Surgeon, Physician and Pioneer Dermatologist: The Man Seen in the Pages of His Book on the Skin," *International Journal of Dermatology* 21, no. 3 (Apr. 1982): 163.

117 Pierre François Olive Rayer et al., *A Theoretical and Practical Treatise on the Diseases of the Skin* (Philadelphia, PA: Carey and Hart, 1845), 17.

118 Hare, *Daniel Turner*, 661.

119 Lyell, *Daniel Turner*, 168.

120 Alan Lyell, "Daniel Turner, and the First Controlled Therapeutic Trial in Dermatology," *Clinical and Experimental Dermatology* 11, no. 2 (1986): 193.

121 Lyell, *Daniel Turner*, 193.

Chapter 10: The Enlightenment

1 Isaac Kramnick, *The Portable Enlightenment Reader* (United States: Penguin Publishing Group, 1995), x.

2 Kors, *Birth of the Modern Mind*, 239.

3 Francis Bacon, *The Philosophical Works of Francis Bacon: Reprinted from the Texts and Translations, with the Notes and Prefaces, of Robert Ellis and James Spedding* (United Kingdom: Routledge, 1905), 288.

4 Kors, *Birth of the Modern Mind*, 146–147.

5 Kors, *Birth of the Modern Mind*, 145.

6 Kors, *Birth of the Modern Mind*, 145.

7 Kors, *Birth of the Modern Mind*, 151.

8 Kors, *Birth of the Modern Mind*, 149.

9 Theodore M. Brown, "Medicine in the Shadow of 'The Principia,'" *Journal of the History of Ideas* 48, no. 4 (1987): 629–648.

10 Brown, *Medicine in the Shadow of 'The Principia,'* 648.

11 Denis Diderot and Jean le Rond d'Alembert, eds. *Encyclopédie, ou dictionnaire raisonné des sciences, des arts et des métiers, etc.* (Chicago, IL: University of Chicago ARTFL Encyclopédie Project (online), 2019), no page, preface.

12 Diderot and d'Alembert, *Encyclopédie*, no page, preface.

13 Voltaire, *The Works of Voltaire: A Contemporary Version*, ed. John Morley and Tobias Smollett, rev. and trans. William F. Fleming and Oliver H.G. Leigh, 21 vols. (New York, NY: E. R. DuMont, 1901), Vol. XIX, 197.

14 "Peau." *Encyclopédie, ou dictionnaire raisonné des sciences, des arts et des métiers, etc.*, ed. Denis Diderot and Jean le Rond d'Alembert (Chicago, IL: University of Chicago ARTFL Encyclopédie Project (online), 2019), no page. Translated by the author.

15 Dennis Fletcher, "The Chevalier de Jaucourt and the English Sources of the Encyclopedic Article 'Patriote,'" *Diderot Studies* 16 (1973): 23.

16 Louis Jaucourt, "Pores de la Peau," in *Encyclopédie, ou dictionnaire raisonné des sciences, des arts et des métiers, etc.*, ed. Denis Diderot and Jean le Rond d'Alembert (Chicago, IL: University of Chicago ARTFL Encyclopédie Project (online), 2019), no page. Translated by the author.

17 Menuret Chambaud, "Maladies de la Peau," in *Encyclopedie*, ed. Denis Diderot et al. (Chicago, IL: University of Chicago ARTFL *Encyclopédie Project*, 2019), no page. Translated by the author.

18 Chambaud, *Maladies de la Peau*.

19 Chambaud, *Maladies de la Peau*.

20 John Lesch, "Systematics and the Geometrical Spirit," in Tore Frängsmyr, J.L. Heilbron, and Robin E. Rider, *The Quantifying Spirit in the 18th Century* (United States: University of California Press, 1990), 75.

21 John Lyon, "The 'Initial Discourse' to Buffon's *Histoire Naturelle*: The First Complete English Translation," *Journal of the History of Biology* 9, no. 1 (1976): 164.

22 Anthony Serafini, *The Epic History of Biology* (New York, NY: Springer, 2013), 149.

23 Leo Damrosch, *Jean-Jacques Rousseau: Restless Genius* (Boston, MA: Houghton Mifflin Harcourt, 2007), 471.

24 John Wright, *The Naming of the Shrew: A Curious History of Latin Names* (London: Bloomsbury, 2015), 29.

25 Wright, *Naming of the Shrew*, 29–30.

26 Lesch, *Systematics*, 96.

27 Crissey and Parish, *Dermatology and Syphilology*, 24.

28 Crissey and Parish, *Dermatology and Syphilology*, 24.

29 Porter, *Greatest Benefit*, 260.

30 William A. Smeaton, "Herman Boerhaave (1668–1738): Physician, Botanist, and Chemist," *Endeavour* 12, no. 3 (1988): 139–140.

31 Gillian Hull, "The Influence of Herman Boerhaave," *Journal of the Royal Society of Medicine* 90, no. 9 (1997): 512–514.

32 Strathern, *A Brief History of Medicine*, 159–160.

33 Strathern, *A Brief History of Medicine*, 159–160.

34 Strathern, *A Brief History of Medicine*, 159–160.

35 Sanjib K. Ghosh, "Giovanni Battista Morgagni (1682–1771): Father of Pathologic Anatomy and Pioneer of Modern Medicine," *Anatomical Science International* 92, no. 3 (June 2017): 305–312.

36 Giambattista Morgagni and Benjamin Alexander, *The Seats and Causes of Diseases Investigated by Anatomy in Five Books* … (Birmingham, AL: Classics of Medicine Library, 1983), Letter XXX, Article 2.

37 Ghosh, *Giovanni Battista Morgagni*, 305.

38 Ghosh, *Giovanni Battista Morgagni*, 311.

39 Malcolm O. Perry, "John Hunter—Triumph and Tragedy," *Journal of Vascular Surgery* 17, no. 1 (1993): 9.

40 Strathern, *A Brief History of Medicine*, 181.

41 John Ayrton Paris, *A Treatise on Diet: With a View to Establish, on Practical Grounds, a System of Rules, for the Prevention and Cure of the Diseases Incident to a Disordered State of the Digestive Functions* (United Kingdom: T. & G. Underwood, 1826). Cover page (cited as manuscript note from Hunter's lectures).

42 Wendy Moore, *The Knife Man: Blood, Body Snatching, and the Birth of Modern Surgery* (New York, NY: Broadway Books, 2005), 273.

43 John Hunter, *A Treatise on the Blood, Inflammation, and Gun-Shot Wounds, by the Late John Hunter, to Which Is Prefixed a Short Account of the Author's Life* (London: Georg Nichol, 1794), 275.

44 Moore, *Knife Man*, 275.

45 Catherine Price, "The Age of Scurvy," *Distillations* 3, no.2 (Summer 2017), 4th para.

46 Stephen Bown, *Scurvy: How a Surgeon, a Mariner, and a Gentlemen Solved the Greatest Medical Mystery of the Age of Sail* (New York, NY: St. Martin's Press, 2005), 5.

47 James Lind, "A Treatise on the Scurvy, in Three Parts, Containing an Inquiry Into the Nature, Causes, and Cure, of that Disease, Together with a Critical and Chronological View of What Has Been Published on the Subject (London: S. Crowder, 1772), 149.

48 Ted J. Kaptchuk, "Placebo Controls, Exorcisms, and the Devil." *Lancet* 374, no. 9697 (2009): 1234.

49 Kaptchuk, *Placebo Controls, Exorcisms, and the Devil*, 1234.

50 Benjamin Franklin, "Franklin's Description of his Ailments," *The Papers of Benjamin Franklin* 25 (New Haven, CT: Yale University Press, 1986): 77–80.

51 Mark A. Everett, "Anne Charles Lorry, the First French Dermatologist," *International Journal of Dermatology* 18, no. 9 (1979): 762.

52 Everett, *Anne Charles Lorry*, 762.

53 Anne-Charles Lorry, *Tractatus de morbis cutaneis* (Paris, 1777), 2. Translated by the author and Althea Ashe.

54 Everett, *Anne Charles Lorry*, 764.

55 Crissey, Holubar, and Parish, *Historical Atlas*, 11.

56 Rayer et al., *Treatise on the Diseases of the Skin*, 17.

57 J.H. Cohen and E. Cohen, "Doctor Marat and His Skin," *Medical History* 2, no. 4 (Oct. 1958), 282.

58 Cohen and Cohen, *Doctor Marat*, 282–283.

59 Cohen and Cohen, *Doctor Marat*, 284–286.

60 Tony de-Dios et al., "Metagenomic Analysis of a Blood Stain from the French Revolutionary Jean-Paul Marat (1743–1793)," *Infection, Genetics and Evolution* 80 (2020), 104209.

61 Reuben Friedman, "The Emperor's Itch: The Legend Concerning Napoleon's Affliction with Scabies," *JAMA* 115, no. 23 (1940): 2020.

62 Friedman, *Emperor's Itch*, 2020.

63 Seguin Henry Jackson, *Dermato-Pathologia* (London: H. Reynell and J. Robson, 1792), xiv.

64 Jackson, *Dermato-Pathologia*, 64.

65 Jackson, *Dermato-Pathologia*, v–vi.

66 Diederick Janssen, "Dermatology: Coinage of the Term by Johann Heinrich Alsted (1630)," *International Journal of Dermatology* 60, no. 7 (2021): 877.

67 Lavoisien, Jean-François, *Dictionnaire portatif de médecine, d'anatomie, de chirurgie, de pharmacie, de chymie, d'histoire naturelle, de botanique et de physique* (France: P.Fr. Didot le Jeune, 1764), 200.

68 Leonard J Hoenig and Lawrence Charles Parish, "How Dermatology Got Its Name." *Clinics in Dermatology* 39, no. 2 (2021): 353.

69 Jackson, *Dermato-Pathologia*, 27–28.

70 Jackson, *Dermato-Pathologia*, 181–183.

71 Jackson, *Dermato-Pathologia*, vi.

72 John E. Lane, "Joseph Jacob Plenck, 1738?–1807," *AMA Archives of Dermatology and Syphilology* 28, no. 2 (1933), 193.

73 Karl Holubar and Joseph Frankl, "J. Joseph Plenck (1735–1807). A Forerunner of Modern European Dermatology," *Journal of the American Academy of Dermatology* 10, no. 2 (1984): 326–332.

74 Lane, *Joseph Jacob Plenck*, 195–196.

75 Lane, *Joseph Jacob Plenck*, 197.

76 Lane, *Joseph Jacob Plenck*, 197.

77 Lane, *Joseph Jacob Plenck*, 197.

78 Joseph Jacob Plenck, *Doctrina De Morbis Cutaneis* (Vienna: Apud Rudolphum Græffer, 1783), 3. Translated by the author and Dr. Althea Ashe.

79 Robert Weston, *Medical Consulting by Letter in France, 1665–1789* (United Kingdom: Taylor & Francis, 2016), 48.

80 Lane, *Joseph Jacob Plenck*, 193.

81 Lane, *Joseph Jacob Plenck*, 199.

82 Lane, *Joseph Jacob Plenck*, 199.

83 Lane, *Joseph Jacob Plenck*, 201.

84 Lane, *Joseph Jacob Plenck*, 200.

85 Lane, *Joseph Jacob Plenck*, 206.

86 Lane, *Joseph Jacob Plenck*, 201.

87 Friday King and Laura King. "Josef Plenck—Grandfather of Modern Dermatology," *Journal of the American Academy of Dermatology* 11, no. 1 (1984): 145.

88 Percivall Pott, *The Chirurgical Works in Three Volumes* (United Kingdom: Lowndes, Johnson, Robinson, Cadell, 1783), 225–227.

89 John R. Brown and John L. Thornton, "Percivall Pott (1714–1788) and Chimney Sweepers' Cancer of the Scrotum," *British Journal of Industrial Medicine* 14, no. 1 (1957): 70.

90 Personal email from Dr. Stephen J. Greenberg, National Library of Medicine.

91 Personal email from Dr. Stephen J. Greenberg, National Library of Medicine.

92 Siena, *Moral Biology of 'the Itch,'* 82.

93 Thomas A. Spooner, *A Compendious Treatise of the Diseases of the Skin from the Slightest Itching Humour in Particular Parts Only, to the Most Inveterate Itch* (London: J. Roberts, 1728), 1.

94 Spooner, *Diseases of the Skin*, 3.

95 Spooner, *Diseases of the Skin*, 9–11.

96 Spooner, *Diseases of the Skin*, 33.

97 Siena, *Moral Biology of 'the Itch,'* 8.

Interlude 3: Syphilis

1 Thomas A. Peterman and Sarah E. Kidd, "Trends in Deaths Due to Syphilis, United States, 1968–2015," *Sexually Transmitted Diseases* 46, no. 1 (2019): 37.

2 Justin D. Radolf et al., "*Treponema pallidum*, the Syphilis Spirochete: Making a Living as a Stealth Pathogen," *Nature Reviews Microbiology* 14, no. 12 (2016): 744.

3 John J. Ross, "Shakespeare's Chancre: Did the Bard Have Syphilis?" *Clinical Infectious Diseases* 40, no. 3 (Feb. 2005): 399.

4 Claude Quétel, *History of Syphilis* (Baltimore, MD: John Hopkins University Press, 1992), 10.

5 Quétel, *History of Syphilis*, 10.

6 Quétel, *History of Syphilis*, 11, 16.

7 Quétel, *History of Syphilis*, 12.

8 Quétel, *History of Syphilis*, 15.

9 Quétel, *History of Syphilis*, 17.

10 Quétel, *History of Syphilis*, 19.

11 Quétel, *History of Syphilis*, 20.

12 Louis Pelner, "Narration: Francisco Lopez de Villalobos (1474?–1542?)," *Journal of the American Medical Association* 211, no. 2 (1970): 348

13 Pelner, *Francisco Lopez de Villalobos*, 348.

14 Arrizabalaga et al., *Great Pox*, 72.

15 Arrizabalaga et al., *Great Pox*, 56–87.

16 Arrizabalaga et al., *Great Pox*, 74.

17 Arrizabalaga et al., *Great Pox*, 75.

18 Arrizabalaga et al., *Great Pox*, 79.

19 Quétel, *History of Syphilis*, 26.

20 Kohn, *Encyclopedia of Plague and Pestilence*, 114.

21 Quétel, *History of Syphilis*, 17.

22 Jared M. Diamond, *Guns, Germs, and Steel: The Fates of Human Societies* (New York, NY: W. W. Norton, 1999), 210.

23 Girolamo Fracastoro, *Hieronymus Fracastor's Syphilis: From the Original Latin: A Translation in Prose of Fracastor's Immortal Poem* (United States: Philmar Company, 1911), 55.

24 Leo Spitzer, "The Etymology of the Term Syphilis." *Bulletin of the History of Medicine* 29, no. 3 (1955): 269–273.

25 Harry Keil, "The Evolution of the Term Chancre and Its Relation to the History of Syphilis," *Journal of the History of Medicine and Allied Sciences* 4, no. 4 (Autumn 1949), 413.

26 Richard M. Swiderski, *Quicksilver: A History of the Use, Lore and Effects of Mercury* (Jefferson, NC: McFarland, 2008), 96.

27 Quétel, *History of Syphilis*, 33–34.

28 Quétel, *History of Syphilis*, 34–35.

29 Bruce Rothschild et al., "First European Exposure to Syphilis: The Dominican Republic at the Time of Columbian Contact," *Clinical Infectious Diseases* 31, no. 4 (Oct. 2000), 936.

30 Warren R. Heymann, "The History of Syphilis," *Journal of the American Academy of Dermatology* 54, no. 2 (2006): 322.

31 Quétel, *History of Syphilis*, 44.

32 Mircea Tampa et al., "Brief History of Syphilis," *Journal of Medical Life* 7, no. 1 (2014): 7.

33 Quétel, *History of Syphilis*, 38.

34 Pusey, *History of Dermatology*, 37–38.

35 Ellis H. Hudson, "Christopher Columbus and the History of Syphilis," *Acta Tropica* 25, no. 1 (1968), 12.

36 Crane-Kramer, *Confusion between Leprosy and Syphilis?* 113.

37 Ellis H. Hudson, "Historical Approach to the Terminology of Syphilis," *Archives of Dermatology* 84, no. 4 (1961): 548.

38 Hudson, *Christopher Columbus and the History of Syphilis*, 12.

39 Heymann, *History of Syphilis*, 322; Kristin N. Harper, "The Origin and Antiquity of Syphilis Revisited: An Appraisal of Old World Pre-Columbian Evidence for Treponemal Infection," *American Journal of Physical Anthropology* 146, sup. 53 (2011): 99.

40 Harper, *Origin and Antiquity of Syphilis Revisited*, 99.

41 Crane-Kramer, *Confusion between Leprosy and Syphilis?* 113.

42 Tampa et al., *Brief History of Syphilis*, 5.

43 Charles Scott Sherrington, *The Endeavour of Jean Fernel: With a List of the Editions of His Writings* (Cambridge: Cambridge University Press, 1946), 130–131.

44 Norman Himes, *Medical History of Contraception* (United States: Schocken Books, 1970), 190.

45 Fahd Khan et al. "The Story of the Condom," *Indian Journal of Urology* 29, no. 1 (2013): 14.

46 Khan, *Story of the Condom*, 14.

47 Andrzej Grzybowski, Piotr Kanclerz, and Lawrence C. Parish, "Daniel Turner (1667–1740)," *Clinics in Dermatology* 38, no. 2 (2020): 265–269.

48 Daniel Turner, *Syphilis: A Practical Dissertation on the Venereal Disease* (London, 1737), 84.

49 Nate Pedersen and Lydia Kang, *Quackery: A Brief History of the Worst Ways to Cure Everything* (New York, NY: Workman, 2017), 5.

50 Pedersen and Kang, *Quackery*, 10.

51 Quétel, *History of Syphilis*, 85.

52 Pedersen and Kang, *Quackery*, 13.

53 Patrick Eppenberger, Francesco Galassi, and Frank Rühli, "A Brief Pictorial and Historical Introduction to Guaiacum—from a Putative Cure for Syphilis to an Actual Screening Method for Colorectal Cancer," *British Journal of Clinical Pharmacology* 83, no. 9 (2017): 2119.

54 Quétel, *History of Syphilis*, 60.

55 Moore, *The Knife Man*, 135.

56 John Hunter and George Babington, *A Treatise on the Venereal Disease.* (Philadelphia, PA: Haswell, Barrington, and Haswell, 1839), 269.

57 Moore, *Knife Man*, 136.

58 George Qvist, "John Hunter's Alleged Syphilis," *Annals of the Royal College of Surgeons of England* 59, no. 3 (1977): 205–208.

59 Qvist, *John Hunter's Alleged Syphilis*, 208.

60 Qvist, *John Hunter's Alleged Syphilis*, 208.

61 Philip K. Wilson, "Exposing the Secret Disease: Recognizing and Treating Syphilis in Daniel Turner's London," in Linda Evi Merians, *The Secret Malady: Venereal Disease in Eighteenth-Century Britain and France* (Lexington, KY: University Press of Kentucky, 1996), 68.

62 Quétel, *History of Syphilis*, 89.

63 Wilson, *Secret Disease*, 70.

64 Turner, *Syphilis*, preface iii.

65 Wilson, *Secret Disease*, 70–71.

66 Turner, *Syphilis*, 10.

67 Turner, *Syphilis*, 3.

68 Wilson, *Secret Disease*, 73.

69 Wilson, *Secret Disease*, 81.

70 John J. Ross, "Shakespeare's Chancre: Did the Bard Have Syphilis?" *Clinical Infectious Diseases* 40, no. 3 (Feb. 2005): 399.

71 Ross, *Shakespeare's Chancre*, 400.

72 Ross, *Shakespeare's Chancre*, 400.

73 Ross, *Shakespeare's Chancre*, 400.

74 Ross, *Shakespeare's Chancre*, 401–402.

75 Ross, *Shakespeare's Chancre*, 403.

76 Goodman, *Notable Contributors*, 73.

77 Daniel Turner, *Aphrodisiacus: Containing a Summary of the Ancient Writers on the Venereal Disease … Extracted from the Two Tomes of Aloysius Luisinus* (London: John Clarke, 1736), preface.

78 Jean Astruc, *A Treatise of Venereal Diseases: in Nine Books; Containing an Account of the Origin, Propagation, and Contagion of This Distemper …Together with a Short Abstract of the Lives of the Authors Who Have Wrote on Those Diseases, and a List of Their Works*, Book II (Paris: W. Innys, 1754), 267.

79 Weston, *Medical Consulting*, 48.

80 Astruc, *Venereal Diseases*, I, 31, 75.

81 Astruc, *Venereal Diseases*, I, 118.

82 Astruc, *Venereal Diseases*, I, 118.

83 Astruc, *Venereal Diseases*, I, 123.

84 Astruc, *Venereal Diseases*, I, 123.

85 Astruc, *Venereal Diseases*, I, 126.

86 Astruc, *Venereal Diseases*, I, 207.

87 Astruc, *Venereal Diseases*, I, 306–404.

88 Astruc, *Venereal Diseases*, I, 135.

89 Astruc, *Venereal Diseases*, II, 1.

90 Astruc, *Venereal Diseases*, II, 36.

91 Astruc, *Venereal Diseases*, II, 36.

92 Astruc, *Venereal Diseases*, II, 37–47.

93 Pusey, *History of Dermatology*, 47.

94 Astruc, *Venereal Diseases*, IV, 12–13.

95 Crissey and Parish, *Dermatology and Syphilology*, 11–12.

96 Crissey and Parish, *Dermatology and Syphilology*, 12.

97 Quétel, *History of Syphilis*, 85.

98 Quétel, *History of Syphilis*, 111.

99 Robert S. Morton, "Dr. William Wallace (1791–1837) of Dublin," *Medical History* 10, no. 1 (1966): 42.

100 George Weisz, *Divide and Conquer: A Comparative History of Medical Specialization* (Oxford: Oxford University Press, 2006), 213.

101 Quétel, *History of Syphilis*, 137.

102 M.A. Waugh, "Alfred Fournier, 1832–1914: His Influence on Venereology," *British Journal of Venereal Disease* 50, no. 3 (1974): 234.

103 Weisz, *Divide and Conquer*, 23.

104 Waugh, *Alfred Fournier, 1832–1914*, 232.

105 Goodman, *Notable Contributors*, 159.

106 Mohammed Alsaidan et al., "Jonathan Hutchinson—The Eponyms Physician," *JAMA Dermatology* 151, no. 6 (2015): 634.

107 Pusey, *History of Dermatology*, 130.

108 Crissey and Parish, *Dermatology and Syphilology*, 225.

109 Crissey and Parish, *Dermatology and Syphilology*, 192–194.

110 Anne Kveim Lie, "Abominable Ulcers, Open Pores and a New Tissue: Transforming the Skin in the Norwegian Countryside, 1750–1850," in Kevin P. Siena, *A Medical History of Skin: Scratching the Surface* (London, Routledge, 2016), 31–42.

111 Kveim Lie, *Abominable Ulcers*, 34–36.

112 Kveim Lie, *Abominable Ulcers*, 37.

113 Kveim Lie, *Abominable Ulcers*, 39.

114 James Moran, "Protecting the Skin of the British Empire: St Paul's Bay Disease in Quebec," in Kevin P. Siena, *A Medical History of Skin: Scratching the Surface* (London: Routledge, 2016), 45.

115 Moran, *Protecting the Skin of the British Empire*, 45.

116 Anne Hanley, "Syphilization and Its Discontents: Experimental Inoculation against Syphilis at the London Lock Hospital," *Bulletin of the History of Medicine* 91, no. 1 (2017): 1–32.

117 Jesper Kragh, "Malaria Fever Therapy for General Paralysis of the Insane in Denmark," *History Psychiatry* 21, no. 84, pt. 4 (2010): 472.

118 Kragh, *Malaria Fever Therapy*, 478.

119 Wolfgang Regal and Michael Nanut, *Vienna—A Doctor's Guide: Walking Tours through Vienna's Medical History* (Vienna: Springer, 2007), 75.

120 Melissa Hope Ditmore, *Prostitution and Sex Work* (Westport, CT: Greenwood, 2011), 53.

121 Ruth Rosen, *The Lost Sisterhood: Prostitution in America, 1900–1918* (Baltimore, MD: Johns Hopkins University Press, 1994), 35.

122 Oliver Kim and Lois Magner, *A History of Medicine* (Boca Raton, FL: CRC Press, 2017), 138.

123 Charlotte Paul and Barbara Brookes, "The Rationalization of Unethical Research: Revisionist Accounts of the Tuskegee Syphilis Study and the New Zealand 'Unfortunate Experiment,'" *American Journal of Public Health* 105, no. 10 (2015): e12–e19.

124 E. Gurney Clark and Niels Danbolt, "The Oslo Study of the Natural History of Untreated Syphilis; An Epidemiologic Investigation Based on a Restudy of the Boeck-Bruusgaard Material; A Review and Appraisal," *Journal of Chronic Diseases* 2, no. 3 (Sept. 1955): 311.

125 Adewole Adamson and Jules Lipoff, "Reconsidering Named Honorifics in Medicine—The Troubling Legacy of Dermatologist Albert Kligman," *JAMA Dermatology* 157, no. 2. (2021): 153.

126 https://www.med.upenn.edu/evpdeancommunications/2021-08-20-283.html.

127 Elemir Macedo de Souza, "A Hundred Years Ago, the Discovery of *Treponema pallidum*," *Anais Brasileiros de Dermatologia* 80, no. 5 (2005): 547.

128 Souza, *Discovery of Treponema Pallidum*, 547.

129 https://www.cdc.gov/std/statistics/2019/tables/1.htm.

130 Crissey, Holubar, and Parish, *Historical Atlas*, xx.

Chapter 11: The Nineteenth Century: An Introduction

1   Porter, *Greatest Benefit*, 366.
2   Porter, *Greatest Benefit*, 366–367.
3   Ramon F. Martin and Sukumar P. Desai, "An Appraisal of the Life of Charles Thomas Jackson as Attention Deficit Hyperactivity Disorder," *Journal of Anesthesia History* 1, no. 2 (2015): 40.
4   Richard J. Wolfe and Richard W. Patterson, *Charles Thomas Jackson, "The Head behind the Hands": Applying Science to Implement Discovery and Invention in Early Nineteenth Century America*, History of Science.com, 2007, v.
5   Julie M. Fenster, *Ether Day: The Strange Tale of America's Greatest Medical Discovery and the Haunted Men Who Made It* (New York, NY: HarperCollins, 2001), 230–239.
6   Porter, *Greatest Benefit*, 367.
7   Porter, *Greatest Benefit*, 367.
8   Porter, *Greatest Benefit*, 368.
9   Lindsey Fitzharris, *The Butchering Art: Joseph Lister's Quest to Transform the Grisly World of Victorian Medicine* (United States: Farrar, Straus and Giroux, 2017), 145.
10 Fitzharris, *The Butchering Art*, 148.
11 Julius Bauer, "The Tragic Fate of Ignaz Philipp Semmelweis." *California Medicine* 98, no. 5 (May 1963): 265
12 Bauer, *Ignaz Philipp Semmelweis*, 265.
13 Hollingham, *Blood and Guts*, 99.
14 Nuland, *Doctors*, 414.
15 Kveim Lie, *Abominable Ulcers*, 36.
16 Fitzharris, *The Butchering Art*, 153.
17 Fitzharris, *The Butchering Art*, 153.
18 Patrick Berche, "Louis Pasteur: From Crystals of Life to Vaccination," *Clinical Microbiology and Infection* 18 (2012): 3.
19 Berche, *Louis Pasteur*, 3.
20 Charles Eliot. *Scientific Papers; Physiology, Medicine, Surgery, Geology* (United States: P. F. Collier & Son, 1910), 373.
21 Thomas M. Rivers, "Viruses and Koch's Postulates," *Journal of Bacteriology* 33, no. 1 (Jan. 1937): 3.
22 G.A. Silver, "Virchow, the Heroic Model in Medicine: Health Policy by Accolade," *American Journal of Public Health* 77, no. 1 (1987): 86.
23 Castiglioni, *History of Medicine*, 835.
24 Cushing, Harvey, *The Life of Sir William Osler* (Oxford: Clarendon Press, 1925).
25 Charles S. Bryan, "New Observations Support William Osler's Rationale for Systemic Bloodletting," *Proceedings* (Baylor University Medical Center) 32, no. 3 (2019): 372–373.
26 Bryan, *New Observations*, 375.
27 Castiglioni, *History of Medicine*, 835.
28 Porter, *Greatest Benefit*, 357.
29 Sepideh Ashrafzadeh, et al. "Gender Differences in Dermatologist Practice Locations in the United States: A Cross-Sectional Analysis of Current Gender Gaps." *International Journal of Women's Dermatology* 7, no. 4 (May 3, 2021): 435; Albert Wu, Shari Lipner, "National Trends in Gender and Ethnicity in Dermatology Training: 2006 to 2018." *Journal of the American Academy of Dermatology* 86, no. 1 (Jan. 2022): 212.
30 Weisz, *Divide and Conquer*, xix.
31 George Weisz, "The Emergence of Medical Specialization in the Nineteenth Century," *Bulletin of the History of Medicine* 77, no. 3 (Fall 2003): 536.
32 Roy Porter, *Quacks: Fakers and Charlatans in English Medicine* (Stroud, Gloucestershire: Tempus, 2003), 24.
33 Porter, *Quacks*, 15–92.
34 Porter, *Quacks*, 133.
35 Sheldon L. Mandel, "Of Asklepiads, Quacks, and Early Caretakers of the Skin," *International Journal of Dermatology* 26, no. 9 (Nov. 1987): 613.

36 Porter, *Quacks*, 139.

37 Porter, *Quacks,* 193–194.

38 Porter, *Quacks*, 208.

39 James Gowing-Middleton, *The Skin and Skin Quacks* (Paris: Clarke and Bishop, 1904), v–vi.

40 Nooshin Bagherani, Bruce Smoller, and Torello Lotti, "History of Novel Dermatology and Dermatopathology in Different Countries—Italy," *Global Dermatology* 2 (2016): S55.

41 David Gentilcore, "'Italic Scurvy,' 'Pellarina,' 'Pellagra': Medical Reactions to a New Disease in Italy, 1770–1830," in K. Siena et al. ed. *A Medical History of Skin: Scratching the Surface* (London: Routledge, 2016), 68.

42 Gentilcore, *'Italic Scurvy,' 'Pellarina,' 'Pellagra,'* 69.

43 Vincenzo Chiarugi, *Delle malattie cutanee sordide in genere e in specie: Trattato teorico-pratico ...* vol. 1 (Florence: Giovacchino Pagani, 1807), 2.

Chapter 12: The British School

1 Christopher C. Booth, "Robert Willan, MD FRS (1757–1812): Dermatologist of the Millennium," *Journal of the Royal Society of Medicine* 92, no. 6 (1999): 313.

2 Booth, *Robert Willan*, 313–314.

3 Thomas Bateman, "The Biographical Memoir of the Late Robert Willan," *Edinburgh Medical and Surgical Journal* 8 (October 1812): 510.

4 Bateman, *Robert Willan*, 510.

5 Amanda Swank, Andrzej Grzybowski, and Lawrence Charles Parish, "Robert Willan: A Quaker Physician Who Founded the Morphologic Approach to Modern Dermatology," *Clinical Dermatology* 29, no. 5 (September–October 2011): 568.

6 Walter B. Shelley and John Thorne Crissey, *Classics in Clinical Dermatology: With Biographical Sketches*, 2nd ed. (Boca Raton, FL: Parthenon, 2003): 3.

7 *Plan of the Publick Dispensary in Carey-Street, Lincoln's Inn: Instituted 1783, for the Relief of the Sick Poor, with Advice, Medicines, and Attendance, when Necessary, at Their Own Habitations* (Printed at the Philanthropic Reform, St. George's Fields, 1794): 7.

8 Irvine S.L. Loudon, "The Origins and Growth of the Dispensary Movement in England," *Bulletin of the History Medicine* 55, no. 3 (Fall 1981): 324.

9 Mabel C. Buer, *Health, Wealth and Population in the Early Days of the Industrial Revolution* (London: Routledge, 2013): 136.

10 *Plan of the Publick Dispensary*, 10.

11 Loudon, *Dispensary Movement*, 324.

12 Loudon, *Dispensary Movement*, 329.

13 Sampson Low, *The Charities of London in 1852–3: Presenting a Report of the Operation, Resources, and General Condition of the Charitable and Religious Institutions of London* (London: Sampson Low, 1854): 31.

14 *Plan of the Publick Dispensary*, 9–10.

15 Booth, *Robert Willan*, 315.

16 Franz Ehring, *Skin Diseases: Five Centuries of Scientific Illustration* (Stuttgart: Gustav Fischer, 1989): 73.

17 Andrzej Grzybowski and Lawrence C. Parish, "Robert Willan: Pioneer in Morphology," *Clinical Dermatology* 29, no. 2 (March–April 2011): 128.

18 Robert Willan, *On Cutaneous Diseases,* vol. I (Philadelphia, PA: Kimber and Conrad, 1809): 7–8

19 Thomas Bateman, *A Practical Synopsis on Cutaneous Diseases According to the Arrangement of Dr. Willan* (Philadelphia, PA: Crissy, 1824): viii–ix.

20 Willan, *Cutaneous Diseases*, 8.

21 Bateman, *Practical Synopsis*, x.

22 Gérard Tilles and Daniel Wallach, "Robert Willan and the French Willanists," *British Journal of Dermatology* 140, no. 6 (June 1999): 1123.

23 Nick Levell, "Thomas Bateman MD FLS 1778–1821," *British Journal of Dermatology* 143, no. 1 (2000): 11.

24   Goodman, *Notable Contributors*, 149.

25   Bateman, *Practical Synopsis*, xv.

26   Bateman, *Practical Synopsis*, viii.

27   Bateman, *Practical Synopsis*, ix.

28   Tilles and Wallach, *Robert Willan*, 1123.

29   Bateman, *Robert Willan*, 504.

30   Rayer et al., *Treatise on the Diseases of the Skin*, 18.

31   Andrzej Grzybowski, "Robert Willan—A Versatile Physician and Scholar," *International Journal of Dermatology* 48, no. 8 (August 2009): 533.

32   Nick Levell, "Robert Willan," in *Pantheon of Dermatology: Outstanding Historical Figures*, eds. Christoph Löser, Gerd Plewig, and Walter H.C. Burgdorf (Berlin: Springer, 2013): 1189.

33   Pusey, *History of Dermatology*, 64.

34   Willan, *Cutaneous Diseases*, 82.

35   Willan, *Cutaneous Diseases*, 115.

36   Brian Russell, "Lepra, Psoriasis, or the Willan-Plumbe Syndrome," *British Journal of Dermatology* 62 (1950): 360.

37   Swank, Grzybowski, and Parish, *Robert Willan*, 569.

38   Margaret R. O'Leary, *Dr. Thomas Addison, 1795–1860: Agitating the Whole Medical World* (Bloomington, IN: iUniverse, 2014): 51.

39   JAMA, 533.

40   Robert Willan, *Miscellaneous Works of the Late Robert Willan*, ed. Ashby Smith (London: T. Cadell, 1821): 390.

41   Bateman, *The Biographical Memoir*, 507.

42   John E. Lane, "Robert Willan," *AMA Archives of Dermatology and Syphilology* 13, no. 6 (1926): 744.

43   O'Leary, *Dr. Thomas Addison, 1795–1860*, 52.

44   Bateman, *Robert Willan*, 504.

45   Obituary, "Robert Willan," *Gentleman's Magazine* 82, part 1 (1812):595.

46   Bateman, *Robert Willan*, 507–508.

47   Nick J. Levell, "Thomas Bateman MD FLS, 1778–1821," *British Journal of Dermatology* 143 (2000): 9.

48   Bateman, *Practical Synopsis*, v.

49   Bateman, *Practical Synopsis*, v–vi.

50   Levell, *Thomas Bateman*, 11–12.

51   Pusey, *History of Dermatology*, 67.

52   James Rumsey, *Some Account of the Life and Character of the Late Thomas Bateman* (London: Longman, Rees, Orme, Brown, and Green, 1826): 220–221.

53   James Rumsey, *A Brief Memoir of the Late Thomas Bateman, etc.* (London: J. Butterworth & Son, 1822): 8–9.

54   Geoffrey L. Asherson, "Bateman, Thomas (1778–1821), Physician and Dermatologist," in *Oxford Dictionary of National Biography* (Oxford: Oxford University Press, 2004).

55   Rumsey, *Life and Character of the Late Thomas Bateman*, 218–219.

56   O'Leary, *Dr. Thomas Addison, 1795–1860*, xv.

57   Samuel J. Zakon, "The Centenary of Thomas Addison (1793–1860): His Contributions to Dermatology," *Archives of Dermatology* 83, no. 6 (1961): 935.

58   Zakon, *Thomas Addison*, 935.

59   John M. Pearce, "Thomas Addison (1793–1860)," *Journal of the Royal Society of Medicine* 97, no. 6 (June 2004): 297.

60   Horatio G. Adamson, "Erasmus Wilson: His Predecessors and His Contemporaries," *British Journal of Dermatology* 45 (1933): 443.

61   Pearce, *Thomas Addison*, 299.

62   Pearce, *Thomas Addison*, 299.

63   Pearce, *Thomas Addison*, 300.

64   Arthur Rook, "James Startin, Jonathan Hutchinson and the Blackfriars Skin Hospital," *British Journal of Dermatology* 99, no. 2 (August 1978): 215.

65   Rook, *James Startin*, 215.

66   Adamson, *Erasmus Wilson*, 440.

67 Russell, *Lepra, Psoriasis, or the Willan-Plumbe Syndrome*, 359.

68 Adamson, *Erasmus Wilson*, 439.

69 John Wilson, *A Familiar Treatise on Cutaneous Diseases*, 2nd ed. (London: J. Callow, 1814): 55–56.

70 Wilson, *Familiar Treatise*, 2.

71 Wilson, *Familiar Treatise*, 1–2.

72 Wilson, *Familiar Treatise*, 3–4.

73 Wilson, *Familiar Treatise*, 6–7.

74 Theodore Rosenthal, "Samuel Plumbe," *AMA Archives of Dermatology and Syphilology* 36, no. 2 (1937): 349.

75 Rosenthal, *Samuel Plumbe*, 348.

76 Samuel Plumbe, *A Practical Treatise on Diseases of the Skin* (Philadelphia: Haswell, Barrington, and Haswell, 1837): 40.

77 Plumbe, *Practical Treatise*, vi.

78 Adamson, *Erasmus Wilson*, 440.

79 Plumbe, *Practical Treatise*, from Plumbe's five section headings.

80 Wolfgang Weyers, "Samuel Plumbe," in *Pantheon of Dermatology: Outstanding Historical Figures*, eds. Christoph Löser, Gerd Plewig, and Walter H.C. Burgdorf (Berlin: Springer, 2013): 885.

81 Tilles and Wallach, *Robert Willan*, 1123.

82 "The French Schools-Paris," *Lancet* 11 (Thetford: J. Onwhyn, 1827): 570.

83 Robert M.B. MacKenna, "Samuel Plumbe, 1795 to 1837," *British Journal of Dermatology* 69, no. 6 (1957): 219.

84 Plumbe, *Practical Treatise on Diseases of the Skin*, 47.

85 MacKenna, *Samuel Plumbe*, 218.

86 Crissey and Parish, *Dermatology and Syphilology*, 100.

87 Rosenthal, *Samuel Plumbe*, 351.

88 Rosenthal, *Samuel Plumbe*, 353.

89 Ehring, *Skin Diseases*, 90.

90 Ehring, *Skin Diseases*, 96.

91 Jean De Bersaques, "Wilhelm Gottlieb Tilesius," in *Pantheon of Dermatology: Outstanding Historical Figures*, eds. Christoph Löser, Gerd Plewig, and Walter H.C. Burgdorf (Berlin: Springer, 2013): 1098.

92 De Bersaques, *Wilhelm Gottlieb Tilesius*, 1098.

93 Adamson, *Erasmus Wilson*, 437.

94 Adamson, *Erasmus Wilson*, 441.

95 Everett, *Erasmus Wilson*, 347.

96 Peter W. Copeman, "Choosing a Dermatological Hero for the Millennium: Erasmus Wilson (1809–1884)," *Clinical and Experimental Dermatology* 25, no. 1 (January 2000): 82.

97 Copeman, *Choosing a Dermatological Hero*, 83.

98 Copeman, *Choosing a Dermatological Hero*, 83.

99 Erasmus Wilson, *On Diseases of the Skin*, 3rd American ed. (Philadelphia, PA: Blanchard and Lea, 1852): preface xxxi.

100 Adamson, *Erasmus Wilson*, 444.

101 Adamson, *Erasmus Wilson*, 444.

102 Copeman, *Choosing a Dermatological Hero*, 83.

103 Everett, *Erasmus Wilson*, 350.

104 Everett, *Erasmus Wilson*, 348.

105 Erasmus Wilson, *Healthy Skin: A Popular Treatise on the Skin and Hair, Their Preservation and Management* (London: John Churchill, 1853): 377.

106 Crissey and Parish, *Dermatology and Syphilology*, 140–141.

107 Adamson, *Erasmus Wilson*, 442.

108 Mieneke te Hennepe, "'To Preserve the Skin in Health': Drainage, Bodily Control and the Visual Definition of Healthy Skin 1835–1900," *Medical History* 58, no. 3 (July 2014): 402.

109 Wilson, *Diseases of the Skin*, 3rd American ed., 63–64.

110 Hennepe, *To Preserve the Skin in Health*, 405.

111 Hennepe, *To Preserve the Skin in Health*, 400.

112 Pusey, *History of Dermatology*, 125.

113 Hennepe, *To Preserve the Skin in Health*, 414.

114 Erasmus Wilson, "Letter of the Editor," *Lancet* 2 (1864): 588.

115 Crissey and Parish, *Dermatology and Syphilology*, 134.

116 Everett, *Erasmus Wilson*, 351.

117 Nick Levell, "William James Erasmus Wilson," in *Pantheon of Dermatology: Outstanding Historical Figures*, eds. Christoph Löser, Gerd Plewig, and Walter H.C. Burgdorf (Berlin: Springer, 2013): 1195.

118 Crissey and Parish, *Dermatology and Syphilology*, 143.

119 Wilson, *Diseases of the Skin*, 3rd American ed., xiii.

120 Wilson, *Diseases of the Skin*, 3rd American ed., xvii.

121 Wilson, *Diseases of the Skin*, 3rd American ed., xxvi.

122 Everett, *Erasmus Wilson*, 349.

123 Everett, *Erasmus Wilson*, 347.

124 Erasmus Wilson, *On Diseases of the Skin* (Philadelphia, PA: Lea and Blanchard, 1865): xii–xiii.

125 Alan Lyell, "Erasmus Wilson and the Chair of Pathology at Aberdeen," *British Journal of Dermatology* 100, no. 3 (March 1979): 344.

126 R.M. Hadley, "The Life and Works of Sir William James Erasmus Wilson, 1809–1884," *Medical History* 3, no. 3 (1959): 228.

127 Lyell, *Erasmus Wilson*, 345.

128 "Chronicles in Cartoon," *The Windsor Magazine* (London: Ward, Lock and Bowden, 1906): 557.

129 David I. Williams, "Three British Dermatologists: Arthur Whitfield, Erasmus Wilson, and Henry Radcliffe Crocker," *Archives of Dermatology* 112 (1976): 1656.

130 Williams, *Three British Dermatologists*, 1657.

131 Lyell, *Erasmus Wilson*, 345.

132 Erasmus Wilson, "Lectures on Dermatology," *The Half-Yearly Abstract of the Medical Sciences: Being a Digest of British and Continental Medicine, and of the Progress of Medicine and the Collateral Sciences. No. 74* (Norman, OK: J. & H.G. Langley, 1873): 80.

133 Obituary, "Sir Erasmus Wilson, F.R.C.S.," *Lancet* 2 (1884): 302–303.

134 Lyell, *Erasmus Wilson*, 345.

135 Williams, *Three British Dermatologists*, 1658.

136 John Hayman, "Charles Darwin Returns to the Dermatologist," *International Journal of Dermatology* 50, no. 9 (September 2011): 1162–1165.

137 Hayman, *Charles Darwin*, 1162.

138 Hayman, *Charles Darwin*, 1162.

139 Hayman, *Charles Darwin*, 1163.

140 Hayman, *Charles Darwin*, 1163.

141 Joseph D. Hooker, "Reminiscences of Darwin," *Nature* 60 (1899): 187–188.

142 Mary P. English, "William Tilbury Fox and Dermatological Mycology," *British Journal of Dermatology* 97, no. 5 (May 1977): 573.

143 Nick Levell, "William Tilbury Fox," in *Pantheon of Dermatology: Outstanding Historical Figures*, eds. Christoph Löser, Gerd Plewig, and Walter H.C. Burgdorf (Berlin: Springer, 2013): 339.

144 Crissey, Holubar, and Parish, *Historical Atlas*, 46.

145 G.H. Findlay, "William Tilbury Fox (1836–1879): His Contribution to British Dermatology," *British Journal of Dermatology and Syphilis* 62, no. 5 (May 1950): 222.

146 Pusey, *History of Dermatology*, 126–127.

147 Findlay, *William Tilbury Fox*, 224.

148 Arthur Rook, "William Tilbury Fox (1836–1879): His Contribution to Tropical Dermatology," *International Journal of Dermatology* 20, no. 2 (March 1981): 140.

149 Rook, *William Tilbury Fox*, 142.

150 Findlay, *William Tilbury Fox*, 221.

151 Stephen Gold, "'Emerging Heroes,' *A Biographical History of British Dermatology*," British Association of Dermatologists, https://www.bad.org.uk/about-us/history/biographical.

152 Crissey and Parish, *Dermatology and Syphilology*, 276.

153 Crissey, Holubar, and Parish, *Historical Atlas*, 52.

154 Almut Böer-Auer, "Jonathan Hutchinson," in *Pantheon of Dermatology: Outstanding Historical Figures*, eds. Christoph Löser, Gerd Plewig, and Walter H.C. Burgdorf (Berlin: Springer, 2013): 506.

155 Goodman, *Notable Contributors*, 160; Crissey, Holubar, and Parish, *Historical Atlas*, 55.

156 Jack E. McCleary and Eugene M. Farber, "Dermatological Writings of Sir Jonathan Hutchinson," *AMA Archives of Dermatology and Syphilology* 65, no. 2 (February 1952): 130.

157 Om P. Sharma and Hidenobu Shigemitsu, "A Historical Sketch; Life and Time of Jonathan Hutchinson (1828–1913), the First Sarcoidologist," *Sarcoidosis, Vasculitis, and Diffuse Lung Diseases* 25, no. 2 (December 2008): 73.

158 Sharma and Shigemitsu, *Jonathan Hutchinson*, 74.

159 Robert Jackson, "How Do Physicians React to New Knowledge: The Experience of Jonathan Hutchinson 1828–1913 with Comments on Its Relevance Today," *Journal of Cutaneous Medicine and Surgery* 3, no. 1 (1998): 55.

160 McCleary and Farber, *Writings of Sir Jonathan Hutchinson*, 132.

161 Robert Jackson, "Hutchinson's Archives of Surgery Revisited," *Archives of Dermatology* 113, no. 7 (1977): 961–964.

162 William Osler and Charles N.B. Camac, *Counsels and Ideals from the Writings of William Osler* (Boston, MA: Houghton, Mifflin & Company, 1906): 3–4.

163 Pusey, *History of Dermatology*, 130.

164 Jonathan Hutchinson. "An Address on the Study of Skin Diseases as Illustrating the Doctrines of General Pathology," *British Medical Journal* 2 (1887): 229–232.

165 Jonathan Hutchinson, "The Future of Dermatology," *British Medical Journal* 2, no. 1547 (August 23, 1890): 440.

166 Hutchinson, *Future of Dermatology*, 441.

167 Hutchinson, *Future of Dermatology*, 442

168 Crissey, Holubar, and Parish, *Historical Atlas*, 51.

169 Goodman, *Notable Contributors*, 174.

170 John L. Burton, "Diet and Dermatology in 1888: The Influence of H. Radcliffe Crocker," *British Journal of Dermatology* 119, no. 4 (October 1988): 472.

171 Robert J. Thomsen, "Medical Treatment of Skin Disease in Late Nineteenth Century England: A Review Based on Diseases of the Skin by Henry Radcliffe Crocker," *International Journal of Dermatology* 27, no. 3 (April 1988): 200.

172 Henry Radcliffe Crocker, *Diseases of the Skin: Their Description, Pathology, Diagnosis, and Treatment: With Special Reference to the Skin Eruptions of Children* (Philadelphia, PA: P. Blakiston, Son & Company, 1893): 631–632.

173 J.A. Tibbles and M.M. Cohen Jr., "The Proteus Syndrome: The Elephant Man Diagnosed," *British Medical Journal (Clinical Research Edition)* 293, no. 6548 (September 1986): 683–685.

174 Goodman, *Notable Contributors*, 173.

175 Christopher B. Bunker and Pauline M. Dowd, "Henry Radcliffe Crocker, M.D., F.R.C.P. (1845–1909), Physician to the Skin Department of University College Hospital," *International Journal of Dermatology* 31, no. 6 (June 1992): 448.

176 Daniel Lewis, ed. "Obituary—Henry Radcliffe Crocker," *Medical Review of Reviews* 15 (Austin Flint Association, 1909): 631.

Chapter 13: The French School

1 B. Barker Beeson, "Laurent-Théodore Biett," *AMA Archives of Dermatology and Syphilology* 21, no. 2 (1930): 297–298.

2 Mark A. Everett, "Jean Louis Alibert, the Father of French Dermatology," *International Journal of Dermatology* 23, no. 5 (1984), 351.

3 Everett, *Jean Louis Alibert*, 351.

4 Shelley and Crissey, *Classics in Clinical Dermatology*, 31.

5 Daniel Wallach, "Choosing a Dermatological Hero for the Millennium: Jean-Louis Alibert (1768–1837)," *Clinical and Experimental Dermatology* 25, no. 1 (Jan. 2000): 91.

6 Everett, *Jean Louis Alibert*, 352.

7 Pusey, *History of Dermatology*, 74.

8 Everett, *Jean Louis Alibert*, 352.

9   Shelley and Crissey, *Classics in Clinical Dermatology*, 31.
10 Crissey and Parish, *Dermatology and Syphilology*, 44.
11 B. Barker Beeson, "Alibert," *AMA Archives of Dermatology and Syphilology* 26, no. 6 (1932), 1090.
12 Beeson, *Alibert*, 1090.
13 Everett, *Jean Louis Alibert*, 353.
14 Crissey and Parish, *Dermatology and Syphilology*, 47.
15 Wallach, *Jean-Louis Alibert*, 92.
16 Wallach, Jean-*Louis Alibert*, 92; Thomas Bieber, "Pierre-Antoine-Ernest Bazin," in *Pantheon of Dermatology: Outstanding Historical Figures*, ed. Christoph Löser, Gerd Plewig, and Walter H.C. Burgdorf (Berlin: Springer, 2013), 78.
17 Tilles and Wallach, *Robert Willan*, 1124.
18 Crissey and Parish, *Dermatology and Syphilology*, 48.
19 Crissey, Holubar, and Parish, *Historical Atlas*, 23.
20 Wallach, *Jean-Louis Alibert*, 93.
21 Wallach, *Jean-Louis Alibert*, 93.
22 Douglass W. Montgomery, "Jean Louis Alibert, the Clinician, 1766–1837," *AMA Archives of Dermatology and Syphilology* 20, no. 4 (1929): 506–507.
23 Shelley and Crissey, *Classics in Clinical Dermatology*, 31.
24 Thomas Bieber, "Jean Louis Alibert," in *Pantheon of Dermatology: Outstanding Historical Figures*, ed. Christoph Löser, Gerd Plewig, and Walter H.C. Burgdorf (Berlin: Springer, 2013), 21.
25 Danièle Ghesquier D. "A Gallic Affair: The Case of the Missing Itch-Mite in French Medicine in the Early Nineteenth Century," *Medical History* 43, no. 1 (1999): 34.
26 B. Barker Beeson, "*Acarus scabiei*: Study of Its History," *AMA Archives of Dermatology and Syphilology* 16, no. 3 (1927): 303.
27 Crissey and Parish, *Dermatology and Syphilology*, 389.
28 Everett, *Jean Louis Alibert*, 355.
29 Bateman, *Practical Synopsis*, xi, xiii
30 Montgomery, *Jean Louis Alibert*, 506.
31 Beeson, *Laurent-Théodore Biett*, 298.
32 Beeson, *Laurent-Théodore Biett*, 299.
33 Tilles and Wallach, *Robert Willan*, 1124.
34 Tilles and Wallach, Robert Willan, 1124.
35 Crissey and Parish, *Dermatology and Syphilology*, 57.
36 B. Barker Beeson, "Camille Melchior Gibert," *AMA Archives of Dermatology and Syphilology* 30, no. 1 (1934): 101.
37 R. Díaz Díaz and M. Casado Jiménez, "Camille Melchior Gibert (1797–1866)," *Journal of the European Academy of Dermatology and Venereology* 19 (2005): 785.
38 Pusey, *History of Dermatology*, 81.
39 Shelley and Crissey, *Classics in Clinical Dermatology*, 73.
40 Crissey, Holubar, and Parish, *Historical Atlas*, 34.
41 Friederike Kauer, "Marie-Guillaume-Alphonse Devergie," in *Pantheon of Dermatology: Outstanding Historical Figures*, ed. Christoph Löser, Gerd Plewig, and Walter H.C. Burgdorf (Berlin: Springer, 2013), 230.
42 B. Barker Beeson, "Alphonse Devergie," *AMA Archives of Dermatology and Syphilology* 21, no. 6 (1930): 1032.
43 Rayer et al., *Treatise on the Diseases of the Skin*, 14.
44 Rayer et al., *Treatise on the Diseases of the Skin*, 17.
45 Rayer et al., *Treatise on the Diseases of the Skin*, 17.
46 B. Barker Beeson, "Pierre François Olive Rayer, 1793–1867," *AMA Archives of Dermatology and Syphilology* 22, no. 5 (1930): 895.
47 Pusey, *History of Dermatology,* 80.
48 Crissey, Holubar, and Parish, *Historical Atlas*, 28.
49 Beeson, *Pierre François Olive Rayer*, 897.
50 B. Barker Beeson, "Ernest Bazin: A Sketch of His Life and Works," *AMA Archives of Dermatology and Syphilology* 20, no. 6 (1929): 866–872.

51 Thomas Bieber, "Pierre-Antoine-Ernest Bazin," in *Pantheon of Dermatology: Outstanding Historical Figures*, ed. Christoph Löser, Gerd Plewig, and Walter H.C. Burgdorf (Berlin: Springer, 2013), 78.

52 Beeson, *Ernest Bazin*, 867.

53 Beeson, *Ernest Bazin*, 867.

54 Goodman, *Notable Contributors*, 196.

55 Amiya K. Mukhopadhyay, "Teigne Tondante and Mahon Brothers: Two Laymen 'Physicians' of Hôpital Saint-Louis, Paris," *Indian Dermatology Online Journal* 9, no. 6 (2018): 481–483.

56 Crissey and Parish, *Dermatology and Syphilology*, 105.

57 Beeson, *Ernest Bazin*, 867.

58 Crissey, Holubar, and Parish, *Historical Atlas*, 47.

59 Pusey, *History of Dermatology*, 83.

60 Beeson, *Ernest Bazin*, 869–870.

61 Beeson, *Ernest Bazin*, 870.

62 Crissey and Parish, *Dermatology and Syphilology*, 150.

63 Goodman, *Notable Contributors*, 200.

64 Crissey and Parish, *Dermatology and Syphilology*, 152.

65 Bieber, *Bazin*, 80.

66 Bieber, *Bazin*, 80.

67 Gérard Tilles, "Pierre Louis Philippe Alfred Hardy," in *Pantheon of Dermatology: Outstanding Historical Figures*, ed. Christoph Löser, Gerd Plewig, and Walter H.C. Burgdorf (Berlin: Springer, 2013), 434.

68 Erwin H. Ackerknecht, "Diathesis: The Word and the Concept in Medical History," *Bulletin of the History of Medicine* 56, no. 3 (1982): 317.

69 Ackerknecht, *Diathesis*, 317.

70 Ackerknecht, *Diathesis*, 321–322, 325.

71 Crissey and Parish, *Dermatology and Syphilology*, 154.

72 Crissey, Holubar, and Parish, *Historical Atlas*, 47.

73 Beeson, *Ernest Bazin*, 871–872.

74 B. Barker Beeson, "Alfred Hardy, 1811–1893," *AMA Archives of Dermatology and Syphilology* 21, no. 1 (1930): 109.

75 Crissey and Parish, *Dermatology and Syphilology*, 146.

76 Tilles, *Pierre Louis Philippe Alfred Hardy*, 434.

77 Beeson, *Alfred Hardy*, 109.

78 Crissey, Holubar, and Parish, *Historical Atlas*, 48.

79 Crissey and Parish, *Dermatology and Syphilology*, 147.

80 Alfred Hardy, *The Dartrous Diathesis, or Eczema and Its Allied Affections* (New York, NY: Moorhead, Simpson & Bond, 1868), 2.

81 Crissey and Parish, *Dermatology and Syphilology*, 148.

82 Henry G. Piffard, Preface to *The Dartrous Diathesis, or Eczema and Its Allied Affections*, by Alfred Hardy (New York, NY: Moorhead, Simpson, and Bond, 1868), vii.

83 Crissey and Parish, *Dermatology and Syphilology*, 152.

84 Crissey and Parish, *Dermatology and Syphilology*, 149.

85 Crissey and Parish, *Dermatology and Syphilology*, 156.

86 Crissey and Parish, *Dermatology and Syphilology*, 157–158.

87 Crissey and Parish, *Dermatology and Syphilology*, 158–159.

88 Crissey and Parish, *Dermatology and Syphilology*, 160.

89 Crissey and Parish, *Dermatology and Syphilology*, 391.

90 Tilles, *Pierre Louis Philippe Alfred Hardy*, 439.

91 Beeson, *Alfred Hardy*, 110.

92 Gérard Tilles, "Charles-Philippe Lailler," in *Pantheon of Dermatology: Outstanding Historical Figures*, ed. Christoph Löser, Gerd Plewig, and Walter H.C. Burgdorf (Berlin: Springer, 2013), 635.

93 Tilles, *Charles-Philippe Lailler*, 635.

94 Tilles, *Charles-Philippe Lailler*, 639.

95 Crissey, Holubar, and Parish, *Historical Atlas*, 70.

96 Pusey, *History of Dermatology*, 119.

97 Crissey, Holubar, and Parish, *Historical Atlas*, 73.
98 Crissey, Holubar, and Parish, *Historical Atlas*, 73.
99 Wolfgang Weyers, "Ernest Besnier," in *Pantheon of Dermatology: Outstanding Historical Figures*, ed. Christoph Löser, Gerd Plewig, and Walter H.C. Burgdorf (Berlin: Springer, 2013), 89.
100 Pusey, *History of Dermatology*, 118.
101 Weyers, *Ernest Besnier*, 90.
102 Crissey and Parish, *Dermatology and Syphilology*, 396.
103 B. Barker Beeson, "Ernest Besnier, 1831–1909," *AMA Archives of Dermatology and Syphilology* 20, no. 1 (1929), 97.
104 Weyers, *Ernest Besnier*, 91.
105 Beeson, *Ernest Besnier*, 97–99.
106 Beeson, *Ernest Besnier*, 98.
107 Beeson, *Ernest Besnier*, 97.
108 Beeson, *Ernest Besnier*, 97.
109 John J. Pringle, "Ernest Besnier," *British Journal of Dermatology and Syphilis* 21 (1909), 226.
110 B. Barker Beeson, "Louis Brocq, MD, 1856–1928," *AMA Archives of Dermatology and Syphilology* 19, no. 5 (1929): 808.
111 Lucien M. Pautrier, "The Man behind the Eponym: Jean Louis Brocq (1856–1928)," *American Journal of Dermatopathology* 8, no. 1 (Feb. 1986): 80.
112 E. Graham Little, "Louis Brocq," *British Journal of Dermatology* 41, no. 3 (1929): 117.
113 Bernard Cribier, "Louis Anne Jean Brocq," in *Pantheon of Dermatology: Outstanding Historical Figures*, ed. Christoph Löser, Gerd Plewig, and Walter H.C. Burgdorf (Berlin: Springer, 2013), 128.
114 Beeson, *Louis Brocq*, 809.
115 Pautrier, *Jean Louis Brocq*, 81.
116 Pusey, *History of Dermatology*, 120.
117 Beeson, *Louis Brocq*, 809.
118 Little, *Louis Brocq*, 117.
119 Pautrier, *Jean Louis Brocq*, 79–82.
120 "Manuel pratique de dermatologie: Le diagnostic, la peau et ses réactions, thérapeutique, les dermatoses," *Journal of the American Medical Association* 101, no. 23 (1933): 1824–1825, a book review of A. Desaux et A. Boutelier avec la collaboration de Pierre Brocq. Manuel pratique de dermatologie: Le diagnostic, la peau et ses réactions, thérapeutique, les dermatoses. Paris: Masson, 1932.
121 Jean Civatte, "Jean Darier: A Memoir," *American Journal of Dermatopathology* 1, no. 1 (Spring 1979): 57.
122 Peter Beighton and Greta Beighton, "Darier, Jean," in *The Person Behind the Syndrome* (London: Springer, 1997), 51.
123 Wolfgang Weyers, "Jean Darier," in *Pantheon of Dermatology: Outstanding Historical Figures*, ed. Christoph Löser, Gerd Plewig, and Walter H.C. Burgdorf (Berlin: Springer, 2013), 207.
124 Weyers, *Jean Darier*, 213.
125 Civatte, *Jean Darier*, 59.
126 Weyers, *Jean Darier*, 211.
127 Robert Jackson, "Jean Darier and His Précis," *Journal of Cutaneous Medicine and Surgery* 11, no. 4 (2007): 153, 155.

Interlude 4: Smallpox

1 Jonathan B. Tucker, *Scourge: The Once and Future Threat of Smallpox* (New York, NY: Grove Press, 2002), 2.
2 Gareth Williams, *Angel of Death* (London: Palgrave Macmillan, 2016), 20.
3 Williams, *Angel of Death*, 24.
4 David Shuttleton, "A Culture of Disfigurement: Imagining Smallpox in the Long Eighteenth Century," in *Framing and Imagining Disease in Cultural History*, eds. George S. Rousseau et al. (London: Palgrave Macmillan, 2003), 81.

5   Shuttleton, *Culture of Disfigurement,* 69.

6   Williams, *Angel of Death,* 22.

7   Stefan Riedel, "Edward Jenner and the History of Smallpox and Vaccination," *Baylor University Medical Center Proceedings* 18, no. 1 (2005): 21.

8   Frank Fenner, *Smallpox and Its Eradication* (Geneva: World Health Organization, 1988), 210.

9   Riedel, *Edward Jenner,* 21.

10 Joshua Loomis, *Epidemics: The Impact of Germs and Their Power over Humanity* (Santa Barbara, CA: Praeger, an Imprint of ABC-CLIO, 2018), 41.

11 Robert Willan, *Miscellaneous Works of the Late Robert Willan,* ed. Ashby Smith (London: T. Cadell, 1821), 91–92.

12 Donald R. Hopkins, "Smallpox: Ten Years Gone," *American Journal of Public Health* 78, no. 12 (1988): 1593.

13 Fortuine, *Words of Medicine,* 196.

14 Lenn E. Goodman, "The Greek Impact on Arabic Literature," in *Arabic Literature to the End of the Umayyad Period,* ed. Alfred F.L. Beeston (Cambridge, MA: Cambridge University Press, 1983), 468.

15 Abbas M. Behbehani, "Rhazes: The Original Portrayer of Smallpox," *JAMA* 252, no. 22 (1984): 3156.

16 Abū Bakr Muḥammad ibn Zakarīyā Rāzī, *A Treatise on the Smallpox and Measles (Commonly Called Rhazes),* trans. William Alexander Greenhill (London: Sydenham Society, 1847), 34.

17 Rāzī, *On the Smallpox and Measles,* 72.

18 Rāzī, *On the Smallpox and Measles,* 113.

19 Behbehani, *Rhazes,* 3158.

20 Rāzī, *On the Smallpox and Measles,* 29.

21 Rāzī, *On the Smallpox and Measles,* 29.

22 Rāzī, *On the Smallpox and Measles,* 30.

23 Avicenna, *Canon of Medicine,* 265.

24 Hieronymi Fracastoro, *De contagione et contagiosis morbis et eorum curatorie,* libri III (1548), trans. Wilmer Wright (New York, NY: Putnam, 1930), xix.

25 Arthur M. Silverstein, *A History of Immunology* (Cambridge, MA: Academic Press, 2012), 9.

26 Dewhurst, *Dr. Thomas Sydenham,* 116.

27 Williams, *Angel of Death,* 9.

28 James C. Moore, *The History of the Small Pox* (London: Longman, Hurst, Rees, Orme, and Brown, 1815), 214.

29 Herman Boerhaave et al., *Boerhaave's Aphorisms: Concerning the Knowledge and Cure of Diseases* (London: Printed for B. Cowse and W. Innys in St. Paul's Church-Yard, 1715), 403.

30 Silverstein, *A History of Immunology,* 15.

31 Reiss, *Medicine and the American Revolution,* 103.

32 James Drake, *Anthropologia Nova: Or, a New System of Anatomy,* Volume 1 (London, 1707), 25.

33 Silverstein, *A History of Immunology,* 14.

34 Shuttleton, *Culture of Disfigurement,* 79.

35 Thomas Fuller, *Exanthematologia: Or An Attempt to Give a Rational Account of Eruptive Fevers, Especially the Measles and Smallpox. In Two Parts* (London: Printed for Charles Rivington and Stephen Austen, 1730), 189.

36 Silverstein, *A History of Immunology,* 15.

37 Riedel, *Edward Jenner,* 21.

38 Fenner, *Smallpox and Its Eradication,* 229.

39 Fenner, *Smallpox and Its Eradication,* 236–237; Hopkins, *Smallpox,* 1589.

40 Hopkins, *The Greatest Killer,* 216.

41 Elizabeth A. Fenn, "Biological Warfare in Eighteenth-Century North America: Beyond Jeffery Amherst," *Journal of American History,* 86, no. 4 (2000): 1553–1555.

42 Francis Parkman, *The Conspiracy of Pontiac and the Indian War after the Conquest of Canada* (United States: Little, Brown, 1893), 39–40.

43 Hopkins, *Smallpox,* 1590.

44 Fenner, *Smallpox and Its Eradication*, 213.

45 Ana T. Duggan et al., "17th Century Variola Virus Reveals the Recent History of Smallpox," *Current Biology* 26, no. 24 (2016): 3411.

46 Ann G. Carmichael and Arthur M. Silverstein, "Smallpox in Europe before the Seventeenth Century: Virulent Killer or Benign Disease?" *Journal of the History of Medicine and Allied Sciences* 42, no. 2 (1987): 156.

47 Carmichael and Silverstein, *Smallpox in Europe*, 148.

48 Carmichael and Silverstein, *Smallpox in Europe*, 147–168.

49 Shuttleton, *Culture of Disfigurement*, 68.

50 Fenner, *Smallpox and Its Eradication*, 229.

51 Riedel, *Jenner*, 21.

52 Hopkins, *Smallpox*, 1589–1595.

53 Hopkins, *Smallpox*, 1590.

54 Hany E. Emson, "For the Want of an Heir: The Obstetrical History of Queen Anne," *British Medical Journal* 304, no. 6838 (1992): 1366.

55 Williams, *Angel of Death*, 49.

56 Hopkins, *Smallpox*, 1590.

57 Shuttleton, *Culture of Disfigurement*, 76.

58 Williams, *Angel of Death*, 36.

59 Hopkins, *Smallpox*, 1592.

60 Huckbody, *Dermatology throughout the Dark Ages*, 346.

61 Fenner, *Smallpox and Its Eradication*, 228.

62 Niels R. Finsen, "The Red Light Treatment of Small-Pox," *British Medical Journal* 2, no. 1823 (1895): 1414.

63 Fenner, *Smallpox and Its Eradication*, 228.

64 Riedel, *Jenner*, 22.

65 Hopkins, *Smallpox*, 1591.

66 Riedel, *Jenner*, 22.

67 Riedel, *Jenner*, 23.

68 Riedel, *Jenner*, 23.

69 Mark Best, Achilles Katamba, and Duncan Neuhauser, "Making the Right Decision: Benjamin Franklin's Son Dies of Smallpox in 1736," *Quality and Safety in Health Care* 16, no. 6 (2007): 478.

70 Thomas Jefferson, *The Papers of Thomas Jefferson*, Volume 31, 1799 Feb 1–1800 May 31 (Princeton, NJ: Princeton University Press, 2004).

71 Armond S. Goldman and Frank C. Schmalstieg Jr., "Abraham Lincoln's Gettysburg Illness," *Journal of Medical Biography* 15, no. 2 (May 2007): 104–110.

72 Riedel, *Jenner*, 23.

73 Voltaire, *Works*, 19.

74 Arthur W. Boylston, "The Myth of the Milkmaid," *New England Journal of Medicine* 378, no. 5 (2018): 414.

75 Boylston, *Myth of the Milkmaid*, 414.

76 Riedel, *Jenner*, 24.

77 Riedel, *Jenner*, 24.

78 Edward Jenner, *On the Origin of the Vaccine Inoculation* (United Kingdom: G. Elsick, 1863), 8.

79 Thomas Jefferson, "To George C. Jenner, 14 May 1806," *Founders Online*, National Archives, https://founders.archives.gov/documents/Jefferson/99-01-02-3718.

80 Lisa Rosner, *Vaccination and Its Critics: A Documentary and Reference Guide* (Santa Barbara, CA: ABC-CLIO, 2017), 7.

81 Williams, *Angel of Death*, 11.

82 Williams, *Angel of Death*, 10.

83 Hopkins, *Smallpox*, 1593.

84 Stephen B. Greenberg, "'Bacilli and bullets': William Osler and the Antivaccination Movement," *Southern Medical Journal* 93, no. 8 (2000): 764.

85 Greenberg, *Bacilli and bullets*, 764–765.

86 Greenberg, *Bacilli and bullets*, 765.

87 Richard B. Kennedy et al., "Smallpox Vaccines for Biodefense," *Vaccine* 27, no. suppl. 4 (2009): D73–D79.

88 Robert J. Thornton, "Second Letter to Mr. Tilloch on the Cow-Pock," *Philosophical Magazine* 20, no. 79 (1804): 146–147.

Chapter 14: The Vienna School and the German Schools

1 Alfred Vogl, "Six Hundred Years of Medicine in Vienna: A History of the Vienna School of Medicine," *Bulletin of the New York Academy Medicine* 43, no. 4 (April 1967): 282.

2 Vogl, *Six Hundred Years,* 290.

3 Vogl, *Six Hundred Years,* 290.

4 Ronald Batt, *History of Endometriosis* (London: Springer, 2014), 17.

5 Vogl, *Six Hundred Years,* 291.

6 Clark W. Finnerud, "Ferdinand von Hebra and the Vienna School of Dermatology," *AMA Archives of Dermatology and Syphilology* 66, no. 2 (1952): 223.

7 Carl Wunderlich, *Wien und Paris: Ein Beitrag zur Geschichte und Burteiling den gegenwärtigen Heilkunde in Deutschland und Frankreich* (Stuttgart, 1841; new ed., Bern: H. Huber, 1974) 35, trans. by Erwin Ackerknecht, *Medicine at the Paris Hospital,* 179.

8 Finnerud, *Ferdinand von Hebra,* 225.

9 Crissey, Holubar, and Parish, *Historical Atlas,* 41.

10 Finnerud, *Ferdinand von Hebra,* 226, 229.

11 Finnerud, *Ferdinand von Hebra,* 224.

12 Pusey, *History of Dermatology,* 102.

13 Pusey, *History of Dermatology,* 102.

14 Goodman, *Notable Contributors,* 225.

15 Ernest Spitzer, "Ferdinand von Hebra: In Commemoration of His Appointment One Hundred Years Ago as Professor of Dermatology at the University of Vienna," *AMA Archives of Dermatology and Syphilology* 64, no. 3 (1951): 283.

16 John T. Crissey and Lawrence C. Parish, "Ferdinand Hebra: A Reexamination of his Contributions to Dermatology," *International Journal of Dermatology* 19, no. 10 (1980): 587.

17 Shelley and Crissey, *Classics in Clinical Dermatology,* 100.

18 Crissey and Parish, *Dermatology and Syphilology,* 123.

19 Crissey and Parish, *Dermatology and Syphilology,* 123.

20 Finnerud, *Ferdinand von Hebra,* 229.

21 Crissey and Parish, *Ferdinand Hebra,* 585.

22 Shelley and Crissey, *Classics in Clinical Dermatology,* 101.

23 Crissey and Parish, *Ferdinand Hebra,* 586.

24 Finnerud, *Ferdinand von Hebra,* 229.

25 Goodman, *Notable Contributors,* 229.

26 Crissey and Parish, *Ferdinand Hebra,* 587.

27 D. Friday King, "Gustav Simon: The Father of Dermatopathology," *American Journal of Dermatopathology* 1, no. 3 (Fall 1979): 225–226.

28 Hans M. Buley, "German Schools of Dermatology in the Past Century," *AMA Archives of Dermatology and Syphilology* 66, no. 4 (1952): 445.

29 Marianna Karamanou et al., "The Eminent Dermatologist Moriz Kaposi (1837-1902) and the First Description of Idiopathic Multiple Pigmented Sarcoma of the Skin," *Journal of Balkan Union of Oncology* 18, no. 4 (2013): 1102.

30 Filippo Pesapane et al., "Mór Cohen, better known as Moriz Kaposi," *JAMA Dermatology* 150, no. 3 (March 2014): 265.

31 Karl Holubar and Joseph Frankl, "Moriz (Kohn) Kaposi," *American Journal of Dermatopathology* 3, no. 4 (Winter 1981): 352.

32 Karamanou, *Moriz Kaposi,* 1102.

33 Arty R. Zantinga and Max J. Coppes, "Moriz Kaposi (1837–1902): Great Master of the Viennese School of Dermatology," *Medical and Pediatric Oncolology* 27, no. 2 (August 1996): 130.

34 Karamanou, *Moriz Kaposi,* 1103.
35 Goodman, *Notable Contributors,* 239–240.
36 Max Hundeiker, "Moriz Kaposi," in *Pantheon of Dermatology: Outstanding Historical Figures,* ed. Christoph Löser, Gerd Plewig, and Walter H.C. Burgdorf (Berlin: Springer, 2013), 578.
37 Franz Trautinger, "Isidor Neumann von Heilwart," in *Pantheon of Dermatology: Outstanding Historical Figures,* ed. Christoph Löser, Gerd Plewig, and Walter H.C. Burgdorf (Berlin: Springer, 2013), 798.
38 Trautinger, *Isidor Neumann von Heilwart,* 800.
39 Goodman, *Notable Contributors,* 244.
40 Crissey, Holubar, and Parish, *Historical Atlas,* 60; P. Arenberger, "Filipp Josef Pick," in *Pantheon of Dermatology: Outstanding Historical Figures,* ed. Christoph Löser, Gerd Plewig, and Walter H.C. Burgdorf (Berlin: Springer, 2013), 858.
41 Goodman, *Notable Contributors,* 244.
42 Goodman, *Notable Contributors,* 244.
43 Pusey, *History of Dermatology,* 110; Goodman, *Notable Contributors,* 234.
44 Max Hundeiker, "Heinrich Auspitz," in *Pantheon of Dermatology: Outstanding Historical Figures,* ed. Christoph Löser, Gerd Plewig, and Walter H.C. Burgdorf (Berlin: Springer, 2013), 51.
45 Hundeiker, *Heinrich Auspitz,* 52.
46 Hundeiker, *Heinrich Auspitz,* 50.
47 Hundeiker, *Heinrich Auspitz,* 50; Karl Holubar, "The Man Behind the Eponym. Remembering Heinrich Auspitz," *American Journal of Dermatopathology* 8, no. 1 (1986): 84.
48 Crissey, Holubar, and Parish, *Historical Atlas,* 61.
49 Rafal Białynicki-Birula, "Heinrich Köbner (1838–1904)—The Founder of the Wroćaw (Breslau) School of Dermatology and One of the Founders of German Dermatology," *Dermatologia Kliniczna* 8, no. 3 (2006): 154.
50 Crissey, Holubar, and Parish, *Historical Atlas,* 64.
51 Marco Diani, Chiara Cozzi, and Gianfranco Altomare, "Heinrich Koebner and His Phenomenon," *JAMA Dermatology* 152, no. 8 (2016): 919.
52 Crissey and Parish, *Dermatology and Syphilology,* 368.
53 Gunter W. Korting, "Some Aspects of the Genesis and Development of German Dermatology," in *On the History of German Dermatology,* ed. Herzberg et al. (Berlin: Grosse, 1987), 120.
54 Albrecht Scholz, "Albert Neisser," in *Pantheon of Dermatology: Outstanding Historical Figures,* ed. Christoph Löser, Gerd Plewig, and Walter H.C. Burgdorf (Berlin: Springer, 2013), 771.
55 Scholz, *Albert Neisser,* 773.
56 Albrecht Scholz and G. Sebastian, "Albert Neisser and His Pupils," in *On the History of German Dermatology,* ed. Herzberg et al. (Berlin: Grosse, 1987), 167.
57 Scholz and Sebastian, *Albert Neisser,* 170.
58 Scholz and Sebastian, *Albert Neisser,* 170.
59 Scholz and Sebastian, *Albert Neisser,* 176.
60 Scholz and Sebastian, *Albert Neisser,* 176.
61 Scholz and Sebastian, *Albert Neisser,* 170.
62 Scholz and Sebastian, *Albert Neisser,* 171.
63 Leyre A. Falto-Aizpurua, Robert. D. Griffith, Keyvan Nouri, "Josef Jadassohn: A Dermatologic Pioneer," *JAMA Dermatology* 151, no. 1 (2015): 41.
64 Falto-Aizpurua, Griffith, and Nouri, *Josef Jadassohn,* 41.
65 Buley, *German Schools,* 442.
66 Buley, *German Schools,* 446.
67 K. Winkler, "Dermatology in Berlin—A Retrospective View," in *On the History of German Dermatology,* ed. Herzberg et al. (Berlin: Grosse, 1987), 135.
68 Winkler, *Dermatology in Berlin,* 135.
69 Winkler, *Dermatology in Berlin,* 135.
70 Sam Shuster, "The Nature and Consequence of Karl Marx's Skin Disease," *British Journal of Dermatology* 158, no. 1 (January 2008): 1.
71 Shuster, *Karl Marx's Skin Disease,* 2.
72 Shuster, *Karl Marx's Skin Disease,* 2–3.
73 Norman Walker and H.L. Roberts, "Paul Gerson Unna," *British Journal of Dermatology* 41 (1929): 159.

74 Fabrizio Vaira, Gianluca Nazzaro, and Stefano Veraldi, "The Men or Women behind Nevi: Paul Gerson Unna," *JAMA Dermatology* 150, no. 2 (February 2014): 176.

75 H. Leslie Roberts and Norman Walker, "Paul Gerson Unna," *British Journal of Dermatology* 41 (1929): 157.

76 Crissey, Holubar, and Parish, *Historical Atlas*, 66.

77 Wolfgang Weyers, "Paul Gerson Unna," in *Pantheon of Dermatology: Outstanding Historical Figures*, ed. Christoph Löser, Gerd Plewig, and Walter H.C. Burgdorf (Berlin: Springer, 2013), 1133.

78 Weyers, *Paul Gerson Unna*, 1133.

79 Roberts and Walker, *Paul Gerson Unna*, 158.

80 Sigmund Pollitzer, "Paul Gerson Unna, M.D., 1850–1929," *AMA Archives of Dermatology and Syphilology* 19, no. 4 (1929): 676.

81 Weyers, *Paul Gerson Unna*, 1133.

82 Paul G. Unna, *Histopathology of Diseases of the Skin*, trans. Norman Walker (Edinburgh: W. F. Clay, 1896), v.

83 Unna, *Histopathology*, vi.

84 Unna, *Histopathology*, vii.

85 Unna, *Histopathology*, vii, viii.

86 Pollitzer, *Paul Gerson Unna*, 676.

87 Alfred Hollander, "Scientific Work of Paul Gerson Unna," *AMA Archives of Dermatology and Syphilology* 62, no. 3 (September 1950): 357.

88 Pollitzer, *Paul Gerson Unna*, 677.

89 Crissey and Parish, *Dermatology and Syphilology*, 219.

90 Hollander, *Scientific Work of Paul Gerson Unna*, 353.

91 Hollander, *Scientific Work of Paul Gerson Unna*, 352.

92 Crissey and Parish, *Dermatology and Syphilology*, 378.

93 Pusey, *History of Dermatology*, 164; Weyers, 1138.

94 Goodman, *Notable Contributors*, 260.

95 Weyers, *Paul Gerson Unna*, 1135.

96 Pollitzer, *Paul Gerson Unna*, 677–678.

97 Pollitzer, *Paul Gerson Unna*, 678.

98 Weyers, *Paul Gerson Unna*, 1132.

99 Hollander, *Scientific Work of Paul Gerson Unna*, 361.

100 Pusey, *History of Dermatology*, 160.

Chapter 15: American Dermatology in the Nineteenth Century

1 William A. Pusey, "Noah Worcester, A.M., M.D., Pioneer Internist and Dermatologist in the Middle West," *AMA Archives of Dermatology and Syphilology* 27, no. 5 (1933): 827.

2 James Q. Gant, "One Hundredth Anniversary of the First American Textbook of Dermatology," *AMA Archives of Dermatology and Syphilology* 52, no. 2 (1945): 117; Pusey, *Noah Worcester*, 828.

3 Noah Worcester, *A Synopsis of the Symptoms, Diagnosis and Treatment of the More Common and Important Diseases of the Skin* (Philadelphia, PA: Cowperthwait, 1845): iii, 9.

4 Pusey, *Noah Worcester*, 832.

5 Pusey, *Noah Worcester*, 831.

6 Worcester, *Synopsis*, 22.

7 Worcester, *Synopsis*, 22.

8 Worcester, *Synopsis*, 18–19.

9 Worcester, *Synopsis*, 13–17.

10 Worcester, *Synopsis*, 23–24.

11 Worcester, *Synopsis*, 28.

12 Gant, *One Hundredth Anniversary of the First American Textbook of Dermatology*, 117.

13 Anthony C. Cipollaro, "Henry Daggett Bulkley, 1804 to 1872: Pioneer American Dermatologist," *Archives of Dermatology* 99, no. 5 (May 1969): 523.

14 Lucius D. Bulkley, *Manual of Diseases of the Skin*, 4th ed. (New York, NY: G, Putnam's Sons, 1898): 1

15 Cipollaro, *Henry Daggett Bulkley*, 527–528.

16 Crissey, Holubar, and Parish, *Historical Atlas*, 81.

17 Lawrence Parish, "Lucius Duncan Bulkley," in *Pantheon of Dermatology: Outstanding Historical Figures*, eds. Christoph Löser, Gerd Plewig, and Walter H.C. Burgdorf (Berlin: Springer, 2013): 135.

18 Crissey, Holubar, and Parish, *Historical Atlas*, 81.

19 Lawrence C. Parish, "How Did Dermatology Develop in the United States?" *Clinics in Dermatology* 29, no. 3 (2011): 341.

20 Malcolm Morris, "In Memoriam: James Clarke White," *British Journal of Dermatology* 28 (1916): 4.

21 Gwen Kay, "James Clarke White," *American National Biography* (New York, NY: Oxford University Press, 1999, online version): 2.

22 Kay, *James Clarke White*, 2.

23 Wolfgang Koenen, "James Clarke White," in *Pantheon of Dermatology: Outstanding Historical Figures*, eds. Christoph Löser, Gerd Plewig, and Walter H.C. Burgdorf (Berlin: Springer, 2013): 1175.

24 Morris, *James Clarke White*, 7.

25 Morris, *James Clarke White*, 5.

26 Morris, *James Clarke White*, 6.

27 Morris, *James Clarke White*, 7.

28 Paul E. Bechet, "Henry Granger Piffard: A Great Factor in the Progress of American Dermatology," *AMA Archives of Dermatology and Syphilology* 37, no. 5 (1938): 781.

29 Crissey, Holubar, and Parish, *Historical Atlas*, 84.

30 Bechet, *Henry Granger Piffard*, 784.

31 Barbara Burrall, "A Brief History of the Department of Dermatology, New York University," *Dermatology Online Journal* 7, no. 1 (2001): 7.

32 Thomas G. Cropley, "Henry G. Piffard," in *Pantheon of Dermatology: Outstanding Historical Figures*, eds. Christoph Löser, Gerd Plewig, and Walter H.C. Burgdorf (Berlin: Springer, 2013): 866.

33 Cropley, *Henry G. Piffard*, 866.

34 Bechet, *Henry Granger Piffard*, 784.

35 Frederick C. Gaede, "Henry Granger Piffard, MD and His Photogenic Pistol Cartridges," *Clinical Dermatology* 37, no. 3 (May–Jun. 2019): 286.

36 Christoph Löser, "George Henry Fox," in *Pantheon of Dermatology: Outstanding Historical Figures*, eds. Christoph Löser, Gerd Plewig, and Walter H.C. Burgdorf (Berlin: Springer, 2013): 328.

37 William A. Pusey, "George Henry Fox, M.D., 1846–1937," *AMA Archives of Dermatology and Syphilology* 36, no. 2 (1937): 361.

38 Löser, *George Henry Fox*, 329.

39 Löser, *George Henry Fox*, 329.

40 Pusey, *George Henry Fox*, 363.

41 Jean Strouse, *Morgan: American Financier* (New York, NY: Random House, 2014): 265–266.

42 Strouse, *Morgan*, 265.

43 Vincent J. Derbes, "Louis A. Duhring, MD—Pathfinder for Dermatology," *Archives of Intern Medicine* 121, no. 6 (1968): 578.

44 Christopher Hoolihan, "Louis Adolphus Duhring," in *American National Biography* (New York, NY: Oxford University Press, 2000, online version): 1.

45 Lawrence C. Parish, "Dermatology at Blockley—100 Years Ago," *Archives of Dermatology* 96, no. 3 (1967): 329.

46 Paul E. Bechet, "Louis Adolphus Duhring: A Great American Dermatologist," *AMA Archives of Dermatology and Syphilology* 30, no. 3 (1934): 369.

47 Bechet, *Louis Adolphus Duhring*, 372.

48 Bechet, *Louis Adolphus Duhring*, 373.

49 Hoolihan, *Louis Adolphus Duhring*, 2.

50 Bechet, *Louis Adolphus Duhring*, 374.

51 W.R.B., "Centenary. Louis Adolphus Duhring," *British Journal of Dermatology* 58 (1946): 34.

52 Bechet, *Louis Adolphus Duhring*, 376.

53 Bechet, *Louis Adolphus Duhring*, 370.

54 Pusey, *History of Dermatology*, 146.

55 Bechet, *Louis Adolphus Duhring*, 371.

56 Bechet, *Louis Adolphus Duhring*, 371.
57 Bechet, *Louis Adolphus Duhring*, 371.
58 Bechet, *Louis Adolphus Duhring*, 371.
59 Louis A. Duhring, "The Scope of Dermatology," Chairman's Address Read in Section of Dermatology and Syphilography at the Forty-Fourth Annual Meeting of the American Medical Association, *JAMA* 22, no. 7 (1894): 207–210.
60 Duhring, *Scope of Dermatology*, 207.
61 Duhring, *Scope of Dermatology*, 207.
62 Duhring, *Scope of Dermatology*, 207–208.
63 Duhring, *Scope of Dermatology*, 208.
64 Duhring, *Scope of Dermatology*, 208.
65 Duhring, *Scope of Dermatology*, 208.
66 Duhring, *Scope of Dermatology*, 208–209.
67 Duhring, *Scope of Dermatology*, 209.
68 Duhring, *Scope of Dermatology*, 209.

Chapter 16: The Twentieth Century and Beyond

1   Oumeish Yousef Oumeish. "Congressus Mundi Dermatologiae, Paris 1889–Paris 2002." *Clinics in Dermatology* 22, no. 6 (2004): 453.
2   Thomsen, *Medical Treatment of Skin Disease*, 198–203. Thomsen's excellent review of dermatological therapeutics in Crocker's *Diseases of the Skin* is the source of the following information.
3   Francis Adams, *The Genuine Works of Hippocrates* (London: Sydenham Society, 1849), VII, 87.
4   Vito W. Rebecca, Vernon K. Sondak, Keiran S.M. Smalley, "A Brief History of Melanoma: From Mummies to Mutations," *Melanoma Research* 22, no. 2 (Apr. 2012): 115.
5   Rebecca, Sondak, and Smalley, *Brief History of Melanoma*, 115.
6   D.C. Bodenham, "A Study of 650 Observed Malignant Melanomas in the South-West Region," *Annals of the Royal College of Surgeons of England* 43, no. 4 (Oct. 1968): 218.
7   Rebecca, Sondak, and Smalley, *Brief History of Melanoma*, 114–115.
8   H. Elizabeth Crouch, "History of Basal Cell Carcinoma and Its Treatment," *Journal of the Royal Society of Medicine* 76, no. 4 (1983): 304.
9   Carl Thiersch, *Der Epithelialkrebs, namentlich der Haut; eine anatomisch-klinische Untersuchung* (Leipzig: Engelmann, 1865).
10 Crouch, *History of Basal Cell Carcinoma*, 303.
11 Crouch, *History of Basal Cell Carcinoma*, 304.
12 Willard Marmelzat. "'Noli-Me-Tangere' Circa 1754: Jacques Daviel's Forgotten Contribution to Skin Cancer." *Archives of Dermatology* 90, no. 3 (1964): 283.
13 Scott M. Jackson and Lee T. Nesbitt, *Differential Diagnosis for the Dermatologist* (Heidelberg: Springer, 2012).
14 Christoph Löser, Gerd Plewig, and Walter H.C. Burgdorf, ed., *Pantheon of Dermatology: Outstanding Historical Figures* (Berlin: Springer, 2013).
15 Martin M. Black, Geoffrey Barrow Dowling, in *Pantheon of Dermatology: Outstanding Historical Figures*, ed. Christoph Löser, Gerd Plewig, and Walter H.C. Burgdorf (Berlin: Springer, 2013), 246.
16 Clarence S. Livingood, "History of the American Board of Dermatology, Inc. (1932–1982)," *Journal of the American Academy of Dermatology* 7, no. 6 (Dec. 1982): 821.
17 NRMP Results and Data: 2020 Main Residency Match (https://www.nrmp.org/match-data-analytics/residency-data-reports/).
18 Aram A. Namavar et al., "US Dermatology Residency Program Rankings Based on Academic Achievement," *Cutis* 101, no. 2 (Feb. 2018):146–149.
19 Peter C. Gøtzsche, "Niels Finsen's Treatment for Lupus Vulgaris," *Journal of the Royal Society of Medicine* 104, no. 1 (2011): 41.
20 Herbert Hönigsmann, "History of Phototherapy in Dermatology," *Photochemical and Photobiological Sciences* 12, no. 1 (Jan. 2013): 16.

21 Rishu Gupta et al., "The Goeckerman Regimen for the Treatment of Moderate to Severe Psoriasis." *Journal of Visualized Experiments* 77 (2013), 3.

22 Adam Aldahan et al., "The History of Sunscreen," *JAMA Dermatol* 151, no. 12 (2015): 1316.

23 Yangmyung Ma and Jinah Yoo. "History of Sunscreen: An Updated View." *Journal of Cosmetic Dermatology* 20, no. 4 (2021): 1045.

Conclusion

1 Weisz, *Divide and Conquer*, 5.

2 Weisz, *Divide and Conquer*, 12.

3 Weisz, *Divide and Conquer*, 11–12.

4 Weisz, *Divide and Conquer*, 63.

5 Weisz, *Divide and Conquer*, 27.

6 T. McCall Anderson, "The Progress of Dermatology during the Last Quarter Century," *British Medical Journal* 2 (1879): 399–400.

7 Weisz, *Divide and Conquer*, 23.

8 Weisz, *Divide and Conquer*, 215.

9 Weisz, *Divide and Conquer*, 216–217.

10 M. Morris, "An Address Delivered at the Opening of the Section of Dermatology. The Rise and Progress of Dermatology," *British Medical Journal* 2, no. 1916 (1897): 699–700.

Index

Printed in the USA
CPSIA information can be obtained
at www.ICGtesting.com
LVHW081143221223
766782LV00084B/147

9 781032 226606